Diabetes Mellitus
Diagnosis and Treatment
Fourth Edition

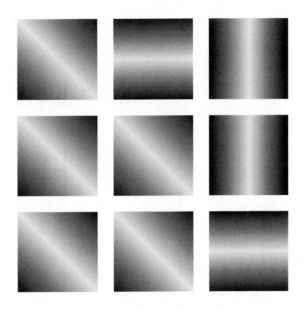

Mayer B. Davidson, M.D.
Associate Director, Clinical Diabetes
City of Hope National Medical Center
Duarte, California
Clinical Professor of Medicine
University of California, Los Angeles
UCLA School of Medicine
Los Angeles, California

W.B. SAUNDERS COMPANY
A Division of Harcourt Brace & Company
Philadelphia   London   Toronto   Montreal   Sydney   Tokyo

W.B. SAUNDERS COMPANY
A Division of Harcourt Brace & Company

The Curtis Center
Independence Square West
Philadelphia, Pennsylvania 19106

Library of Congress Cataloging-in-Publication Data

Davidson, Mayer B.
Diabetes mellitus: diagnosis and treatment / Mayer B. Davidson.—4th ed.

p.   cm.

Includes bibliographical references and index.

ISBN 0–7216–6403–2

1. Diabetes.   I. Title.   [Diabetes Mellitus—diagnosis.   2. Diabetes
Mellitus—therapy.   WK 810 D253d 1998]

RC660.D37   1998   616.4′62—DC21

DNLM/DLC   97-50320

DIABETES MELLITUS: DIAGNOSIS AND TREATMENT   ISBN 0-7216-6403-2

Printed in the United States of America.

Last digit is the print number: 9   8   7   6   5   4   3   2   1

To Roseann, with much gratitude for her loving support

CONTRIBUTORS

Marion Franz, M.S., C.D.E., R.D.
International Diabetes Center, Minneapolis, Minnesota

John L. Kitzmiller, M.D.
Director, Maternal-Fetal Medicine, Good Samaritan Hospital, San
Jose, California

Anne L. Peters, M.D.
Associate Professor of Medicine, UCLA School of Medicine, Los
Angeles, California

Carol S. Rosenberg, R.N., M.S.N., C.D.E.
Diabetes Clinical Nurse Specialist, HealthCare Partners Medical
Group, Torrance, California; Assistant Clinical Professor, UCLA
School of Nursing, Los Angeles, California

PREFACE

Diabetes mellitus has a far-reaching impact on both the health of individuals and the health care system in the United States. It affects 6 to 7% of the total population, or approximately 16 million people. The prevalence in people over 65 years of age, a rapidly increasing segment of the population, is estimated to be 20%, half of whom remain undiagnosed. Compared with a 6% prevalence in Caucasians, the prevalence of diabetes is approximately 10% in African Americans and Asian Americans, 15% in Hispanics (especially in Mexican Americans), and 20 to 50% in Native American populations. Diabetes is the leading cause of new cases of blindness in this country in people between the ages of 20 and 74. Over one third of patients on dialysis have end-stage renal disease secondary to diabetic nephropathy. Fifty to seventy-five percent of nontraumatic lower extremity amputations take place in people with diabetes. If deaths caused by vascular disease in diabetic patients are ascribed to diabetes, it ranks as the fourth leading cause of death in the United States. The estimated direct medical costs of caring for patients with diabetes have escalated rapidly: 5 billion dollars in 1974, 8 billion dollars in 1979, 20 billion dollars in 1987, and 45 billion dollars in 1992. Fifteen percent of total medical costs in this country is spent on diabetic patients, most of it for the complications of diabetes. (And most of these complications could be prevented with appropriate treatment.)

The key factor in improving the quality of life and medical outcomes for diabetic patients lies in the hands of their physicians and other diabetes health care providers.

Many aspects of diabetic therapy, however, remain controversial. As is often the case in medicine, physicians are called upon to make decisions that are based on fragmentary and inconclusive evidence but that may have a profound influence on patients. Of these decisions, those related solely to the diabetic component of care fall into only a few areas. In other words, most of the clinical judgments required in the care of diabetic patients are not very different from those required in the treatment of nondiabetic patients. Problems associated with infection, heart disease, renal disease, cerebrovascular disease, and neuropathy, among others, are similar in diabetic and nondiabetic patients alike. Although the onset and clinical course of some conditions (such as bacterial and fungal infections) may have certain distinctive features in diabetic patients, the basic decisions regarding diagnosis and treatment do not differ appreciably.

On the other hand, several types of clinical judgments are limited to the treatment of patients with diabetes. Some obvious examples are insulin therapy, prescribing special diets, education of patients and their families about diabetes, using oral antidiabetes medications, and treatment of diabetic ketoacidosis. As heretical as it may sound, my feeling is that much of the information in textbooks and review articles on diabetes mellitus is not pertinent to these kinds of clinical decisions. For instance, in muscle, insulin increases glucose transport and has an independent stimulatory effect on glycogen synthesis. In the liver, insulin does not affect glucose transport but does affect the rate-limiting enzymes of glycolysis and gluconeogenesis in a manner that limits hepatic glucose production. The intricate biochemical mechanisms involving phosphorylation and dephosphorylation of the insulin receptor, substrates, and enzymes by which insulin exerts its myriad pleiotropic effects are slowly coming to light through the efforts of basic research investigations. These facts, however, do not really help the physician to decide how to use insulin in a diabetic patient. Other examples of data that contribute to an understanding of the pathogenesis and ramifications of diabetes mellitus but are not important (as yet) in the actual care of diabetic patients are those involving autoantibodies against islet cells, insulin and glutamic acid decarboxylase (GAD), histocompatibility leukocyte antigen (HLA) typing, basement membranes, and mechanisms of insulin secretion.

The purpose of this book is to offer guidance in making only those clinical decisions that are restricted to the treatment of diabetic patients. My personal approach, which has evolved during 30 years of caring for these patients, is presented. Where scientific data are available that permit a better understanding of the problem and/or provide support for the approach used, they are briefly discussed and referenced so that interested readers can avail themselves of more information. In many instances, however, there are no firm data on which to choose the superiority of one method over another. In these situations, my personal reasons for using a particular approach are presented.

This book is intended not only for physicians but also for other health care professionals (e.g., dietitians and nurses) involved in the care and education of people with diabetes. It is important to realize that over 90% of diabetic patients are cared for by primary care physicians (i.e., internists, pediatricians, family practitioners, and general practitioners) rather than by endocrinologists or diabetologists. The level of care offered, however, should be no different among these groups. Evidence-based guidelines of

diabetes care are provided in Chapter 7 and should be met in all diabetic patients regardless of who is caring for them. After all, the patient's health should not be held hostage to the training and the specialty of his or her physician. In several instances, however, I have included additional information that may be of more interest to the specialist, since these data are not readily available from other sources. For example, an explanation of the different methodologies and the clinical interpretation of the various tests for glycated hemoglobins and albumin are provided in Chapter 7.

The first edition of this book was published 16 years ago. Since that time, many important developments have occurred in the field of diabetes. Although they have been welcomed, some have not necessarily led to better care for diabetic patients. I would place in that category the introduction of second-generation sulfonylurea agents and the commercial development of human insulins. Other developments have the potential to improve diabetic care but have yet to do so. This category should include the new information concerning the pathogenesis of types 1 and 2 diabetes, the development of new classes of antihypertensive agents, and continued refinement of beta cell transplantation techniques. Although much more data have been collected concerning the roles of various dietary components on diabetes, these may have complicated the prescribing of diets for people with diabetes.

Some developments have had a positive impact on the care of diabetic patients. In that category, I would place the evolving technologies and use of both self-monitoring of blood glucose and glycated hemoglobin measurements; the treatment of diabetic nephropathy with angiotensin-converting enzyme inhibitors; the introduction of new classes of oral antidiabetes drugs and ultra–short-acting insulin; and the advances in renal transplantation.

In my view, we are now at a crossroads in diabetes care. With the publication of the results of the Diabetes Control and Complications Trial (DCCT) in type 1 diabetes and the Kumamoto Trial in type 2 diabetes (see Chapter 2), there can no longer be any doubt that near euglycemia will certainly ameliorate and possibly prevent the microvascular and neuropathic complications of diabetes. Furthermore, a number of prospective observational studies have shown that better diabetic control is associated with a significant lowering of cardiovascular events and mortality (also in Chapter 2). Yet, the evidence to date is that very few patients are being treated intensively. In the absence of a cure (which seems to me to still be a long way off), we are going to have to use the current tools at our disposal to effect a marked turnaround in the diabetic outcomes in our patients. This, of course, involves the education and motivation of patients as well as of ourselves.

The fourth edition of this book has been updated or rewritten to reflect the changes that have occurred in diabetes care since the last edition. Chapter 1 describes the new classification and diagnostic criteria recently adopted by the American Diabetes Association and the World Health Organization. Chapter 2 incorporates the latest evidence that now unequivocally shows the benefit of attaining near euglycemia. Chapter 3 has been completely rewritten by Marion J. Franz, R.D., C.D.E., M.S., and discusses (among other new information) how to apply the recent American Diabetes Association changes in nutritional therapy involving sucrose, other carbohydrates, and fat content in the diet. Chapter 4 describes the use of the new rapid-acting lyspro (Humalog) insulin and utilizing the bedtime insulin, daytime sulfonylurea (BIDS) approach in patients failing to improve with maximal tolerated doses of oral antidiabetes medication. Chapter 5 describes the use of metformin (Glucophage) and acarbose (Precose). Although the diagnosis and treatment of diabetic ketoacidosis and hyperosmolar nonketotic syndrome have not changed much in recent years (Chapter 6), there is now evidence that cerebral edema probably occurs prior to treatment and is not simply a consequence of therapy. Chapter 7 discusses new evidence-based guidelines for diabetes care and recent information concerning hypoglycemia unawareness, suggesting that much of it may be iatrogenic and reversible. Chapter 8 discusses the Insulin Resistance Syndrome (Syndrome X), new approaches to microalbuminuria and clinical proteinuria, and hypertension, and hyperlipidemia and updates the treatments for diabetic neuropathy. Chapter 9 is a completely new one, Diabetes and Pregnancy, cowritten with John L. Kitzmiller, M.D. Finally, Chapter 10, written by Carol Rosenberg, R.N., C.D.E., M.S., and Anne L. Peters, M.D., describes in detail the information and approaches necessary for effective patient education, the cornerstone of effective diabetes management.

Dietitians and nurses should find all the information they need in Chapters 3 and 10, respectively. Reference is made in these chapters to other parts of the book for more detailed information in specific areas. This book can serve as a reasonably complete textbook on diabetes for all providers caring for such patients, whether they are generalists or specialists. It is my continued hope that the practical information contained in this volume will be used by enough physicians and allied health professionals to significantly improve the health of people with diabetes. We still have a long way to go.

MAYER B. DAVIDSON, M.D.

ACKNOWLEDGMENTS

I am grateful to Anne L. Peters, M.D., for her meticulous review and critique of this volume.

CONTENTS

Diagnosis and Classification of Diabetes Mellitus

DEFINITION

Diabetes mellitus is a syndrome with metabolic, vascular, and neuropathic components that are interrelated. The metabolic syndrome is characterized by alterations in carbohydrate, fat, and protein metabolism secondary to absent or markedly diminished insulin secretion and/or ineffective insulin action. Hyperglycemia is the sine qua non of the metabolic syndrome and is the parameter most closely monitored to make the diagnosis and to judge therapy. The vascular syndrome consists of abnormalities in both large vessels (macroangiopathy) and small vessels (microangiopathy). The macroangiopathic changes cause cerebrovascular accidents, myocardial infarctions, and peripheral vascular disease. Although these large vessel sequelae all occur in people without diabetes, they appear earlier and are more severe in diabetic patients. The clinical expressions of the microangiopathic changes are diabetic retinopathy and nephropathy. Finally, various abnormalities in the peripheral and autonomic nervous systems are also part of the diabetic syndrome. Most of these neuropathic changes are due to metabolic alterations, although a few of them may be secondary to vascular causes.

HISTORICAL BACKGROUND

The difficulty with making a diagnosis of diabetes with certainty is that with the exception of a few populations with markedly increased prevalences of diabetes and conse-

quently a bimodal distribution of glucose concentrations, the distribution of glucose concentrations across most populations is a continuum or unimodal. Thus, the choice of cutoff values for the diagnosis is somewhat arbitrary.[1] It is not surprising, therefore, that before 1979, many different criteria were suggested for the diagnosis of diabetes mellitus.[2] In that year, the National Diabetes Data Group (NDDG) proposed the criteria listed in Table 1-1 for the diagnosis of diabetes.[3] They based their approach on the reasonable assumption that a level of hyperglycemia that subsequently produced the microvascular complications associated with diabetes should be the basis for the diagnosis of diabetes. The criteria in Table 1-1 were based on prospective studies in which approximately 1,500 individuals underwent an oral glucose tolerance test (OGTT) and were evaluated for diabetic retinopathy 3 to 8 years later. Nearly 100 subjects developed retinopathy; 85% of these had values commensurate with a fasting plasma glucose (FPG) concentration $\geq$140 mg/dl and/or a plasma glucose concentration $\geq$200 mg/dl 2 hours after a glucose challenge.[4] (Whole blood glucose concentrations, which are approximately 12% less than plasma values, were measured in some of these studies and converted to FPG levels by the NDDG.) The NDDG[3] also defined normal and impaired glucose tolerance (IGT) (see Table 1-1). The latter is associated with macrovascular disease (see Chapter 8 for discussion of the Insulin Resistance Syndrome) but not the microvascular or neuropathic complications of diabetes. The World Health Organization (WHO)

Table 1–1. National Diabetes Data Group Criteria

	Diabetes Mellitus	Impaired Glucose Tolerance	Normal Glucose Tolerance
Fasting	≥140 (7.8)*	<140 (7.8)*	<115 (6.4)*
	or	*and*	*and*
OGTT (2 hour)	≥200 (11.1)	140–199 (7.8–11.1)	<140 (7.8)
	and	*and*	
OGTT (0.5, 1, or 1.5 hour)	>200 (11.1)	>200 (11.1)	Not part of criteria
	or		
Random	"Gross and unequivocal elevation" of glucose levels with classic symptoms of uncontrolled diabetes	Not part of criteria	Not part of criteria

OGTT, oral glucose tolerance test.
*Venous plasma glucose concentrations in mg/dl (mmol/L).
From National Diabetes Data Group: Classification and diagnosis of diabetes mellitus and other categories of glucose intolerance. Diabetes 28:1039, 1979

adopted similar criteria[5] for the diagnosis of diabetes and IGT except that a glucose concentration during the OGTT before 2 hours was not included (Table 1–2). They did not define normal glucose tolerance. The omission of a glucose concentration before the 2-hour value in the OGTT as part of the criteria simplified the diagnosis because approximately 20% of OGTT results were nondiagnostic by NDDG criteria[4]—that is, the results did not fit into any of the three categories defined in Table 1-1.

CURRENT RECOMMENDED CRITERIA

The criteria for the diagnosis of diabetes have been reevaluated, mainly because the cutoff points of an FPG concentration of 140 mg/dl and a 2-hour value in the OGTT of 200 mg/dl are not equivalent.[6] Nearly everyone with an FPG ≥140 mg/dl has a 2-hour OGTT value ≥200 mg/dl, whereas fewer than half of those not previously known to have diabetes but with 2-hour OGTT values ≥200 mg/dl have FPG concentrations ≥140 mg/dl.[7, 8] Thus, individuals receiving an OGTT would be more likely to be diagnosed with diabetes than if only an FPG concentration were used to evaluate glycemic status. Several large studies have determined that the FPG concentration that is equivalent to a 2-hour OGTT value of 200 mg/dl is approximately 7 mmol/L or 126 mg/dl.[6] Furthermore, OGTTs are poorly reproducible, inconvenient, more costly, and, importantly, not

Table 1–2. Previous Criteria of the World Health Organization

	Diabetes Mellitus	Impaired Glucose Tolerance
Fasting	≥140 (7.8)*	<140 (7.8)*
	or	*and*
OGTT (2 hour)	>200 (11.1)	140–199 (7.8–11.1)
	or	
Random	>200 (11.1)	Not part of criteria

OGTT, oral glucose tolerance test.
*Venous plasma glucose concentrations in mg/dl (mmol/L).
From World Health Organization: Diabetes Mellitus: Report of a WHO Study Group (Tech Rep Series 626). WHO, Geneva, 1980

often used clinically to diagnose diabetes.[4, 8] Based on these considerations, new criteria for the diagnosis of diabetes, which rely heavily on FPG concentrations, have been adopted by the American Diabetes Association and the WHO (Table 1–3). Note that OGTTs are not recommended for routine clinical use. If one is performed (sampling only before and 2 hours after a 75-g glucose load under conditions described by the NDDG[3] and the WHO[5]), the 2-hour value of the NDDG criteria (see Table 1–1) determines the glycemic status.

The new criteria also identify FPG concentrations that do not meet the criteria for diabetes but are higher than the normal value of 110 mg/dl. These individuals are considered to have *impaired fasting glucose* (IFG). IFG is not considered a clinical entity in its own right but is a risk factor for the future development of diabetes (and macrovascular disease). The new classification for etiologic disorders of glycemia (discussed later) does not recognize IGT. Therefore, if

an OGTT is performed and the 2-hour value meets the older criterion for IGT (see Table 1–2), this entity is now considered only a risk factor for the development of diabetes (and macrovascular disease). The risk for diabetes in individuals who had been diagnosed in the past with IGT has been evaluated in nearly 3,000 subjects monitored from 1 to 28 years. Approximately 25% developed diabetes, 25% reverted to normal glucose tolerance, and half remained with IGT (references furnished on request). The rate of progression from IGT to diabetes was <5% per year in Caucasian populations[3] but higher in ethnic groups predisposed to type 2 diabetes (discussed later). One would assume that a similar prognosis would hold for IFG, although data to substantiate this statement are not easily available.

ALTERNATIVE APPROACH

The following is a personal approach to the diagnosis of diabetes, not one sanctioned by either the American Diabetes Association or the WHO. The new FPG concentration for the diagnosis of diabetes defines a new group of individuals who now are considered to have diabetes (i.e., those with FPG concentrations of 126 to 139 mg/dl). Sixty percent of these newly identified diabetic patients have normal glycated hemoglobin levels.[9] In my view, this is incompatible with the diagnosis of diabetes that has been based on a level of hyperglycemia that subsequently produces retinopathy, as discussed earlier. Because glycation of proteins has such a prominent role in the development of the microvascular and neuropathic complications of diabetes,[10] it is difficult (in my opinion) to justify labeling individuals with normal glycated hemoglobin levels as having diabetes. Defining a level of hyperglycemia that optimally diagnoses diabetes requires balancing the insurance, employment, and social costs of making this diagnosis in those who are not at risk for the complications of

Table 1–3. Official Criteria for the Diagnosis of Diabetes Mellitus

1. Symptoms of diabetes plus casual plasma glucose concentration ≥200 mg/dl (11.1 mmol/L). [Casual = any time of day without regard to time since last meal. The classic symptoms of diabetes include polyuria, polydipsia, and unexplained weight loss.]
   or
2. Fasting plasma glucose (FPG) ≥126 mg/dl (7.0 mmol/L). Fasting is defined as no caloric intake for at least 8 hours.
   or
3. Two-hour plasma glucose (2hPG) ≥200 mg/dl during an oral glucose tolerance test (OGTT). The test should be performed as described in reference 3 or 5 using a load of 75 g anhydrous glucose.

In the absence of unequivocal hyperglycemia with acute metabolic decompensation, these criteria should be confirmed by repeat testing on a different day.
The third measure (OGTT) is not recommended for routine clinical use.

Adapted from Report of the Expert Committee on the Diagnosis and Classification of Diabetes Mellitus. Diabetes Care 20:1183, 1977

diabetes against failing to make the diagnosis in those who are.[1] It seems to me that giving subjects with normal glycated hemoglobin levels the diagnosis of diabetes leads to more negative costs than positive benefits. I am unaware of any evidence to support the argument that giving individuals with mild degrees of hyperglycemia a diagnosis of diabetes makes them more compliant with the life style changes (diet and exercise) that are the cornerstone of treatment for them.

An alternative approach to diagnosing diabetes that has clinical relevance uses measurements of FPG concentrations followed by measurement of glycated hemoglobin levels in those with FPG concentrations that neither are normal (<110 mg/dl) nor meet the older criteria for diabetes (≥140 mg/dl)—that is, those with FPG concentrations of 110 to 139 mg/dl. Fewer than 2% of subjects with an FPG concentration <110 mg/dl have a 2-hour OGTT value ≥200 mg/dl.[8] Conversely, approximately 95% of individuals with an FPG concentration ≥140 mg/dl have a 2-hour OGTT value ≥200 mg/dl.[8] Thus, these FPG levels accurately reflect an OGTT that is either normal or diagnostic of diabetes. FPG concentrations between 110 and 139 mg/dl do not accurately predict the results of an OGTT. The 2-hour value is normal (<140 mg/dl), consistent with the older diagnosis of IGT (140 to 199 mg/dl), or diagnostic of diabetes (≥200 mg/dl) in approximately equal proportions (i.e., one third each).[8]

I use a glycated hemoglobin determination (see Chapter 7 for discussion of glycated hemoglobin) to decide whether an individual with an FPG concentration of 110 to 139 mg/dl has diabetes or a milder degree of hyperglycemia. A glycated hemoglobin level ≥1% above the upper limit of normal (ULN) for the assay used (if confirmed) establishes the diagnosis of diabetes. A lower value places subjects in a higher risk category to develop diabetes (and possibly cardiovascular disease) but does not label them as having diabetes at this time. This glycated hemoglo-

bin value was selected for four reasons. First, a strong clinical argument can be made for maintaining a glycated hemoglobin level <1% above the ULN. The mean glycated hemoglobin level in the intensively treated patients in both the Diabetes Control and Complications Trial[11] (evaluating type 1 patients) and the Kumamoto study[12] (evaluating type 2 patients) (see Chapter 2 for description of these) was approximately 1% above the ULN for the assays used. This group of patients in both of these long-term studies had a marked decrease in the development and progression of the microvascular and neuropathic complications of diabetes compared with the control group, whose mean glycated hemoglobin levels were approximately 3% above the ULN. Furthermore, in a large study[13] evaluating the development of microalbuminuria (the earliest evidence of diabetic nephropathy [see Chapter 8]), the risks were minimal in patients with glycated hemoglobin levels <1% above the ULN for their assay. Second, patients with glycated hemoglobin levels ≥1% above the ULN for the assay used had a 90% to 95% chance of meeting the OGTT criteria for diabetes.[4, 8] Third, individuals with lesser degrees of hyperglycemia (e.g., IFG) almost always have normal or only slightly elevated glycated hemoglobin levels. Fourth, a glycated hemoglobin level ≥1% above the ULN is high enough to keep the false-positive rate for the diagnosis of diabetes to 5% to 10%, and most of these individuals would have IFG.[4, 8]

What would be lost by not making the diagnosis of diabetes in an individual with an FPG of 126 to 139 mg/dl (the new cohort of diabetic patients by the revised criteria) but with a glycated hemoglobin level <1% above the ULN for the assay used? Most clinicians would agree that if a patient's glycated hemoglobin level is <1% above the ULN, control is satisfactory and no change in therapy is necessary. Therefore, these patients are given nutritional counseling and exercise advice, not pharmacologic agents, irrespective of whether they carried the diagnosis of diabetes or IFG. An analogy might be made to obese individuals who have FPG concentrations <110 mg/dl and who are also at risk for diabetes, hypertension, and certain dyslipidemias. The clinical approach is the same in both groups. In addition to nutritional and exercise counseling, blood pressure, lipid levels, and glycemic status should be closely monitored and each treated pharmacologically if necessary. Thus, no therapeutic advantage is gained by giving patients the diagnosis of diabetes, but there are potential employment, insurance, and social disadvantages.[14]

To summarize my alternative approach to diagnosing diabetes, the initial test is an FPG concentration. If the value is <110 mg/dl, the individual has normal glycemia. If the value is ≥140 mg/dl, the individual has diabetes if that value is confirmed. If the FPG concentration is 110 to 139 mg/dl, a glycated hemoglobin level is measured. If the level is ≥1% above the ULN for the assay used, the individual has diabetes if that value is confirmed. If the glycated hemoglobin level is <1% above the ULN, the individual has a degree of hyperglycemia that is less than

diabetes and would be included in the new category of IFG (realizing that according to the new official criteria,[6] those individuals with FPG concentrations of 126 to 139 mg/dl would be considered to have diabetes regardless of their glycated hemoglobin levels).

An algorithm for using this alternative approach for diagnosing diabetes, taking into account the various possibilities on repeat testing to confirm the diagnosis, is shown in Figure 1-1. Although the assay for glycated hemoglobin has not yet been standardized,[15] its imperfections would lead (in my view) to many fewer misdiagnoses in individuals with FPG concentrations of 126 to 139 mg/dl. These patients, by the new criteria, are now considered to have diabetes. For example, if the results of the glycated hemoglobin test were falsely low, leading to a false-negative diagnosis of diabetes, the initial treatment with diet and exercise would be the same if the patient had been correctly diagnosed with diabetes. If the results of the glycated hemoglobin test were falsely high, a false-positive diagnosis of diabetes would be made. However, this would assuredly occur in many less than 60% of the new cohort of

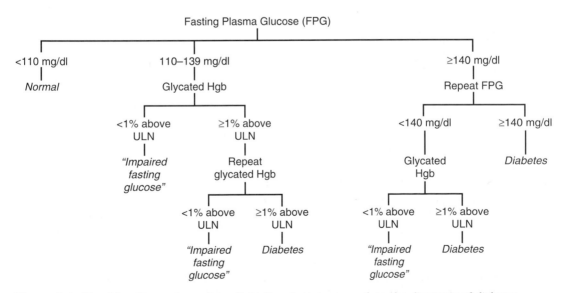

Figure 1–1. Algorithm for an alternative, clinically relevant approach to the diagnosis of diabetes mellitus. ULN, upper limit of normal for assay used; FPG, fasting plasma glucose; Hgb, hemoglobin.

Table 1–4. Criteria for Testing for Diabetes in Asymptomatic, Undiagnosed Individuals

1. Testing for diabetes should be considered in all individuals at age 45 years and older. If results are normal, it should be repeated at 3-year intervals.
2. Testing should be considered at a younger age or should be carried out more frequently in individuals who
   * are obese (≥120% desirable body weight or a body mass index ≥27 kg/m²)
   * have a first-degree relative with diabetes
   * are members of a high-risk ethnic population (e.g., African American, Hispanic, Native American)
   * delivered a baby weighing >9 pounds or who have been diagnosed with gestational diabetes mellitus (GDM)
   * are hypertensive (≥140/90)
   * have an HDL-C level ≤35 mg/dl and/or a triglyceride level ≥250 mg/dl
   * had impaired fasting glucose (IFG) or impaired glucose tolerance (IGT) on previous testing

The FPG test or OGTT may be used to diagnose diabetes; however, the FPG test is greatly preferred because of its ease of administration, convenience, acceptability to patients, and lower cost. The OGTT is not recommended in clinical settings.

OGTT, oral glucose tolerance test.

Adapted from Report of the Expert Committee on the Diagnosis and Classification of Diabetes Mellitus. Diabetes Care 20:1183, 1977

patients diagnosed with diabetes. Therefore, if one agrees that making the diagnosis of diabetes in a person whose glycated hemoglobin level is normal is inappropriate, the approach depicted in Figure 1–1, for the reasons discussed earlier, is a reasonable alternative.

Persons who should be screened for diabetes are listed in Table 1–4.

GESTATIONAL DIABETES MELLITUS

Pregnancy presents an exception to the previous discussion about the diagnosis of diabetes. Because even minor abnormalities of glucose tolerance in pregnant women can be associated with increased risk to the fetus at delivery or in the neonatal period, it was previously recommended that screening for gestational diabetes mellitus (GDM) be carried out for all pregnant women. This recommendation has been altered to exclude from screening those women in a low-risk group for GDM because it is unlikely to be very cost-effective.[6] Women in this low-risk group are younger than 25 years, are of normal body weight, have no first-degree relatives with diabetes, and are not members of an ethnic/racial group with a high prevalence of type 2 diabetes (Hispanic, African American, Native American, Asian). Pregnant women who fulfill *all* of these criteria usually do not need to be screened for GDM unless they have other high-risk characteristics for a poor obstetric outcome (see Chapter 9).

Screening is usually carried out between 24 and 28 weeks of gestation (unless other high-risk factors indicate an earlier evaluation). The oral glucose load is 50 g, and the test does not have to be performed in the fasting state. If the glucose concentration measured 1 hour later is ≥140 mg/dl, a full OGTT should be carried out. This OGTT differs from the OGTT performed in the nonpregnant state in three respects. First, the recommended oral glucose load is 100 g. Second, blood samples are collected before and 1, 2, and 3 hours after the oral challenge. Third—and most importantly—the criteria (Table 1-5) for making the diagnosis of diabetes in pregnancy are much more sensitive than in nongravid women.[3] When screening was carried out in all pregnant women, GDM was found in approximately 2% to 4%.[16] This prevalence should remain unchanged if low-risk women are excluded from screening. (Diabetes and pregnancy are discussed in Chapter 9.)

CLASSIFICATION

In 1979, the NDDG (in addition to proposing diagnostic criteria) also classified diabetes and its related disorders.[3] The WHO adopted this classification (with minor modifications)

**Table 1–5. Screening* and Diagnosis†
Scheme for Gestational Diabetes Mellitus**

	50-g Screening Test	100-g Diagnostic Test
Fasting	—	105 mg/dl
1 hour	140 mg/dl	190 mg/dl
2 hour	—	165 mg/dl
3 hour	—	145 mg/dl

*Screening for gestational diabetes mellitus (GDM) should *not* be performed in pregnant women who meet *all* of the following criteria: <25 years of age, normal body weight, no first-degree relative with diabetes, *and* not Hispanic, Native American, Asian, or African-American.

†The 100-g diagnostic test is performed on patients who have a positive result of a screening test. The diagnosis of GDM requires any two of the four plasma glucose values obtained during the test to meet or exceed the values shown above.

Adapted from Report of the Expert Committee on the Diagnosis and Classification of Diabetes Mellitus. Diabetes Care 20:1183, 1997

the next year[5] and added malnutrition-related diabetes in 1985.[17] Given the state of knowledge at that time, the classification was based on a combination of clinical manifestations or treatment requirements—for example, insulin-dependent diabetes mellitus (IDDM, type 1), non-insulin-dependent diabetes mellitus (NIDDM, type 2), and pathogenesis (e.g., "other types" [secondary], gestational). When the earlier classification was formulated, a definitive cause of any of the categories of diabetes had not been established except for some of the secondary types (e.g., steroid induced, pancreatitis). Some of the genetic markers for type 1 diabetes had just been discovered, but an in-depth understanding of the immunologic basis for type 1 diabetes was in its infancy.

In the past decade and a half, a much firmer understanding of the pathogenesis and, in some cases, the etiology of the various categories of diabetes has been attained. On the basis of these new findings, both the Expert Committee on the Diagnosis and Classification of Diabetes[6] (constituted by the American Diabetes Association) and the WHO[18] have proposed a new classification of diabetes and its related disorders (Table

1–6). The main features of the changes are as follows:

1. The terms *insulin-dependent diabetes mellitus* and *non-insulin-dependent diabetes mellitus* and their acronyms (IDDM and NIDDM) have been eliminated. Many physicians, allied health professionals, and patients have been confused by this nomenclature and mistakenly classified all individuals receiving insulin as having IDDM. The terms *type 1* and *type 2* diabetes are retained.

2. The category of diabetes named *type 1* includes all forms of diabetes that are either *primarily* caused by autoimmune destruction of the pancreatic β-cells or due to a *primary* defect in β-cell function secondary to another (nonautoimmune) cause.

3. The category of diabetes named *type 2* includes the most common form of diabetes, which results from insulin resistance combined with inadequate insulin secretion.

4. IGT is removed as a distinct clinical entity and is considered to be a risk factor only.

5. The category of gestational diabetes is retained but has been defined differently by the Expert Committee on the Classification and Diagnosis of Diabetes[6] (who retained the criteria of the NDDG[3]) and the WHO.[18]

6. Malnutrition-related diabetes has been deleted by the WHO.

It is important to realize that in this new classification, patients with any form of diabetes may require insulin treatment at some stage of their disease. The use of insulin per se does not help to designate which category of diabetes a patient has.

TYPE 1 DIABETES

The *autoimmune* form is by far the most common. It was previously called type 1 diabetes, IDDM, or juvenile-onset diabetes. It results from a cell-mediated autoimmune destruction of the pancreatic β-cells. The rate of destruction is variable but is generally more rapid in children than in adults. Some

Table 1–6. Etiologic Classification of Diabetes Mellitus

I. Type 1 diabetes* (β-cell destruction usually leading to absolute insulin deficiency)
  A. Autoimmune
  B. Idiopathic
II. Type 2 diabetes* (insulin resistance with relative insulin deficiency)
III. Other specific types
  A. Genetic defects of β-cell function
    1. Mitochondrial DNA defect
    2. Wolfram's syndrome
    3. Maturity-onset diabetes of the young (MODY)
      a. Chromosome 20q (MODY-1)
      b. Chromosome 7p (MODY-2)
      c. Chromosome 12q (MODY-3)
  B. Genetic defects in insulin action
    1. Type A insulin resistance
    2. Leprechaunism
    3. Rabson-Mendenhall syndrome
    4. Lipodystrophy
  C. Diseases of the exocrine pancreas
    1. Pancreatitis (including fibrocalculous pancreatopathy)
    2. Pancreatectomy
    3. Trauma (severe)
    4. Neoplasia
    5. Cystic fibrosis
    6. Hemochromatosis
  D. Endocrinopathies
    1. Cushing's syndrome
    2. Acromegaly
    3. Pheochromocytoma
    4. Glucagonoma
    5. Aldosteronoma
    6. Hyperthyroidism
    7. Somatostatinoma
  E. Drug or chemical induced
    1. Nicotinic acid
    2. Glucocorticoids
    3. Thyroid hormone
    4. β-Adrenergic agonists
    5. Thiazides
    6. Phenytoin (Dilantin)
    7. Pentamidine (intravenous)
    8. Diazoxide
    9. Vacor
    10. Interferon-α
  F. Infections
    1. Congenital rubella
    2. Cytomegalovirus
    3. Coxsackie B
    4. Mumps
    5. Adenovirus
  G. Uncommon forms of immune-mediated diabetes
    1. Anti-insulin receptor antibodies
    2. Stiff-man syndrome
  H. Other genetic syndromes sometimes associated with diabetes
    1. Down's syndrome
    2. Klinefelter's syndrome
    3. Turner's syndrome
    4. Prader-Willi syndrome
    5. Myotonic dystrophy
    6. Laurence-Moon-Biedl syndrome
    7. Friedreich's ataxia
    8. Huntington's chorea
    9. Porphyria
    10. Others†
IV. Gestational diabetes mellitus (GDM)

*Patients with any form of diabetes may require insulin at some stage of their disease. Such use of insulin does not, per se, classify the patient.

†A more complete listing of genetic syndromes sometimes associated with diabetes can be found in Table 24-3 in reference 71.

Adapted from Report of the Expert Committee on the Diagnosis and Classification of Diabetes Mellitus. Diabetes Care 20:1183, 1997

patients, particularly children and adolescents, may present with ketoacidosis as the first manifestation of the disease. Others have modest fasting hyperglycemia that can rapidly change to severe hyperglycemia or ketoacidosis in the presence of infection or other stress. Still others, particularly adults, may retain residual β-cell function for many years. When β-cell reserves of insulin are depleted, these patients are ketosis prone—that is, they develop ketosis and eventually ketoacidosis in the absence of insulin treatment (see Chapter 2) and cannot survive without it. Markers of immune destruction (autoantibodies to islet cells, insulin, glutamic acid decarboxylase [GAD] in the islets, and tyrosine phosphatases in the islets) are present in 85% to 90% of individuals when fasting hyperglycemia is initially detected. The peak incidence of this form of type 1 diabetes occurs in childhood and adolescence. Approximately 75% of individuals who develop this type of diabetes do so before 30 years of age. The onset in the remaining patients may occur at any age, even in the eighth and ninth decades of life. Autoimmune destruction of β-cells has a genetic predisposition (that can be identified by human leukocyte antigen [HLA] typing) but is also related to environmental factors that are still poorly understood (see Chapter 2). Although these patients are characteristically lean, this form of type 1 diabetes can occasionally occur in obese individuals as well. These patients are also prone to other autoimmune disorders, such as Graves' disease, Hashimoto's thyroiditis, Addison's disease, and vitiligo.

Some forms of type 1 diabetes are *idiopathic*. Only a small minority of patients with type 1 diabetes fall into this category. Of these, not all have permanent insulinopenia and are prone to ketoacidosis. This is a form of type 1 diabetes, most common among African Americans,[19, 20, 20a] in which patients may present with diabetic ketoacidosis but their subsequent requirements for insulin may wax and wane. The lesion seems to be decreased insulin secretion rather than insulin resistance.[21] This form of diabetes is strongly inherited, lacks immunologic evidence for autoimmunity, and is not associated with any particular types of HLA.

TYPE 2 DIABETES

In type 2 diabetes, NIDDM, or adult-onset diabetes, affected individuals have insulin resistance in combination with a relative (rather than an absolute) deficiency of insulin secretion. Initially and sometimes throughout their lifetimes, these patients do not require insulin to achieve satisfactory diabetic control. There are almost certainly many different causes of type 2 diabetes (as defined here), and it is likely that the number of patients in this currently most common form of diabetes will decrease in the future as identification of specific pathogenic processes and genetic defects permits better dif-

ferentiation and a more definitive classification. Indeed, the major differences between the older classification[3] and this new one (see Table 1-6) reflect just that evolution. Although the specific causes of this form of diabetes are not known, autoimmune destruction of pancreatic β-cells does not occur and patients do not have any other known causes of diabetes or association with other diseases listed in Table 1-6.

Eighty to 90% of patients with this form of diabetes are obese. Obesity itself adds additional insulin resistance. Even those patients who are not obese by traditional weight criteria—for example, percent of desirable body weight (see appendix to Chapter 7 for estimation) or body mass index (kilograms of weight per meters of height^2)—may have an increased percentage of body fat distributed predominantly in the abdominal region (see the discussion of Insulin Resistance Syndrome in Chapter 8). Ketoacidosis can rarely occur in type 2 diabetes, but it is almost always precipitated by the stress of another illness (e.g., infection). Type 2 diabetes is frequently undiagnosed for many years because the elevated glucose concentrations are not high enough to elicit the classic symptoms of uncontrolled diabetes. It has been estimated that the length of time between the onset of hyperglycemia and the diagnosis of type 2 diabetes is 9 to 12 years.[22] Unfortunately, these patients are at increased risk of developing the microvascular, neuropathic, and macrovascular complications of diabetes (see Chapter 8) during this period. This delay in diagnosis explains why approximately 20% of patients have one or more of the microvascular and neuropathic complications when the diagnosis of diabetes is first made.

Although patients with this form of diabetes may have insulin concentrations that appear to be normal or even high, the elevated glucose levels would be expected to result in even higher insulin concentrations if β-cell function were normal. Thus, insulin secretion is defective in these patients and is insufficient to compensate for their insulin resistance. Although their insulin resistance diminishes with weight reduction and lowering of glucose concentrations by either nonpharmacologic or pharmacologic means (reversal of glucose toxicity[23]), the genetic component of insulin resistance remains. Because some effective insulin also remains in these patients, they are ketosis resistant —that is, even in the absence of treatment, ketonuria is very unlikely (see Chapter 2 for metabolic explanation).

The risk of developing type 2 diabetes increases with obesity, age, and a sedentary life style. It is estimated that the chances double for every 20% increase over desirable body weight and for each decade after the fourth (the latter regardless of weight). The prevalence of diabetes in persons 65 to 74 years of age is nearly 20%[7] and probably is higher in people in the 9th and 10th decades. Type 2 diabetes is more common in certain ethnic groups. Compared with a 6% prevalence in Caucasians, the prevalence in African Americans and Asian Americans is estimated to be 10%, in Hispanics 15%, and in certain Native American tribes 20% to 50%.[24, 25] Finally, it occurs much more frequently in women with prior GDM (25% to 50%)[26] compared with those going through pregnancy with normal glucose tolerance (see Chapter 9). Type 2 diabetes is often associated with a strong familial, probably genetic predisposition, much more so, in fact, than with the autoimmune form of type 1 diabetes. However, the genetics of type 2 diabetes are complex and not clearly defined (see Chapter 2). This is at least partly because of the heterogeneity of this form of diabetes, as mentioned earlier.

OTHER SPECIFIC TYPES

Genetic Defects of the β-Cell

A point mutation in mitochondrial DNA (which is therefore maternally transmitted) has been found to be associated with diabe-

tes and deafness.[27, 28] This occurs at position 3243 in the transfer RNA of the leucine gene leading to an A-to-G substitution. An identical lesion occurs in the MELAS syndrome (*mito*chondrial myopathy, *e*ncephalopathy, *l*actic acidosis, and *s*trokelike syndrome); however, diabetes is not part of this syndrome, suggesting different phenotypic expressions of this genetic lesion.

Wolfram's syndrome is an autosomal recessive disorder characterized by insulin-deficient diabetes and the absence of β-cells at autopsy.[29] Other manifestations include diabetes insipidus, hypogonadism, optic atrophy, and neural deafness.

Maturity-onset diabetes of the young (MODY) is characterized by onset of hyperglycemia at an early age (generally before age 25 years).[30] It is inherited in an autosomal dominant pattern. Individuals with MODY have impaired insulin secretion rather than decreased insulin action.[31-33] Abnormalities at three genetic loci in separate families have been identified. The lesion on chromosome 7p (MODY-2) results in a defective glucokinase gene.[34, 35] Glucokinase converts glucose to glucose-6-phosphate, the metabolism of which in the β-cell stimulates insulin secretion. Thus, glucokinase serves as the glucose sensor for the β-cell. Because of this defect in the glucokinase gene, increased concentrations of glucose are necessary to elicit normal insulin secretion. A second lesion that has been identified is on chromosome 20q (MODY-1) and is tightly linked to the adenosine deaminase locus.[36, 37] A third identified lesion is on chromosome 12q (MODY-3) and is linked to microsatellite markers.[38, 39] The mechanisms by which the latter two genetic abnormalities cause hyperglycemia are unknown, although both affected genes produce hepatic transcription factors.

Genetic Defects in Insulin Action

Many unusual causes of diabetes result from genetically determined abnormalities of insulin action. The metabolic abnormalities associated with mutations of the insulin receptor[40] may range from hyperinsulinemia and modest hyperglycemia to frank diabetes. Some individuals with these mutations may have acanthosis nigricans. Women may be virilized and have enlarged, cystic ovaries. In the past, this syndrome was termed *type A insulin resistance*.[41] Leprechaunism[42, 43] and the Rabson-Mendenhall syndrome[44] are two pediatric syndromes that have mutations in the insulin receptor gene with subsequent alterations in insulin receptor function and extreme insulin resistance. The former is distinguished by characteristic facial features, and the latter is associated with abnormalities of teeth and nails and pineal gland hyperplasia. Patients with these syndromes and other patients with alterations in insulin receptor function may have defects[40] in (1) receptor synthesis, (2) transport of the receptor to the plasma membrane, (3) binding of the receptor to the insulin molecule, (4) transmembrane signaling, or (5) endocytosis-recycling-degradation of the receptor.

Patients with both total[45] and partial[46] congenital lipodystrophy have insulin resistance but normal insulin receptor genes.[47, 48] Therefore, it is assumed that the lesions must reside in the postreceptor signal transduction pathways in these conditions.

Diseases of the Exocrine Pancreas

Any process that diffusely injures enough of the pancreas can cause diabetes. Acquired processes include pancreatitis,[49] pancreatectomy, and severe trauma. A unique combination of pancreatitis and diabetes, termed *fibrocalculous pancreatic diabetes*[50] or *fibrocalculous pancreatopathy*,[6] is a form of diabetes with a high prevalence in tropical and developing countries. It most often affects young and malnourished individuals. It is characterized by abdominal pain radiating to the back, pancreatic calcifications on radiographs, and, frequently, exocrine insufficiency.[50, 51] It had been considered part of malnutrition-related diabetes[50] until recently,

when that category of diabetes was deleted.[18] Inherited processes include cystic fibrosis[52] and hemochromatosis[53] (bronze diabetes). An exception to the statement that diffuse injury is necessary to cause diabetes is the increased association of diabetes with adenocarcinoma of the pancreas[54, 55] (which is usually localized to a small part of the pancreas).

Endocrinopathies[56]

Hormonal secretion by some endocrine tumors can cause diabetes. Excess secretion of glucocorticoids (Cushing's syndrome, in which Cushing's disease is one cause), growth hormone (acromegaly), and catecholamines (pheochromocytoma) impairs insulin action. The main effect of hyperthyroidism is to increase glucose turnover, although insulin action is also mildly impaired.[57] Diabetes does not occur in hyperthyroidism unless β-cell reserve is also decreased. Catecholamines (pheochromocytoma), somatostatinomas,[58] and aldosteronomas (via hypokalemia)[59] impair insulin secretion. Glucagonomas cause mild diabetes by increasing hepatic glucose production. Diabetes generally disappears with successful treatment of the endocrinopathies, although in my experience it may persist even after resolution of Cushing's syndrome and acromegaly.

Drug or Chemical Induced[60, 61]

Drugs can cause diabetes by either impairing insulin secretion or enhancing insulin resistance. Those that affect insulin secretion are intravenous (not inhaled) pentamidine,[61a] Vacor[62] (a rat poison, not a drug), phenytoin (Dilantin), interferon-α[63, 64] (probably by an autoimmune mechanism), diazoxide, and thiazides (secondary to potassium deficiency). Those that affect insulin action are nicotinic acid (niacin), glucocorticoids, β-adrenergic agonists, thyroid hormones, and estrogens. Estrogens and thyroid hormones usually precipitate diabetes only in those who have impaired β-cell reserves, who in the absence of these two drugs are able to maintain normoglycemia.

Infections

The role of viruses in causing diabetes is controversial.[65] They may be involved in the pathogenesis of diabetes in one of two ways: either by directly infecting and destroying pancreatic β-cells or by precipitating or contributing to the autoimmune process that underlies immune-mediated type 1 diabetes. Although evidence for direct pancreatic involvement has been obtained in several patients,[66, 67] it has been conspicuously absent in almost all others in which it was sought.[68] Thus, the viruses listed in Table 1–6 are most likely to be involved in the pathogenesis of diabetes by participating somehow in the autoimmune process, because circulating autoantibodies are found in the majority of patients whose diabetes has been linked to viruses.

Uncommon Forms of Immune-Mediated Diabetes

Two known conditions are currently in this category. The stiff-man syndrome is an autoimmune disorder involving the central nervous system and is characterized by painful stiffness of the axial muscles and painful spasms.[69] Patients often have high titers of autoantibodies to GAD, and approximately one third develop diabetes.

Autoantibodies to the insulin receptor compete with insulin for binding to the receptor, thereby blocking the action of the hormone and causing diabetes.[41] As in other states of extreme insulin resistance (listed earlier under Genetic Defects of Insulin Action), patients with antibodies to the insulin receptor often have acanthosis nigricans. This syndrome was originally termed *type B insulin resistance*.[41] These antibodies can sometimes activate the insulin receptor,

causing hypoglycemia. Anti-insulin receptor antibodies are also occasionally found in other autoimmune states (e.g., systemic lupus erythematosus, Hashimoto's thyroiditis, scleroderma, primary biliary cirrhosis, immune thrombocytopenia purpura) as well as in Hodgkin's lymphoma.[70] In these instances, hypoglycemia is the clinical problem.

Other Genetic Syndromes Sometimes Associated with Diabetes

Many genetic syndromes are accompanied by an increased incidence of diabetes mellitus.[71] The chromosomal abnormalities of only a few have been identified (e.g., Down's syndrome, Klinefelter's syndrome, Turner's syndrome). In none of these genetic syndromes, however, has the mechanism of diabetes been elucidated. Other genetic syndromes sometimes associated with diabetes are listed in Table 1–6.

REFERENCES

1. Knowler WC: Screening for NIDDM: opportunities for detection, treatment, and prevention. Diabetes Care 17:445, 1994
2. Valleron AJ, Eschwege E, Papoz L, Rosselin GE: Agreement and discrepancy in the evaluation of normal and diabetic oral glucose tolerance test. Diabetes 24:585, 1975
3. National Diabetes Data Group: Classification and diagnosis of diabetes mellitus and other categories of glucose intolerance. Diabetes 28:1039, 1979
4. Davidson MB, Peters AL, Schriger DL: An alternative approach to the diagnosis of diabetes with a review of the literature. Diabetes Care 18:1065, 1995
5. World Health Organization (WHO): Diabetes Mellitus: Report of a WHO Study Group (Tech Rep Series 646). WHO, Geneva, 1980
6. Report of the Expert Committee on the Diagnosis and Classification of Diabetes Mellitus. Diabetes Care 20:1183, 1997
7. Harris MI, Hadden WC, Knowler WC et al: Prevalence of diabetes and impaired glucose tolerance and plasma glucose levels in U.S.

population aged 20-74 yr. Diabetes 36:523, 1987

8. Peters AL, Davidson MB, Schriger DL et al: A clinical approach for the diagnosis of diabetes mellitus. JAMA 15:1246, 1996

9. Peters AL, Schriger DL: Impact of new diagnostic criteria on the diagnosis of diabetes (abstract). Diabetes 46(suppl I): 7A, 1997

10. Bucala R, Cerami A, Vlassara H: Advanced glycosylation end products in diabetic complications. Diabetes Rev 3:258, 1995

11. The Diabetes Control and Complications Trial Research Group: The effect of intensive treatment of diabetes on the development and progression of long-term complications in insulin-dependent diabetes mellitus. N Engl J Med 329:977, 1993

12. Ohkubo Y, Kishikawa H, Araki E et al: Intensive insulin therapy prevents the progression of diabetic microvascular complications in Japanese patients with non-insulin-dependent diabetes mellitus: a randomized prospective 6-year study. Diabetes Res Clin Pract 28:103, 1995

13. Krolewski AS, Laffel LMB, Krolewski M et al: Glycosylated hemoglobin and the risk of microalbuminuria in patients with insulin-dependent diabetes mellitus. N Engl J Med 332:1251, 1995

14. Tattersall RB, Jackson JGL: Social and emotional complications of diabetes. In Keen H, Jarrett J (eds): Complications of Diabetes. Year Book Medical Publishers, Chicago, 1982, p 271

15. American Diabetes Association: Tests of glycemia in diabetes (Position Statement). Diabetes Care 20 (Suppl 1) S18–S20, 1997

16. Coustan DR: Diagnosis of gestational diabetes. Diabetes Rev 3:614, 1995

17. World Health Organization: Diabetes Mellitus: Report of a WHO Study Group (WHO Tech Rep Series 727). WHO, Geneva, 1985

18. World Health Organization: Diabetes mellitus (WHO Tech Rep Series). WHO, Geneva, December 1997

19. Winter WE, Maclaren NK, Riley WJ et al: Maturity-onset diabetes of youth in black Americans. N Engl J Med 316:285, 1987

20. Banerji MA, Lebovitz HE: Remission in non-insulin-dependent diabetes mellitus: clinical characteristics of remission and relapse in black patients. Medicine 69:176, 1990

20a. Umpierrez GE, Casals MMC, Gebhar SSP et al: Diabetic ketoacidosis in obese African-Americans. Diabetes 44:790, 1995

21. Banerji MA, Chaiken RL, Lebovitz HE: Long-term normoglycemic remission in black newly diagnosed NIDDM subjects. Diabetes 45:337, 1996

22. Harris MI, Klein R, Welborn TA et al: Onset of NIDDM occurs at least 4-7 yr before clinical diagnosis. Diabetes Care 15:815, 1992

23. Yki-Jarvinen H: Glucose toxicity. Endocr Rev 13:415, 1992

24. Carter JS, Pugh JA, Monterrosa A: Non-insulin-dependent diabetes mellitus in minorities in the United States. Ann Intern Med 125:221, 1996

25. Fujimoto WY, Leonetti DL, Kinyoun J et al: Prevalence of diabetes mellitus and impaired glucose tolerance among second-generation Japanese-American men. Diabetes 36:721, 1987

26. O'Sullivan JB: Body weight and subsequent diabetes mellitus. JAMA 248:949, 1982

27. Gerbitz K-D, Gempel K, Brdiczka D: Genetic, biochemical and clinical implications of the cellular energy circuit. Diabetes 45:113, 1996

28. Maassen JA, Kadowaki T: Maternally inherited diabetes and deafness: a new diabetes subtype. Diabetologia 39:375, 1996

29. Karasik A, O'Hara C, Srikanta S et al: Genetically programmed selective islet β cell loss in diabetes mellitus of Wolfram syndrome. Diabetes Care 12:135, 1989

30. Fajans SS: Scope and heterogeneous nature of MODY. Diabetes Care 13:49, 1990

31. Herman WH, Fajans SS, Ortiz FJ et al: Abnormal insulin secretion, not insulin resistance, is the genetic or primary defect of MODY in the RW pedigree. Diabetes 43:40, 1994

32. Wajngot A, Alvarsson M, Glaser A et al: Glucose potentiation of arginine-induced secretion is impaired in subjects with a glucokinase Glu256Lys mutation. Diabetes 43:1402, 1994

33. Pueyo ME, Clement K, Vaxillaire M et al: Arginine-induced insulin release in glucokinase-deficient subjects. Diabetes Care 17:1015, 1994

34. Hattersley AT, Turner RC, Permutt MA et al: Linkage of type 2 diabetes to the glucokinase gene. Lancet 339:1307, 1992

35. Froguel P, Zouali H, Vionnet N et al: Familial

hyperglycemia due to mutations in glucokinase. N Engl J Med 328:697, 1993

36. Bell GI, Xian K-S, Newman MV et al: Gene for non-insulin-dependent diabetes mellitus (maturity-onset diabetes of the young subtype) is linked to DNA polymorphism on human chromosome 20q. Proc Natl Acad Sci USA 88:1484, 1991

37. Bowden DW, Gravius TC, Akots G et al: Identification of genetic markers flanking the locus for maturity-onset diabetes of the young on human chromosome 20. Diabetes 41:88, 1992

38. Vaxillaire M, Boccio V, Philippi A et al: A gene for maturity onset diabetes of the young (MODY) maps to chromosome 12q. Nature Genet 9:418, 1995

39. Menzel S, Yamagat K, Trabb JB et al: Localization of MODY3 to a 5-cM region of human chromosome 12. Diabetes 44:1408, 1995

40. Taylor SI: Molecular mechanisms of insulin resistance: lessons from patients with mutations in the insulin-receptor gene. Diabetes 41:1473, 1992

41. Kahn CR, Flier JS, Bar RS et al: The syndromes of insulin resistance and acanthosis nigricans. N Engl J Med 294:739, 1976

42. Yoshimasa Y, Seino S, Whittaker J et al: Insulin-resistant diabetes due to a point mutation that prevents insulin proreceptor processing. Science 240:784, 1988

43. Kadowaki T, Bevins CL, Cama A et al: Two mutant alleles of the insulin receptor gene in a patient with extreme insulin resistance. Science 240:787, 1988

44. Muller-Wieland D, van der Vorm ER, Streicher R et al: An in-frame insertion in exon 3 and a nonsense mutation in exon 2 of the insulin receptor gene associated with severe insulin resistance in a patient with Rabson-Mendenhall syndrome. Diabetologia 36:1168, 1993

45. Senior B, Gellis SS: The syndromes of total lipodystrophy and of partial lipodystrophy. Pediatrics 33:593, 1964

46. Davidson MB, Young RT: Metabolic studies in familial partial lipodystrophy of the lower trunk and extremities. Diabetologia 11:561, 1975

47. van der Vorm ER, Kuipers A, Bonenkamp JW et al: Patients with lipodystrophic diabetes mellitus of the Seip-Berardineli type express normal insulin receptors. Diabetologia 36:172, 1993

48. Desbois-Mouthon C, Magre J, Amselem S et al: Lipoatrophic diabetes: genetic exclusion of the insulin receptor gene. J Clin Endocrinol Metab 80:314, 1995

49. Sjoberg RJ, Kidd GS: Pancreatic diabetes mellitus. Diabetes Care 12:715, 1989

50. Hoet JJ, Tripathy BB, Rao RH et al: Malnutrition and diabetes in the tropics. Diabetes Care 19:1014, 1996

51. Mohan V, Premalatha G, Padma A et al: Fibrocalculous pancreatic diabetes. Diabetes Care 11:1274, 1996

52. Handwerger S, Roth J, Gorden P et al: Glucose intolerance in cystic fibrosis. N Engl J Med 281:451, 1969

53. Phelps G, Chapman I, Hall P et al: Prevalence of genetic haemochromatosis among diabetic patients. Lancet 2:925, 1989

54. Morris DV, Nabarro JDN: Pancreatic cancer and diabetes mellitus. Diabetes Med 1:119, 1984

55. Gullo L, Pezzilli R, Morselli-Labate AM et al: Diabetes and the risk of pancreatic cancer. N Engl J Med 331:81, 1994

56. Berelowitz M, Eugene HG: Non-insulin dependent diabetes mellitus secondary to other endocrine disorders. In LeRoith D, Taylor S, Olefsky JM (eds): Diabetes Mellitus. A Fundamental and Clinical Text. Lippincott-Raven, 1996, pp 496–502

57. Shen D-C, Davidson MB, Kuo S-W et al: Peripheral and hepatic insulin antagonism in hyperthyroidism. J Clin Endocrinol Metab 66:565, 1988

58. Konomi K, Chijiiwa K, Katsuta T et al: Pancreatic somatostatinoma: a case report and review of the literature. J Surg Oncol 43:259, 1990

59. Conn JW: Hypertension, the potassium ion and impaired carbohydrate tolerance. N Engl J Med 273:1135, 1965

60. Pandit MK, Burke J, Gustafson AB et al: Drug-induced disorders of glucose tolerance. Ann Intern Med 118:529, 1993

61. Bressler P, DeFronzo RA: Drugs and diabetes. Diabetes Rev 2:53, 1994

61a. Bouchard P, Sai P, Reach G et al: Diabetes mellitus following pentamidine-induced hypoglycemia in humans. Diabetes 31:40, 1982

62. Gallanosa AG, Spyker DA, Curnow RT: Diabetes mellitus associated with autonomic and peripheral neuropathy after Vacor poisoning: a review. Clin Toxicol 18:441, 1981

63. Fabris P, Betterle C, Floreani A et al: Development of type I diabetes mellitus during interferon alpha therapy for chronic HCV hepatitis. Lancet 340:548, 1992

64. Shiba T, Morino Y, Tagawa K et al: Onset of diabetes with high titer anti-GAD antibody after IFN therapy for chronic hepatitis. Diabetes Res Clin Pract 30:237, 1996

65. Yoon J-W: A new look at viruses in type 1 diabetes. Diabetes Metab Rev 11:83, 1995

66. Yoon JW, Austin M, Onodera T et al: Virus-induced diabetes mellitus: isolation of a virus from the pancreas of a child with diabetic ketoacidosis. N Engl J Med 300:1173, 1979

67. Champsaur H, Bottazzo G, Bertrams J et al: Virologic, immunologic and genetic factors in insulin-dependent diabetes mellitus. J Pediatr 100:15, 1982

68. Foulis AK, McGill M, Farquharson MA et al: A search for evidence of viral infection in pancreases of newly diagnosed patients with IDDM. Diabetologia 40:53, 1997

69. Solimena M, Folli F, Aparisi R et al: Autoantibodies to GABA-nergic neurons and pancreatic beta cells in stiff-man syndrome. N Engl J Med 41:347, 1992

70. Taylor SI, Barbetti F, Accili D et al: Syndrome of autoimmunity and hypoglycemia. Endocrinol Metab Clin North Am 18:123, 1989

71. Raffel LJ, Scheuner MT, Rotter JI: Genetics of diabetes. In Porte D, Sherwin RS (eds): Diabetes Mellitus, 5th ed. Appleton & Lange, Norwalk, CT, 1997, p 401

CHAPTER 2

TREATMENT—GENERAL PRINCIPLES

METABOLIC PRINCIPLES

In the postabsorptive state (usually 4 or more hours after eating), the plasma glucose concentration remains relatively constant and reflects the balance between glucose production by the liver and glucose utilization by peripheral tissues. The sources of hepatic glucose production are glycogenolysis (the breakdown of glycogen, the storage form of glucose) and gluconeogenesis (the synthesis of new glucose from noncarbohydrate precursors). After 8 to 12 hours without food intake, hepatic glycogenolysis decreases markedly, and gluconeogenesis by the liver is the main source of circulating glucose. At this time, glucose is utilized mainly by the brain and red blood cells, whereas the rest of the tissues use free fatty acids (FFA). The role of basal insulin levels in the fasting state is to oppose the effect of glucagon on the liver and to restrain hepatic glucose production. Insulin does not affect glucose utilization by the brain or red blood cells.

In the 4-hour period after an oral glucose challenge, approximately 70% is taken up by peripheral tissues (primarily muscle) and the remainder is used by splanchnic tissues (probably mostly by the liver). Insulin is secreted in response to the carbohydrate and protein contents of a meal. It increases the amount of glucose transported into muscle. Its effects on hepatic carbohydrate metabolism are complex. Essentially, insulin stimulates glucose utilization by enhancing its storage as glycogen or by increasing glycolysis.

The latter can lead to the conversion of hepatic glucose into adipose tissue triglycerides through a complicated series of reactions. Insulin also inhibits gluconeogenesis and glycogenolysis. The overall results of insulin action on the liver are an increase in glucose utilization after meals and a restraint on glucose production in the postabsorptive state, the period after which meal nutrients have been stored.

Insulin also has a profound influence on fat metabolism. Ingested fat is stored as triglycerides in adipose tissue. Excess carbohydrate calories also form part of the triglyceride molecule. Insulin promotes triglyceride synthesis by helping the dietary fat gain access into the fat cell and by stimulating the conversion of glucose to glycerol, the backbone of the triglyceride molecule. Most importantly, once adipose tissue triglycerides are formed, insulin has a critical role in inhibiting their breakdown. This effect is extremely critical because the FFA released as a result of triglyceride hydrolysis (lipolysis) can be converted to ketone bodies in the liver. In fact, the most important determinant of the rate of formation of ketone bodies is the amount of FFA delivered to the liver. If excess FFA are released from adipose tissue, increased production of ketone bodies by the liver follows. Although these ketone bodies can be utilized to some extent by peripheral tissues, they soon start to accumulate in the circulation and spill over into the urine.

The quantitative relation among the effects of insulin on selected aspects of carbohydrate and fat metabolism is depicted in Figure 2–1. Approximately 25 to 50 μU of insu-

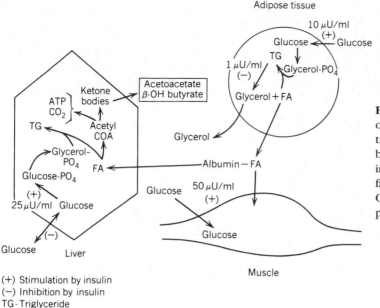

Figure 2–1. Pathophysiology of ketosis. ATP, adenosine triphosphate; (+), stimulation by insulin; (−), inhibition by insulin; TG, triglyceride; FA, fatty acid; β-OH, beta-hydroxy; CO_2, carbon dioxide; PO_4, phosphate; μU, microunit.

lin per milliliter is necessary to affect glucose metabolism by liver and muscle; 10 μU/ml is required to stimulate glucose uptake into fat. However, the inhibition of lipolysis requires only 1 to 2 μU of active insulin per milliliter. Therefore, as the amount of effective insulin diminishes from normal, the first biochemical abnormality to develop is postprandial hyperglycemia. Enough insulin remains to maintain normal fasting glucose concentrations and to prevent ketosis. As the process continues, fasting hyperglycemia develops but the patient still does not become ketotic. Only when virtually no effective insulin is available does ketosis occur. In other words, if an untreated diabetic patient does not manifest ketonuria, the pancreatic β-cells of that patient are still able to secrete some insulin. Alternatively, if a diabetic patient has ketonuria, very little if any effective insulin remains at that time. In patients with type 1 diabetes, the lack of insulin remains because the pancreatic β-cells have been destroyed (see next section), although in a minority of patients some insulin secretion may

return for a brief period (see the discussion of the honeymoon phase in Chapter 7). In severely decompensated type 2 diabetic patients, some (albeit not normal) insulin secretion returns after correction of the marked hyperglycemia and the ketonuria disappears. (This discussion refers to diabetic ketosis and not to starvation ketosis, which is discussed in Chapter 7.)

DISTINGUISHING CLINICAL AND PATHOGENETIC FEATURES OF TYPES 1 AND 2 DIABETES MELLITUS

The distinction between ketosis-resistant and ketosis-prone diabetes has important implications for therapy. Because ketosis-prone (type 1) diabetic patients have virtually no effective endogenous insulin, they require exogenous insulin. Although the need for insulin is not as imperative in ketosis-resistant (type 2) diabetic patients (because without it they do not become ketotic and slip into acidosis), these patients may require insulin because diet and oral medications (sulfonylurea agents and metformin) fail to control their hyperglycemia. Approximately 40% of ketosis-resistant diabetic patients take insulin (see Chapter 4), 40% use sulfonylurea agents (see Chapter 5), and the remaining 20% are treated by diet (see Chapter 3) alone.[1]

Other differences between them are summarized in Table 2–1. Ketosis-prone diabetes has classically been called *juvenile-onset diabetes*. This term is not accurate, however, because a small percentage of diabetic patients whose disease starts in adulthood may be ketosis prone. Furthermore, an increasing number of patients in their teens or at the end of the first decade of life have been found to have ketosis-resistant diabetes, especially in African American, Native Ameri-

can, and Hispanic populations. Patients who have ketosis-prone diabetes usually present with a short history of the symptoms of hyperglycemia (polyuria, polydipsia, lethargy, weight loss), and if their condition is not recognized quickly, it may develop into ketoacidosis.

The events leading up to destruction of the pancreatic β-cell in type 1 diabetes can be divided into five stages. These are depicted in Figure 2–2, in which the hypothetical pancreatic β-cell mass is plotted against time. Genetic, immunologic, and probably environmental (e.g., possibly viral) influences are involved, and these eventually lead to total exhaustion of the β-cell. The major genetic risk factor for the development of type 1 diabetes is the human leukocyte antigen (HLA) genes located on the short arm of

Table 2–1. Metabolic and Clinical Characteristics of the Two Major Types of Diabetes Mellitus

Characteristic	Ketosis-Prone (Type 1)	Ketosis-Resistant (Type 2)
Synonyms	Juvenile-onset diabetes, growth-onset diabetes, IDDM	Adult-onset diabetes, maturity-onset diabetes, NIDDM
Age of onset	Usually during childhood (growth) but sometimes occurs in adults	Usually during adulthood (maturity) but occasionally diagnosed in children and adolescents[a]
Precipitating factors	Altered immune response; environmental "stresses"	Age, obesity
Pancreatic insulin	Very low to absent	Present
Insulin responses to glucose	Little or none	Decreased when weight and glucose levels taken into account
Insulin responses to meals	Little or none	Normal in absolute terms, but nondiabetic persons with this degree of hyperglycemia would have higher levels
Insulin resistance	Present only when diabetes is out of control	Present (independent of obesity and control)
Response to prolonged fast	Hyperglycemia, ketoacidosis	Glucose returns toward normal
Response to stress	Ketoacidosis	Hyperglycemia without ketosis
Associated obesity	Absent	Commonly present (~80%)
Sensitivity to insulin	Usually sensitive	Relatively resistant
Response to diet alone	Negligible	Always present to some degree
Response to sulfonylurea agents and metformin	Absent	Present

IDDM, insulin-dependent diabetes mellitus; NIDDM, non–insulin-dependent diabetes mellitus.
[a]Especially in African American, Native American, and Hispanic populations.

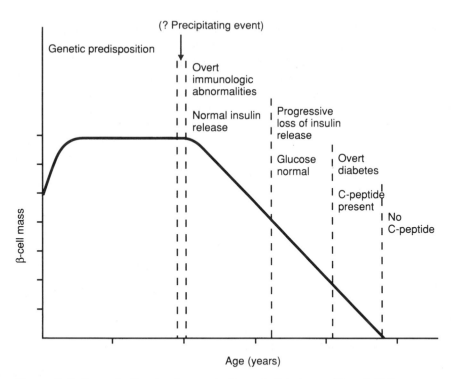

Figure 2–2. Stages in the development of type 1 diabetes mellitus. β-Cell mass (hypothetical) is plotted against time. (From Eisenbarth GS: Type 1 diabetes mellitus: a chronic autoimmune disease. Triangle 23:111, 1984)

the sixth chromosome. Their identification requires testing of white blood cells, which accounts for their name. These genes determine which surface antigens are produced by nucleated cells. The surface antigens are involved in a host of cell-to-cell interactions, one of which includes the rejection process (i.e., the reaction when tissue from one host is transplanted into another). Because many different surface antigens are possible in a population, a large number of separate genes are responsible for them. Two HLA types, DR3 and/or DR4, are present in 95% of Caucasian patients with type 1 diabetes, in contrast to approximately 50% of the general population without type 1 diabetes. This means that certain genes, the ones whose expression produces these HLA types, are also common in these patients and provide a marker for the genetic background that increases susceptibility to type 1 diabetes.

The HLA system in humans is the analogue of the major histocompatibility system that occurs in all animals. This chromosomal region consists of loci that not only control the synthesis of transplantation (surface) antigens but also have fundamental roles in the immune process. Indeed, strong evidence suggests that an immune process is active at the onset of type 1 diabetes. Lymphocytic infiltrates are seen in the islets of Langerhans of patients on whom an autopsy is performed soon after the diagnosis. Autoantibodies against islet cells are present in the sera of more than 80% of type 1 patients if they are tested near the onset of their disease; a gradual reduction in antibody titers occurs during the ensuing year in most patients. Autoantibodies against other antigens are also present.[2] Many patients have autoantibodies against the insulin molecule at the time of diagnosis. (Although it is common for patients treated with insulin to develop antibodies against the hormone [see Chapter 4], new-onset type 1 diabetic patients have not been exposed to exogenous insulin, and their antibodies have been generated against their own insulin.) A third autoantibody that has received much attention in recent years is one produced against glutamic acid decarboxylase (GAD), also known as the 64K antigen until it was correctly identified. This enzyme is located in the β-cell of the pan-

creas. Autoantibodies against antigens between 37,000 and 40,000 molecular weight (commonly called the 37K antigen) have also been found. Some or all of these autoantibodies precede the clinical appearance of type 1 diabetes, sometimes for a period of years. The higher the titer of these autoantibodies (Fig. 2–3) and the more of them present (Fig. 2–4), the more likely the individual is to develop type 1 diabetes.

During this preceding period before the

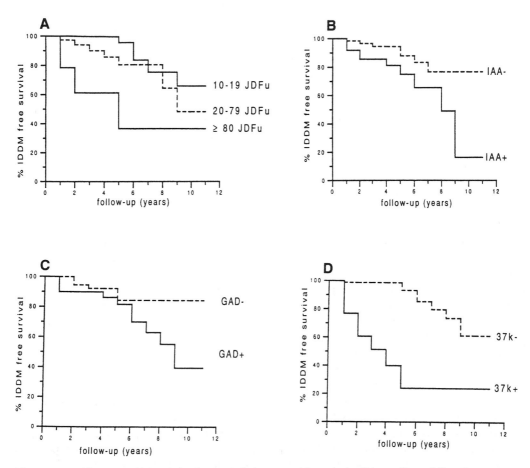

Figure 2–3. The cumulative risk of type 1 diabetes at 10 years in 101 unaffected first-degree relatives of children with type 1 diabetes by *(A)* level of islet cell autoantibodies measured in Juvenile Diabetes Foundation units (JDFu); *(B)* insulin autoantibodies (IAA); *(C)* autoantibodies to glutamic acid decarboxylase (GAD); and *(D)* autoantibodies to the 37K antigen. (From Bingley PJ for the Icarus Group: Interactions of age, islet cell antibodies, insulin autoantibodies, and first-phase insulin response in predicting risk of progression to IDDM in ICA+ relatives: the Icarus data set. Diabetes 45:1720, 1996)

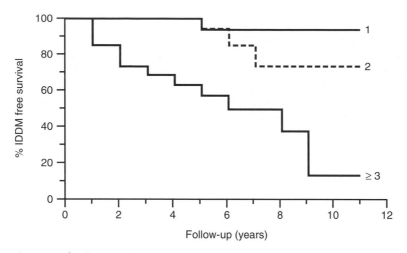

Figure 2–4. The cumulative risk of type 1 diabetes after 10 years in 101 unaffected first-degree relatives of a child with type 1 diabetes by the number of autoantibodies detected. (From Bingley PJ for the Icarus Group: Interactions of age, islet cell antibodies, insulin autoantibodies, and first-phase insulin response in predicting risk of progression to IDDM in ICA+ relatives: the Icarus data set. Diabetes 45:1720, 1996)

development of diabetes in which high titers of these autoantibodies are often present, oral glucose tolerance is normal, and the insulin response to oral glucose is either normal or only subtle changes can be detected. However, the insulin response to intravenous glucose may show a progressive decline. After a bolus of glucose is injected, a rapid (within 1 to 2 minutes) rise of insulin is noted. This acute phase of insulin release falls below 5% of the response in a normal population in those individuals destined to develop type 1 diabetes (even though they still maintain relatively normal glucose and insulin responses to oral glucose). Type 1 diabetes can appear soon afterward (within weeks to months). Even with overt diabetes, these patients initially retain some insulin secretion (as assessed by measurement of C-peptide, a polypeptide packaged with insulin in β-cell granules and secreted along with insulin). Within a year, however, the β-cell is completely exhausted and incapable of secreting any C-peptide or insulin.

Controversy surrounds the possible environmental "stresses" that may trigger the events leading to type 1 diabetes. Although viral infections may have a role, the evidence that viruses precipitate the *acute* clinical onset of type 1 diabetes is much weaker than the case for the importance of an appropriate genetic background and the involvement of immunologic factors. However, evidence suggests that exposure to certain enteroviruses, most commonly Coxsackie B4, may initiate the β-cell destruction starting in the months to years preceding the clinical onset of type 1 diabetes.[2a] The mechanism may involve immunologic cross-reactivity between viral and β-cell antigens. Specifically, one part of the GAD molecule is structurally very similar to a portion of the Coxsackie B4 virus. It seems certain, however, that whatever initiates the chronic auto-immune process, be it viral agent, toxin, or random immunologic event, it occurs because of genetic susceptibility.

Type 2 or ketosis-resistant diabetes was often called *maturity-onset* or *adult-onset* diabetes. As was stated previously, however, ketosis-prone diabetes can start in adults, and ketosis-resistant diabetes (rarely progressing to ketosis) occurs in children and adolescents. The latter is much more common in African American, Native American, and Hispanic populations. Nevertheless, the majority of cases of ketosis-resistant diabetes do begin after the age of 40 years. Aging and obesity have been recognized as two associated factors. Diabetes is diagnosed in approximately 75% of type 2 patients on either a routine physical examination or during the work-up for another medical problem. Only 25% present to their physicians with symptoms.[3]

The pathogenesis of type 2 diabetes involves both relative insulin deficiency and impairment of insulin action. The insulin response to intravenous and oral glucose is decreased, although insulin concentrations after meals are normal or only slightly decreased. Because postprandial glucose levels are elevated, one might expect higher insulin concentrations, and hence a relative insulin deficiency exists. On the other hand, the combination of normal insulin concentrations and hyperglycemia implies the presence of insulin resistance. (The term *insulin resistance* is used here, but this relatively minor degree of insulin ineffectiveness must be distinguished from the clinical syndrome of insulin resistance, in which patients require more than 200 U of insulin per day [see Chapter 4]). Indeed, sophisticated methods of evaluating insulin action have directly shown that insulin works ineffectively in the target tissues (muscle and liver) in patients with type 2 diabetes mellitus. Studies of insulin action in a large number of normal (nondiabetic) subjects have revealed a wide range of sensitivity to insulin. Some normal individuals have as much insulin resistance as those with type 2 diabetes. The former, however, are able to secrete more insulin than the latter.

The following temporal relationship between insulin secretion and sensitivity to insulin is now accepted by most investigators.[4]

Insulin resistance occurs in those patients who may develop type 2 diabetes mellitus. In those in whom pancreatic β-cell reserve is sufficient, normal glucose levels are preserved at the expense of hyperinsulinemia. In those in whom the β-cell reserve is inadequate to maintain normal glucose levels, impaired glucose tolerance (IGT) appears. Hyperinsulinemia initially continues. However, as the β-cell starts to fail, glucose concentrations increase to values consistent with diabetes, and insulin concentrations decline to "normal" or below. Presumably, those individuals who progress from hyperinsulinemia and normal glucose tolerance through hyperinsulinemia and IGT to overt diabetes have a genetic susceptibility for a decreased β-cell reserve. Those with an adequate reserve for insulin secretion maintain normal tolerance or IGT at the expense of continued hyperinsulinemia. This scenario is supported by considering two groups of individuals who are at an increased risk for type 2 diabetes (i.e., the obese and the elderly). Not only has insulin resistance and hyperinsulinemia been documented in both, but IGT is also more common. If enhanced insulin secretion were unable to continue to overcome their insulin resistance, diabetes would ensue, thus accounting for the fact that 80% of type 2 patients are obese, and the prevalence of diabetes in people over 65 years of age may be as high as 15% to 20%.

Why β-cell reserve is not maintained in those individuals developing type 2 diabetes is completely unknown. The mechanism of the insulin resistance is almost as enigmatic. The critical first step of insulin action is binding to receptors located on the cell surface. This triggers a signal (or signals) within the cell that enables insulin to carry out a myriad of effects. However, insulin binding is normal in type 2 diabetic patients. Therefore, the site of the insulin resistance must be at a postbinding step. At the moment, that is all that can be said with certainty for the great majority (probably >95%) of type 2 diabetic patients.

However, in a small number of type 2 diabetic patients, the cause of their diabetes has been pinpointed. These fall into two general groups, maturity-onset diabetes of the young (MODY) and syndromes of extreme insulin resistance. As discussed in Chapter 1, type 2 diabetes can occur in families in an autosomal dominant pattern of inheritance (i.e., it will be present in three successive generations). In many (but not all) of these families, various abnormalities occur in the gene coding for glucokinase, an enzyme important for glucose-induced insulin secretion.[4] In the rare cases of extreme insulin resistance (e.g., babies with leprechaunism, women with hyperandrogenism and acanthosis nigricans), genetic mutations of the insulin receptor have been found.[5]

In contrast to the situation in ketosis-prone diabetes, decreased food intake in the absence of drugs (insulin or sulfonylurea agents) results in improved carbohydrate metabolism in ketosis-resistant patients, especially the obese ones. Similarly, with rare exceptions, the response to stress is hyperglycemia without ketosis or ketoacidosis. If insulin is required, relatively large amounts are needed by obese patients but usually not by lean ones. Ketosis-resistant patients always respond to some extent either to dietary therapy alone or to dietary therapy supplemented with sulfonylurea agents or metformin (see Chapter 5). Thus, the functional distinction between ketosis-prone and ketosis-resistant patients delineates certain metabolic characteristics with important clinical ramifications. Furthermore, the pathogenesis of each is completely different.

The prevalence of ketosis-prone and ketosis-resistant diabetes is shown in Figure 2–5. Of a hypothetical 100 patients, a small minority (5% to 10%) will have ketosis-prone diabetes. An unknown number, but certainly a small proportion, will be young (<20 years of age), ketosis-resistant diabetic patients. The great majority will have diabetes with onset in adulthood, mostly after the age of 40. Of these patients, most will be obese and ketosis resistant. Normal-weight adults with diabetes can be either ketosis prone or keto-

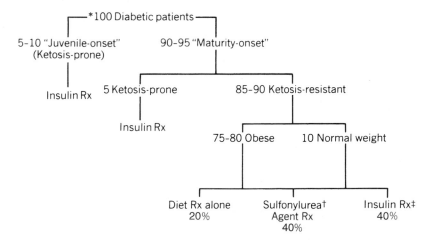

Figure 2–5. Distribution of ketosis-prone versus ketosis-resistant diabetes in a hypothetical population of 100 diabetic patients. *Ketosis-resistant diabetes occurs in older children and adolescents; the prevalence of this phenomenon is unknown at present. †Metformin was introduced into the United States in May 1995; this affects the percent of patients treated with diet, oral medication, or insulin. ‡Patients taking both a sulfonylurea agent plus insulin are included here.

sis resistant. Treatment for each of these subsets of patients is also indicated in Figure 2–5.

RELATION OF DIABETIC CONTROL TO DIABETIC COMPLICATIONS

The causes of death in the diabetic population changed drastically after the introduction of insulin therapy by Banting and Best in 1922. Today, the vast majority of diabetic patients die of one of the vascular complications. These complications usually do not develop until many years after the onset of diabetes mellitus. Thus, there is ample time in which to prevent or at least ameliorate these complications. The complications of diabetes mellitus can be divided into three general categories: macroangiopathy (coronary artery, cerebrovascular, and peripheral vascular disease), microangiopathy (retinopathy, nephropathy), and neuropathy (peripheral and autonomic neuropathy). At present, little evidence shows that controlling glucose levels lessens the risk of the macrovascular diseases. However, a number of other interventions have a beneficial effect (see Chapter 8).

In contrast, extremely strong (and in my view and those of others[6] incontrovertible) evidence now shows that tight diabetic control delays and might possibly prevent the onset of diabetic retinopathy, nephropathy, and neuropathy. (*Good, tight,* and *strict* diabetic control are terms denoting lower glucose concentrations with a goal of near euglycemia.) By 1980, a quite convincing case for this statement could be built on the available animal data.[7] Thus, diabetic nephropathy, retinopathy, and neuropathy are found in monkeys, dogs, rats, or mice who develop diabetes whether occurring spontaneously or induced by chemical, viral, or dietary means. The morphologic hallmark of diabetic microangiopathy is increased thickness of the basement membrane surrounding capillaries, not only in the eyes and kidneys but in most other tissues throughout the body. Increased basement membrane thickness is seen in all of these animal models of diabetes as well. Near euglycemia, whether accomplished by intensive insulin injection regimens or by transplantation of pancreatic β-cells in genetically identical animals, mostly prevents these complications.

A strong clinical impression is that tight control early in the disease is most important for retarding the development of diabetic retinopathy. This has been proved in a 5-year study of diabetic dogs.[8] (Because of the different life expectancies, 5 years in a dog corresponds to approximately 35 years of human life.) Three groups of diabetic dogs were treated as follows: (1) controlled tightly for 5 years; (2) controlled poorly for 5 years; or (3) controlled poorly for the first 2.5 years and tightly for the second 2.5 years. The animals well controlled and poorly controlled for 5 years developed minimal and severe diabetic retinopathy, respectively. Eye changes were also minimal after 2.5 years of poor control in the third group, but despite near euglycemia for the next 2.5 years, diabetic retinopathy was almost as severe as in the animals in poor control for the entire 5-year period. This suggests that the development of diabetic retinopathy in patients and animals follows a similar course.

The increased basement membrane width of capillaries as well as other retinal, nephropathic, and neuropathic changes is reversible by near euglycemia in these animal models of diabetes mellitus. Furthermore, transplanting a normal kidney into a diabetic rat leads to diabetic nephropathy. Conversely, a damaged kidney from a diabetic rat becomes healthy when transplanted into a normal rat. These latter observations strongly suggest that the hyperglycemic environment is the cause of these complications.

All of these findings in animals have now been documented in diabetic patients. The literature contains many cross-sectional studies in which investigators attempted to correlate diabetic complications at the time of study with a retrospective assessment of diabetic control. The majority of these reports support a relation between strict control and less diabetic retinopathy, nephropathy, and neuropathy. However, retrospective studies (especially older ones before the availability of glycated hemoglobin measurements and self-monitoring of glucose) suffer from imprecise evaluations of diabetic control and difficulty in attaining near euglycemia. Discussed here are only prospective studies in which assessment of diabetic control and development of diabetic complications are evaluated concurrently over the same period of time. The degree of diabetic control attained is presented where possible so that physicians (and their patients) will have a realistic view of what is required to forestall these diabetic complications.

RETINOPATHY

In Miki and colleagues' study,[9] the progression of diabetic retinopathy was correlated with fasting blood glucose levels during a 6-year period in 356 diabetic patients (mostly ketosis resistant). Degrees of control were defined as follows: good control, at least 80% of the fasting glucose levels of <140 mg/dl; poor control, more than 50% of the fasting glucose concentrations >170 mg/dl; and fair control, between good and poor control. Retinopathy was graded at least once per year after bilateral dilation of the pupils and examination with magnifying lenses by an ophthalmologist who had no knowledge of the metabolic status of the patient. Two, 4, and 6 years after the study began, the percentage of eyes in which new lesions appeared and older lesions progressed was lowest in patients with good control, intermediate in those with fair control, and highest in those with poor control. Conversely, the percentage of eyes in which old lesions improved was highest in patients with good control, intermediate in those with fair control, and lowest in those with poor control.

Patients receiving one dose of NPH insulin per day were randomly allocated into two groups, one to continue to receive one injection of insulin and the other to receive repeated doses of insulin.[10, 11] Annual fluorescein angiography of the posterior pole was performed, and the number of microaneurysms measured. The two groups had similar baseline characteristics, including duration of diabetes, age at both diagnosis of diabetes and onset of the trial, daily dose of insulin, urinary excretion of glucose (g/24 h), and fasting blood glucose level. Twenty-one patients in each group were monitored for 2 to 5 years, with mean durations of follow-up of 49.1 months for the single-injection group and 51.1 months for the multiple-injection group. Most of the patients in the latter group received intermediate-acting insulin before breakfast and supper. The mean fasting glucose concentration (mg/dl $\pm$ SEM) during the study was significantly lower (P < 0.05) in the multiple-injection group (166 $\pm$ 9) than in the single-injection group (192 $\pm$ 8). Glucosuria (g/24 h $\pm$ SEM) decreased (by 5 $\pm$ 3) from baseline values in patients taking multiple injections, whereas in those receiving one injection it increased (by 5 $\pm$ 4). This difference was also significant (P < 0.05). These modest differences in two parameters of diabetic control were associated with a threefold decrease in the rate of appearance of new microaneurysms in the eyes of patients taking more than one injection of insulin per day, compared with those who remained on one injection [3 $\pm$ 1 (SEM) vs. 9 $\pm$ 1, P < 0.001]. Although the number of microaneurysms fluctuated widely over time and some criticism was leveled at the statistical handling of the data,[12] these results support the association between good diabetic control and a lessening of the severity of diabetic retinopathy.

Another prospective study was a prodigious effort by Belgian physician Dr. Jean Pirart.[13] In 1947, Pirart began to enroll diabetic patients from two university hospitals (964 patients), a diabetic clinic (2,302 patients), and two private practices (1,132 patients) in a longitudinal study. One purpose of the study was to assess the relation between diabetic control and complications. The 4,398 patients in the study were monitored closely by the same personnel for as long as 25 years. The majority (2,795 patients) entered the study at the time of onset of their disease. The remaining 1,603 patients joined the study at various times after the diagnosis of diabetes had been made.

The patients were seen frequently, and much attention was paid to the accuracy of urine tests performed at home at least daily but most often two to four times throughout the day. Blood glucose levels were measured at each office visit, and the time of sampling was purposefully varied in order to avoid a systematic bias due to the interval after eating and/or insulin injection. The criteria used for assessing the annual degree of control are shown in Table 2-2. The records were reviewed each year, and a score was assigned. There was excellent agreement between observers, who judged the same record independently. A cumulative score estimating the degree of control during the entire period in which the patient was monitored was obtained by calculation of the arithmetic mean of consecutive yearly scores.

Each patient was evaluated for diabetic complications at least yearly. A patient was considered to have diabetic retinopathy if microaneurysms plus hemorrhages or exudates were found. In the absence of microaneurysms, hemorrhages and/or exudates were considered diagnostic of diabetic retinopathy only if major hypertension or thrombosis of a vein whose area corresponded to the area of damaged retina was not discovered. Retinopathy was considered absent if neither eye contained microaneurysms, hemorrhages, exudates, or neovascularization. Retinopathy was graded as follows: grade 1, microaneurysms and/or small waxy exudates; grade 2, any hemorrhage and/or nonhypertensive soft exudates even in the absence of microaneurysms or waxy exudates; and grade 3, areas of hemorrhage or exudates larger than the size of the disc. Proliferative retinopathy was diagnosed separately if even a slight degree of neovascularization was noted.

The relation between cumulative diabetic control and the prevalence of retinopathy is shown in Figure 2-6. Three degrees of control were arbitrarily designed as follows, according to cumulative (c) scores: 1.5 or less, fairly good control; 1.5 through 2, intermediate control; and more than 2, poor control. Because duration of diabetes has a marked effect on these complications, the prevalence of retinopathy is also related to dura-

Table 2–2. Criteria Used for Annual Ratings of the Degree of Control of Diabetes in 4,398 Patients Studied by Pirart

Degree of Glycemic Control	Score[a]	Criteria for Scoring			
		Degree of glucosuria during the day	*Postprandial blood glucose (mg/dl)*	*Fasting blood glucose (mg/dl)*	*Ketosis and/ or symptoms*
Good	1	None or exceptionally few	≤200	≤120	None
Fair	2	Variable or constant but moderate	200–300	120–200	Rare and brief
Poor	3	Usually high and prolonged	≥300	≥200	Possible

[a]The score is based on the criteria in the last four columns.

From Pirart J: Diabetes mellitus and its degenerative complications: a prospective study of 4,400 patients observed between 1947 and 1973. Diabetes Care 1:168, 1978.

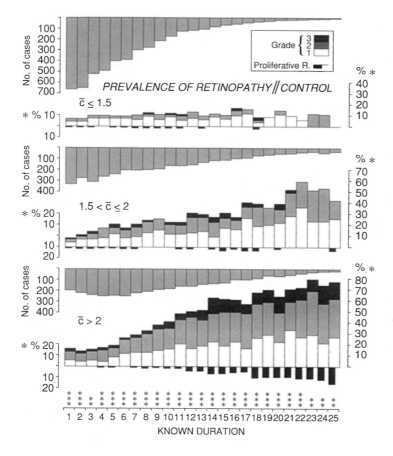

Figure 2–6. Relation between degree of diabetic control and the prevalence of retinopathy in a population of 4,398 diabetic patients monitored by one group of physicians for up to 25 years. Light-colored bars represent the number of patients who were evaluated at each interval and who fall into the respective categories of control. Dark bars show the cumulative frequency (%) of a complication at each year of duration. c̄, Cumulative scores indicating degree of diabetic control. (From Pirart J: Diabetes mellitus and its degenerative complications: a prospective study of 4,400 patients observed between 1947 and 1973. Diabetes Care 1:168, 1978)

tion, which is shown on the abscissa of each graph. The frequency (in percent) of a given complication at each year of duration is represented on the ordinate of each graph (dark bars). The number of patients evaluated at each interval who fall into the respective categories of control (i.e., the denominator on which the percentage of complications is calculated) is shown by the light-colored bars suspended from the top of the graphs. As would be expected, the number of subjects monitored decreases as the duration of diabetes increases. The slope of the histograms depicting prevalence (dark bars) represents the rate of increase of each complication. Only 15% or fewer of the patients in the best-controlled group had retinopathy, and of those who did, very few developed either grade 3 or proliferative changes. In

the intermediate group, the prevalence of retinopathy gradually increased to significant proportions, but the number with grade 3 or proliferative changes remained small. The poorly controlled group had the greatest increase in prevalence of retinopathy over time, and grade 3 and proliferative changes were not uncommon in this group.

Studies have used levels of glycated hemoglobin (Hgb A_{1c}) (see Chapter 7 for a detailed discussion of this method of assessing long-term diabetic control) to evaluate the relation between diabetic complications and control. Fluorescein angiography was used to assess diabetic retinopathy in 231 type 1 diabetic patients who were monitored for 5 years.[14] Incipient retinopathy was diagnosed if only microaneurysms were present in the worst eye, whereas background retinopathy required the presence of hemorrhages or exudates as well. Life-table analysis revealed that the median latency periods between the diagnosis of diabetes and the appearance of incipient and background retinopathy were 9.1 and 14.1 years, respectively. Diabetic control influenced these latency periods.[15] The latency period for incipient retinopathy was significantly (P < 0.01) longer in those with Hgb A_{1c} levels <10% compared with those >10% (10.8 vs. 8.0 years).

Klein and colleagues[16] evaluated 1,878 diabetic patients with stereoscopic fundus photographs at baseline and 4 years later. Hgb A_{1c} levels were measured at baseline. The patients were divided into three groups: (1) those diagnosed before 30 years of age, all of whom were taking insulin; (2) those diagnosed at 30 years of age or older and taking insulin; and (3) those diagnosed at 30 years of age or older but not taking insulin. All of the patients were stratified according to their Hgb A_{1c} levels and comparisons made among each quartile. In patients who did not have any diabetic retinopathy at baseline, the percent who developed it 4 years later progressively increased from the lowest to the highest quartile. In patients with diabetic retinopathy at baseline, there was a similar progressive increase in worsening of retinopathy from the lowest to the highest quartile

in all three groups. Furthermore, the chances of developing proliferative retinopathy increased as the Hgb A_{1c} levels rose. A comparison of the results between the lowest and highest quartiles in the three groups of patients regardless of the duration of diabetes is shown in Table 2-3. These striking differences were evident at each duration of diabetes analyzed at 5-year intervals. The results in 1,298 of these subjects after 10 years[17] are shown in Figure 2-7, which depicts all quartiles of Hgb A_{1c}. As expected, retinopathy has increased substantially in all three groups compared with the results after 4 years (see Table 2-3), but the progressive rise across all quartiles is obvious. Again, striking differences were noted at each duration of diabetes analyzed at 5-year intervals.

Diabetic retinopathy, assessed by direct ophthalmoscopy through dilated pupils, color retinal photography, intravenous fluorescein photography, and slit lamp examinations, was correlated with Hgb A_{1c} levels measured during the previous 6.5 years in 230 patients.[18] Most patients had three or four laboratory tests per year. Long-term good control was defined as a mean Hgb A_{1c} value within 1.33 times the upper limit of normal. Long-term poor control was defined as a mean Hgb A_{1c} level exceeding 1.5 times the upper limit of normal. Retinopathy was

Table 2–3. **Comparison of the Onset of Retinopathy, Progression of Established Retinopathy, and Development of Proliferative Retinopathy over 4 Years in Three Groups of Diabetic Patients in the Lowest and Highest Quartiles of Initial Hemoglobin A_{1c} Levels**

Group	Onset (%)	Progression (%)	Proliferative (%)
Younger onset			
Lowest quartile	45	17	1
Highest quartile	74	68	24
Older onset (insulin Rx)			
Lowest quartile	39	24	4
Highest quartile	74	52	15
Older onset (no insulin)			
Lowest quartile	13	8	2
Highest quartile	52	49	7

Adapted from Klein R, Klein BEK, Moss SE et al: Glycosylated hemoglobin predicts the incidence and progression of diabetic retinopathy. JAMA 260:2864, 1988.

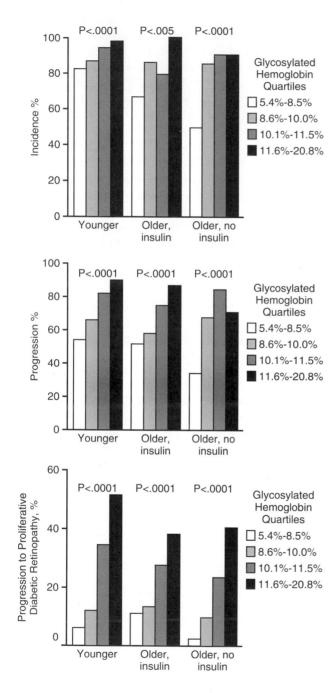

Figure 2–7. The relationship of onset of retinopathy (i.e., in those who did not have it at baseline) (top), progression of background retinopathy present at baseline (center), and progression of background retinopathy to proliferative retinopathy (bottom) in persons with younger-onset diabetes, persons with older-onset diabetes taking insulin, and persons with older-onset diabetes not taking insulin to Hgb A_{1c} levels at baseline by quartiles over the following 10-year period. (From Klein R, Klein BEK, Moss SE et al: Relationship of hyperglycemia to the long-term incidence and progression of diabetic retinopathy. Arch Intern Med 154:2169, 1994)

classified as absent (no changes), mild (microaneurysms only), and moderate to severe (more than microaneurysms present). Patients with long-term poor control had 2.5 times the prevalence of moderate to severe retinopathy as those with long-term good control.

A 5-year longitudinal study[19] of 114 type 2 patients over the age of 60 years revealed that the progression of diabetic retinopathy was directly related to the Hgb A_{1c} levels measured every 2 months (Fig. 2–8). Retinopathy was evaluated by fundus photographs of the right eye at the beginning and end of the study and diagnosed as no lesions (grade 0), nonproliferative (grade 1), preproliferative (grade 2), and proliferative (grade 3) (see Chapter 8 for characteristics of each grade). Progression of retinopathy was defined as an increase of at least one grade during the 5-year study. Similarly, in 346 type 1 diabetic patients evaluated by fluorescein angiopathy every 1 to 2 years, the rate of development of background retinopathy was

directly related to Hgb A_{1c} levels.[20] A 10-fold increase was noted in patients whose mean Hgb A_{1c} values were >11%, compared with those with values <7%.

A longitudinal study[21] of 927 Pima Indians with type 2 diabetes without retinopathy at baseline and monitored for an average of 4.5 years revealed that almost all of the patients who developed it had Hgb A_{1c} levels above the 80th percentile of the distribution of all values. Patients with Hgb A_{1c} levels below these values rarely developed retinopathy during the period of the study.

Reichard and colleagues[22] randomized 48 type 1 diabetic patients to receive intensive insulin therapy and compared them with 54 type 1 diabetic patients receiving standard treatment. Both groups were evaluated for microvascular complications 1.5, 3.0, 5.0, and 7.5 years later. At entry, the Hgb A_{1c} levels were similar in the two groups, 9.5% versus 9.4%, respectively. The mean value throughout the study was significantly (P < 0.001) lower in the intensively treated group, 7.1% versus 8.5%. Retinopathy was assessed by fundus photography and funduscopy during the first 5 years and thereafter by a detailed funduscopic examination through dilated pupils. Serious retinopathy requiring photocoagulation occurred in 27% of the intensively treated patients, compared with 54% of those in the standard treatment group (P < 0.01). Decreased visual acuity (a decrement of at least two lines on the eye chart) occurred in 14% of the patients receiving intensive therapy, compared with 35% of the patients in the standard treatment group (P < 0.02).

All of these data concerning the impact of strict diabetic control on ameliorating the development of diabetic retinopathy provide a strong base of support for the goal of achieving near euglycemia in diabetic patients. The results of the Diabetes Control and Complications Trial (DCCT) have irrefutably clinched the argument.[23] This study enrolled 1441 type 1 diabetic patients, 726 of whom had no diabetic retinopathy (by

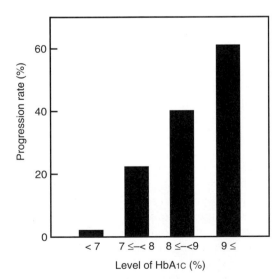

Figure 2–8. Rate of progression of diabetic retinopathy over 5 years as a function of Hgb A_{1c} level. (From Morisaki N, Watanabe S, Kobayashi J et al: Diabetic control and progression of retinopathy in elderly patients: five-year follow-up. J Am Geriatr Soc 42:142, 1994)

seven-field stereoscopic fundus photographs), whereas 715 had mild to moderate nonproliferative (also called *background* —see Chapter 8) retinopathy at baseline. Half of the patients were randomly assigned to intensive treatment (goals—premeal blood glucose concentrations of 70 to 120 mg/dl, postprandial blood glucose concentrations of <180 mg/dl, and normal Hgb A_{1c} levels [Hgb A_{1c} < 6.05%]), and the other half remained on their conventional treatment. The fundus photographs, repeated every 6 months, were evaluated for severity of retinopathy over a 25-step scale. Clinically important changes were defined as a change of at least three steps that was sustained for at least 6 months.

The patients were monitored for a mean of 6.5 years (range, 3 to 9). The planned 10-year study was ended a year early because it was deemed unethical to continue in view of the favorable results. Compared with the conventionally treated group, the intensively treated patients did achieve highly statistically significant decreases in glucose levels (averaging both preprandial and postprandial) concentrations (155 mg/dl vs. 231 mg/dl) and Hgb A_{1c} levels (7.2% vs. 9.0%). The development of retinopathy in the patients without it at baseline (called the *primary prevention cohort*) is shown in Figure 2-9*A*. The incidence curves begin to separate after 3 years—that is, it took that long for effects of near euglycemia to begin to show benefit. Overall, intensive treatment reduced the risk of developing clinically important (≥3 step change) diabetic retinopathy by 76% over the mean 6.5 years that these patients were studied. The progression of established nonproliferative retinopathy at baseline (called the *secondary intervention cohort*) is shown in Figure 2-9*B*. The intensively treated group had a higher cumulative incidence during the first year (it has been repeatedly demonstrated that bringing a patient from poor control to near euglycemia may cause transient worsening of retinopathy) but a lower cumulative incidence of

clinically important retinopathy beginning again at 3 years. Overall, intensive treatment reduced the risk of progression of nonproliferative retinopathy by 54% for the duration of the DCCT. The early worsening of diabetic retinopathy during the first year (which occurred in 22% of the intensively treated patients and 13% of the conventionally treated ones) should not deter physicians from instituting tight control. These changes often disappeared by 18 months in the DCCT. Furthermore, analyzing just those patients with transient worsening, intensive treatment caused a 74% reduction in subsequent progression compared with conventional therapy.

A much smaller randomized study in lean Japanese type 2 diabetic patients carried out for 6 years in a similar manner as the DCCT yielded comparable results. In the Kumamoto study,[23a] 110 patients were enrolled and divided into two cohorts, 55 in a primary prevention group and 55 in a secondary prevention group. The primary prevention cohort had no diabetic retinopathy, whereas the secondary prevention cohort had mild background retinopathy evaluated by fundus photography through dilated pupils. Half of the patients were randomly assigned to intensive treatment with preprandial regular insulin and intermediate-acting insulin at bedtime (goals—fasting blood glucose concentration of <140 mg/dl, postprandial blood glucose concentrations of <200 mg/dl, and a Hgb A_{1c} level <7.0%). The other half remained on their conventional therapy of one or two daily injections of intermediate-acting insulin (goals—fasting blood glucose concentration of <140 mg/dl and avoidance of hypoglycemia and hyperglycemia). Development (in the primary prevention group) or progression (in the secondary prevention group) of diabetic retinopathy was defined as at least a 2-step change in a 19-step scale when the eyes were reevaluated after 6 years.

During periodic 1-day hospitalizations, 11 preprandial and postprandial glucose con-

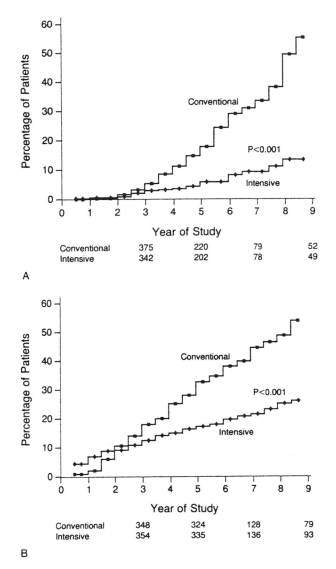

Figure 2–9. *A*: Cumulative incidence of developing diabetic retinopathy in the primary prevention cohort (no retinopathy at baseline). Change in retinopathy status defined as a change of at least three steps in seven-field stereoscopic fundus photographs that was sustained for at least 6 months. The numbers of patients in each therapy group who were evaluated at years 3, 5, 7, and 9 are shown below the graph. *B*: Cumulative incidence of progression of diabetic retinopathy in the secondary intervention cohort (nonproliferative retinopathy present at baseline). Change in retinopathy status defined as a change of at least three steps in seven-field stereoscopic fundus photographs that was sustained for at least 6 months. The numbers of patients in each therapy group who were evaluated at years 3, 5, 7, and 9 are shown below the graph. (From The Diabetes Control and Complications Trial Research Group: The effect of intensive treatment of diabetes on the development and progression of long-term complications in insulin-dependent diabetes mellitus. N Engl J Med 329:977, 1993)

centrations were measured. Compared with the conventionally treated cohort, the intensively treated group had significantly lower fasting blood glucose concentrations (126 mg/dl vs. 164 mg/dl), mean blood glucose concentrations throughout the day (157 mg/dl vs. 221 mg/dl), and Hgb A_{1c} levels (7.1% vs. 9.4%). Twenty-five or 26 patients remained in each of the four groups at the end of the study. In the primary prevention cohort, intensive treatment resulted in a significant decrease in the development of diabetic retinopathy (7.7% vs. 32.0%). Likewise, in the secondary prevention cohort, intensive treatment resulted in a significant decrease in the progression of diabetic retinopathy (19.2% vs. 44.0%). Overall, repeated injections of insulin and the resultant near euglycemia reduced the risk of worsening of diabetic retinopathy by 69% over 6 years in these lean type 2 diabetic patients.

NEPHROPATHY

Fewer prospective studies have evaluated diabetic control and development or progression of nephropathy concurrently. In one,[24] serial renal biopsy specimens were taken of 23 patients whose fasting plasma glucose levels were measured every 2 weeks or more frequently. Good control was defined as values never exceeding 120 mg/dl, poor control as values of more than 150 mg/dl on "all or many occasions," and fair control as between good and poor control. The presence and degree of diabetic nephropathy in the biopsy specimens were evaluated independently by three nephrologists who had no knowledge of the patient's clinical course. Of 13 patients with poor control, 10 showed progression of nephropathy; 3 of 4 with fair control showed progression; and none of the 6 patients with good control showed progression. The duration of diabetes at the time of the first biopsy (approximately 4.5 years) and the follow-up period (approximately 4 years) was similar for patients whose lesions did not progress and for those showing pro-

gression. The age of onset (years ± SEM) of diabetes in the 13 patients whose nephropathy progressed was significantly lower (36.3 ± 3.9) than the age of onset of the 10 patients who showed no progression (52.6 ± 1.9). However, these results do not support the supposition that good control and a relative absence of renal lesions are associated only because ketosis-resistant patients, in whom alteration of carbohydrate metabolism may be less severe than in ketosis-prone individuals, have a genetic constitution that is less subject to nephropathy. In fact, two of the four type 2 diabetic patients with poor control in this study showed progression of renal lesions.

The general format of Miki and colleagues' study[9] was discussed earlier. After 4 and 6 years, proteinuria had progressed much less in patients with good control than in those with fair and poor control.[25]

The general outline of the Pirart study[13] was also described earlier. The diagnosis of diabetic nephropathy was made if unexplained proteinuria was discovered on several occasions. Although the prevalence of this complication (Fig. 2–10) is much less than that of diabetic retinopathy (see Fig. 2–6), the same relation between diabetic control and prevalence of nephropathy holds. Extremely few well-controlled patients had it, approximately 20% of the poorly controlled patients eventually developed it, and the prevalence was approximately half in the intermediate group.

Normal subjects excrete a very small amount of albumin (<30 mg/24 h). Excretion of >300 mg of albumin per 24 hours results in a positive test result for urinary protein by standard semiquantitative (i.e., dipstick) methods and is classified as clinical proteinuria reflecting renal damage. Patients excreting between 30 and 300 mg of albumin per 24 hours are considered to have "microalbuminuria." Prospective studies[26-29] lasting from 6 to 14 years have shown that 75% to 100% of type 1 diabetic patients with microalbuminuria subsequently develop clin-

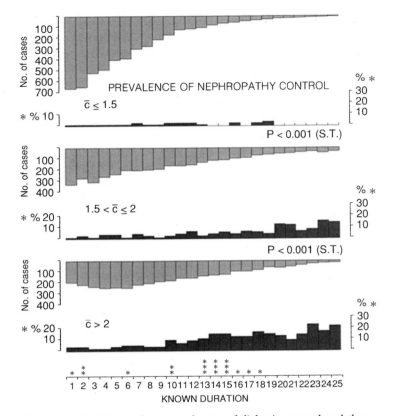

Figure 2–10. Relation between degree of diabetic control and the prevalence of nephropathy in a population of 4,398 diabetic patients monitored by one group of physicians for up to 25 years. Light-colored bars represent the number of patients who were evaluated at each interval and who fall into the respective categories of control. Dark bars show the cumulative frequency (%) of a complication at each year of duration. c̄, Cumulative scores indicating degree of diabetic control. (From Pirart J: Diabetes mellitus and its degenerative complications: a prospective study of 4,400 patients observed between 1947 and 1973. Diabetes Care 1:168, 1978)

ical nephropathy, in contrast to 0% to 13% without it. Thus, microalbuminuria serves as an extremely powerful predictor for the eventual development of overt diabetic nephropathy. Patients with long-term poor control defined by a mean Hgb A_{1c} level 1.5 times the upper normal limit had 3.6 times the prevalence of microalbuminuria than those with long-term good control whose mean Hgb A_{1c} for the previous 6.5 years was within 1.33 times the upper limit of normal.[18]

The development of diabetic nephropathy, defined as proteinuria of at least 1 g/day, was assessed in the longitudinal study of Pima Indians.[21] The vast majority of patients who developed nephropathy had Hgb A_{1c} levels above the 80th percentile of the distribution.

In the study by Reichard and colleagues[22] described earlier, nephropathy (defined as a level of protein excretion that would be dipstick positive) developed in nine patients in the standard treatment group, compared with only one in those treated intensively

(P < 0.01). In the DCCT,[23] intensive treatment reduced the development of microalbuminuria by 34% (P < 0.04) in the primary prevention cohort and by 43% (P < 0.001) in the secondary intervention cohort. The risk of dipstick proteinuria was reduced by 56% (P < 0.01) in the secondary intervention cohort. In the Kumamoto study,[23a] intensive compared with conventional treatment significantly reduced the development of diabetic nephropathy (defined as an albumin excretion of >30 mg/24 h) in the primary prevention group (7.7% vs. 28.0%). Likewise, intensive treatment in the secondary prevention group significantly reduced the progression of diabetic nephropathy (11.5% vs. 32.0%). Overall, repeated injections of insulin and the resultant near euglycemia reduced the risk of worsening of diabetic nephropathy by 70%.

Finally, morphologic changes in the kidneys are favorably influenced by strict control. Eighteen type 1 diabetic patients with microalbuminuria were randomized (nine each) to receive insulin pump therapy or to remain on conventional treatment.[30] Renal biopsies were performed before randomization and after 2 years. Initial Hgb A_{1c} levels (10.1%) were identical in the two groups. The mean Hgb A_{1c} levels were significantly (P < 0.04) lower in the pump patients (8.7%) compared with the conventional group (9.9%). Renal biopsy samples at the end of the study revealed only minimal changes in the patients treated intensively, whereas the conventionally treated patients showed much more progression.

Similarly, 99 patients receiving kidney transplants were randomized either into a standard treatment group (n = 47) or into a maximized treatment group (n = 52).[31] Renal biopsies were performed at the time of transplant and 5 years later. The goals of standard treatment were to avoid both hypoglycemia and symptomatic hyperglycemia and to maintain the Hgb A_{1c} level at <12%. The maximized treatment group was treated intensively in an attempt to achieve a normal Hgb A_{1c} level (5.1% to 7.3%). As might be expected, Hgb A_{1c} levels were significantly (P < 0.001) lower during the study in the patients receiving intensive treatment (9.6% vs. 11.7%). Various morphologic changes that characterize the development and progression of diabetic nephropathy were statistically significantly greater in the transplanted kidneys of the standard treatment group compared with those receiving maximized treatment.

NEUROPATHY

The Pirart study[13] also evaluated diabetic control and the development of neuropathy concurrently. A diagnosis of diabetic neuropathy was made if Achilles and/or patellar reflexes were lost in conjunction with a clear decrease in vibratory sensation. The prevalence of this complication (Fig. 2–11) lies between that of retinopathy (see Fig. 2–6) and nephropathy (see Fig. 2–10). Once again, a similar relation holds between diabetic control and neuropathy. The initial low prevalence of neuropathy (see Fig. 2–11) did not change much as the duration of diabetes increased in the fairly well-controlled group. In sharp contrast, the prevalence increased considerably over time in the other two groups, with the most poorly controlled patients experiencing a faster deterioration of peripheral neurologic function than did the intermediate group.

In the study by Reichard and colleagues[22] described earlier, nerve conduction velocities (which are a sensitive measure of neurologic function) in the lower extremity deteriorated more significantly (P < 0.02) in the standard treatment group than in the intensively treated group.

In the DCCT,[31a] neuropathy was assessed at 5 years. Abnormal results of neurologic examinations (P < 0.001), nerve conduction studies (P < 0.001), and autonomic nerve studies (P < 0.04) all were significantly higher in the conventionally treated group. More specifically, intensive therapy reduced

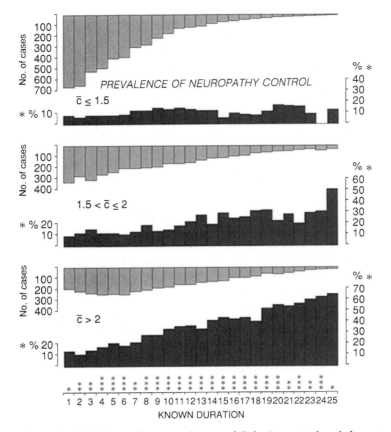

Figure 2–11. Relation between degree of diabetic control and the prevalence of neuropathy in a population of 4,398 diabetic patients monitored by one group of physicians for up to 25 years. Light-colored bars represent the number of patients who were evaluated at each interval and who fall into the respective categories of control. Dark bars show the cumulative frequency (%) of a complication at each year of duration. $\bar{c}$, Cumulative scores indicating degree of diabetic control. (From Pirart J: Diabetes mellitus and its degenerative complications: a prospective study of 4,400 patients observed between 1947 and 1973. Diabetes Care 1:168, 1978)

the appearance of neuropathy in the primary prevention cohort by 69% and in the secondary intervention cohort by 57%.

In the Kumamoto study,[23a] indices of peripheral nerve function significantly improved during intensive treatment but remained unchanged or deteriorated during conventional treatment.

In another study,[32] the development of neurologic dysfunction during the first 5 years after the diagnosis of type 1 diabetes in 32 patients was correlated with Hgb A_{1c} levels during that same period. Thirteen patients maintained normal (<8.3%) Hgb A_{1c} levels, and the remaining 19 had an average value of 10.0%. Nerve conduction velocities and tests of peripheral and autonomic neuropathy were significantly ($P < 0.05$) impaired in those with elevated Hgb A_{1c} levels. Furthermore, none of the patients with normal Hgb A_{1c} levels developed clinical neuropathy, whereas six of the other group did. Finally, nerve conduction velocities were measured at the beginning and 8 years later in 45 type 1 patients randomized to receive conventional treatment or intensive therapy with repeated injections or insulin pumps.[33] After 4 years, patients were allowed to choose which therapy they preferred. Only two remained on conventional treatment during the final half of the study. Twelve patients whose average Hgb A_{1c} level exceeded 10% (normal 5.4% to 7.6%) had a significant ($P < 0.05$ or better) decrease in nerve conduction velocities compared with the 33 whose average Hgb A_{1c} level was <10%. The means of the two groups were 10.9% and 9.0%. Although not measured at baseline, autonomic nerve function was also significantly ($P < 0.05$ or better) decreased in the more poorly controlled group at 8 years.

These prospective studies in which diabetic control and retinopathy, nephropathy, and neuropathy were assessed concurrently clearly show that tight control has a beneficial influence on the development and progression of these complications. The data of Pirart,[13] who monitored the largest number of patients for the longest time (summarized in Table 2–4), show the eventual prevalence of diabetic retinopathy, nephropathy, and neuropathy and the impact of control on each.

REVERSAL OF EARLY CHANGES

The most recent evidence linking strict diabetic control with a favorable effect on diabetic retinopathy, nephropathy, and neuropathy indicates that the *early* lesions are reversible if near euglycemia can be achieved with either repeated injections of insulin or insulin infusion pumps. As mentioned previously, increased capillary basement membrane thickness is the morphologic characteristic of the microvascular changes in diabetes mellitus. Because this occurs in all tissues, muscle biopsies afford an opportunity to monitor the effect of improving diabetic control. Capillary basement membrane thickness decreases considerably, almost to normal (Fig. 2–12), after near euglycemia is achieved by repeated insulin injection[34] or insulin pump therapy.[35, 36]

The earliest ocular abnormality in diabetes is increased leakage of the retinal vessels, which can be measured by vitreous fluorophotometry following injection of a fluorescein dye. These changes are evident years before retinal changes can be seen by ophthalmoscopic examination. In many patients, near euglycemia decreased the leakage of the fluorescein dye to normal.[37–39] Abnormal macular recovery time and oscillatory potential, two parameters of retinal function, have been shown in prospective studies[40, 41] to have a highly predictive value for the eventual development of proliferative retinopathy. These two retinal functions improved significantly when strict diabetic control was implemented.[38, 39] The situation in regard to retinal morphology (i.e., the result of photographic or ophthalmoscopic evaluation of the retina) was more complex. An initial worsening can occur during the first year of

Table 2–4. Impact of Diabetic Control on the Prevalence (%) of Diabetic Retinopathy, Nephropathy, and Neuropathy after 25 Years of Diabetes Mellitus

Condition	Overall	Good Control[a]	Poor Control[a]
Retinopathy	60	10	80
(proliferative)		(<1)	(20)
Nephropathy	20	<1	20
Neuropathy	50	10	65

[a]See text for definitions.

Adapted from Gerich JE: Insulin-dependent diabetes mellitus: pathophysiology. Mayo Clin Proc 61:787, 1986.

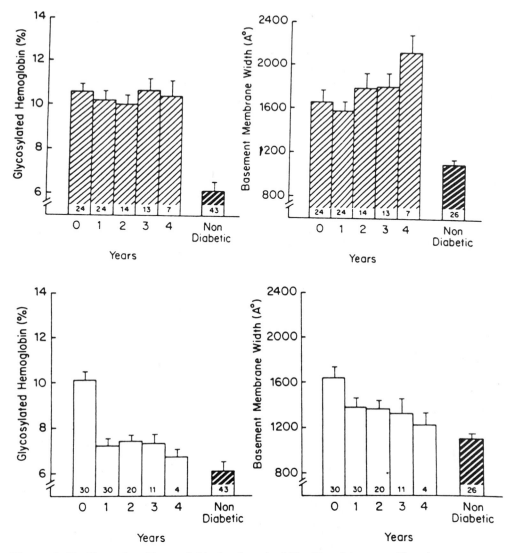

Figure 2–12. Glycosylated hemoglobin levels and width of quadriceps capillary basement membrane in patients with type 1 diabetes under conventional insulin therapy (top) or intensive therapy with insulin pumps (bottom). (From Rosenstock J, Challis P, Stowig S, Raskin P: Improved diabetes control reduces skeletal muscle capillary basement membrane width in insulin-dependent diabetes mellitus. Diabetes Res Clin Pract 4:167, 1988)

near euglycemia,[23, 38, 39, 42–46] with subsequent stabilization or improvement such that at 2 years or beyond, diabetic retinopathy is less advanced than in control patients who had remained on their usual (suboptimal) insulin therapy.[23, 35, 47, 48]

Microalbuminuria and its ability to predict the eventual development of overt diabetic nephropathy was discussed earlier. Strict diabetic control decreases and in some patients entirely reverses microalbuminuria,[43, 49, 50] suggesting (but certainly not proving) that future development of diabetic nephropathy may be delayed or possibly even avoided.

In regard to neuropathy, near euglycemia diminished pain,[51] decreased the vibratory perception threshold[42, 51, 52] (i.e., patients were able to appreciate less intense vibrations), and increased motor nerve conduction velocities.[45, 51-55]

However, once morphologic changes have occurred in the eyes (i.e., retinopathy can be discerned with the ophthalmoscope) or clinical proteinuria is present, strict diabetic control does not prevent the continued deterioration of the retina[39, 42, 43, 56, 57] or kidneys.[56, 58] These latter data emphasize the importance of instituting strict control at the onset of diabetes in an attempt to prevent these devastating complications.

The debate concerning the impact of hyperglycemia and diabetic complications has been raging for more than half a century. With the advent of glucose self-monitoring to help achieve near euglycemia and the availability of measuring Hgb A_{1c} levels to document it, reports clearly indicate that tight diabetic control has a major role in forestalling diabetic retinopathy, nephropathy, and neuropathy. The only serious objection raised to this conclusion is that genetic influences may also be important in the development of these complications.[59] It is true that in diabetic patients with poor control for 25 years, 20% will not develop retinopathy, 80% will not develop nephropathy, and 35% will not develop neuropathy (see Table 2-4). Perhaps genetic factors are protecting these patients. However, the overriding importance of hyperglycemia in the interplay between metabolic and genetic influences is evident in that (1) renal basement membrane thickness is normal at the onset of diabetes[60]; (2) patients with secondary diabetes have the same prevalence of diabetic complications as those with "genetic" diabetes[7, 61]; (3) normal kidneys transplanted into diabetic patients develop nephropathy[7]; and, conversely, (4) morphologic changes of diabetic nephropathy are reversible after transplantation into nondiabetic individuals.[62] Regardless of the genetic background,

diabetic retinopathy, nephropathy, or neuropathy does not occur in the absence of hyperglycemia. Furthermore, in those who are unlikely to have a genetic background for diabetes (patients with secondary diabetes and the nondiabetic recipients of diabetic kidneys), these complications occur in a high percentage.

Clinically, it is critical to recognize that one cannot predict whether or not a patient may be protected from diabetic retinopathy, nephropathy, or neuropathy. Therefore, it behooves us to control their diabetes as tightly as possible without causing serious disruptions in their life styles. Which level of control to aim for and how to achieve it are discussed in detail in Chapter 7.

I have described in some detail the overwhelming evidence concerning the impact of near euglycemia on the development and progression of diabetic retinopathy, nephropathy, and neuropathy. This is because physicians need to be convinced of the importance of tight control so that they vigorously pursue near euglycemia. This entails not only convincing patients but taking the time and exerting the effort in working with patients to achieve it. This is not an easy task. Because most patients are asymptomatic, motivating them to do the necessary work and to continue doing it can be difficult. Physician time and motivation can also be a factor, especially because the rewards are not immediate and accrue only years later in the continued health of patients. Certain patients are not candidates for strict control—for example, the elderly, those with hypoglycemia unawareness (see Chapter 7), those with advanced microvascular and neuropathic complications, or those with severe cardiovascular disease. Some physicians believe that many other patients with type 2 diabetes should not be tightly controlled because of the theoretic risk of hyperinsulinemia.[63] Compensatory hyperinsulinemia, as a response to insulin resistance, is one of a cluster of risk factors (in which glucose intolerance or, in some cases, type 2 diabetes can also occur) for coronary artery disease. In my view,[64] this cluster of risk factors, known as either *syndrome X* or the *insulin resistance syndrome*, should not preclude a patient from being considered for tight control. This issue is discussed more thoroughly in Chapter 7.

REFERENCES

1. Hiss RG, Anderson RM, Hess GE et al: Community diabetes care: a 10-year perspective. Diabetes Care 17:1124, 1994

2. Atkinson MA, Maclaren NK: Islet cell autoantigens insulin-dependent diabetes. J Clin Invest 92:1608, 1993

2a. Hyoty H, Hiltunen MK, Laakkonen M et al: A prospective study of the role of Coxsackie B and other enterovirus infections in the pathogenesis of IDDM. Diabetes 44:652, 1995

3. Pfizer Laboratories: A study among type 2 diabetics. Survey conducted by the Gallup Organization, 1983

4. Matschinsky F, Liang Y, Kesavan P et al: Glucokinase as pancreatic β cell glucose sensor and diabetes gene. J Clin Invest 92:2092, 1993

5. Taylor SI: Lilly lecture: molecular mechanisms of insulin resistance. Lessons from patients with mutations in the insulin-receptor gene. Diabetes 41:1473, 1992

6. Hanssen KF, Dahl-Jorgensen K, Lauritzen T et al: Diabetic control and microvascular complications: the near-normoglycaemic experience. Diabetologia 29:677, 1986

7. Davidson MB: The case for control in diabetes mellitus. West J Med 129:193, 1978

8. Engerman RL, Kern TS: Progression of incipient diabetic retinopathy during good glycemic control. Diabetes 36:808, 1987

9. Miki E, Fukuda M, Kuzuya T et al: Relation of the course of retinopathy to control of diabetes, age, and therapeutic agents in diabetic Japanese patients. Diabetes 18:773, 1969

10. Job D, Eschwege E, Guyot-Argenton C et al: Effect of multiple daily injections on the course of diabetic retinopathy. Diabetes 25:463, 1976

11. Eschwege E, Job D, Guyot-Argenton C et al: Delayed progression of diabetic retinopathy by divided insulin administration: a further follow-up. Diabetes 16:13, 1979

12. Ashikaga T, Borodic G, Sims EAH: Multiple daily insulin injections in the treatment of diabetic retinopathy. The Job Study revisited. Diabetes 27:592, 1978

13. Pirart J: Diabetes mellitus and its degenerative complications: a prospective study of 4,400 patients observed between 1947 and 1973. Diabetes Care 1:168, 1978

14. Burger W, Hovener G, Dusterhus R, Hartmann R et al: Prevalence and development of retinopathy in children and adolescents with type 1 (insulin-dependent) diabetes mellitus. A longitudinal study. Diabetologia 29:17, 1986

15. Weber B, Burger W, Hartmann R et al: Risk factors for the development of retinopathy in children and adolescents with type 1 (insulin-dependent) diabetes mellitus. Diabetologia 29:23, 1986

16. Klein R, Klein BEK, Moss SE et al: Glycosylated hemoglobin predicts the incidence and progression of diabetic retinopathy. JAMA 260:2864, 1988

17. Klein R, Klein BEK, Moss SE et al: Relationship of hyperglycemia to the long-term incidence and progression of diabetic retinopathy. Arch Intern Med 154:2169, 1994

18. Chase HP, Jackson WE, Hoops SL et al: Glucose control and the renal and retinal complications of insulin-dependent diabetes. JAMA 261:1155, 1989

19. Morisaki N, Watanabe S, Kobayashi J et al: Diabetic control and progression of retinopathy in elderly patients: five-year follow-up study. J Am Geriatr Soc 42:142, 1994

20. Danne T, Weber B, Hartmann R et al: Long-term glycemic control has a nonlinear association to the frequency of background retinopathy in adolescents with diabetes. Diabetes Care 17:1390, 1994

21. McCance DR, Hanson R, Charles MA et al: Comparison of tests for glycated haemoglobin and fasting and two hour plasma glucose concentrations as diagnostic methods for diabetes. BMJ 308:1323, 1994

22. Reichard P, Nilsson B-Y, Rosenqvist U: The effect of long-term intensified insulin treatment on the development of microvascular complications of diabetes mellitus. N Engl J Med 329:304, 1993

23. The Diabetes Control and Complications Trial

Research Group: The effect of intensive treatment of diabetes on the development and progression of long-term complications in insulin-dependent diabetes mellitus. N Engl J Med 329:977, 1993

23a. Ohkubo Y, Kishikawa H, Araki E et al: Intensive insulin therapy prevents the progression of diabetic microvascular complications in Japanese patients with non-insulin-dependent diabetes mellitus: a randomized prospective 6-year study. Diabetes Res Clin Pract 28:103, 1995

24. Takazakura E, Nakamoto Y, Hayakawa H et al: Onset and progression of diabetic glomerulosclerosis. A prospective study based on serial renal biopsies. Diabetes 24:1, 1975

25. Miki E, Kuzuya T, Ide T, Nakao K: Frequency, degree, and progression with time of proteinuria in diabetic patients. Lancet 1:922, 1972

26. Viberti GC, Jarrett RJ, Mahmud U et al: Microalbuminuria as a predictor of clinical nephropathy in insulin-dependent diabetes mellitus. Lancet 1:1430, 1982

27. Parving HH, Oxenboll B, Svendsen PA et al: Early detection of patients at risk of developing diabetic nephropathy: a longitudinal study of urinary albumin excretion. Acta Endocrinol (Copenh) 100:550, 1982

28. Mogensen ER, Christiansen CK: Predicting diabetic nephropathy in insulin-dependent patients. N Engl J Med 311:89, 1984

29. Mathiesen ER, Oxenboll B, Johansen K et al: Incipient nephropathy in type 1 (insulin-dependent) diabetes. Diabetologia 16:406, 1984

30. Bangstad H-J, Osterby R, Dahl-Jorgensen K et al: Improvement of blood glucose control in IDDM patients retards the progression of morphological changes in early diabetic nephropathy. Diabetologia 37:483, 1994

31. Barbosa J, Steffes MW, Sutherland DER et al: Effect of glycemic control on early diabetic renal lesions: a 5-year randomized controlled clinical trial of insulin-dependent diabetic kidney transplant recipients. JAMA 272:600, 1994

31a. The Diabetes Control and Complications Trial Research Group: The effect of intensive diabetes therapy on the development and progression of neuropathy. Ann Intern Med 122:561, 1995

32. Ziegler D, Mayer P, Muhlen H et al: The natural history of somatosensory and autonomic nerve dysfunction in relation to glycaemic control during the first 8 years after diagnosis of type 1 (insulin-dependent) diabetes mellitus. Diabetologia 34:822, 1991

33. Amthor K-F, Dahl-Jorgensen K, Berg TJ et al: The effect of 7 years of strict glycaemic control on peripheral nerve function in IDDM patients: the Oslo study. Diabetologia 37:579, 1994

34. Peterson CM, Jones RL, Esterly JS et al: Changes in basement membrane thickening and pulse volume concomitant with improved glucose control and exercise in patients with insulin-dependent diabetes mellitus. Diabetes Care 3:586, 1980

35. Rosenstock J, Friberg T, Raskin P: Effect of glycemic control on microvascular complications in patients with type 1 diabetes mellitus. Am J Med 81:1012, 1986

36. Rosenstock J, Challis P, Stowig S, Raskin P: Improved diabetes control reduces skeletal muscle capillary basement membrane width in insulin-dependent diabetes mellitus. Diabetes Res Clin Pract 4:167, 1988

37. White NH, Waltman SR, Krupin T et al: Reversal of abnormalities in ocular fluorophotometry in insulin-dependent diabetes after five to nine months of improved metabolic control. Diabetes 31:30, 1982

38. Steno Study Group: Effect of 6 months of strict metabolic control on eye and kidney function in insulin-dependent diabetics with background retinopathy. Lancet 1:121, 1982

39. Lauritzen R, Larsen H-W, Frost-Larsen K et al: Effect of 1 year of near-normal blood glucose levels on retinopathy in insulin-dependent diabetics. Lancet 1:200, 1983

40. Simonsen SE: The value of the oscillatory potential in selecting juvenile diabetics at risk of developing proliferative retinopathy. Acta Ophthalmol 58:865, 1980

41. Frost-Larsen K, Larsen H-W, Simonsen SE: Oscillatory potential and nyctometri in insulin-dependent diabetics. Acta Ophthalmol 58:879, 1980

42. Holman RR, Mayon-White V, Orde-Peckar C et al: Prevention of deterioration of renal and sensory-nerve function by more intensive management of insulin-dependent diabetic patients. A two-year randomised prospective study. Lancet 1:204, 1983

43. The Kroc Collaborative Study Group: Blood glucose control and the evolution of diabetic retinopathy and albuminuria. A preliminary multicenter trial. N Engl J Med 311:365, 1984

44. Beck-Neilsen H, Richelsen B, Mogensen CE et al: Effect of insulin pump treatment for one year on renal function and retinal morphology in patients with IDDM. Diabetes Care 8:585, 1985

45. Dahl-Jorgensen K, Brinchmann-Hansen O, Hanssen KF et al: Effect of near normoglycaemia for two years on progression of early diabetic retinopathy, nephropathy, and neuropathy: the Oslo study. BMJ 293:1195, 1986

46. Helve E, Laatikainen L, Merenmies L, Koivisto VA: Continuous insulin infusion therapy and retinopathy in patients with type 1 diabetes. Acta Endocrinol (Copenh) 115:313, 1987

47. Lauritzen T, Frost-Larsen K, Larsen H-W et al: Two-year experience with continuous subcutaneous insulin infusion in relation to retinopathy and neuropathy. Diabetes 34(suppl 3):74, 1985

48. The Kroc Collaborative Study Group: Diabetic retinopathy after two years of intensified insulin treatment: follow-up of the Kroc Collaborative Study. JAMA 260:37, 1988

49. Viberti GC, Pickup JC, Bilous RW et al: Correction of exercise-induced microalbuminuria in insulin-dependent diabetics after 3 weeks of subcutaneous insulin infusion. Diabetes 30:818, 1981

50. Feldt-Rasmussen B, Mathiesen ER, Deckert T: Effect of two years of strict metabolic control on progression of incipient nephropathy in insulin-dependent diabetes. Lancet 2:1300, 1986

51. Boulton AJM, Drury J, Clarke B: Continuous subcutaneous insulin infusion in the management of painful diabetic neuropathy. Diabetes Care 5:386, 1982

52. Service FJ, Rizza RA, Danube JR: Near normoglycaemia improved nerve conduction and vibration sensation in diabetic neuropathy. Diabetologia 28:722, 1985

53. Pietri A, Ehle AL, Raskin P: Changes in nerve conduction velocity after six weeks of glucoregulation with portable insulin infusion pumps. Diabetes 29:668, 1980

54. Chiasson JL, Ducros F, Poliquin-Hamet M et al: Continuous subcutaneous insulin infusion (Mill-Hill Infuser) versus multiple injections (Medi-Jector) in the treatment of insulin-dependent diabetes mellitus and the effect of metabolic control on microangiopathy. Diabetes Care 7:331, 1984

55. Fedele D, Negrin P, Cardone C, et al: Influence of continuous subcutaneous insulin infusion (CSII) treatment on diabetic somatic and autonomic neuropathy. J Endocrinol Invest 7:623, 1984

56. Tamborlane WV, Puklin JE, Bergman M et al: Long-term improvement of metabolic control with the insulin pump does not reverse diabetic microangiopathy. Diabetes Care 5:58, 1982

57. Lawson PM, Champion MC, Canny C et al: Continuous subcutaneous insulin infusion (CSII) does not prevent progression of proliferative and preproliferative retinopathy. Br J Ophthalmol 66:762, 1982

58. Viberti GC, Bilous RW, Mackintosh D et al: Long-term correction of hyperglycaemia and progression of renal failure in insulin dependent diabetes. BMJ 286:598, 1983

59. Raskin P, Rosenstock J: Blood glucose control and diabetic complications. Ann Intern Med 105:254, 1986

60. Osterby R: Morphometric studies of the peripheral glomerular basement membrane in early juvenile diabetes—1. Development of initial basement membrane thickening. Diabetologia 8:84, 1972

61. Couet C, Genton P, Pointel JP et al: The prevalence of retinopathy is similar in diabetes mellitus secondary to chronic pancreatitis with or without pancreatectomy and in idiopathic diabetes mellitus. Diabetes Care 8:323, 1985

62. Arouna GM, Kremer GD, Daddah SK et al: Reversal of diabetic nephropathy in human cadaveric kidneys after transplantation into nondiabetic recipients. Lancet 2:1274, 1983

63. Nathan DM: Inferences and implications. Diabetes Care 18:251, 1995

64. Davidson MB: Why the DCCT applies to NIDDM patients. Clin Diabetes 12:141, 1994

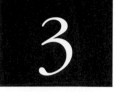

MEDICAL NUTRITION THERAPY

MARION J. FRANZ

Medical nutrition therapy is essential to total diabetes care and management. However, to integrate nutrition effectively into overall management of diabetes requires a coordinated team effort including a knowledgeable dietitian who is skilled in implementing current nutrition recommendations for diabetes.[1, 2] For a person with diabetes, medical nutrition therapy requires an individualized approach and effective self-management education. Furthermore, monitoring of glucose and glycated hemoglobin levels, lipids, blood pressure, weight, and quality of life issues is essential to evaluate the success of nutrition-related recommendations. If desired outcomes (i.e., target blood glucose goals) have not been met as a result of nutrition-related changes, it is the responsibility of the dietitian to notify the physician so that changes in the overall diabetes management (i.e., medication additions or changes) can be made.[3]

Today, just as one insulin regimen or one form of therapy no longer applies to all persons with diabetes, one nutrition prescription no longer applies to everyone with diabetes. Nutrition recommendations and principles from the American Diabetes Association (ADA) underscore the importance of individualized nutrition care.[1, 2] The recommendations depart from previous guidelines by not setting optimal levels for macronutrient intake (Table 3–1); instead, they recommend that macronutrient intake should be based on nutrition assessment, modification of usual eating habits, treatment goals, and monitoring of desired outcomes. Nutrition interventions, including the nutrition prescription and educational tools, should be based on a thorough assessment of each person's usual and customary intake and nutritional status. Of major concern is what an individual with diabetes is able and willing to do. To facilitate adherence, cultural, ethnic, and financial considerations are of prime importance. The guidelines also emphasize the primary goal of nutrition therapy, which is to assist persons with diabetes to keep their blood glucose levels in the near normal range, as well as to implement strategies that can assist individuals in achieving this goal. They incorporate the latest medical and nutrition research and allow for greater individualization and flexibility to help individuals with diabetes make planning food intake easier.

Health care professionals and persons with diabetes report adherence to nutrition and meal-planning principles as the most challenging aspect of diabetes care.[4] Successful integration of nutrition into diabetes management requires a person with diabetes to make some challenging life style changes. In 1993, the Diabetes Control and Complications Trial (DCCT) reaffirmed the importance of compliance with nutrition principles in type 1 (insulin-dependent) diabetes mellitus in order to achieve optimal glycemic control.[5] The 1995 Diabetes Nutrition Guidelines study documented the effectiveness of

Table 3–1. Historical Perspective on Nutrition Recommendations for Diabetes Mellitus

Year	Distribution of Calories from Carbohydrate (%)	Distribution of Calories from Protein (%)	Distribution of Calories from Fat (%)
Before 1921	Starvation diets		
1921	20	10	70
1950	40	20	40
1971	45	20	35
1986	up to 60	12–20	<30
1994	a	10–20	a, b

a Based on nutrition assessment and treatment goals
b <10% saturated fat
From American Diabetes Association: Nutrition recommendations and principles for people with diabetes mellitus (position statement). Diabetes Care 20(suppl 1):S17, 1997

nutrition therapy in type 2 (non–insulin-dependent) diabetes mellitus.[6]

GOALS AND STRATEGIES OF NUTRITION THERAPY

The goals of nutrition therapy are summarized in Table 3–2. Nutrition therapy is essential for keeping blood glucose levels in the near normal range and for achieving optimal lipid levels. Persons with diabetes need individualized target blood glucose ranges that are reasonable for them to achieve. They should understand that the primary goal of nutrition therapy is to balance food intake with insulin (exogenous or endogenous) and exercise to reach and maintain target glucose goals. Nutrition also has an important role in achieving desirable blood lipid levels.[7]

Although carbohydrates are the major determinant of blood glucose levels after food is ingested, caloric content of the meal plan cannot be ignored. This is true for persons using exogenous insulin, for whom weight gain is often an issue,[8, 9] and for persons with type 2 diabetes, for whom weight control is important. For a person with type 2 diabetes, it is important, however, to emphasize a reasonable body weight. Reasonable body weight is defined as that level of weight that individuals, both patients and professionals, acknowledge as achievable and maintainable

in both the short and long term.[1] This is usually not the same as traditionally defined desirable or ideal body weight.

Calories should be prescribed to provide for normal growth and development of children and adolescents. The meal plan is not a

Table 3–2. Goals of Medical Nutrition Therapy for Diabetes Mellitus

- Maintenance of as near normal blood glucose levels as possible
- Achievement of optimal lipid levels
- Provision of adequate calories
    For maintaining or attaining reasonable weights for adults
    For normal growth and development for children and adolescents
    To meet pregnancy and lactation needs
    For recovery from catabolic illness
- Prevention and treatment of the acute complications of insulin-treated diabetes
    Hypoglycemia
    Short-term illnesses
    Exercise-related problems
- Prevention and treatment of the long-term complications of diabetes
    Renal disease
    Autonomic neuropathy (gastrointestinal)
    Hypertension
    Cardiovascular disease
- Improvement of overall health through optimal nutrition

Adapted from American Diabetes Association: Nutrition recommendations and principles for people with diabetes mellitus (position statement). Diabetes Care 20(suppl 1):S14, 1997

restriction of calories but is intended to ensure a reasonably consistent intake and a nutritionally balanced diet. Parents of young children and adolescents need to learn to adjust insulin doses rather than restrict food to control blood glucose levels.

Adequate calories are also needed to meet increased metabolic needs during pregnancy, lactation, and catabolic illnesses. Monitoring of blood glucose levels, urine ketones, appetite, and weight allows appropriate calorie adjustments to be made.

Other nutritional goals are similar for individuals with diabetes as well as for nondiabetic persons. *Dietary Guidelines for Americans*[10] and the *Food Guide Pyramid*[11] outline and illustrate guidelines and nutrient needs for all healthy Americans and can also be used for persons with diabetes and their family members. Family members and significant others are encouraged to follow the same life style recommendations as a person with diabetes.

NUTRITION STRATEGIES FOR INSULIN-REQUIRING PERSONS

To assist persons who require insulin in achieving target blood glucose goals, it is important to integrate the insulin regimen into usual eating and exercise habits. Figure 3-1 illustrates this concept. Unfortunately, even though the ADA nutrition recommendations have stated this since 1979,[12] the insulin regimen is often still established first and then the individual must try to fit the necessary food changes into his or her life style. It is not surprising that adherence has often been less than desired.

Persons receiving two daily injections of short-acting and intermediate-acting insulins fare best if they maintain consistency in the timing and amount of their food intake, monitor their blood glucose levels, identify blood glucose patterns, and learn to adjust their insulin doses. For example, if noon blood glucose levels are higher than the target range for several days in a row, the morning short-acting insulin is increased. If the supper blood glucose levels are higher than the target range, the morning intermediate-acting insulin is adjusted, and so on. It is not necessary to divide meals and snacks into any artificial or unnatural division; however, food intake must be synchronized with the time actions of insulin. To prevent hypoglycemia and wide swings in blood glucose levels, individuals with type 1 diabetes generally fare better with three meals and two to three small snacks. However, individuals using very rapidly acting insulin, such as lispro (Humalog), must take the insulin immediately before eating and do not need snacks. If they wish to eat a snack, they may need

Figure 3–1. Strategies for integrating nutrition therapy for type 1 diabetes into overall diabetes management. Conventional therapy is defined as prebreakfast and presupper injections of short- and intermediate-acting insulins. Intensive therapy consists of three or more injections of insulin or use of an insulin pump. (From American Diabetes Association: Maximizing the Role of Nutrition in Diabetes Management. American Diabetes Association, Alexandria, VA, 1994, p. 33)

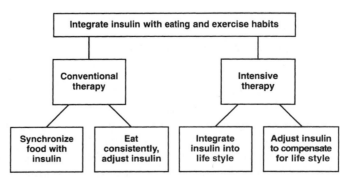

an injection of lispro immediately before eating the snack.

Patients need to be constantly reminded that blood glucose tests before meals and at bedtime (before evening snack) reflect what has happened during the previous 3 to 4 hours and that what they eat at this time affects blood glucose levels during the following 3 to 4 hours. If they react to elevated blood glucose levels by skipping or cutting back on meals or snacks, they do not solve their problems. In fact, they often make the problem worse—because of not eating appropriately, their blood glucose levels become too low.

Persons using intensive insulin therapy, such as multiple injections (three or more insulin injections per day) or infusion pump therapy have more flexibility in when and what they eat. Patients can be taught to adjust premeal insulin doses to compensate for departures from their meal plan and exercise programs, to delay premeal insulin for meals that are late, to make adjustments in the short-acting insulin for blood glucose values that are not in target range, and, if needed, to administer insulin for snacks that are not part of their meal plan. However, even for persons receiving intensive insulin therapy, consistency in food intake and following a meal plan were shown to be related to improved glycemic control. Other nutrition-related strategies linked to improved control included appropriate treatment of hypoglycemia, prompt changes for hyperglycemia, adjusting insulin doses for meal plan deviations, and consistently eating the planned evening snack.[5]

NUTRITION STRATEGIES FOR TYPE 2 DIABETES

In previous diabetes nutrition recommendations, weight loss was the primary goal for persons with type 2 diabetes; however, traditional dietary strategies have usually been ineffective for achieving long-term weight loss. Therefore, a major change in the cur-rent guidelines is to emphasize the importance of helping individuals to achieve and maintain near normal blood glucose levels as opposed to attaining a desirable body weight. A number of strategies for achieving target blood glucose goals are available for individuals to use. Today there is no clear-cut answer as to which strategy should be the first priority.[2] Monitoring of blood glucose levels to determine if target blood glucose goals have been met or if medications need to be added or doses adjusted is essential.

Although weight loss can increase insulin sensitivity and normalize hepatic glucose production, this nutrition strategy has been the most difficult to implement successfully. Furthermore, weight loss may be most beneficial early in the diagnosis of type 2 diabetes, when insulin secretion is the greatest. Genetic predisposition to obesity[13, 14] and possible impaired metabolic and appetite regulation[15, 16] contribute to the difficulty of losing weight and, more importantly, maintaining weight loss. Unfortunately, patients are often told to lose 40 to 60 pounds when even the best treatment programs for obesity (those programs using behavior modification, nutrition, exercise, and extended-length programs) report that individuals who complete weight-loss programs lose approximately 10% of their body weight (average 20 to 22 pounds), only to regain two thirds of it back within 1 year and almost all of it back within 5 years. Because of the psychologic and physiologic impact of "dieting," authorities in the obesity field recommend that the goal of obesity treatment should be refocused from weight loss alone, which is aimed at appearance, to weight management, achieving a reasonable weight in the context of overall health.[17]

Furthermore, moderate weight loss (10% to 15% of body weight) decreases health risks and medical problems in 90% of obese persons.[17] Evidence suggests that this is also true for persons with diabetes. Several studies[18, 19] report that losing as few as 10 to

20 pounds may be enough to improve blood glucose control. Watts and colleagues[19] reported that if blood glucose levels are not <180 mg/dl after a loss of 5 to 10 pounds, the chance that additional weight loss will lead to improved blood glucose control is unlikely. They speculate that because type 2 diabetes results from both insulin resistance and insulin deficiency, individuals who are insulin resistant benefit from moderate weight loss, whereas individuals who are insulin deficient may lose weight too easily owing to decompensated diabetes and require medication for successful diabetes management.

For persons with type 2 diabetes, a nutritionally adequate, moderate caloric restriction (250 to 500 kcal less than average daily intake as calculated from the nutrition assessment) and an emphasis on blood glucose control and reasonable weight rather than weight loss should be used. Exercise, behavior modification, and psychologic support are important if weight management is to be effective. Patients should not be made to feel guilty if they cannot lose weight. The idea that if patients would just lose weight, they would not need a medication should be abandoned. Therapies to assist the majority of patients in long-term weight loss are currently not available.

A hypocaloric diet (independent of much weight loss) is also associated with significantly increased sensitivity to insulin.[18, 20] These studies illustrate the important point that the most significant improvements in blood glucose levels occur before much weight is actually lost. Therefore, improved food choices, especially a reduction in fat intake, should be encouraged. High-fat diets are reported to aggravate insulin resistance, although the exact mechanism for how this occurs is unknown.[21]

Other strategies that can be used include spreading food intake throughout the day (five to six small meals and snacks instead of only three meals).[22, 23] Increasing physical activity can also contribute to improvements in blood glucose control.[24] Figure 3–2 summarizes strategies that can be used to improve metabolic control in persons with type 2 diabetes.

Blood glucose monitoring provides the necessary feedback to make adjustments in nutrition and medications. As duration of diabetes increases, medication use changes. Nearly 64% of adults with type 2 diabetes use oral therapy during the first 5 years after diagnosis, but this is reduced to 37% after 20 years of diabetes duration. Among adults with type 2 diabetes, insulin use increases from 22% at diagnosis to at least 58% be-

Nutrition therapy for type 2

Figure 3–2. Nutrition-related strategies for improved glucose control in persons with type 2 diabetes. (From American Diabetes Association: Maximizing the Role of Nutrition in Diabetes Management. American Diabetes Association, Alexandria, VA, 1994, p. 34)

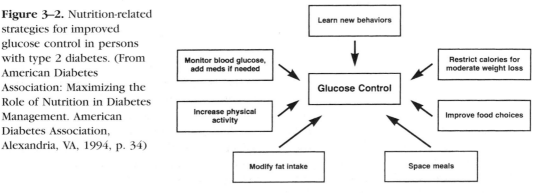

tween 10 and 15 years' duration.[25] These changes should not be viewed as a diet failure but instead reflect that as β-cell function becomes progressively impaired, the insulin secretory response becomes deficient.[26] Patients should be encouraged to take whatever steps are necessary to maintain euglycemia and prevent the destructiveness of glucose toxicity. (High levels of blood glucose impair insulin secretion and, to a lesser extent, insulin action as well.) Frequent follow-up with a dietitian can provide the problem-solving techniques, encouragement, and support that life style changes require.[6]

MACRONUTRIENT DISTRIBUTION

Table 3-1 outlines past recommendations for the distribution of macronutrients. In 1986, the ADA advised that 12% to 20% of daily calories be from protein, up to 55% to 60% from carbohydrate, and <30% from fat. The current guidelines reject such mandatory and rigid percentages. Instead, the protein intake continues to be 10% to 20% of the calories, leaving 80% to 90% of daily calories to be divided between carbohydrate and fat. Exactly how these calories are divided depends on individual treatment goals for glucose and lipid levels, weight management goals, and the nutrition assessment of what a patient is willing and able to do. Critics have suggested that this does not provide enough guidance for professionals. However, evidence does not justify such predetermined recommendations. Studies have shown that individuals with diabetes can reach treatment goals using varying macronutrient percentages.[27]

PROTEIN

No available evidence suggests that persons with uncomplicated diabetes have increased or decreased protein requirements compared with those of the general public.[28]

Average protein intake for most Americans is ~12% to 20% or more of daily calories. At present, scientific evidence does not support either a higher or lower protein intake in diabetes, and protein intake in the range of 10% to 20% of daily calories is recommended.[1] Although 20% of the calories from protein is approximately double the recommended daily allowance (RDA) for protein, no evidence shows that protein intake correlates with the development of nephropathy.[28, 29]

The rate of protein degradation and conversion of protein to glucose in individuals with type 1 diabetes may depend on the state of insulinization and degree of glycemic control. With less than optimal insulinization, conversion of protein to glucose can occur rapidly and can adversely influence glycemic control. In persons with poorly controlled type 2 diabetes, gluconeogenesis is also accelerated and may account for the majority of increased glucose production in the postabsorptive state. However, the independent influence of dietary protein on glycemia and insulin sensitivity in individuals with well-controlled type 1[30] and type 2[31] diabetes appears to be minimal.

Other than the two cited studies,[30, 31] minimal research delineates the effects of protein ingestion on blood glucose levels. Even if ~50% is converted to glucose, it appears not to have much influence on overall blood glucose levels. Although patients have traditionally been taught to have a food source of protein before bedtime (or with other snacks), it is doubtful that this protein has much clinical effect. In a study by Peters and Davidson,[30] 50g of protein (~7 ounces of meat) was added to a standard meal. Five hours after the ingestion of both meals, blood glucose levels were similar, although a small increase in postprandial glucose response and late insulin requirements was noted. The effects of protein and fat on blood glucose levels and insulin sensitivity are clearly issues that demand additional research.

With the onset of incipient nephropathy (i.e., microalbuminuria), restricted protein diets may modify the underlying glomerular injury and, along with controlling hypertension and hyperglycemia, delay the progression of renal failure.[32] Although the benefits of protein restriction in renal disease are controversial,[33] the general response to low-protein diets in studies with subjects with diabetes has been beneficial in terms of progression of renal disease.[34, 35] Therefore, with the onset of nephropathy, a protein intake of not less than 0.8 g/kg/day, or ~10% of calories, is recommended.[1] With a lower protein intake of 0.6 g/kg/day, protein malnutrition becomes evident. Decreased muscle strength and an increase in body fat with no change in total body weight were reported during just 12 weeks of severe protein restriction.[36]

An unresolved issue is the type of protein to restrict. Several studies suggest that animal rather than vegetable protein may be an important determinant in the progression of renal disease. Studies, although preliminary, are based on evidence that vegetable proteins have significantly different renal effects than animal proteins.[37-39] No definitive mechanisms for these differences have been identified, although differences in amino acid composition or the resulting hormone and vasodilatory prostaglandin production may mediate the effects on renal hemodynamics and function.

FAT

It is generally agreed that a reduction in saturated fat (<10% of total calories) and dietary cholesterol (<300 mg/day) is an important goal of nutrition,[1, 2] but the recommended distribution of dietary carbohydrate and fat (monounsaturates and polyunsaturates) remains controversial.

The percentage of calories from fat in the diet depends on the goals established for glucose levels, lipid levels, and weight. If obesity and weight loss are the primary concerns, a reduction in dietary fat should be considered.[40] People who are at a healthy weight and who have normal lipid levels are encouraged to follow the recommendations of the National Cholesterol Education Program (NCEP).[41, 42] The NCEP recommends that all individuals older than 2 years limit fat intake to <30% of calories, with saturated fat intake restricted to <10% of total calories. Polyunsaturated fat intake should be <10% of calories, with monounsaturated fat in the range of 10% to 15% of calories. Dietary cholesterol intake should be <300 mg/day. If low-density lipoprotein (LDL) cholesterol levels are elevated, further restriction of saturated fat to 7% of total calories and dietary cholesterol to <200 mg/day (NCEP step II diet) is recommended.

If triglycerides and very low-density lipoprotein (VLDL) cholesterol are the primary concerns, one approach that may be tried is a moderate increase in monounsaturated fat intake with <10% of the calories from saturated fats and a more moderate carbohydrate intake.[1] Several studies[43-45] suggest that a moderately higher fat diet (up to 40% of daily calories) can lower triglyceride levels as well as or better than fat restriction, provided the additional fat is predominantly monounsaturated fatty acids (MUFAs). However, caloric intake in these studies is kept at a level to prevent weight loss, and the beneficial effect on triglyceride levels may result from the reduced carbohydrate intake as much as from the increased intake of MUFAs. Because major sources of MUFAs are canola, olive, and peanut oils, increasing fat intake beyond substituting these oils in cooking may be difficult. Another option is a low-fat, low-calorie diet. When Pascale and colleagues[46] compared a lower-calorie, high-carbohydrate, low-fat diet with a lower-calorie, lower-carbohydrate, higher-fat diet, no detrimental effect on triglycerides was found.

Lipid levels in persons with type 1 diabetes are not that different from those of matched nondiabetic persons, although the first group is at increased risk for cardiovascular disease.[47] Therefore, the NCEP recommendations are appropriate for most individuals who have type 1 diabetes and who are at a healthy weight and have normal lipid values. Persons with type 2 diabetes have a two- to fourfold increase in the prevalence of dyslipidemia, including increased triglyceride levels, decreased high-density lipoprotein (HDL) cholesterol, and total cholesterol and LDL cholesterol levels similar to age-matched nondiabetic persons.[48] Treatment goals dictate nutrition recommendations for this population. The first priority for treatment of dyslipidemia is improved glucose control. Other strategies that can be used include moderate weight loss, increased physical activity, avoidance of alcohol (if this is a problem), and then the actual composition of the diet. The key is individualization. If patients have been eating 45% of daily calories from fat, lowering fat to even 40% can be helpful and important.

CARBOHYDRATE

Traditional nutrition treatment of diabetes has emphasized avoiding sugars (especially sucrose and often naturally occurring sugars as well) and replacing them with starch. Belief that sugars must be restricted was based on the assumption that sugars are more rapidly digested and absorbed than starches and thereby aggravate hyperglycemia. Starches or complex carbohydrates, although metabolized into glucose, were assumed to break down more slowly, thus producing a slower, steadier rise in blood glucose levels. However, scientific evidence does not justify restriction of sugars because of the foregoing belief.[1, 2]

Research conducted in the past decade has consistently shown that sucrose and other sugars, when consumed separately or as a part of a meal or snack, do not have a greater impact on blood glucose levels than other carbohydrates.[49-55] Figure 3-3 shows examples of results from studies comparing

sucrose and starch as the source of carbohydrate. In subjects with type 1 and type 2 diabetes, 45 g (~20% of calories) of starch was replaced with 45 g of sucrose for 6 weeks, with no significant differences in glycemic or lipid responses.[52] Starches that are polymers of glucose rapidly break down to 100% glucose owing to the presence of enzymes in the intestinal tract, whereas sucrose is metabolized to 50% glucose and 50% fructose. Fructose has a lower glycemic response, which has been attributed to its slow rate of absorption and to its rapid removal by the liver and storage as glycogen rather than conversion to glucose.[56] However, from a clinical perspective, first priority should be given to the total amount of carbohydrate consumed, not the source.[2]

The recommendation to substitute sucrose for starch does not mean that individuals with diabetes can indulge in cookies, cake, and sugar. Portion sizes containing equal grams of carbohydrates are often small compared with other carbohydrates, especially starches, but this does mean that sweets containing sucrose can be substituted for another carbohydrate in an individual's meal plan. For example, a small cookie containing 15 g of carbohydrate can be substituted for a starch or fruit that also contributes 15 g of carbohydrate, and either choice would be expected to have approximately the same effect on blood glucose levels. However, many desserts contain fat as well and therefore add extra calories to the diet.

Individuals previously were instructed to read carefully the ingredient listing on labels and, if sugar was the first, second, or third ingredient, to avoid eating that food. Instead they should be taught to look at the serving size and the total grams of carbohydrate on the Nutrition Facts label (Fig. 3-4). Fifteen grams of carbohydrate is considered to be one carbohydrate choice. They should ignore the grams of sugars (this is included in the total grams of carbohydrate) and the ingredient listing. Persons with diabetes too often assume that if sugar is not an ingredient of food, the food will not affect their

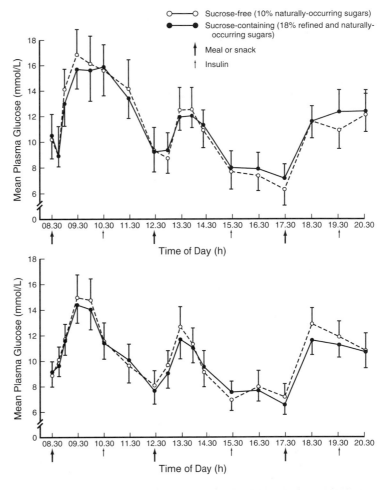

Figure 3-3. In the sucrose-containing diet, 45 g of starch was replaced with 45 g of sucrose at meal times for 6 weeks; total grams of carbohydrate are similar in each test diet. Top panel: 12 persons with type 1 diabetes. Bottom panel: 11 persons with type 2 diabetes. (From Peterson DD, Lambert J, Gerrig S, et al: Sucrose in the diet of diabetic patients—just another carbohydrate? Diabetologia 29:218, 1986)

blood glucose levels, and they eat unlimited quantities of these foods.

Alternative Sweeteners

Additionally, no evidence shows that nutritive sweeteners such as fructose, fruit juice concentrates, corn syrup, honey, starch hydrolysates, or sugar alcohols such as sorbitol or mannitol have advantages or disadvantages over sucrose in decreasing amounts of carbohydrate or calories in the diet or in improving overall diabetes control.[1] Fructose provides 4 kcal/g, as do other carbohydrates, and even though it does have a lower glycemic response than sucrose and other starches, large amounts (double usual intake) of fructose have been reported to have an

adverse effect on cholesterol levels, especially LDL cholesterol.[57] However, there is no reason to recommend that persons with diabetes avoid fructose, which occurs naturally in fruits or is in foods sweetened with fructose.

Calories from sugar alcohols, sorbitol, mannitol, and xylitol vary but average ~2 kcal/g compared with the 4 kcal/g from other carbohydrates.[58] Individuals with diabetes should look at the total grams of carbohydrate and calories in the food product and substitute appropriately in their meal plan. Some individuals report gastric discomfort after eating food sweetened with these products, and consumption of large quantities may cause diarrhea. Starch hydrolysates are formed by the partial hydrolysis of edible

Nutrition Facts

Serving Size 1 cup (228g)
Servings Per Container 2

Amount Per Serving

Calories 90   Calories from Fat 30

	% Daily Value*
Total Fat 3g	**5%**
Saturated Fat 0g	**0%**
Cholesterol 0mg	**0%**
Sodium 300mg	**13%**
Total Carbohydrate 13g	**4%**
Dietary Fiber 3g	**12%**
Sugars 3g	
Protein 3g	

Vitamin A 80%	•	Vitamin C 60%
Calcium 4%	•	Iron 4%

* Percent Daily Values are based on a 2,000 calorie diet. Your daily values may be higher or lower depending on your calorie needs:

		Calories:	2,000	2,500
Total Fat	Less than		65g	80g
Sat Fat	Less than		20g	25g
Cholesterol	Less than		300mg	300mg
Sodium	Less than		2,400mg	2,400mg
Total Carbohydrate			300g	375g
Dietary Fiber			25g	30g

Calories per gram:
Fat 9 • Carbohydrate 4 • Protein 4

Figure 3–4. Nutrition Facts food label.

starches. Their reducing activity can then be eliminated by hydrogenation, and the product becomes a polyol.

Saccharin, aspartame, and acesulfame K are noncaloric sweeteners currently approved for use in the United States by the Food and Drug Administration (FDA). FDA approval is being sought for sucralose, alitame, and cyclamates, other noncaloric sweeteners. All of these sweeteners must undergo rigorous testing by the manufacturer and scrutiny from the FDA before they are approved and marketed to the public.[59] The

FDA determines an acceptable daily intake (ADI) for products it approves; this is defined as a safe amount for daily consumption over a lifetime. The ADI includes a 100-fold safety factor and greatly exceeds average consumption levels. For example, aspartame consumption (14-day average) in persons with diabetes is 2 to 4 mg/kg/day, well below the FDA's ADI of 50 mg/kg/day.[60] All FDA-approved nonnutritive sweeteners can be used by individuals with diabetes, including pregnant women (because saccharin can cross the placenta, other sweeteners are better choices during pregnancy).[1]

Fiber

Although soluble fiber (fiber from legumes, oats, fruits, some vegetables) is capable of inhibiting absorption of glucose from the small intestine, the clinical significance of this effect is probably not important.[1] Previous recommendations theorized that soluble fiber would form a gel in the intestine and would slow the absorption of glucose. However, the original studies used unreasonably large amounts of fiber[61] or had several variables, and all the benefits were assumed to be from fiber. A beneficial effect on blood glucose control was not observed in studies based on usual amounts of soluble fiber.[62, 63] Dietary fiber may be beneficial in treating or preventing several benign gastrointestinal disorders and colon cancer. Diets containing 20 g/day of soluble fiber may be capable of producing modest reductions in fasting circulating total and LDL cholesterol when administered in conjunction with a diet containing at least 50% of the calories from carbohydrate.[2] It is difficult to consume that amount of soluble fiber in foods alone. The recommendation for fiber intake for persons with diabetes is similar to the recommendation for the general public: approximately 20 to 35 g/day of dietary fiber from both soluble and insoluble fibers.[1]

OTHER NUTRIENTS

SODIUM

Individuals differ in their sensitivity to sodium and its effect on blood pressure. However, there does appear to be a relationship between diabetes and hypertension, and evidence suggests that persons with type 2 diabetes are more sodium sensitive than the general public.[64] Even though in type 2 diabetes an association between hypertension and obesity is noted, the association of hypertension with diabetes exists even in the absence of obesity in both type 1 and type 2 diabetes.

Because sodium-sensitive individuals are not easy to identify, intake recommendations for sodium range from approximately 2,400 mg/day to 3,000 mg/day. For persons who are hypertensive, <2,400 mg/day of sodium is recommended.[1, 65] Single servings of foods that contain >400 mg of sodium or entrees with >800 mg of sodium are significant sources of sodium in the diet.

OTHER VITAMINS AND MINERALS

There is no justification for routine prescription of vitamin and mineral supplements for the majority of persons with diabetes.[66] Antioxidant therapy is a possible consideration in the future. A person's response to supplements is largely determined by nutritional state, and thus only persons with micronutrient deficiencies are likely to respond favorably. Persons who are at greatest risk of deficiency and who may benefit from prescription of vitamin and mineral supplements include the following: patients on extremely low-calorie diets, strict vegetarians, the elderly, pregnant or lactating women, those taking medications known to alter micronutrient metabolism, persons in poor metabolic control (with glucosuria), or patients in critical care environments. Magnesium replacement may be needed for pa-

tients with poor glycemic control or for those receiving diuretics. Magnesium depletion has been associated with insulin insensitivity, which may improve with oral supplementation.[67]

Chromium picolinate is probably the most frequently asked about supplement. Chromium in the form of "glucose tolerance factor" is thought to enhance the action of insulin. Chromium supplements are poorly absorbed by the body and are absorbed better if combined with picolinic acid (made naturally in the liver and kidneys), which binds with minerals. This binding is necessary to move minerals quickly and effectively into cells where they are needed.

Rabinowitz and colleagues[68] studied chromium in persons with and without diabetes and could not identify any deficiencies or any differences between the two groups. They concluded that most persons with diabetes are not chromium deficient. Although a severe chromium deficiency can lead to elevated blood glucose levels, its role in causing diabetes is not significant. In three double-blind placebo-controlled studies in which persons with diabetes received a chromium supplement, the supplement had no effect on blood glucose control.[66]

Chromium supplementation is useful only for those with a chromium deficiency, the incidence of which is probably small and not a concern for well-nourished individuals. Reliable testing for chromium deficiency is not currently available, and chromium supplementation provides no proven benefit for people with diabetes.[2, 66]

ALCOHOL

The same precautions that apply to everyone in regard to the use of alcohol also apply to persons with diabetes. The effect of alcohol on blood glucose levels depends not only on the amount of alcohol ingested but also on the relationship to food intake. For persons taking exogenous insulin in a fasting state, alcohol consumption may produce hypoglycemia. In the liver, the main pathway for the oxidation of alcohol to acetaldehyde and then to energy involves the enzyme alcohol dehydrogenase. Alcohol is not converted to glucose, blocks gluconeogenesis, and augments or increases the effects of insulin by interfering with the counterregulation to insulin-induced hypoglycemia.[69]

For most individuals, blood glucose levels are not affected by moderate use of alcohol when diabetes is well controlled.[70] If they choose, persons with diabetes can have as many as two drinks (1 drink equals 12 ounces of beer, 5 ounces of wine, or 1 1/2 ounces of distilled spirits) of an alcoholic beverage with and in addition to their regular meal plan. No food should be omitted because of the possibility of alcohol-induced hypoglycemia and because alcohol does not require insulin to be metabolized. For persons concerned with calories, alcohol is best substituted for fat exchanges or fat calories (alcohol contributes 7 kcal/g).[1] Persons with elevated triglyceride levels and pregnant women should avoid consumption of alcohol.

SELF-MANAGEMENT EDUCATION

Managing diabetes is a team effort. Dietitians, nurses, physicians, and other health care providers contribute their expertise to the development of therapeutic regimens that assist persons with diabetes to achieve the best metabolic control that is possible. The person with diabetes must be at the center of the team because he or she has the responsibility for day-to-day implementation of management. The goal is to provide persons with the knowledge, skills, and motivation to incorporate self-management into their daily life style. Education is a planned process that requires time, materials, space, and professional expertise to individualize.

The knowledge and skills needed to implement nutrition recommendations cannot be acquired in one session, and nutrition education must be an ongoing component of diabetes care.

For patients whose diabetes is newly diagnosed, a staged approach to education should be used. Initial education focuses on the skills needed for survival. In-depth information and additional topics are added after a patient has had time to adjust to the diagnosis of diabetes. Topics are numerous and vary according to the type of diabetes and the individual characteristics and needs of the patient with diabetes. Tables 3-3 and 3-4 outline the topics addressed at each stage.

IMPLEMENTING NUTRITION SELF-MANAGEMENT

The five components of nutrition education are as follows: assessment for the development of the nutrition care plan and prescription, establishment of clinical and behavioral goals, implementation of education, evaluation of the outcomes, and documentation. At the beginning and throughout the relationship, the person with diabetes and the health care team must have rapport if the nutrition plan is to be successful.[71]

Table 3–3. Basic and Initial Nutrition Therapy: Self-Management Education (Survival Skills) for All Persons with Diabetes

Basic meal plan guidelines
Exercise guidelines
Signs, symptoms, treatment, and prevention of hypoglycemia
Nutritional management during short-term illness
Blood glucose monitoring skills, if needed
Plan for continuing care

From Monk A, Barry B, McClain K, et al: Practice guidelines for medical nutrition therapy by dietitians for persons with non–insulin-dependent diabetes mellitus. J Am Diet Assoc 95:999, 1995

Table 3–4. Essential Nutrition Topics for Self-Management

Essential education for ongoing nutrition self-management. Topics emphasized based on patient's life style, level of nutrition knowledge, and experience in planning, purchasing, and preparing food and meals	Sources of carbohydrate, protein, fat
	Nutrition labels
	Grocery shopping guidelines
	Eating out, restaurant, cafeteria, and fast-food choices
	Modifying fat intake
	Use of sugar-containing foods
	Alcohol guidelines
	Snack choices
	Using blood glucose monitoring for problem solving and identification of blood glucose patterns
	Adjusting meal times
	Making meal planning more flexible
	Dietetic foods and sweeteners
	Exchanges
	Recipes, menu ideas, cookbooks
	Adjusting food for exercise
	Behavior modification techniques
	Problem-solving tips
	Birthdays, special occasions, holidays
	Brown bag lunches
	Travel, schedule changes
	Vitamin, mineral, other nutritional supplements
	Working rotating shifts, if needed

From Monk A, Barry B, McClain K, et al: Practice guidelines for medical nutrition therapy by dietitians for persons with non–insulin-dependent diabetes mellitus. J Am Diet Assoc 95:999, 1995

Responsibilities of the physician and the dietitian are outlined in Table 3-5. The ADA recommends that every person with diabetes have an individual consultation with a registered dietitian to tailor a food plan to his or her life style and health needs.[72] Individualized meal plans should *not* begin with a predetermined calorie level and ideal macronutrient distribution. Figure 3–5 illustrates this well. It is the responsibility of the dietitian or nutrition counselor to determine the nutrition prescription based on the food/nutrition history. Outcomes must be identified, and the effectiveness of nutrition interventions continually documented.

Assessment

When a nutrition care plan and prescription are developed, the following parameters are assessed: anthropometric measures, biochemical indices and laboratory data, clinical signs, food/nutrition history, learning style, cultural heritage, and socioeconomic status. Minimum referral data needed from a physician before beginning an assessment are listed in Table 3-6.

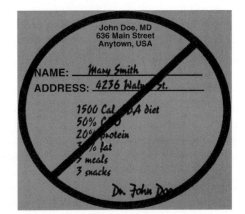

Figure 3–5. Outdated description of an ADA diet. (From American Diabetes Association: Maximizing the Role of Nutrition in Diabetes Management. American Diabetes Association, Alexandria, VA, 1994, p. 54)

Table 3–5. Physician and Dietitian Responsibilities for Medical Nutrition Therapy

Physician responsibilities	Refer patient to dietitian for nutrition therapy
	Provide referral data (see Table 3–6)
	Communicate medical treatment goals for patient care to dietitian
	Provide medical clearance for exercise as appropriate
	Based on outcomes of nutrition intervention, adjust medications for diabetes control if needed
	Reinforce nutrition self-management education
Dietitian responsibilities	Obtain referral data and treatment goals before the initial nutrition intervention
	Obtain and assess food, exercise, monitoring of blood glucose, psychosocial and economic issues
	Evaluate patient's knowledge, skill level, and readiness to learn
	Identify patient's goals
	Determine and implement an appropriate nutrition prescription
	Provide education on meal planning and self-management using appropriate teaching tools
	Evaluate the effectiveness of nutrition therapy on medical outcomes and adjust nutrition therapy as needed
	Make recommendations to the physician based on the outcomes of the nutrition interventions
	Communicate outcomes to all team members
	Decide number of visits patient requires for initial education
	Make recommendations for ongoing nutrition therapy and self-management education

Adapted from Monk A, Barry B, McClain K, et al: Practice guidelines for medical nutrition therapy by dietitians for persons with non–insulin-dependent diabetes mellitus. J Am Diet Assoc 95:999, 1995

A complete food/nutrition history should be taken at the onset of nutrition therapy to familiarize the health care team with an individual's life style and eating habits. A nutrition history form with key questions (Fig. 3–6) can be useful for recording the data. It is essential first to learn about an individual's daily routine and schedule. The following information is needed: (1) the time that individual wakes up, (2) usual meal and eating times, (3) work schedule or school hours, (4) type, amount, and timing of exercise, and (5) usual sleep habits. The history can also reveal other useful information: (1) usual caloric intake, (2) quality of the usual diet, (3) times, size, and content of meals and snacks, (4) food idiosyncrasies, (5) frequency of eating at restaurants, (6) who usually prepares food, (7) ethnic food preferences, (8) eating problems (dental, gastrointestinal, and so on), and (9) alcoholic beverage usage.

Nutrition histories can be taken in several ways. The objective is to determine a schedule and pattern of eating that are the least disruptive to the life style of the individual with diabetes and that at the same time facilitate improved glycemic control. With this objective in mind, asking an individual either to record or to report what, how much, and when he or she typically eats during a 24-hour period may be the most useful. An alternative approach is to solicit from the individual a 24-hour recall of exactly what was eaten during that period. This provides specific objective information but may not be representative of a typical day's intake. Individuals can also be asked to keep 3-day or weekly food diaries. Assessment of the most typical daily pattern can then be made.

A preliminary meal plan can then be designed by using the nutrition history information and a form such as that in Figure 3–6. The nutrition prescription is determined by

Table 3–6. Minimum Referral Data Before Nutrition Assessment

	Data Needed
Diabetes treatment regimen	Nutrition therapy alone
	Nutrition therapy and oral glucose-lowering agents
	Nutrition therapy and insulin or combination therapy
Laboratory data	Glycated hemoglobin
	Fasting or nonfasting plasma glucose level
	Cholesterol and fractionations
	Fasting triglyceride value
	Blood pressure
	Microalbumin
Physician goals for patient care	Target blood glucose levels
	Target glycated hemoglobin
	Method and frequency of self-monitoring of blood glucose (SMBG)
	Plans for instruction and evaluation of SMBG
Medical history	Dyslipidemia and/or cardiovascular disease
	Hypertension
	Renal disease
	Autonomic neuropathy, especially gastrointestinal
Medications that affect nutrition therapy	Diabetes medications
	Hypertension medications
	Lipid-lowering medications
	Gastrointestinal medications
	Others
Guidelines for exercise	Medical clearance for exercise
	Exercise limitations, if any

Adapted from Monk A, Barry B, McClain K, et al: Practice guidelines for medical nutrition therapy by dietitians for persons with non–insulin-dependent diabetes mellitus. J Am Diet Assoc 95:999, 1995

modifying the usual food intake as necessary. Figure 3-7 is an example of an individual's reported food intake, and Figure 3-8 is the modified preliminary meal plan. The nutrient information from the exchange lists can be a useful tool for evaluating nutrition assessments. Table 3-7 lists the macronutrient and caloric values for the exchange lists. By totaling the number of exchanges from each list and multiplying the grams of carbohydrate and protein by 4 and the grams of fat by 9, total calories and percentage of calories from each macronutrient can be determined.

The next step is to evaluate the preliminary meal plan. First and foremost, does the individual with diabetes feel it is feasible to implement for his or her life style? Second, are the calories appropriate? Third, is it appropriate for diabetes management? Fourth, does it encourage healthful eating?

Is the meal plan feasible for the individ- *ual with diabetes to implement?* The meal plan is reviewed with the individual in terms of general food intake. Timing of meals and snacks and approximate portion sizes and types of foods are covered. A meal-planning approach is selected later to assist the individual in making his or her own food choices. At this point, it needs to be determined if this meal plan is reasonable for the individual.

Are the calories appropriate? Next determine if the number of calories is appropriate for the individual. Caloric requirement is dependent on several factors, such as age, gender, height, weight, and activity level. Table 3-8 outlines a simple method for determining approximate caloric requirements based on current weight.

It should be emphasized that methods for determining caloric requirements are only approximate. On a practical basis, however, *Text continued on page 64*

NUTRITION ASSESSMENT

Date _____
Dietitian _____
Chart # _____
Physician _____

Name _____ Age _____

Diagnosis of Diabetes _____ Present Diabetes Treatment _____
Medical History _____ Other Medications_____
_____ _____

Lab Data
  HbA1c _____ BG_____
  Cholesterol _____ HDL-C_____ Triglycerides_____ LDL-C_____
  BP_____ Microalbumin _____ Other _____

Target Goals
  Target BG's _____ mg/dl to _____ mg/dl
  Target HbA1c _____ %

SMBG: Frequency_____ Times of day _____ Method_____
Medical clearance for exercise: Y / N   Exercise limitations _____

	Bkft	Snack	Lunch	Snack	Dinner	Snack	Total serving /day	CHO (g)	Protein (g)	Fat	Calories
Time											
Starch								15	3	1	80
Fruit								15			60
Milk								12	8	1	90
Veg.								5	2		25
Meat/ Sub									7	5(3)	75(55)
Fat										5	45
Other							Total g				
							Calories	x4	x4	x9	Total =
							Percent calories				

Ht _____ (_____ %) Wt History _____
Wt _____ (_____ %) Reasonable Wt _____
Estimated calorie expenditure + Activity factor = Total calorie needs
_____

History

Occupation _____
Lives with _____
Hypoglycemia _____
Alcohol use_____
Hours worked _____
Meal preparation _____
Eating out _____
Travel _____
Schedule changes/Weekends/School schedule _____
Exercise: Type/Frequency _____
Appetite/GI problems/Allergies/Intolerances _____
Vitamin & mineral supplements _____
Psychosocial/Economic _____
Assessment

_____
_____
_____
_____

Goals (Nutrition/Exercise/SMBG)

_____
_____
_____
_____

Figure 3–6. Example of a nutrition history form for persons with diabetes.

<u>ONE DAY FOOD RECORD</u>

NAME _Judy Smith_

HEIGHT _5'5"_   WEIGHT _165#_

(INSTRUCTION ON REVERSE SIDE)

INDICATE ACTUAL TIME FOOD IS EATEN	AMOUNT	FOOD & BEVERAGE	METHOD OF PREPARATION	DO NOT WRITE IN THIS SPACE
When you get up 7 AM	1 cup	orange juice		2 fruit ⑤ CHO
Breakfast 7:30	Large bowl 1 cup 2 cups	cereal milk coffee		2 starch 1 milk
Middle of the morning snack 10 AM	1 2 cups	Donut or Danish coffee		1-2 starch 1-2 fat ② CHO
Lunch 12:15 PM	2 slices 2 slices ¾ oz. pkg. 1 Large	Sandwich bread luncheon meat chips cookie Diet soda		4-5 starch 2-3 meat 2-3 fat ④⑤ CHO
Middle of the afternoon snack 3:10	1	cookie or apple Diet soda		1-2 starch 1-2 fat ② CHO
Supper 6:30	3-4 oz. 1 cup 1 1 cup	Chicken/pork chop/spaghetti potatoes/rice/corn roll or bread veg. or salad 2% milk fruit	broiled with Margarine with Margarine with dressing	3-4 meat 3 starch 1-2 veg 1 milk 1 fruit 2-3 fat ⑤⑥ CHO
Evening snack 10:30		ice cream/cookie/fruit		2 starch 1-2 fat ② CHO

What has your doctor told you to do about eating?

Eat on time and don't eat Sugar

300 g CHO   46%
105 g protein   16%
110 g fat   38%
2600-2700 kcal

Figure 3–7. Example of a completed 1-day food history form.

Judy Smith

Meal/Snack/Time

Food Group	Breakfast 7:00–7:30	Snack 10:00	Lunch 12:15	Snack 3:10	Dinner 6:30	Snack 10:30	Total Servings/day	CHO (g)	Protein (g)	Fat (g)	Calories
Starch	1–2	1	2–3		2–3	1–2	10	15 / 150	3 / 30	1 / 10	80
Fruit	1		0–1	1	1		3	15 / 45			60
Milk 1%	1		–		1		2	12 / 24	8 / 16	2+ / 4	90
Vegetables			✓		1–2		2	5 / 10	2 / 4		25
Meats/ Substitutes			2–3		3–4		5		7 / 35	5(3) / 25	75(55)
Fats	0–1	0–1	1–2	0–1	1–2	0–1	6			5 / 30	45

	3–4 CHO	1 CHO	3–4 CHO	1 CHO	4–5 CHO	1–2 CHO	Total	229	85	69	
							Calories	X4= 916	X4= 340	X9= 621	Total = 1800–1900
							Percent calories	49%	18%	33%	

Meal Plan

Meal Plan for: Judy Smith   Date: 8-30-95

Dietitian: Harriet James   Phone: 825-1244

	Grams	Percent
Carbohydrate	230	49%
Protein	85	18%
Fat	70	33%
Calories	1800–1900	

Time	Number of Exchanges/Choices	Menu Ideas	Menu Ideas
7:00–7:30	**3–4** Carbohydrate group / 1–2 Starch / 1 Fruit / 1 Milk 1% / ___ Meat group / 0–1 Fat group	½ cup orange juice / 1 cup cereal / 1 cup 1% milk	
10:00	**1** Carbohydrate / 0–1 fat	½ bagel / 1 Tbsp reduced-fat cream cheese	
12:15	**3–4** Carbohydrate group / 2–3 Starch / 0–1 Fruit / ___ Milk / ✓ Vegetables / 2–3 Meat group / 1–2 Fat group	2 sliced bread – 2 oz. lowfat luncheon meat / 1 Tbsp light mayonnaise / lettuce & tomato slices / 1 cup vegetable beef soup / 1 cookie	
3:10	**1** Carbohydrate / 0–1 fat	1 small apple	
6:30	**4–5** Carbohydrate group / 2–3 Starch / 1 Fruit / 1 Milk 1% / ✓ Vegetables / 3–4 Meat group / 1–2 Fat group	1 medium baked potato / 1 dinner roll / 3 oz baked chicken breast / ½ cup broccoli – small dinner salad / ¾ cup mandarin oranges / 2 Tbsp regular sour cream 2 Tbsp light salad dressing	
10:30	**1–2** Carbohydrate / 0–1 fat	½ cup light ice cream / ½ cup strawberries	

Figure 3–8. Example of a meal plan and sample menu calculated from the sample food history.

Table 3–7. Macronutrient and Caloric Values for Exchange Lists

Groups/Lists	Carbohydrate (g)	Protein (g)	Fat (g)	Calories
Carbohydrate Group				
Starch	15	3	1 or less	80
Fruit	15	—	—	60
Milk				
Skim	12	8	0–3	90
2%	12	8	5	120
Whole	12	8	8	150
Other carbohydrates	15	Varies	Varies	Varies
Vegetables	5	2	—	25
Meat and Meat Substitute Group				
Very lean	—	7	0–1	35
Lean	—	7	3	55
Medium fat	—	7	5	75
High fat	—	7	8	100
Fat Group	—	—	5	45

From American Diabetes Association: Exchange Lists for Meal Planning. American Diabetes Association, Alexandria, VA, 1995

Table 3–8. Estimating Caloric Requirements for Adults

Approximate caloric requirements for adults:
10 kcal/pound (20 kcal/kg) = kcal for obese or very inactive persons and chronic dieters
13 kcal/pound (25 kcal/kg) = kcal for persons >55 years, active women, sedentary men
15 kcal/pound (30 kcal/kg) = kcal for active men or very active women
20 kcal/pound (40 kcal/kg) = kcal for very active men or athletes

they do provide a starting point for evaluating the caloric adequacy of the meal plan. Adjustments in calories can be made during follow-up visits. Parameters that should be taken into account are weight changes, feelings of satiety and hunger, and concerns about palatability.

The determination of a calorie level and a nutrition prescription for a child or adolescent is also based on the nutrition assessment. The appropriate calorie needs can be calculated in various ways. Probably the best method is to ascertain what the child usually eats to maintain his or her weight, because children have a natural ability to know just how much to eat for normal growth and development. Several formulas that can be used to confirm that a child is receiving the minimum necessary calories are shown in Table 3–9. Whatever the method used, it is essential that the meal plan provide sufficient calories. As mentioned earlier, adolescents and parents of young children need to learn to adjust insulin intake rather than restrict food to control blood glucose levels.

Is the meal plan appropriate for diabetes management? This involves assessing both distribution of the meals and snacks as well as the macronutrient percentages. Appropriateness is based on the types of medications prescribed as well as the treatment goals.

For insulin-requiring individuals, the timing of eating is extremely important. Food consumption must be synchronized with the time actions of insulin. Individuals who have type 1 diabetes and who take intermediate-acting insulin usually require an afternoon snack, and all patients should have a bedtime snack. Many adults, even though they use a short-acting insulin at breakfast, find they do not require a morning snack (probably because blood glucose levels tend to be the highest during this period). Children and adolescents generally require a morning snack and often fare better with two afternoon snacks, especially if their school lunch is early and their dinner relatively late. Carbohydrate may also need to be ingested before or after physical activities. For activities performed on a regular basis, this can be a part of the regular meal plan. For activities performed more sporadically, this carbohydrate should be in addition to the usual nutrition prescription.

Persons with type 2 diabetes often fare better with smaller meals and with snacks. However, snacks cannot be in addition to the usual meals. A portion of their meal should be saved to be eaten as a snack between meals. Extra food is usually not needed for increased physical activity. In fact, eating extra food can be counterproduc-

Table 3–9. Estimating Caloric Requirements for Youth

- Base calories on nutrition assessment
- Validate caloric needs

Method 1:   1,000 kcal for first year
Add 100 kcal/year up to age 11
Girls 11–15 years, add 100 kcal or less per year after age 10
Girls >15 years, calculate as for an adult
Boys 11–15 years, add 200 kcal/year after age 10
Boys >15 years, 23 kcal/pound (50 kcal/kg) if very active
18 kcal/pound (40 kcal/kg) usual
15–16 kcal/pound (30–35 kcal/kg) if sedentary

Method 2:   1,000 kcal for first year
Add 125 kcal × age for boys
Add 100 kcal × age for girls
Add up to 20% more kcal for activity
(For toddlers between 1–3 years, 40 kcal per inch length)

From American Diabetes Association: Maximizing the Role of Nutrition in Diabetes Management. American Diabetes Association, Alexandria, VA, 1994

tive to the benefits of the exercise. Persons who have type 2 diabetes and who are taking medications generally have fewer problems with hypoglycemia as well.

Does the meal plan encourage healthful eating? The best way to ensure nutritional adequacy is to encourage patients to eat various foods from all of the food groups. The *Food Guide Pyramid,* with its suggested number of servings from each food group, can be used to compare a patient's meal plan with the nutrition recommendations for all Americans.

Short- and Long-Term Medical and Behavioral Goals

Both short- and long-term medical and behavioral goals should be mutually identified by both the individual with diabetes and the professional. Short-term (days/weeks) behavioral goals usually relate to life style changes (i.e., for food, exercise, and self-monitoring of blood glucose). The primary behavioral goals are consistent and appropriate food intake, regular physical activity, correct medication dosage (if needed), and frequent blood glucose monitoring. Long-term goals (months/years) are generally diabetes management goals for desired outcomes (i.e., blood glucose and lipid levels, weight) that lead to improved and maintained metabolic control. In addition, even a modest weight loss for persons with type 2 diabetes may make a significant difference in levels of blood glucose and lipids, and weight loss should be viewed as a means to an end rather than an end in itself.

Education

An appropriate meal-planning approach should be selected, and strategies for behavior change that enhance motivation and adherence to necessary life style changes identified. A number of meal-planning approaches are available.[73] They range from simple guidelines or menus to more complex

counting methods (Table 3–10). None of the meal-planning approaches has been shown to be more effective than any other, and the tool selected depends on a patient's stage of learning and his or her needs. *Exchange Lists for Meal Planning,*[74] developed by the ADA and the American Dietetic Association, has been a common approach. The exchange lists' macronutrient values are a useful tool for evaluating nutrition assessments. However, exchange lists may not be the most appropriate tool for many persons with diabetes.

EXCHANGE LISTS | The food exchange system has the advantage of facilitating the widest possible selection of foods, thereby offering variety and versatility to the diet. It is viewed as the most complex system and therefore should be used only with persons who can understand it and put it into practice. The 1995 *Exchange Lists for Meal Planning* booklet is available from the ADA and the American Dietetic Association. The word *exchange* refers to the fact that each item on a particular list, in the portion listed, may be interchanged with any other item on the same list. An exchange can be explained to the patient as a substitution, choice, or serving. Patients should have a basic understanding of what types of categories foods are divided into (i.e., carbohydrates, meat and meat substitutes, and fat) and approximate portion sizes. Their meal plan outlines for them the number of choices they should be making from each list at meal times and snack times on a daily basis.

The exchange lists (see Table 3–7) were revised in 1995, the primary changes being made in the order and the grouping of the lists. The three basic lists are carbohydrates, meat and meat substitutes, and fat. Starch, fruit, milk, and other carbohydrates are now listed under carbohydrates. Although some foods have been listed in one particular exchange list, they could just as appropriately fit into another group. For example, the starch, fruit, and milk list all are based on

Table 3–10. Meal-Planning Approaches for Diabetes

Diabetes nutrition guidelines	*The First Step in Diabetes Meal Planning* (American Diabetes Association, American Dietetic Association). A pamphlet that promotes healthy eating. Designed to be given to patients to use until an individualized meal plan can be implemented by a dietitian.
	Health Eating (International Diabetes Center, Minneapolis, MN). A low-literacy booklet with illustrated food lists divided into two categories: Good for You and Not As Good for You. General information on the role of meal planning in diabetes is also covered.
	Eating Healthy Foods (American Diabetes Association, American Dietetic Association). Booklet designed specifically for persons with minimal reading skills. The amount of text is limited; symbols and color codes are used, and concepts and foods are presented visually.
Menu approaches	*Month of Meals 1, Month of Meals 2, Month of Meals 3, Month of Meals 4, Month of Meals 5* (American Diabetes Association). Separate booklets; each booklet contains 28 days of complete menus for breakfast, lunch, dinner, and snacks. Menus are written for a basic meal plan of 1,500 kcal daily with instructions on how to adjust the calorie level upward or downward. Although certain elements are consistent in each volume, each volume has unique features: *Month of Meals 1* includes a special occasion section; *2* adds more ethnic foods; *3* emphasizes time-saving meals; *4* features family favorites; and *5* is vegetarian.
Exchange list approaches	*Exchange Lists for Meal Planning* (American Diabetes Association, American Dietetic Association). Each list is a group of measured foods that contribute approximately the same number of calories and the same amount of carbohydrate, protein, and fat. The 1995 revision divides foods into three basic lists: carbohydrates, meat and meat substitutes, and fat. An individualized meal plan that outlines the number of choices from each list for each meal and for snacks is needed.
	My Food Plan (International Diabetes Center, Minneapolis, MN). Simplified groups of carbohydrates, meat and meat substitutes, and fats containing approximate portions of common foods. A personalized food plan panel provides for individualization. General guidelines are included for making healthful food choices.
Counting approaches	*Carbohydrate Counting Booklets (Getting Started; Moving On; Using Carbohydrate/Insulin Ratios)* (American Diabetes Association). *Getting Started* is an introduction to carbohydrate counting; *Moving On* focuses on identifying patterns in blood glucose levels as related to food intake, medications (if used), and exercise; *Using Carbohydrate/Insulin Ratios* introduces the carbohydrate-to-insulin ratio and is designed for use in intensive diabetes management.
	Carbohydrate Counting (International Diabetes Center, Minneapolis, MN). A booklet that explains carbohydrate counting and how it can be added to the exchange system of meal planning to give persons with diabetes more flexibility in food choices. A meal plan outlines the number of carbohydrate choices each person can select for meals and for snacks.

Adapted from Pastors JG, Holler JJ (eds): Diabetes Care and Education Practice Group of The American Dietetic Association: Meal Planning Approaches for Diabetes Management, 2nd ed. American Dietetic Association, Chicago, 1994.

food portions that contribute approximately 15 g of carbohydrate. In addition, foods on the other carbohydrate list (dessert type or snack foods that do not fit into the starch or starch plus one fat list) also contribute 15 g of carbohydrate and may be interchanged with the foregoing three lists. There are small differences between the starch, fruit, and milk lists. Foods on the starch list contribute 15 g of carbohydrate, ~3 g of protein, a trace of fat, and therefore 80 kcal per serving. Foods on the fruit list contribute 15 g of carbohydrate and 60 kcal per serving, whereas foods on the milk list contribute 12 g of carbohydrate, 8 g of protein, ~1 g fat (skim or nonfat milk, which is recommended), and 90 kcal per serving.

Vegetables are listed after the carbohydrates and, unless eaten in very large amounts (such as a very large salad or vegetable plate), can be considered free. Half-cup servings of cooked vegetables contribute ~5 g of carbohydrate, 2 g of protein, and only 25 kcal per serving.

Meats are divided into very lean, lean, medium fat, and high fat, based on their fat content. An exchange is 1 ounce of cooked meat, fish, or poultry; 1 ounce of cheese; one egg; or 2 tablespoons of peanut butter. It contributes ~7 g of protein (see Table 3–7 for fat values). The type of meat an individual generally eats should be calculated when designing the meal plan (this usually is lean or medium-fat meat). Individuals are encouraged to use lean meat as much as possible but do not need to add or subtract fat exchanges when using different meat categories.

Foods from the fat list contribute 5 g of fat and 45 kcal per serving. This list is divided into saturated, monounsaturated, and polyunsaturated fat choices. A free food list is based on servings of foods that contribute 20 kcal or less per serving. It has been updated to include many fat-free or nonfat foods. The final lists are combination and fast foods that are commonly eaten by individuals.

CARBOHYDRATE COUNTING | Carbohydrate counting either can be used as a basic meal-planning approach or can be used to add more flexibility and choices to the exchange lists. The DCCT used various meal-planning approaches. They all worked equally well, and none was shown to be superior, although carbohydrate counting was a popular approach.[75] Several carbohydrate-counting educational tools are available.[76, 77] All are based on the concept that after eating, it is the carbohydrate in foods that has the major impact on blood glucose levels and one carbohydrate choice contributes 15 g of carbohydrate.

The ADA and the American Dietetic Association have developed three levels of carbohydrate-counting tools—*Carbohydrate Counting. Getting Started; Moving On;* and *Using Carbohydrate/Insulin Ratios.*[77] *Getting Started* is an introduction to carbohydrate counting. It focuses on what foods contain carbohydrate, how to count carbohydrates, keeping simple food records, and how to eat consistent amounts of carbohydrate at meals and snacks. *Moving On* is intended for individuals who have mastered the basics of carbohydrate counting. It focuses on identifying patterns in blood glucose levels as related to food intake, diabetes medication (if used), and physical activity. The individual is taught to interpret records and take action based on blood glucose patterns (pattern control or management). *Using Carbohydrate/Insulin Ratios* is designed for people who take insulin and have chosen intensive diabetes management using multiple daily insulin injections or an insulin pump. Food and blood glucose records are used to fine-tune diabetes management by adjusting short-acting insulins according to anticipated carbohydrate intake and physical activity. The relationship between food eaten and insulin injected can be shown as a carbohydrate-to-insulin ratio. This ratio gives an individual a good idea of how much short-acting insulin to take when eating more or less than usual. Before a carbohydrate-to-insulin ratio can be established, blood glucose levels must be under good control and the usual dose of both the basal insulin and short-acting insulin determined. Level 3 requires that an experienced team of professionals be available to provide individualized instruction and follow-up care.

SIMPLIFIED MEAL-PLANNING TOOLS | *My Food Plan*[78] combines both carbohydrate counting and calorie control in a more simplified approach than *Exchange Lists for Meal Plan-*

ning. It groups carbohydrate choices by approximate portion sizes for general categories of starches, fruits, milk, and more carbohydrate choices. Meat and meat substitutes and fat are also listed by approximate portion sizes. General guides for food planning are listed, as well as tips for choosing healthful foods. A form for filling in an individualized meal plan is available. Figure 3–9 pictures the inside pages of this educational tool.

The First Step in Diabetes Meal Planning[79] is available from the ADA and the

CARBOHYDRATE CHOICES

Foods with carbohydrate affect your blood glucose levels the most. Pay special attention to the carbohydrate in your food plan. A food plan usually includes three to four carbohydrate choices at each meal, and one to two choices at each snack.

Starch/Bread Group

1 choice = 15 grams carbohydrate, variable protein, 60-90 calories (each item listed is 1 choice)

Bagel or English muffin	1 half or 1 oz.	Pasta, cooked (macaroni,	1/2 cup
Bread, slice or roll	1 or 1 oz.	noodles, spaghetti)	
Cereal, cooked	1/2 cup	Peas, cooked	1/2 cup
Cereal, dry, unsweetened	3/4 cup	Popcorn, plain, unbuttered	3 cups
Corn, cooked	1/2 cup	Potato, small	1 (3 oz.)
Crackers, snack♦	4-5	Potato, mashed	1/2 cup
Dried beans, cooked	1/2 cup	Rice, cooked	1/3 cup
Graham crackers	3 squares	Squash, winter, cooked	1 cup
Hamburger or hot dog bun	1 half or 1 oz.	Taco shells, 6" across♦	2
Lima beans, cooked	2/3 cup	Tortilla, 6" across	1
Muffin, small♦	1 (1 1/2 oz.)	Waffles, 4 1/2" across♦	1
Pancakes, 4" across♦	2		

Fruit Group

1 choice = 15 grams carbohydrate, 60-90 calories (each item listed is 1 choice)

Banana	1/2 medium	Fresh fruit	1 medium
Berries or melon	1 cup	Fruit juice	1/3 to 1/2 cup
Canned fruit in juice	1/2 cup	Grapes or cherries	12 to 15
or water		Raisins	2 Tbsp.
Dried fruit	1/4 cup		

Milk Group

1 choice = 12-15 grams carbohydrate, 8 grams protein, 60-90 calories (each item listed is 1 choice)

Milk, skim or lowfat	1 cup (8 oz.)
Yogurt, lowfat, artificially	3/4 to 1 cup (6-8 oz.)
sweetened	
Yogurt, plain, lowfat	3/4 to 1 cup (6-8 oz.)

More Carbohydrate Choices

1 choice = 15 grams carbohydrate, variable protein, fat, and calories (each item listed is 1 choice)

Cake, no icing, 2" square♦	1 piece	Nonfat frozen yogurt	1/3 cup
Casserole or hot dish★	1/2 cup	Pizza, thin-crust★	1 slice
Chili★	1/2 cup	Soup, broth based♣	1 cup
Cookie, 3" across♦	1	Soup, milk based♦♣	1 cup
Granola bar♦	1 bar	Soup, bean based♣	1 cup
Ice cream or light ice cream♦	1/2 cup	Spaghetti or pasta	1/2 cup
Maple syrup, honey,	1 Tbsp.	sauce, canned ♦♣	
or table sugar			

MEAT AND MEAT SUBSTITUTES

1 ounce = 7 grams protein, 3-8 grams fat, 50-100 calories (average serving is 3 ounces)

Meats

Beef	Lamb	Seafood
Fish	Pork	Veal
Ham♣	Poultry (no skin)	

Meats should be baked, broiled, roasted or grilled. One serving is:
- about the size of a deck of cards
- 1 small pork chop
- 1 leg and 1 thigh, or 1/2 whole breast of chicken
- 1/4 pound (weight before cooking) ground meat
- 1 medium unbreaded fish fillet

Meat Substitutes

Each item equals 1 ounce meat

Cottage cheese	1/4 cup	Peanut butter♦	2 Tbsp.
Cheese	1 oz.	Tuna, salmon	1/4 cup
Egg	1	(water packed)	

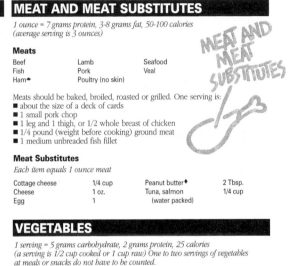

VEGETABLES

1 serving = 5 grams carbohydrate, 2 grams protein, 25 calories (a serving is 1/2 cup cooked or 1 cup raw) One to two servings of vegetables at meals or snacks do not have to be counted.

Asparagus
Beets
Broccoli
Cabbage
Carrots
Cauliflower
Celery
Cucumbers
Green beans
Greens (collard, kale, mustard, spinach, turnip)
Mixed vegetables (without corn, peas, or pasta)
Mushrooms
Onions
Pea pods
Peppers
Radishes
Salad greens (lettuce, spinach)
Tomatoes
Turnips
Zucchini

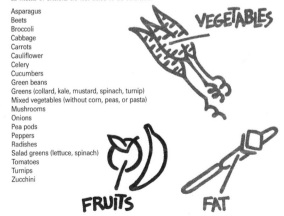

♦ also has 1 fat   ★ also has 1 fat and 1 meat   ♣ high sodium content

Figure 3–9. *See legend on opposite page*

American Dietetic Association. It is designed to be given to patients by their physician or by other team members to use for meal planning *until* an individualized meal plan can be implemented by a dietitian. It lists general guidelines based on the *Food Guide Pyramid*.

BEHAVIORAL CHANGES | The transtheoretical model as outlined in Table 3–11 has been proposed by Prochaska as a general model of intentional behavior change. It includes a sequence of stages along a continuum of behavior change. It can help professionals to identify their clients' readiness to change. Different intervention strategies are needed for individuals at different stages of the change process. Professionals far too often assume that patients are ready for action when in actuality they are still stuck in pre-contemplation. Motivational interventions may work best with individuals who are in the earlier contemplative stages, whereas specific skill-training interventions may be most appropriate for persons who have de-

FATS

1 serving = 5 grams fat, 45 calories (each item listed is 1 serving)

Butter+	1 tsp.	Peanut butter	2 tsp.
Cream cheese+	1 Tbsp.	Salad dressing	1 Tbsp.
Cream, table or light+	2 Tbsp.	Salad dressing, reduced-fat	2 Tbsp.
Gravy+	2 Tbsp.	Sour cream+	2 Tbsp.
Margarine	1 tsp.	Sunflower seeds	1 Tbsp.
Margarine, lower-fat	1 Tbsp.		
Mayonnaise	1 tsp.		
Mayonnaise, reduced-fat	1 Tbsp.		
Nuts	1 Tbsp.		
Oil	1 tsp.	+ saturated fat	

FREE FOODS

Free foods are foods or beverages with less than 20 calories or less than 5 grams carbohydrate per serving. They have little or no effect on blood glucose levels.

Unlimited

Beverages	**Seasonings**	**Sweet Substitutes**
Bouillon♦	Butter-flavored sprinkles	Gelatin desserts, sugar-free
Broth♦	Butter-flavored sprays	Gum, sugar-free
Club soda	Flavoring extracts	Popsicles, sugar-free
Coffee	Herbs and spices	Sugar substitutes
Drink mixes, sugar-free	Mustard, prepared	
Mineral water	Nonstick cooking spray	
Soft drinks, diet	Soy sauce♦	
Tea	Vinegar	
Tonic water, sugar-free	Wine, used in cooking	

Limit to 2-3 Times a Day

Fat-free Foods		**Sweet Substitutes**	
Cream cheese, fat-free	1 Tbsp.	Cocoa powder	1 Tbsp.
Creamers, non-dairy	1 Tbsp.	Jam or jelly, low sugar	1 to 2 tsp.
Mayonnaise, fat-free	1 Tbsp.	or light	
Salad dressing, fat-free	1 Tbsp.	Syrup, sugar-free	2 Tbsp.
Salsa	1/4 cup	Whipped topping	1 Tbsp.
Sour cream, fat-free	1 Tbsp.	Yogurt, plain	2 Tbsp.

Condiments

Catsup	1 Tbsp.
Dill pickle♦	1 large
Taco sauce	1 Tbsp.

COMMENTS

_____

_____

_____

_____

Dietitian _____ Phone _____

PERSONALIZED FOOD PLAN

Calories _____

Carbohydrate_____ gms (___%) Protein_____ gms (___%) Fat_____ gms (___%)

Breakfast Time: _____

☐ Carbohydrate Choices (or ___ starch ___ fruit ___ milk)

_____

☐ Meat _____
☐ Fat _____

Morning Snack Time: _____

☐ Carbohydrate Choices (or ___ starch ___ fruit ___ milk)

☐ _____

Lunch Time: _____

☐ Carbohydrate Choices (or ___ starch ___ fruit ___ milk)

_____

☑ Vegetable _____
☐ Meat _____
☐ Fat _____

Afternoon Snack Time: _____

☐ Carbohydrate Choices (or ___ starch ___ fruit ___ milk)

☐ _____

Dinner Time: _____

☐ Carbohydrate Choices (or ___ starch ___ fruit ___ milk)

_____

☑ Vegetable _____
☐ Meat _____
☐ Fat _____

Evening Snack Time: _____

☐ Carbohydrate Choices (or ___ starch ___ fruit ___ milk)

☐ _____

Figure 3–9. Inside pages of *My Food Plan*. (From International Diabetes Center, with permission)

Table 3–11. The Transtheoretical Model of Intentional Behavior Change

Stages of Change Model	Description
Precontemplation	Individuals have no intention of changing behavior in the foreseeable future. They are usually unaware that they have a problem and are resistant to efforts to modify the behavior.
Contemplation	Individuals are aware they have a problem and are seriously thinking about change, but they have not yet made a commitment to take action in the near future.
Preparation	This is the stage of decision making. A commitment to take action within the next 30 days has been made, and small behavioral changes are already being made.
Action	Notable overt efforts are being made to change. Individuals have modified the target behavior to an acceptable criterion.
Maintenance	Individuals are working to stabilize their behavior change and to avoid relapse. In general, maintenance is sustaining action for at least 6 months.

Adapted from Ruggerio L, Prochaska JO (eds): Readiness for change: application of the transtheoretical model to diabetes. Diabetes Spectrum 61:21, 1993

cided to change. Relapse and recycling through the stages occur quite frequently as individuals attempt to modify behaviors.[80]

EVALUATION AND DOCUMENTATION

The effectiveness of the nutrition intervention should be evaluated throughout the entire education process. Medical and clinical outcomes should be monitored after the second or third visit (approximately 6 weeks after the initial nutrition consultation) to determine whether the individual is making progress toward his or her goals. If no progress is evident, the individual and educator need to reassess and consider possible revisions of the nutrition care plan. If the patient has done all that he or she can do or is willing to do and if blood glucose levels are not in the target range, the dietitian should notify the physician that medications need to be added or adjusted.[3]

Finally, documentation is essential for communication and reimbursement. Table 3–12 lists the areas of the nutrition intervention that require documentation.

FOLLOW-UP AND ONGOING NUTRITION THERAPY

In the long term, individuals and team members need to understand that diabetes is a chronic disease and persons with diabetes need continued or follow-up nutrition care at least every 6 to 12 months.[6] Asking a patient to keep 3-day or weekly food records between visits provides invaluable informa-

Table 3–12. Nutrition Care Documentation Areas

Short- and long-term goals
Nutrition prescription
Meal plan
Educational topics covered
Patient acceptance and understanding
Anticipated compliance
Successful behavioral changes
Additional needed skills or information
Additional recommendations
Plans for ongoing care

From Monk A, Barry B, McClain K, et al: Practice guidelines for medical nutrition therapy by dietitians for persons with non–insulin-dependent diabetes mellitus. J Am Diet Assoc 95:999, 1995

tion. Food records can be compared with the meal plan and assist in assessing whether the initial meal plan is actually feasible for the patient to implement. Furthermore, food records can be integrated with the blood glucose monitoring records, and changes in eating patterns that can lead to improved glycemic control can be assessed. For patients on insulin, it can be determined if blood glucose values outside target ranges can be corrected by adjustments in the meal plan or if it would be more appropriate to make insulin adjustments. Patients should be encouraged to speak freely about problems they are having with food and with the meal plan. An extremely rigid attitude of the physician or dietitian only leads to a patient's not being able to follow the meal plan.

Patients on hypocaloric diets must also be warned that most of the weight loss during the first 1 or 2 weeks is a result of fluid losses, not loss of fat tissue. Patients may also need to be warned that they may actually gain some weight as control improves, even though they have reduced their food intake. Many patients have become very dehydrated as a result of the frequent urination accompanying the elevated blood glucose levels and, as hydration improves with control, discover that they have gained several pounds. They can be assured this does not usually continue unless they begin to overeat consistently, and they need to continue following their meal plan.

NUTRITION STRATEGIES FOR BRIEF ILLNESSES

Acute illnesses such as upper respiratory tract infections or gastroenteritis with vomiting and diarrhea can lead to the development of diabetic ketoacidosis (DKA) in persons with type 1 diabetes if not handled appropriately. Table 3–13 outlines the steps patients need to know and implement on days of acute illness to prevent DKA. Patients taking insulin have a special problem when

Table 3–13. Sick Day Guidelines

Diabetes and Brief Illness: Guidelines for Persons with Diabetes

1. During acute illnesses, usual doses of insulin should be given. The need for insulin continues or may increase during illness. Fever, dehydration, infection, or the stress of illness can trigger the release of the counterregulatory or "stress" hormones, raising blood glucose levels.
2. Monitoring of blood glucose levels and urine testing for ketones should be done at least four times a day—before each meal and before bedtime. Blood glucose readings >250 mg/dl and moderate to large urine ketones are a danger signal. Additional insulin is needed.
3. If regular foods cannot be tolerated, liquid or soft carbohydrate-containing foods should be eaten. At least 45 to 50 g of carbohydrate should be consumed every 3 to 4 hours. This should be done in small, frequent feedings. The following are examples of foods that often can be tolerated when ill and that provide 15 g of carbohydrate:
   - ½ cup (4 ounces) regular soft drinks
   - ½ cup regular Jell-O
   - 1 cup soup
   - 1 slice toast or 6 soda crackers
   - 1 popsicle (3 ounces)
   - ½ cup ice cream or frozen yogurt
   - ½ cup fruit juice
4. A large glass of liquid should be ingested every hour. If nausea or vomiting occurs, small sips—1 or 2 tablespoons every 15 to 30 minutes—should be consumed. If vomiting continues, the health care team should be notified.
5. The health care team should be called if illness continues for more than 1 day.

Adapted from Franz MJ, Joynes JO: Diabetes and Brief Illness. IDC Publishing, Minneapolis, 1993, p. 4

an illness affects their appetite or their ability to retain what they have eaten. Although patients often assume that they need less insulin when food intake is less than normal, infection and stress are associated with an increase in the counterregulatory hormones, and therefore the need for insulin continues and is often increased. The first step is to remind patients to take at least their usual dose of insulin during illness. Blood glucose and urine ketone monitoring is essential, and if blood glucose levels are >300 mg/dl with moderate to large ketones, additional insulin is needed.

Besides taking insulin and testing blood glucose and urine for ketones, it is also important for a patient to ingest carbohydrate, especially if blood glucose levels are <200 mg/dl. This is done to prevent not only hypoglycemia but also "starvation ketosis" (see Chapter 7). In general, 45 to 50 g of carbohydrate is needed during every 3- to 4-hour period. Patients should have a list of easily digestible carbohydrate-containing foods that are often tolerated during acute illnesses. It is important to do this with small, frequent feedings (see Table 3–13).

Patients should also be instructed to drink liquids, especially those that are calorie free. A large glass of liquid should be ingested at least every hour to replace lost body fluids and to prevent dehydration. If patients are nauseated or are vomiting, they should take sips of liquid—1 or 2 tablespoons every 15 to 30 minutes—and call their health care team.

Furthermore, patients should call their health care team if their blood glucose levels are elevated with moderate to large ketones and if they need advice on how to adjust their insulin dose, if they are unable to retain any type of food or liquids, or if they develop any of the symptoms of DKA.

Persons with type 2 diabetes need to test their blood glucose levels more frequently when ill. If blood glucose levels are elevated, they also need to call their health care team.

NUTRITION STRATEGIES FOR EXERCISE

Given appropriate guidelines, persons with diabetes can exercise safely. The exercise plan varies for each person depending on interest, age, general health, and level of physical fitness. The goals of an exercise program for persons with diabetes are (1) to allow individuals with diabetes to experience the same benefits and enjoyment that those without diabetes gain from a regular exercise program; (2) to maintain or improve cardiovascular fitness to prevent or minimize the long-term cardiovascular complications of diabetes; (3) to improve flexibility, which is impaired as muscle and joint collagen becomes glycated (attachment of glucose to the collagen, which makes it stiffer); (4) to allow people with type 1 diabetes to participate safely in and enjoy physical and/or sport activities; and (5) to assist in glucose control and weight management in people with type 2 diabetes.

TYPE 1 DIABETES AND EXERCISE

In exercising persons, insulin levels fall while counterregulatory hormones (primarily glucagon) rise, so increased glucose utilization of exercising muscle is matched by increased glucose production by the liver. In persons with type 1 diabetes, the glycemic response to exercise varies, depending on overall diabetes control, glucose and insulin levels at the start of exercise, intensity and duration of the exercise, previous food intake, and previous conditioning. An important variable is the level of plasma insulin during and after exercise. Excessive insulin levels can potentiate hypoglycemia because of insulin-enhanced muscle glucose uptake and inhibition of the release of glucose from the liver. In contrast, in a poorly controlled (underinsulinized) exerciser, insulin levels are too low; thus, with the rise in counterregulatory hormones during exercise, production of glucose by the liver continues and free fatty acid release by adipose tissue is enhanced, whereas muscle glucose uptake is minimal. This can result in large increases in plasma glucose and ketone levels. If blood glucose levels are >250 mg/dl and urine ketones are present or if blood glucose is >300 mg/dl, irrespective of whether ketones are present, it is generally advisable to increase insulin doses and delay exercising in people with type 1 diabetes.[81] Exercise of high intensity can also result in hyperglycemia. This more than likely is due to the effects of the counterregulatory hormones.[82, 83]

Hypoglycemia, however, is the most common potential problem of acute exercise for persons taking insulin or oral glucose-lowering agents. When monitoring blood glucose, it is important to consider not only the absolute glycemic levels but also the rate at which change in glycemia occurs. For example, a glucose level that is stable at 100 mg/dl may reflect a safe situation for exercise, but if the immediately preceding glucose was 150 mg/dl, a value of 100 mg/dl may indicate rapidly decreasing blood glucose levels and may require glucose ingestion.[81] Hypoglycemia is more common after exercise than during exercise because of the need to replete muscle glycogen, which can take 24 to 30 hours.[84]

Blood glucose monitoring, both before and after exercise, is the key to safety and understanding how exercise affects diabetes control. Furthermore, it provides feedback to help with insulin and carbohydrate adjustments. The choices between increasing carbohydrate or decreasing medication need to be individualized.

Moderate-intensity exercise increases whole body glucose uptake by 2 to 3 mg/kg/min. This means that in a 150-pound (70-kg) individual, an added 8.4 to 12.6 g of carbohydrate is required for every hour of exercise. During high-intensity exercise, the rate of whole body glucose uptake may increase by 5 to 6 mg/kg/min. Despite this increased rate of glucose use, the demand on glucose stores and the risk of hypoglycemia is less because exercise of this intensity cannot be sustained for long intervals.[81] General guidelines that can be given to persons with diabetes include the following: One hour of increased exercise requires an additional 15 g of carbohydrate, either before or after exercise. For more strenuous exercise, 30 g of carbohydrate per hour may be required. Moderate exercise of <30 minutes rarely requires any additional carbohydrate or insulin adjustment; however, a small snack may be needed if blood glucose is <80 mg/dl. Table 3–14 lists general guidelines on how to increase carbohydrate with exercise.

It is often necessary to adjust the insulin dose to prevent hypoglycemia. This occurs most often with strenuous activity of >45 to 60 minutes' duration. For most persons, a modest decrease (~20%) in the insulin component corresponding to the period of exercise is sufficient to prevent hypoglycemia. For very prolonged vigorous exercise, a larger decrease in the total daily insulin dose (by as much as one third to one half) may be necessary to prevent repeated hypoglycemic episodes. In contrast to these acute reductions in insulin doses, individuals participating in regular exercise programs (at least every other day) often do not need to adjust their insulin doses. In the process of training, they may have already decreased their total insulin by as much as 15% to 20%, and their bodies have adjusted to the regular exercise.[81]

TYPE 2 DIABETES AND EXERCISE

Persons with type 2 diabetes can achieve improved blood glucose control with exercise. This is because of increased insulin sen-

Table 3–14. Carbohydrate Adjustments for Exercise

Type of Activity	If Blood Glucose Is:	Carbohydrate Adjustment
Short duration, low intensity (30 minutes or less: e.g., walking half-mile, leisurely biking)	Less than 100 mg/dl Over 100 mg/dl	10–15 g carbohydrate (CHO) (1 carbohydrate choice) No extra CHO needed
Moderate duration, moderate intensity (30–60 minutes: e.g., tennis, swimming, bicycling jogging)	Less than 100 mg/dl 100–180 mg/dl 180–300 mg/dl*	30–45 g CHO (2–3 carbohydrate choices) 15 g CHO (1 carbohydrate choice) No extra CHO needed
Long duration, moderate intensity 1 hour or more: e.g., football, hockey, basketball, strenuous bicylcing)	Less than 100 mg/dl 100–180 mg/dl 180–300 mg/dl*	45 g CHO (3 carbohydrate choices) 30–45 g CHO (2–3 carbohydrate choices) 15 g CHO per hour (1 carbohydrate choice)

*If blood glucose level is higher than 250 mg/dl before exercise, check urine for ketones. If urine ketones are present (moderate to high), wait to exercise until blood glucose is better controlled.

Adapted with permission from Franz MJ, Barry B: Diabetes and Exercise. Guidelines for Safe and Enjoyable Activity. IDC Publishing, Minneapolis, MN, 1993, p. 16

sitivity, which results in increased peripheral use of glucose not only during but after their exercise as well. Because enhanced insulin sensitivity is lost within 48 hours after exercise, repeated bouts of physical activity at regular intervals are needed to reduce the glucose intolerance associated with type 2 diabetes. This exercise-induced enhanced sensitivity to insulin occurs without changes in body weight.

Timing of the exercise session for persons with type 2 diabetes can be used advantageously. For example, exercise performed later in the day has been shown to reduce hepatic glucose output and decrease fasting glycemia.[85] Exercise after eating can also be beneficial because it reduces postprandial hyperglycemia, common in type 2 diabetes.

EXERCISE PROGRAMS

The type of exercise that individuals choose to perform should be tailored to their physical capacity and interest. A complete exercise program includes warm-up and cool-down periods composed of flexibility-type stretches. These not only prepare muscles for an aerobic workout but also promote improved range of motion. Cardiovascular conditioning is also helpful. Most persons can, at a minimum, undertake a walking program safely. Ideally, the aerobic portion of an exercise session should last at least 20 minutes, with a goal of 30 to 40 minutes. However, even three sessions of 10 minutes of activity performed at different times during the day can lead to improved physical fitness.[86] Muscle-strengthening exercises, such as lifting light weights, are also an important component of an exercise session. Muscles dispose of glucose, and this type of exercise can also contribute to improvement in glucose control.[87]

NUTRITION STRATEGIES FOR TREATING HYPOGLYCEMIA

Hypoglycemia is a common side effect of insulin therapy. In general, treatment begins with 15 g of carbohydrate. Commercially available glucose tablets have the advantage of being premeasured to help prevent overtreatment. Table 3-15 outlines steps for treatment of hypoglycemia. Patients have traditionally been taught to ingest 15 g of a

Table 3–15. Treatment of Hypoglycemia

- Immediate treatment with carbohydrate is essential
- If blood glucose falls below 70 mg/dl, treat with 15 g of carbohydrate:
  three glucose tablets
  ½ cup fruit juice or regular soft drink (4 ounces)
  1 cup milk
  seven hard candies
- Wait 15 minutes; retest, and if blood glucose level is <70 mg/dl, treat with another 15 g of carbohydrate
- Repeat testing and treating until blood glucose level returns to normal range
- Evaluate timing to next meal or snack to determine the need for additional food. If >1 h to next meal, eat an additional small snack

Adapted from Santiago J (ed): Medical Management of Insulin-Dependent (Type 1) Diabetes, 2nd ed. American Diabetes Association, Alexandria, VA, 1994, p. 27

"quick" or "fast-acting" simple sugar; however, there really are no quick or fast-acting foods. The reason foods such as regular soft drinks, fruit juice, honey, hard candies, and commercial glucose products remain good choices is not because they are absorbed so rapidly but because they are convenient, readily available, easily and quickly consumed, and do not spoil. Even though many of these foods have a relatively low glycemic response (probably because of their fructose content), they are still absorbed rapidly enough to treat hypoglycemia effectively.

Slama and colleagues[88] studied the use of 15 g of carbohydrates in tablets or solution from glucose and sucrose, glucose gel, orange juice, and a hydrolyzed polysaccharide solution for the correction of artificially induced hypoglycemia. Ten minutes after their ingestion, treatment with glucose or sucrose in solution or tablets or the hydrolyzed polysaccharide solution resulted in a similar rise in blood glucose levels. However, almost no rise in blood glucose levels was obtained 10 minutes after ingestion of the glucose gel or orange juice. Fifteen and 20 minutes after ingestion, all the carbohydrates had raised blood glucose levels, but glycemic responses

from orange juice and glucose gel still remained consistently lower.

Wiethop and Cryer[89] reported that 10 g of an oral glucose solution raised plasma glucose levels from 60 to 97 mg/dl over 30 minutes and that 20 g raised plasma glucose levels from 58 to 122 mg/dl over 45 minutes. With both treatments, levels began to fall after 60 minutes. They concluded that treatment with glucose is an effective but temporary measure and that persistent hypoglycemia generally requires subsequent ingestion of a more substantial meal to prevent recurrent hypoglycemia.

To determine whether treatment of hypoglycemia with a snack containing both protein and carbohydrate results in more prolonged protection against subsequent hypoglycemia than ingestion of carbohydrate alone, Gray and coworkers[90] studied six persons with type 1 diabetes on two occasions. On both occasions subjects were made hypoglycemic (50 mg/dl) by an insulin infusion and then treated with either bread (15 g carbohydrate) or bread plus protein (meat) (15 g carbohydrate, 18 g protein, 7 g fat). The insulin infusion was continued for the next 3 hours or until glucose levels again fell to 50 mg/dl. Although the bread plus meat resulted in a more marked rise in glucagon than did bread alone, neither the post-treatment peak glucose level nor the subsequent fall of glucose differed. They concluded that treatment of hypoglycemia with a protein-enriched snack merely adds calories rather than prolonged protection against hypoglycemia.

Of interest is that insulin-induced hypoglycemia significantly increases the rate of gastric emptying of solids and liquids to about 15 to 16 minutes during hypoglycemia as compared with about 40 minutes during normoglycemia.[91] Furthermore, the emptying rates for the solid and liquid tests were similar, making it difficult to distinguish between the solids and liquids. This finding provides evidence for the statement that there are no quick or fast-acting carbohydrates.

SUMMARY

Nutrition must be integrated into the overall management plan. Using a team approach is important. The dietitian or nutrition counselor cannot work in isolation from other team members. To assist patients to achieve treatment goals, all team members must be communicating and supporting the same nutrition messages. Goals, not rigid rules and regulations, should be emphasized. Recommendations given to patients must be practical and achievable in the real world. Monitoring of desired outcomes—medical, clinical, educational, psychosocial—is essential and provides the information needed to evaluate how well nutrition therapy has been integrated into the overall management plan.

REFERENCES

1. American Diabetes Association: Nutrition recommendations and principles for people with diabetes mellitus (position statement). Diabetes Care 20(suppl 1):S14, 1997
2. Franz MJ, Horton ES Sr, Bantle JP, et al: Nutrition principles for the management of diabetes and related complications (technical review). Diabetes Care 17:490, 1994
3. Monk A, Barry B, McClain K, et al: Practice guidelines for medical nutrition therapy by dietitians for persons with non–insulin-dependent diabetes mellitus. J Am Diet Assoc 95:999, 1995
4. Lockwood D, Frey ML, Gladish NA, Hiss R: The biggest problem in diabetes. Diabetes Educ 12:30, 1986
5. Delahanty LM, Halford BN: The role of diet behaviors in achieving improved glycemic control in intensively treated patients in the Diabetes Control and Complications Trial. Diabetes Care 16:1453, 1993
6. Franz MJ, Monk A, Barry B et al: Effectiveness of medical nutrition therapy provided by dietitians in the management of non-insulin-dependent diabetes mellitus: a randomized controlled clinical trial. J Am Diet Assoc 95:1009, 1995
7. American Diabetes Association: Detection and management of lipid disorders in diabetes (consensus statement). Diabetes Care 19(suppl 1):S96, 1996
8. Wing RR, Klein R, Moss SE: Weight gain associated with improved glycemic control in population-based sample of subjects with type I diabetes. Diabetes Care 13:1106, 1990
9. The DCCT Research Group: Weight gain associated with intensive therapy in the Diabetes Control and Complications Trial. Diabetes Care 11:567, 1988
10. U.S. Department of Agriculture, U.S. Department of Health and Human Services: Nutrition and Your Health: Dietary Guidelines for Americans, 3rd ed. USDA's Human Nutrition Information Service, Hyattsville, MD, 1990
11. U.S. Department of Agriculture: The Food Guide Pyramid. USDA's Human Nutrition Information Service, Hyattsville, MD, 1992
12. American Diabetes Association: Principles of nutrition and dietary recommendations for individuals with diabetes mellitus: 1979 (special report). Diabetes 28:1027, 1979
13. Bouchard C, Tremblay A, Despres J-P et al: The response to long-term overfeeding in identical twins. N Engl J Med 322:1477, 1990
14. Stunkard AJ, Harris JR, Pedersen NL, McClearn GE: The body-mass index of twins who have been reared apart. N Engl J Med 322:1483, 1990
15. Brownell KD, Wadden TA: Etiology and treatment of obesity: understanding a serious, prevalent, and refractory disorder. J Consult Clin Psychol 60:505, 1992
16. Foreyt JP: Issues in the assessment and treatment of obesity. J Consult Clin Psychol 55:677, 1987
17. National Academy of Sciences Committee to Develop Criteria for Evaluating Outcomes of Approaches to Prevent and Treat Obesity, Food and Nutrition Board, Institute of Medicine: Summary: weighing the options—criteria for evaluating weight-management programs. J Am Diet Assoc 95:96, 1995
18. Wing RR, Koeske R, Epstein LH et al: Long-term effects of modest weight loss in type II diabetic patients. Arch Intern Med 147:1749, 1987
19. Watts NB, Spanheimer RG, DiGirolamo M et al: Prediction of glucose response to weight loss in patients with non–insulin-dependent diabetes mellitus. Arch Intern Med 150:803, 1990

20. Wing RR, Blair EH, Bononi P et al: Caloric restriction per se is a significant factor in improvement in glycemic control and insulin sensitivity during weight loss in obese NIDDM patients. Diabetes Care 17:30, 1994

21. Mayer EJ, Newman B, Quesenberry CP, Selby JV: Usual dietary fat intake and insulin concentrations in healthy women twins. Diabetes Care 16:1459, 1993

22. Jenkins DJA, Ocana A, Jenkins A et al: Metabolic advantages of spreading the nutrient load: effects of increased meal frequency in non-insulin-dependent diabetes. Am J Clin Nutr 55:461, 1992

23. Bertelsen J, Christiansen C, Thomsen C et al: Effect of meal frequency on blood glucose, insulin, and free fatty acids in NIDDM subjects. Diabetes Care 16:3, 1993

24. Schneider SH, Ruderman NB: Exercise and NIDDM (technical review). Diabetes Care 13:785, 1990

25. American Diabetes Association: Diabetes 1996 Vital Statistics. Alexandria, VA, American Diabetes Association, 1996

26. Raskin P (ed): Medical Management of Non-Insulin-Dependent (Type II) Diabetes, 3rd ed. American Diabetes Association, Alexandria, VA, 1994

27. Milne RM, Mann JI, Chisholm AW, Williams SM: Long-term comparison of three dietary prescriptions in the treatment of NIDDM. Diabetes Care 17:74, 1994

28. Henry RR: Protein content of the diabetic diet (technical review). Diabetes Care 17:1502, 1994

29. Jamueel N, Pugh JA, Mitchell BD, Stern MP: Dietary protein intake is not correlated with clinical proteinuria in NIDDM. Diabetes Care 15:178, 1992

30. Peters AL, Davidson MB: Protein and fat effects on glucose response and insulin requirements in subjects with insulin-dependent diabetes mellitus. Am J Clin Nutr 58:555, 1993

31. Nuttall FQ, Mooradian AD, Gannon MC et al: Effect of protein ingestion on the glucose and insulin response to a standardized oral glucose load. Diabetes Care 7:465, 1984

32. American Diabetes Association: The diagnosis and management of nephropathy in patients with diabetes mellitus (consensus statement). Diabetes Care 19(suppl 1):S67, 1996

33. Klahr S, Levey AS, Beck GJ et al: The effects of dietary protein restriction and blood pressure control on the progression of chronic renal disease. N Engl J Med 330:877, 1994

34. Zeller KR, Whittaker E, Sullivan L et al: Effect of restricting dietary protein on the progression of renal disease in patients with insulin-dependent diabetes mellitus. N Engl J Med 324:78, 1991

35. Dullart RR, Beusekamp BJ, Meijer S et al: Long-term effects of protein-restricted diet on albuminuria and renal function in IDDM patients without clinical nephropathy and hypertension. Diabetes Care 16:483, 1993

36. Brodsky IG, Robbins DC, Hiser E et al: Effects of low-protein diets on protein metabolism in insulin-dependent diabetes mellitus patients with early nephropathy. J Clin Endocrinol Metab 75:351, 1992

37. Jibani MM, Bloodworth LL, Foden E et al: Predominantly vegetarian diet in patients with incipient and early clinical diabetic nephropathy: effects on albumin excretion rate and nutritional status. Diabetic Med 8:949, 1991

38. Nakamura H, Ito S, Ebe N, Shibata A: Renal effects of different types of protein in healthy volunteer subjects and diabetic patients. Diabetes Care 16:1071, 1993

39. Pecis M, deAzevdo MJ, Gross JL: Chicken and fish diet reduces glomerular hyperfiltration in IDDM patients. Diabetes Care 17:665, 1994

40. Yost TJ, Eckel RH: Fat calories may be preferentially stored in reduced-obese women: a permissive pathway for resumption of the obese state. J Clin Endocrinol Metab 67:259, 1988

41. Expert Panel on Detection, Evaluation, and Treatment of High Blood Cholesterol in Adults: Summary of the second report of the national cholesterol education program (NCEP) expert panel on detection, evaluation, and treatment of high blood cholesterol in adults (Adult Treatment Panel II). JAMA 269:3015, 1993

42. The Expert Panel on Blood Cholesterol Levels in Children and Adolescents: Report of the expert panel on blood cholesterol levels in children and adolescents. Pediatrics 89(suppl 3):525, 1992

43. Garg A, Bantle JP, Henry RR et al: Effects of varying carbohydrate content of diet in patients with non-insulin dependent diabetes mellitus. JAMA 271:1421, 1994

44. Coulston AM, Hollenbeck CB, Swislock ALM,

Reaven GM: Persistence of hypertriglyceri-demic effect of low fat, high carbohydrate diets in NIDDM patients. Diabetes Care 12:94, 1989

45. Parillo M, Rivellese AA, Ciardullo AV et al: A high-monounsaturated-fat/low carbohydrate diet improves peripheral insulin sensitivity in non-insulin-dependent diabetic patients. Metabolism 41:1371, 1992

46. Pascale RW, Wing RR, Butler B et al: Effects of a behavioral weight loss program stressing calorie restriction versus calorie plus fat restriction in obese individuals with NIDDM or a family history of diabetes. Diabetes Care 18:1241, 1995

47. Dunn FL: Plasma lipid and lipoprotein disorders in IDDM. Diabetes 41(suppl 2):102, 1992

48. Harris M: Hypercholesterolemia in diabetes and glucose intolerance in the U.S. population. Diabetes Care 14:366, 1991

49. Hollenbeck CB, Coulston A, Donner C et al: The effects of variations in percent of naturally occurring complex and simple carbohydrates on plasma glucose and insulin response in individuals with non-insulin-dependent diabetes mellitus. Diabetes 34:151, 1985

50. Loghmani E, Richard K, Washburne L et al: Glycemic response to sucrose-containing mixed meals in diets of children with insulin-dependent diabetes mellitus. J Pediatr 119:531, 1991

51. Bantle JP, Swanson JE, Thomas W, Laine DC: Metabolic effects of dietary sucrose in type II diabetic subjects. Diabetes Care 16:1301, 1993

52. Peterson DB, Lambert J, Gerrig S et al: Sucrose in the diet of diabetic patients—just another carbohydrate? Diabetologia 29:216, 1986

53. Peters AL, Davidson MB, Eisenberg K: Effect of isocaloric substitution of chocolate cake for potato in type I diabetic patients. Diabetes Care 13:888, 1990

54. Wise JE, Keim KS, Huisinga JL, Willmann PA: Effect of sucrose-containing snacks on blood glucose control. Diabetes Care 12:423, 1989

55. Franz MJ: Avoiding sugar: does research support traditional beliefs? Diabetes Educ 19:144, 1993

56. Nuttall FQ, Gannon MC, Burmeister LA et al: The metabolic response to various doses of fructose in type II diabetic subjects. Metabolism 41:510, 1992

57. Bantle JP, Swanson JE, Thomas W, Laine DC: Metabolic effects of dietary fructose in diabetic subjects. Diabetes Care 15:1468, 1992

58. Federal Register 58:2175, 1993

59. Position of The American Dietetic Association: Use of nutritive and nonnutritive sweeteners. J Am Diet Assoc 93:816, 1993

60. Butchko HH, Kotsonis FN: Acceptable intake vs actual intake: the aspartame example. J Am Coll Nutr 10:258, 1991

61. Simpson HCR, Simpson RW, Lously S et al: A high carbohydrate leguminous fibre diet improves all aspects of diabetic control. Lancet 3:1, 1981

62. Hollenbeck CB, Coulston AM, Reaven GM: To what extent does increased dietary fiber improve glucose and lipid metabolism in patients with noninsulin-dependent diabetes mellitus? Am J Clin Nutr 43:16, 1986

63. Nuttall FQ: Dietary fiber in the management of diabetes. Diabetes 42:503, 1993

64. Tuck M, Corry D, Trujillo A: Salt-sensitive blood pressure and exaggerated vascular reactivity in the hypertension of diabetes mellitus. Am J Med 88:210, 1990

65. Tjoa HI, Kaplan NM: Nonpharmacological treatment of hypertension in diabetes mellitus. Diabetes Care 14:449, 1991

66. Mooradian AD, Failla M, Hoogwerf B et al: Selected vitamins and minerals in diabetes mellitus (technical review). Diabetes Care 17:464, 1994

67. American Diabetes Association: Magnesium supplementation in the treatment of diabetes (consensus statement). Diabetes Care 19(suppl 1):S93, 1996

68. Rabinowitz MB, Levin SR, Gonick HC: Comparisons of chromium status in diabetic and normal men. Metabolism 29:355, 1980

69. Franz MJ: Alcohol and diabetes. Part I and Part II. Its metabolism and guidelines for its occasional use. Diabetes Spectrum 3:136, 210, 1990

70. Koivisto VA, Tulokas S, Toivonen M et al: Alcohol with a meal has no adverse effects on postprandial glucose homeostasis in diabetic patients. Diabetes Care 16:1612, 1993

71. Tinker LF, Heins JM, Holler HJ: Commentary and translation: 1994 nutrition recommenda-

tions for diabetes. J Am Diet Assoc 94:507, 1994

72. American Diabetes Association: Standards of medical care for patients with diabetes mellitus (position statement). Diabetes Care 20(suppl 1):S5, 1997

73. Pastors JG, Holler HJ (eds): Diabetes Care and Education Practice Group of The American Dietetic Association: Meal Planning Approaches for Diabetes Management, 2nd ed. American Dietetic Association, Chicago, 1994

74. Exchange Lists for Meal Planning. American Diabetes Association, Alexandria, VA, The American Dietetic Association, Chicago, IL, 1995

75. Diabetes Control and Complications Trial Research Group: Nutrition interventions for intensive therapy in the Diabetes Control and Complications Trial. J Am Diet Assoc 93:768, 1993

76. Barry B, Castle G: Carbohydrate Counting. Adding Flexibility to Your Food Choices. International Diabetes Center, Institute for Research and Education, Health System Minnesota, Minneapolis, MN, 1994

77. Carbohydrate Counting. Getting Started; Moving On; Using Carbohydrate/Insulin Ratios. American Diabetes Association, Alexandria, VA, The American Dietetic Association, Chicago, IL, 1995

78. Monk A: My Food Plan. International Diabetes Center, International Diabetes Center, Institute for Research and Education, Health System Minnesota, Minneapolis, MN, 1996

79. The First Step in Diabetes Meal Planning. American Diabetes Association, Alexandria, VA, The American Dietetic Association, Chicago, IL, 1995

80. Ruggiero L, Prochaska JO (eds): Readiness for change: application of the transtheoretical model to diabetes. Diabetes Spectrum 61:21, 1993

81. Wasserman DH, Zinman B: Exercise in individuals with IDDM (technical review). Diabetes Care 17:924, 1994

82. Mitchell TH, Abraham G, Schiffrin A et al: Hyperglycemia after intense exercise in IDDM subjects during continuous subcutaneous insulin infusion. Diabetes Care 11:311, 1988

83. Purdon C, Brousson M, Nyveen L et al: The roles of insulin and catecholamines in the glucoregulatory response during intense exercise and early recovery in insulin-dependent-diabetic and control subjects. J Clin Endocrinol Metab 76:566, 1993

84. MacDonald MJ: Postexercise late-onset hypoglycemia in insulin-dependent diabetic patients. Diabetes Care 10:584, 1987

85. Devlin JT, Hirshman M, Horton ED, Horton ES: Enhanced peripheral and splanchnic insulin sensitivity in NIDDM men after single bout of exercise. Diabetes Care 36:434, 1987

86. Pate RR, Pratt M, Blair SN et al: Physical activity and public health. A recommendation from the Centers for Disease Control and Prevention and the American College of Sports Medicine. JAMA 273:402, 1995

87. Soukup JT, Kovaleski JE: A review of the effects of resistance training for individuals with diabetes mellitus. Diabetes Educ 19:307, 1993

88. Slama G, Traynard P-Y, Desplanque N et al: The search for an optimized treatment of hypoglycemia. Arch Intern Med 150:589, 1990

89. Wiethop BV, Cryer PE: Alanine and terbutaline in the treatment of hypoglycemia in IDDM. Diabetes Care 16:1131, 1993

90. Gray RO, Butler PC, Beers TR, et al: Comparison of the ability of bread versus bread plus meat to treat and prevent subsequent hypoglycemia in patients with insulin-dependent diabetes mellitus. J Clin Endocrinol Metab 81:1508, 1996

91. Schvaracz E, Palmer M, Aman J et al: Hypoglycemia increases the gastric emptying rate in patients with type I diabetes mellitus. Diabetic Med 10:660, 1993

92. American Diabetes Association: Maximizing the Role of Nutrition in Diabetes Management. American Diabetes Association, Alexandria, VA, 1994

93. Franz MJ, Joynes JO: Diabetes and Brief Illness. Chronimed Publishing, Minneapolis, 1993, p. 4

94. Franz MJ, Barry B: Diabetes and Exercise. Guidelines for Safe and Enjoyable Activity. Chronimed Publishing, Minneapolis, 1993, p. 16

95. Santiago J (ed): Medical Management of Insulin-Dependent (Type I) Diabetes, 2nd ed. American Diabetes Association, Alexandria, VA, 1994, p. 27

INSULIN THERAPY

INSULIN PREPARATIONS

Choosing which insulin preparations to order for a patient can be confusing. Two pharmaceutical firms manufacture insulin preparations sold in the United States. At present, more than 30 different insulin preparations are being marketed in this country.

Four properties characterize insulin preparations used for injection: concentration, species source, purity, and type—that is, certain physicochemical modifications that determine the time course of action. Choosing the concentrations and types of insulin to use usually does not present a problem. Therefore, these two aspects of insulin preparations are discussed at the beginning of this chapter. The choices concerning the species source and purity are more subtle and are related, to a large extent, to some of the side effects of insulin. Therefore, these characteristics of insulin preparations are discussed later in conjunction with a description of the immunologic responses to insulin therapy.

Insulin is marketed in 10-ml vials at a concentration of 100 U/ml (U-100). If a patient injects 0.5 ml, she or he receives 50 U of insulin. From another viewpoint, administration of 20 U of insulin requires injection of 0.2 ml of U-100 insulin. Fortunately, calculations by the patient are obviated by the use of syringes with the number of units marked directly on the barrel.

From a therapeutic point of view, three characteristics of the time course of action of the different types of insulin preparations

are important: onset of action, time of peak activity, and duration of action. These depend on the rate of absorption after the subcutaneous injection. The values listed in Table 4-1 (except for Lispro) were obtained in studies of patients with stable, well-controlled diabetes and relatively low daily insulin requirements.[1] After the patients were admitted to a metabolic ward, insulin therapy was discontinued and the blood glucose level was allowed to rise above 200 mg/dl. At this time, a single large dose of animal insulin (usually about 80 U) was given, and the blood glucose level was determined every 4 hours. One sixth of a patient's total daily caloric intake was ingested after each blood sample was taken, and the study was continued for at least 36 hours. The relations summarized in Table 4-1 may not pertain exactly to the clinical situation in which patients' physical activity and eating patterns differ from conditions imposed by the metabolic ward setting. These ranges are only approximations because of the great variability among patients and because the response of an occasional patient may differ considerably from the values listed. However, these are probably the best data available on the time-activity relations of the various insulin preparations. Some studies using sophisticated measures to analyze kinetics of insulin action have suggested that human insulin preparations may act slightly faster,[3] but clinically this potential difference is not important because of the great variability in the response to insulin, not only between patients but also in the same patient from day to day.[4]

Table 4–1. Approximate Time-Activity Relation of Various Insulin Preparations

Kind of Insulin	Preparation	Onset of Action (h)	Maximal Action (h)	Total Duration of Action (h)
Short-acting	Regular[a]	0.5–1	2–4[b]	4–6
	Lispro	0.25	1	3–4
Intermediate-acting	NPH[c]	3–4	8–14	20–24
	Lente	3–4	8–14	20–24
Long-acting	Ultralente	6–8	14–20	>32

[a]Also called crystalline zinc insulin (CZI).

[b]In some patients, the action of regular insulin may peak later than indicated here (between 4 and 8 hours) and last considerably longer.[2]

[c]Neutral protamine Hagedorn.

Regular insulin has no modifying agent and therefore is the only one that should be administered intravenously. In the lente series, insulin is buffered by acetate, and the size of the crystal determines the rate of absorption. Lente insulin has a time course of action that is indistinguishable from that of neutral protamine Hagedorn (NPH) insulin. The protamine in the NPH preparation (originally formulated by Hagedorn) delays the absorption of insulin. The amount of protamine in NPH insulin is small enough (30 to 50 mg/100 U) that regular insulin added to the same syringe is still rapidly absorbed. Regular insulin can be added to the lente insulins.

The reason for the slight delay in the absorption of regular insulin is a self-association between insulin molecules. Two amino acids in the 28th and 29th positions of the B chain, proline and lysine, respectively, are responsible. When these two amino acids are switched, the insulin molecule no longer self-associates, and after injection, absorption begins immediately. This very rapid-acting insulin, lispro *(Humalog)*, was recently approved by the Federal Drug Administration and was introduced into clinical practice in the fall of 1996. Because of its rapid absorption, it can be injected immediately before eating (unlike regular insulin, which should be injected 30 minutes before a meal to accommodate for the delay in absorption). Initially, the Federal Drug Administration is requiring a prescription for lispro (unlike other insulins in many states), and not sanctioning its use in insulin pumps or in pregnant diabetic patients. It can be substituted for regular insulin in all of the regimens discussed in this chapter.

USE OF INSULINS: GENERAL CONSIDERATIONS

An intermediate-acting* preparation as the sole or major source of insulin is often used for the following reasons. The action of the long-acting insulin has a small peak at times of little or no food intake. Therefore, the maintenance of acceptable glucose concentrations before breakfast and throughout the day often requires amounts of ultralente insulin that pose a risk of hypoglycemia during the night. Because the time courses of action of lente and NPH insulins are indistinguishable and because short-acting insulins can be added to the same syringe, either of these intermediate-acting insulins is theoretically suitable. However, the absorption of regular insulin added to lente or ultralente insulin is delayed compared with its absorption when added to NPH insulin.[5, 6]

The most effective way to use the available insulin preparations necessarily depends on the goals involved. It is obviously much easier to render an insulin-requiring diabetic pa-

---

*Throughout this book, the terms *NPH* and *regular insulin* are used interchangeably with the terms *intermediate-* and *short-acting insulin*, respectively.

tient asymptomatic (i.e., no nocturia, poly-uria, or polydipsia; prevention of weight loss; and avoidance of increased susceptibility to infection) than to return the prevailing glu-cose concentrations to nearly normal levels. The evidence presented in Chapter 2 relating strict diabetic control to amelioration of the microangiopathic and neuropathic complica-tions is a persuasive argument for dedicated efforts to achieve the best possible control in each patient. How can this goal be achieved? In theory, insulin should be used in a manner that maximizes the chances of maintaining nearly normal glucose levels at all times and minimizes disruption in the lives of diabetic patients.

Figure 4–1 shows the usual time course of the activity of a single injection of insulin given before breakfast. Intermediate-acting insulin (NPH or lente) is represented by the solid curve. A lag period of 3 to 4 hours usually intervenes before enough insulin is absorbed to have a measurable effect. Activ-ity peaks around suppertime (8 to 14 hours after injection), and the total duration of the effect is approximately 24 hours. Because of delayed absorption, hyperglycemia often occurs after breakfast. In order to avoid this problem, a small amount of short-acting insu-lin (regular; represented by the dotted line in the figure) can be added to the syringe with the intermediate-acting insulin. This short-acting insulin is absorbed rapidly and starts to work within 30 to 60 minutes; its activity usually peaks at 2 to 4 hours and may last as long as 4 to 6 hours. If it is to prevent hyperglycemia, this single injection must cover the calories consumed at break-fast, lunch, dinner, and a bedtime snack and must also provide enough insulin to control hepatic glucose production throughout the night.

Three responses to a single injection of intermediate-acting insulin in the morning are noted. In a small minority of patients, such an injection satisfactorily controls glu-cose concentrations during the following 24-hour period. Most commonly, however, the amount of intermediate-acting insulin that results in satisfactory control during the day is not adequate to prevent fasting hypergly-cemia the following morning; the patient is also hyperglycemic during much of the night. Less often, the amount of intermedi-ate-acting insulin appropriate for daytime needs is more than adequate for the night, and fasting hypoglycemia occurs. If attempts are made to correct this situation, the patient is hyperglycemic throughout much of the day because the amount of intermediate-act-ing insulin is decreased in order to avoid nighttime hypoglycemia.

A feasible way to achieve the dual goals of controlling glucose levels and minimizing

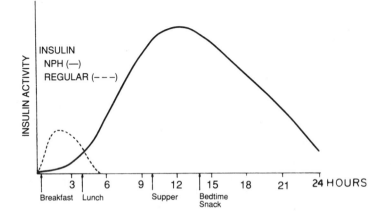

Figure 4–1. Time course of action of one injection of insulin per day before breakfast. (From Davidson MB: The case for control in diabetes mellitus. West J Med 129:193, 1978)

disruptions of daily activity patterns is to inject insulin twice a day—before breakfast and before supper. The usual time course of the activity of insulin given in this manner is depicted in Figure 4-2. The total insulin activity during a given period is the sum of all of the curves operating at that time. The intermediate-acting insulin (NPH or lente) is supplemented as necessary with a short-acting insulin (regular) in the same syringe.

In general, between two thirds and three fourths of the intermediate-acting insulin is given in the morning and the remainder before supper. If regular insulin is also required, 5 to 10 U at each time usually suffices (in nonobese patients). Ideally, *only after the appropriate dose of intermediate-acting insulin has been established should short-acting insulin be added.* Regular insulin is usually necessary in the morning to handle the breakfast calories because of the lag period before NPH insulin starts to work. Even though the intermediate-acting insulin administered in the morning exerts its maximal effect in the late afternoon and early evening, an amount appropriate to cover the interval before supper may be inadequate to cover the caloric intake of the largest meal of the day. In that case, regular insulin should be added to the second insulin injection. The advantage of this approach is that each component of the insulin prescription can

be regulated independently (Table 4-2). Thus, as can be deduced from the intervals of maximal action of the various insulin preparations (see Table 4-1), the blood (or urine) test that best reflects the patient's response to the morning NPH insulin injection is the one before supper; the following morning's test is the best indicator of the effect of NPH insulin given before supper (or bedtime); the test before lunch best reflects the action of regular insulin given before breakfast; and the test at bedtime is the most sensitive indicator of the action of regular insulin received before supper.

Because of the accumulating evidence that strict diabetic control is extremely beneficial in attenuating the microvascular and neuropathic complications of diabetes, an increasing number of physicians and their patients are attempting to achieve near euglycemia. When a split/mixed (i.e., NPH and regular) insulin regimen is used with this goal in mind, patients have relatively limited flexibility in their eating patterns. Not only must their meals not be delayed, but the amount of carbohydrate in each meal must be close to the prescribed amount or hypoglycemia is likely to occur. In addition, extra exercise may also pose a problem because of the enhanced absorption from the large depots of injected insulin (see Chapter 7). Patients have much more flexibility in regard to both

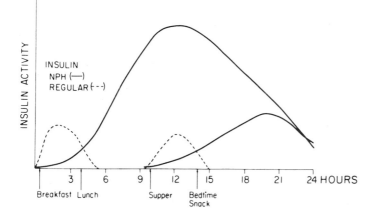

Figure 4–2. Time course of action of two injections of insulin —one before breakfast and one before supper. (From Davidson MB: The case for control in diabetes mellitus. West J Med 129:193, 1978)

Table 4–2. Period During Which Glucose is Controlled by Various Components of the Insulin Regimen and Timing of Tests Reflecting That Activity

Insulin	Time Injected	Period of Activity	Test Reflecting Insulin Action
Regular	Before a meal	Between that meal and either the subsequent one or the bedtime snack (if insulin is taken before supper)	Both following meal before which insulin is injected and before next meal or bedtime snack (if insulin is taken before supper)
NPH	Before breakfast	Between lunch and supper	Before supper
NPH	Before supper *or* before bedtime	Overnight	Before breakfast
Ultralente	Before breakfast *or* before supper *or* half of dose at each time	Mostly overnight because regular overrides its effect during the day	Before breakfast

eating and exercise with three or four injections of insulin each day. With this approach, regular insulin is taken before each meal and the test after the meal or before the next one reflects the effectiveness of that dose. For instance, an injection before lunch is judged by the result of the postprandial lunch test and/or the before supper test. Control of glucose levels overnight is provided by small amounts of ultralente insulin injected before breakfast and before supper or NPH insulin taken either before supper or at bedtime. Obviously, the effectiveness of the long- or intermediate-acting insulin with these approaches is judged by the results of

the fasting test. Achieving tight control in motivated patients using two, three, and four injection regimens is discussed in Chapter 7 in conjunction with self-monitoring of blood glucose (SMBG). Finally, because the onset of regular insulin is usually ½ to 1 hour (see Table 4–1), it should be given 30 minutes before a meal. The insulin absorbed between injection and eating blunts the initial rise of postprandial glycemia.

Seven different insulin regimens are described in Table 4–3. Certain caveats should be kept in mind with each of the regimens listed. In regimens A and B (as already mentioned), patients have the least flexibility

Table 4–3. Various Insulin Regimens

Regimen	Before Breakfast	Before Lunch	Before Supper	Before Bedtime
A	NPH/regular[a]		NPH/regular	
B	NPH/regular		Regular	NPH
C	Regular	Regular	NPH/regular	
D	Regular	Regular	Regular	NPH
E	Ultralente/regular (separate injections)	Regular	Ultralente/regular	
F[b]	Maximal dose of oral agent(s)			NPH
G[c]	Insulin pump (small amounts of regular insulin infused throughout 24-hour period [basal rate] with *boluses* of regular insulin given before each meal)			

[a]Regular insulin should be injected 30 minutes before designated meal.

[b]Before the introduction of the oral agent metformin (see Chapter 5), this regimen was called BIDS (bedtime insulin, daytime sulfonylurea); it is now possible for patients to be on two oral agents at the time bedtime NPH insulin is added, although there are no data on the efficacy of all three.

[c]In my view, only physicians who are experienced with this mode of therapy and who will devote the extra amount of time that it requires should supervise patients on pump therapy.

with regard to the timing and content of meals. Hypoglycemia is most likely to occur with these two regimens if meals are delayed. In regimens A and C, the intermediate-acting insulin taken before supper may have peak activity in the middle of the night rather than toward morning in some patients. In this situation, increasing the dose may lead to hypoglycemic reactions overnight before the target level of glucose before breakfast is achieved. If this should occur, switching the intermediate-acting insulin to before bedtime (regimen B) should solve the problem. In regimens C and D, if the period between lunch and supper is too long (usually >5 to 7 hours), the blood glucose level before supper may be too high because the effect of the regular insulin taken before lunch may have worn off. Ultralente insulin (regimen E) starts to work 6 to 8 hours after administration. If supper is delayed, hypoglycemia may occur in the late afternoon or early evening. Similarly, it may occur overnight if the injection is taken before supper or before breakfast if taken at bedtime. This is usually not a problem when the dose of the long-acting insulin is low (~10 U) but may become one with higher amounts. Another caveat concerning ultralente insulin is that because its duration of action is so long, the effect of changing the dose may not become apparent for 2 to 3 days until a new equilibrium is reached. Finally, with regimen F, late morning or late afternoon hypoglycemia may occur after the fasting glucose level is lowered by bedtime NPH insulin even though the patient had been in poor control with maximal doses of oral agents previously. In that case, the dose of the sulfonylurea agent has to be decreased.

INITIATION OF INSULIN THERAPY IN HOSPITALIZED PATIENTS

Although initiating insulin therapy in an outpatient or office setting is becoming more and more common, how it may be done in the hospital is described first because the general principles are the same regardless of the location. The initial dose of insulin given to a patient is to some extent empirically based. Lean individuals are given 12 to 15 U of NPH insulin: 8 to 10 U before breakfast and 4 to 5 U before supper. Obese patients (>125% of desirable body weight; see appendix in Chapter 7) receive a total of 30 U of NPH insulin: 20 U in the morning and 10 U in the evening. A patient's response is monitored closely, and the amounts of intermediate-acting insulin are adjusted accordingly, usually by 4 or 5 U at a time initially. In extremely obese patients and in any others with plasma glucose levels exceeding 300 mg/dl, increments of 8 to 10 U may initially be advisable to achieve control faster. (An important point to remember is that these results are obtained at times of maximal action of NPH insulin and that glucose concentrations presumably are even higher at other times.) In the early stages of therapy with NPH insulin, amounts are adjusted daily. In contrast, when patients who are outside of the hospital and who are taking stable, established amounts of insulin inexplicably lose control, changes are made only after several days of poor test results. One exception is in cases of moderate to large ketonuria in the presence of glucosuria; these problems require more immediate action (see Chapter 7).

For patients receiving intermediate-acting insulin twice a day, glucose concentrations in specimens measured before breakfast and before supper determine what adjustments should be made in the amounts of NPH insulin administered. If a patient's hospital stay is to be minimized, these test results must be made available in time to change the appropriate NPH insulin dose if necessary. Because the amount of insulin given before breakfast depends on the result of the test before supper on the preceding day, this result must be communicated to the physician during the evening. By the same token, the fasting glucose concentration must be made available to the physician during the day so that the evening NPH insulin dose can be altered if necessary.

The physician should write insulin orders on a continuing basis (rather than repeated orders for one dose only) to ensure that the patient receives insulin at the proper times. Even if an appropriate change in dose is not made, at least the previous dose will automatically be given, and the orderly flow of gradually increasing amounts of insulin will not be interrupted. If the physician orders each insulin dose or each day's insulin prescription separately (with the intent of using the most recent appropriate glucose results to determine the amount of insulin given the next day), he or she may for some reason fail to write a particular order, and valuable time is lost. Even if the error is caught quickly and the patient receives insulin late, the response to that dose may not accurately reflect the efficacy of injected insulin because of the altered relation between the times of peak insulin action and meals. If the patient has been approaching reasonable control and his or her control deteriorates significantly because a dose is missed, the amount of insulin required to return to the control attained previously may exceed the requirement once control has been regained. (For reasons that are not entirely clear, diabetic patients are often less sensitive to insulin when their glucose levels are very high than when these levels are more near normal. This is termed *glucose toxicity*.) In instances such as these, hospitalization is prolonged, and with current daily hospital rates, such errors can be expensive.

Diabetic control should not be too tight in patients who are in the hospital to be started on insulin. Their diets, exercise, and emotional pattern will almost certainly be different when they return to the usual home environment, and these changes will certainly influence the insulin requirements. Therefore, the goal while these patients are in the hospital is to achieve preprandial glucose concentrations of only <200 mg/dl. In-

termediate-acting insulin is used alone until the before breakfast and before supper values are lowered to these levels. At this point, regular insulin is added in small amounts (if necessary) to attain similar levels of glucose before lunch and before the bedtime snack. However, in today's climate of shortened hospital stays, if insulin is started in the hospital, I often routinely add a small, fixed amount (2 to 4 U in lean and obese patients, respectively) of regular insulin to each injection of NPH insulin. In this manner, patients can be taught how to mix insulins while in the hospital; this may be important if outpatient education is difficult to arrange. I do not start to change the doses of regular insulin until the corresponding fasting and before supper glucose concentrations are <200 mg/dl. If one starts to adjust the amounts of regular insulin immediately, more may be required when the before breakfast or supper glucose concentration is higher than when lower. For instance, 20 U of regular insulin before breakfast may not lead to hypoglycemia before lunch if the fasting glucose value is 250 mg/dl but may do so after the before breakfast value has been reduced to 150 mg/dl by increasing evening doses of NPH insulin. (In contrast, if insulin is being started on an outpatient basis or in an office setting, I usually do not add regular insulin to the before breakfast and supper injections of NPH insulin until corresponding glucose levels of <150 mg/dl have been achieved at each of these times.) Once all preprandial and bedtime snack glucose concentrations are <200 mg/dl in the hospital, the patient is discharged and final adjustments of the insulin doses are carried out in the usual home environment. The illustrative case study that follows brings out these points.

PATIENT 1

CASE STUDY

This 48-year-old alcoholic (therefore metformin contraindicated) woman has had type 2 diabetes mellitus for 3 years. She is 5 feet 2 inches tall, has a medium frame, and currently weighs 165 pounds. Despite institution of an 1,100-calorie diet (which, she admits, is difficult for her to follow) and treatment with 10 mg of glyburide twice per day, her fasting plasma glucose levels consistently exceed 250 mg/dl. She refuses to test either blood or urine glucose levels herself. The patient has only mild symptoms of polyuria and polydipsia. Because of her failure to respond to maximal dosages of glyburide, she enters the hospital for initiation of insulin therapy. She arrives in the morning before breakfast, and a blood specimen is taken so that a fasting plasma glucose level can be determined. Because the weight

of the patient exceeds 125% of her desirable body weight (which is approximately 110 pounds), a 20 U–10 U split NPH regimen is initially prescribed. The patient's response to insulin is summarized in the flow sheet in Table 4-4. She is discharged with a prescription for 45 U of NPH and 8 U of regular insulin before breakfast and 20 U of NPH and 8 U of regular insulin before supper.

COMMENT

A simple flow sheet like the one shown in Table 4-4 is extremely helpful in monitoring the progress of a patient in the hospital. Anyone reviewing the chart can quickly and easily determine the patient's degree of dia-

Table 4–4. Flow Sheet Showing Response of Patient 1 to Initiation of Insulin Therapy

Date	Time	Plasma Glucose[a] (mg/dl)	Insulin (U) NPH	Regular	Remarks
9/19	0800	285			
	0920		20		
	1600	306	10		Urine 0.5%
	2200	328			
9/20	0700	254	30		Urine 0.25%
	1100	333			Urine 2%
	1600	278	15		Injected herself
	2200	346			Urine 2%
9/21	0700	222	40		Urine negative
	1100	280			
	1600	232	20		
	2200	302			
9/22	0700	172	45		
	1100	248			
	1600	163	20		
	2200	278			
9/23	0700	178	45	4	
	1100	210			
	1600	152	20	4	
	2200	223			
9/24	0700	165	45	8	
	1100	183			
	1600	157	20	8	
	2200	195			
9/25	0700	172	45	8	
					Discharge

NPH, neutral protamine Hagedorn.

[a]If bedside monitoring is routinely performed, heading should be Blood Glucose because glucose is measured in a drop of blood rather than in plasma.

betic control and response to insulin. The flow sheet should be placed in the records in front of the patient's chart or at the bedside for easy access. Wherever it is located, some member of the health care team (nurse, house staff, attending physician) must be responsible for accurate charting of blood glucose results and insulin doses. The use of a properly kept flow sheet saves time by making it unnecessary to go through the chart to locate the dose of insulin given (medication sheet and/or order sheet), the glucose response (laboratory results), and the patient's subjective response (nurses' notes and physician's progress notes). The flow sheet also saves time in constructing the temporal relations between insulin administration, glucose concentrations, and the patient's reaction. Thus, the flow sheet should be used for all insulin-requiring diabetic patients, regardless of the reason for hospitalization. If, for some reason, urine glucose results rather than plasma or blood glucose concentrations are monitored, the results can be recorded under the column headed "Remarks."

With regard to the patient just described, the initial morning injection of 20 U of NPH insulin was clearly suboptimal because the 1600 glucose level (i.e., at 4 PM) was 306 mg/dl. As the morning dose of NPH insulin was increased, the glucose concentration before supper gradually decreased to acceptable levels. Similarly, the initial amount of NPH insulin (10 U) given before supper was inadequate; the next morning's fasting glucose concentration was 254 mg/dl. Increases over several days to a dose of 20 U in the evening finally brought the fasting glucose level below 200 mg/dl. Note that the morning and evening insulin doses were adjusted independently of each other. For example, on 9/22 the morning dose of NPH insulin was increased, whereas the evening dose remained the same.

It is a common practice to measure glucose levels routinely before meals and the bedtime snack, especially if bedside monitor-

ing on samples produced by a finger stick is ordered. However, in keeping with the approach discussed earlier, the before lunch and bedtime values of 9/20 and 9/21 were ignored (i.e., no regular insulin was added to the appropriate NPH insulin injections). Importantly, no extra regular insulin was given for these elevated glucose levels at the time they were obtained. If that had been done, the subsequent glucose concentrations (i.e., before supper if regular insulin had been given before lunch, and the next day's fasting glucose value if regular insulin had been given at bedtime) would not reflect the effect of the corresponding NPH insulin alone. The action of both the short-acting and intermediate-acting insulins would have coincided. If this had occurred, valuable information about the effect of the dose of NPH insulin would have been lost and hospitalization would have been prolonged. However, once the before breakfast and supper glucose levels fell to below 200 mg/dl on 9/22, the before lunch and bedtime snack values were taken into consideration. A gradual increase of regular insulin added to the morning and evening NPH insulin lowered these concentrations to <200 mg/dl, and the patient was discharged.

Although the patient's glucose concentrations after institution of insulin therapy were much lower than her levels before insulin therapy, the recorded values represent the minimal levels attained during the day, and the patient was probably significantly hyperglycemic at most other times. Her fairly rapid response to insulin was aided by her dietary compliance in the hospital and by the decrease in glucose toxicity—that is, once glucose levels begin to be brought under control, not only does a patient's sensitivity to insulin (exogenous or endogenous) increase but, in type 2 diabetes, insulin secretion improves as well.

The final adjustments of the insulin dose after the patient's discharge from the hospital have to take into account her probable increased level of activity (which will lower insulin requirements) and her probable increased caloric intake, as predicted on the basis of her previous lack of dietary compliance (which will raise insulin requirements). Intermittent determinations of fasting and late afternoon glucose levels will be helpful in the choice of appropriate doses of NPH insulin, and values before lunch and before the bedtime snack will determine the amount of regular insulin necessary.

However, regular insulin should only be increased after the dose of NPH insulin that yields fasting and before supper glucose values of <150 mg/dl has been established. The reason for this is as follows. In essence, the short-acting insulin given before breakfast and supper controls the postprandial rise of glucose concentrations following these meals. The goal is to maintain the preprandial glucose level at a satisfactory value, and the effectiveness of the two injections of regular insulin is determined by the difference between the glucose concentrations before breakfast and lunch and before supper and the bedtime snack, respectively. If the fasting and before supper glucose levels are high, the values before lunch and the bedtime snack will probably also be elevated. The approach to remedy this situation is to lower the before breakfast and before supper glucose concentrations by appropriate manipulations of the NPH insulin. Only then should the effectiveness of the regular insulin be evaluated by examining the results of the before lunch and before bedtime snack tests. Because the role of the regular insulin in this approach is to restrain the postprandial rise of glucose and restore it to suitable preprandial values before the next meal or bedtime (snack), the goal should be a minimal difference between the two preprandial values. If the dose of regular insulin is raised in response to elevated test results before lunch and bedtime (snack) and these were largely the result of high glucose levels before breakfast and supper, the new increased doses of short-acting insulin may be too high once the NPH insulin adjustments had low-

ered the prebreakfast and presupper values. Because of her obesity, this patient may require more than the 5 to 10 U of short-acting insulin that is usually adequate in a lean patient.

INITIATION OF INSULIN THERAPY IN NONHOSPITALIZED PATIENTS

If circumstances permit (i.e., availability of diabetes education, motivated patient, ability to perform urine testing or preferably SMBG, opportunity to return frequently during the first week or so to reinforce insulin injection and monitoring techniques), it is possible to start insulin therapy outside of the hospital. Under the current pressures to decrease medical care costs, starting insulin in the office or outpatient setting should be the usual approach, with hospitalization an exception. An obvious example of an exception is patients who initially present with diabetic ketoacidosis. These patients should be hospitalized for intensive treatment with regular insulin and appropriate fluid replacement. The subsequent transition from regular to NPH insulin is discussed in Chapter 6.

The office or outpatient setting is particularly appropriate for diabetic patients who are switching from another mode of therapy to insulin and who presumably already have a basic knowledge of the pathophysiology of diabetes, diet, urine testing, and/or preferably SMBG. These patients need only to acquire information related to insulin therapy and its possible consequences (e.g., hypoglycemia).

Obviously, a patient must have the opportunity to communicate frequently with the physician and/or other health care personnel about insulin doses and related matters (e.g., SMBG) as appropriate. If this is new-onset diabetes, the patient's reaction to the diagnosis often involves a great deal of anger, depression, and denial. Not only are efforts at education poorly received under such circumstances, but patients often fail to call their physicians regularly for adjustment of insulin doses. In contrast to the situation in the hospital, where the patient is a captive audience and a formal system operates to ensure that insulin orders are reviewed, follow-up on adjustment of insulin doses outside the hospital can be inadequate if neither the patient nor the physician takes the initiative. Thus, when insulin therapy is begun for a nonhospitalized diabetic patient, the physician or office personnel should contact the patient on a prearranged schedule (or vice versa) and should see the patient at frequent intervals. Although initiation of insulin therapy in the office or outpatient setting may be less efficient (and economical) from a physician's point of view, the greatly diminished disruption of a patient's life and the tremendous savings in health care costs make this approach desirable when at all possible.

PATIENT 1 REVISITED

Let us assume that this patient is willing and capable of learning SMBG and that her physician is able to initiate insulin therapy in the office setting. She is seen in the afternoon, and it is decided to place her on a mixed/split insulin regimen (i.e., NPH and regular insulin taken before breakfast and before supper). The nurse teaches her to perform SMBG, and her blood glucose is 295 mg/dl (Table 4-5). By now it is late afternoon, and the timing of the insulin injection is nearly before her usual supper time. Because she is obese, the 20 U-10 U split NPH regimen is initially prescribed. (No regular insulin is given until the before breakfast and before supper SMBG values are lowered to <150 mg/dl.) She is taught to draw up 10 U of NPH insulin into a syringe, and with the help of the nurse, it is injected subcutaneously into the abdomen. The patient is told to discontinue her glyburide. She returns the next morning before breakfast, and the nurse supervises the performance of SMBG. This value is 254 mg/dl. Again under supervision

by the nurse, the patient draws up 20 U of NPH insulin into the syringe and injects it subcutaneously into the abdomen. She is also taught the signs, symptoms, and treatment of hypoglycemia. Because her fasting blood glucose concentration is so high, her before supper NPH insulin dose is increased to 14 U. She is asked to perform SMBG (and record the values in the glucose monitoring book given to her) before breakfast and before supper each day and to return one more time the next morning before breakfast. At that time, the patient's insulin administration and SMBG techniques are reviewed and both her before breakfast and before supper NPH insulin doses are increased based on the corresponding glucose values obtained the evening before (252 mg/dl) and that morning (216 mg/dl) (see Table 4-5). She is instructed in the time course of action of NPH insulin and asked to call the office every 2 to 3 days for adjustment of her NPH insulin doses.

On 4/14, both doses of NPH insulin were raised because of elevated corresponding SMBG values (see Table 4-5). On 4/17, the glucose values for the previous several days before breakfast and supper were >150 mg/dl, and therefore no further increases were made in the NPH insulin doses. The patient was told to start measuring before lunch and before the bedtime snack to ascertain the need for regular insulin. If these were >150 mg/dl, she was to be seen in the office to learn how to mix regular insulin with NPH insulin in the same syringe. This occurred in the afternoon of 4/19, at which time 4 U of regular insulin was added to both NPH doses and she was taught the time course of action of the short-acting insulin. When she called on 4/22, the before supper dose of regular insulin was increased to 6 U because of elevated glucose values before her bedtime snack on the previous three evenings. The dose of morning regular insulin was not changed because the before lunch glucose values were approximately 150 mg/dl. A further increase to 8 U in the before supper

Table 4–5. Flow Sheet Showing Response of Patient 1 to Initiation of Insulin Therapy in an Office Setting (Mixed/Split Regimen)

	Before Breakfast	Before Lunch	Before Supper	Before Bedtime[a]
4/10				
SMBG (mg/dl)			295	
Insulin dose (U)			10 NPH	
4/11				
SMBG (mg/dl)	254		252	
Insulin dose (U)	20 NPH		14 NPH	
4/12				
SMBG (mg/dl)	216		222	
Insulin dose (U)	24 NPH		18 NPH	
4/13				
SMBG (mg/dl)	183		198	
Insulin dose (U)	24 NPH		18 NPH	
4/14[b]				
SMBG (mg/dl)	176		202	
Insulin dose	24 NPH		20 NPH	
4/15				
SMBG (mg/dl)	142		153	
Insulin dose (U)	28 NPH		20 NPH	
416				
SMBG (mg/dl)	138		142	
Insulin dose (U)	28 NPH		20 NPH	
4/17[b]				
SMBG (mg/dl)	146		144	
Insulin dose (U)	28 NPH		20 NPH	
4/18				
SMBG (mg/dl)	132	213	162	247
Insulin dose (U)	28 NPH		20 NPH	

dose of regular insulin was made on 4/25 because the before bedtime snack glucose levels were still >150 mg/dl. When she called on 4/27, she was told to send in her SMBG results in 1 month because almost all of the values were now <150 mg/dl. Final adjustments to achieve goal values of <120 mg/dl with minimal hypoglycemia (see Chapter 7) should be made to analyze glucose patterns occurring over longer periods.

PATIENT 1 (REVISITED AGAIN)

An increasingly popular insulin regimen to use for patients failing to respond to maximal doses of sulfonylurea agents is BIDS —bedtime insulin and daytime sulfonylureas

(see regimen F in Table 4-3). The concept behind BIDS therapy is simple. The evening NPH insulin lowers the fasting blood glucose level to an acceptable value, and the sulfonylurea agent maintains it during the day. For this approach to be successful, the postprandial excursion of glucose would have to be reasonably constant, with a return to baseline regardless of the starting preprandial level (top and bottom curves in Fig. 4-3). On the other hand, if postprandial glucose concentrations failed to return to near the preprandial level, a progressive rise would occur throughout the day (see middle curve in Fig. 4-3) and the BIDS approach would not be very effective. The goal with this

Table 4–5. Flow Sheet Showing Response of Patient 1 to Initiation of Insulin Therapy in an Office Setting (Mixed/Split Regimen) *Continued*

	Before Breakfast	Before Lunch	Before Supper	Before Bedtime[a]
4/19				
SMBG (mg/dl)	142		146	
Insulin dose (U)	28 NPH	208	20 NPH/4 Reg	203
4/20				
SMBG (mg/dl)	129		132	
Insulin dose (U)	28 NPH/4 Reg	154	20 NPH/4 Reg	212
4/21				
SMBG (mg/dl)	135		148	
Insulin dose (U)	28 NPH/4 Reg	142	20 NPH/4 Reg	196
4/22[b]				
SMBG (mg/dl)	128		141	
Insulin dose (U)	28 NPH/4 Reg	139	20 NPH/6 Reg	163
4/23				
SMBG (mg/dl)	119		161	
Insulin dose (U)	28 NPH/4 Reg	145	20 NPH/6 Reg	191
4/24				
SMBG (mg/dl)	132		146	
Insulin dose (U)	28 NPH/4 Reg	151	20 NPH/6 Reg	183
4/25[b]				
SMBG (mg/dl)	135		138	
Insulin dose (U)	28 NPH/4 Reg	142	20 NPH/8 Reg	147
4/26				
SMBG (mg/dl)	121		132	
Insulin dose (U)	28 NPH/4 Reg	148	20 NPH/8 Reg	138
4/27[b]				
SMBG (mg/dl)	133			
Insulin dose (U)	28 NPH/4 Reg	151		

SMBG, Self-monitoring of blood glucose.
[a]Glucose should be measured before snack (if eaten).
[b]Phone call to office during the day.

regimen is to lower the fasting glucose concentration to <120 mg/dl (without causing overnight hypoglycemia). Once this is accomplished, the patient should perform SMBG before supper. High values predict that BIDS therapy will not yield tight control. Alternatively, once fasting glucose concentrations decrease to this low a level, patients may experience late afternoon hypoglycemia on maximal doses of sulfonylurea agents, and the dose of the oral drug will have to be lowered.

Let us assume that patient 1 is to be placed on BIDS therapy. Her maximal dose of gly-buride is continued, and on the afternoon of 4/10 the nurse is able to get her to inject saline into her abdomen and shows her how to draw up insulin into the syringe. The nurse supervises the patient as she draws up 14 U of NPH insulin into an insulin syringe. (I usually start lean and obese patients on 8 to 10 U and 14 to 16 U of NPH insulin, respectively.) The patient takes the syringe home and is instructed to inject the contents subcutaneously into her abdomen at bedtime. The patient is also taught how to perform SMBG and is told to measure her fasting

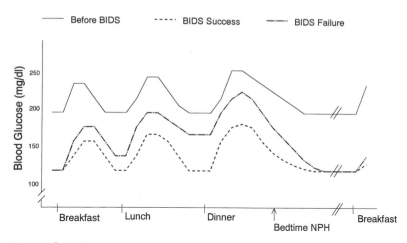

Figure 4–3. Blood glucose response: (——) before initiation of bedtime NPH insulin; (- - - -) BIDS success; (— · —) BIDS failure.

blood glucose value with the machine and strips to be purchased that evening. She returns the next day, at which time the nurse observes both her SMBG and injection (of saline) techniques and teaches her the signs, symptoms, and treatment of hypoglycemia. Because the patient's fasting blood glucose value that morning was 243 mg/dl (Table 4-6), her NPH dose is increased to 18 U. The nurse supervises the drawing up of that amount, and the patient is told to take this dose each evening, to measure her fasting blood glucose, and to call the office with the results in 2 days. Her course is summarized in Table 4-6. She is to return to the office in 1 week for a final review of her SMBG technique and ability to draw up insulin accurately. Note that at this visit (on 4/17) her fasting glucose values were low enough (although not at target) that she was instructed to wait another week before calling the office. The response to that call (on 4/24) was to increase the NPH dose slightly, to begin monitoring before supper, and to send the results to the office in 1 month. To reiterate, to avoid hypoglycemia when a patient is approaching the lower target goals, the final adjustments should be made only after analysis of glucose patterns over longer periods (at least several weeks).

Table 4–6. Flow Sheet Showing Response of Patient 1 to Initiation of BIDS Therapy in an Office Setting

Date	Fasting Blood Glucose (mg/dl)	Bedtime NPH Insulin (U)	Date	Blood Glucose (mg/dl)	Bedtime NPH Insulin (U)
4/10		14	4/18	132	26
4/11	243	18	4/19	135	26
4/12	196	18	4/20	128	26
4/13[a]	208	22	4/21	142	26
4/14	172	22	4/22	137	26
4/15[a]	163	24	4/23	131	26
4/16	148	24	4/24[a]	129	28
4/17[b]	144	26			

[a]Phone call to office.
[b]Office visit.

If a patient is capable of following a simple algorithm, it is possible to reduce the number of calls to the office. I have found the algorithm summarized in Table 4-7 to be very useful in the initial dose adjustments until the fasting blood glucose level decreases to <150 mg/dl. At that point, the patient is asked to send in the results each month.

BIDS therapy is particularly useful in type 2 diabetic patients who fail to respond to maximal doses of oral agents and who are reluctant to start insulin. One injection and (at least initially) one finger stick for SMBG a day is easier to sell than two or more injections per day. Importantly, a patient's life style is less interrupted in terms of eating and exercise patterns with BIDS therapy. Several studics compared BIDS therapy with two or more injections of insulin and found no difference in the level of diabetic control achieved after 3[7] or 6[8, 9] months. In one study,[10] excellent control was maintained for a year with BIDS therapy. To avoid blaming themselves, it is important for patients to understand that once their fasting blood glucose levels are in the target range, the level of control is entirely dependent on the ability of the sulfonylurea agent to control the glucose levels during the day. Because this depends to a large extent on the β-cell response, a patient can do little about it (except lose weight if obese). Although theoretically adjusting two or more injections of insulin should provide improved control in patients with fasting blood glucose concen-

trations <120 mg/dl but still poorly controlled, this has yet to be demonstrated. Patients' compliance and the reluctance of physicians to use the large amounts of insulin required by obese patients may account for this. There is no published experience of adding metformin (see Chapter 5) to a patient failing to respond to BIDS therapy.

PATIENT 2

CASE STUDY

A 27-year-old financial planner reports a 3-week history of increasing urination, thirst, and a 6-pound weight loss despite an increased appetite. He denies blurring of vision or a family history of diabetes. He is 5 feet 11 inches tall and weighs 155 pounds. A glucose value measured on a meter is 420 mg/dl, and his urine shows 2% glucose and strong ketone bodies. His breathing appears normal. It is late morning. The patient has blood drawn for serum electrolyte and acetoacetate measurement, is given 5 U of regular insulin subcutaneously, and is told to return in midafternoon when the results of the laboratory tests will be available. These return as follows: Na, 135 mEq/L; K, 3.6 mEq/L; Cl, 98 mEq/L; HCO$_3$, 22 mEq/L; and acetoacetate, trace positive in the undiluted serum. When he returns that afternoon, he is told that he probably has (slowly evolving) type 1 diabetes and will require insulin therapy. Both mixed/split and multiple injection (regular insulin before each meal and bed-

Table 4–7. Initiation of BIDS Therapy[a] in Patients Able to Follow Simple Algorithm and Self-Adjust NPH Insulin Doses

	Lean	Obese
Initial dose	8–10 U	14–16 U
FBG >200 mg/dl for 2 days in a row	Increase by 2 U	Increase by 4 U
FBG between 150–200 mg/dl for 2 days in a row[b]	Increase by 1 U	Increase by 2 U

[a]Goal is fasting blood glucose (FBG) <150 mg/dl; to lower to <120 mg/dl, glucose pattern over a longer period of time should be analyzed.
[b]Applies if one day >200 mg/dl and the next day between 150–200 mg/dl or vice versa.

time NPH insulin) are described to him. Because of a variable eating schedule (erratic timing of meals due to meeting with clients) as well as an inconstant exercise pattern, he chooses the multiple injection regimen. He is taught SMBG and how to draw up insulin into a syringe. The initial doses for this regimen that I use are as follows: for lean patients, 4 to 5 U of regular insulin and 8 to 10 U of NPH insulin; for obese patients, 8 to 10 U of regular insulin and 14 to 16 U of NPH insulin. Therefore, this patient was supervised to give himself 4 U of regular insulin subcutaneously in the abdomen, drew up 8 U of NPH insulin for the bedtime injection, and was instructed on the signs, symptoms, and treatment of hypoglycemia. He was told to eat supper immediately after leaving the office, to perform and record the results of SMBG before each meal and his bedtime snack, and to return to the office the next day to review and reinforce the material that had just been taught.

His course is summarized in Table 4–8. Note that the NPH insulin dose was increased the next day at the office visit because of the elevated fasting glucose value but that the doses of regular insulin were increased more slowly because the differences between the preprandial levels were fairly low. That is, the amount of regular insulin given before a meal was able to bring the postprandial glucose rise back to the preprandial level. This *delta response* to regular insulin is a useful index of the efficacy of the dose. If the succeeding preprandial glucose concentration (i.e., before the next meal or bedtime snack) was much higher, more regular insulin would be needed. Conversely, if the preprandial level could be lowered (e.g., by increasing the bedtime NPH insulin), an amount of regular insulin that yielded a small delta response between two meals (or between supper and the bedtime snack) would provide near euglycemia throughout the day. Therefore, appropriate doses of regular insulin should be determined only once the preprandial glucose levels are in a satisfactory range. If preprandial glucose values are high and enough regular insulin is given to achieve satisfactory levels before the next meal, hypoglycemia will ensue once the high preprandial glucose concentrations are lowered. For this reason, doses of regular insulin should be raised cautiously when initiating insulin therapy until preprandial glucose concentrations are satisfactory. (I do not find that a delta response between breakfast and supper in a mixed/split regimen is very helpful in adjusting NPH insulin doses.) At his office visit on 6/3, the patient's dose of regular insulin before supper was increased to 8 U and he was told to send in his SMBG results in 1 month.

USE OF URINE TESTS TO INITIATE INSULIN THERAPY

Although SMBG is preferable to urine testing to evaluate glycemia, it is often not feasible for some patients. Reasons may include cost, complexity, pain, fear of blood, and reluctance to interrupt one's life style. Urine testing is much simpler to perform and much less costly (although some patients are reluctant to deal with urine). The obvious drawback of urine testing is the fact that negative tests reflect only blood glucose concentrations below the renal threshold (T_m) for glucose and do not delineate how much below. Conversely, positive test results are not helpful to delineate how much above the T_m the blood glucose level is. On the other hand, a slight advantage to urine testing is that the single voided (discussed later) urine sample tested before a meal reflects a large portion of the preceding postprandial period whereas a SMBG preprandial value is only a single point in time. For instance, elevated postprandial glucose concentrations (exceeding the T_m) decreasing to acceptable subsequent preprandial levels would signal the need for more insulin, which might not be apparent with the results of SMBG. In a study[11] in which urine testing and SMBG

Table 4–8. Flow Sheet Showing Response of Patient 2 to Initiation of Insulin Therapy in an Office Setting (Preprandial Regular/Bedtime NPH)

	Before Breakfast	Before Lunch	Before Supper	Before Bedtime[a]
5/23[b]				
SMBG (mg/dl)		420	333	286
Insulin dose (U)		4 R	4 R	8 NPH
5/24[b]				
SMBG (mg/dl)	243	268	222	193
Insulin (U)	4 R	4 R	4 R	10 NPH
5/25				
SMBG (mg/dl)	208	175	196	200
Insulin (U)	4 R	4 R	4 R	10 NPH
5/26[b]				
SMBG (mg/dl)	183	188	155	182
Insulin (U)	4 R	5 R	5 R	12 NPH
5/27				
SMBG (mg/dl)	152	163	145	175
Insulin (U)	5 R	5 R	5 R	12 NPH
5/28				
SMBG (mg/dl)	148	172	139	163
Insulin (U)	5 R	5 R	6 R	14 NPH
5/29				
SMBG (mg/dl)	135	154	128	148
Insulin (U)	6 R	5 R	6 R	14 NPH
5/30[c]				
SMBG (mg/dl)	129	163	137	162
Insulin (U)	6 R	5 R	6 R	14 NPH
5/31				
SMBG (mg/dl)	131	172	148	182
Insulin (U)	6 R	5 R	6 R	14 NPH
6/1[c]				
SMBG (mg/dl)	125	148	125	151
Insulin (U)	6 R	5 R	7 R	14 NPH
6/2				
SMBG (mg/dl)	133	127	119	147
Insulin (U)	7 R	5 R	7 R	14 NPH
6/3[b]				
SMBG (mg/dl)	121	138		
Insulin (U)	7 R	5 R		

SMBG, self-monitoring of blood glucose.

[a]Glucose should be measured before snack (if eaten).

[b]Office visit.

[c]SMBG results phoned to office.

were compared in the same type 1 diabetic patients, both methods produced the same improvement in glycemic control. In a second study,[12] type 1 diabetic patients were instructed to use either SMBG or (second voided) urine tests three to four times a day and were monitored for 2 years. Glycated hemoglobin levels decreased to a comparable degree in both groups. The incidence of severe hypoglycemia was no different between the two groups. Diabetic ketoacidosis occurred in only one patient (60 patients in each group). In a third study[13] of type 1 patients, intensive treatment was based on the results of urine testing because of the expense of SMBG. Although near euglycemia was not achieved, episodes of diabetic ketoacidosis and hospitalizations for diabetes out of control were markedly reduced. Therefore, if SMBG is not feasible for some patients, urine testing should be encouraged.

Either a single-voided or double-voided urine sample can be tested. To provide a single-voided sample, the patient simply urinates. A double-voided sample is collected by discarding the first-voided sample, drinking approximately 8 ounces of water, and collecting a second sample 30 minutes later. The results of the double-voided sample more closely correlate to the blood glucose value measured at that time. The results of the single-voided sample reflect the average glucose concentration during the time period between collecting the single-voided sample and the preceding urination. Testing the first-voided urine specimen gives results[13] identical to those obtained with the double-voided sample 60% to 80% of the time. Furthermore, the second-voided urine shows more glucosuria than the initial sample only 5% of the time.[14] Therefore, results of the urine collected in the first void are equal to or higher than the results in the second-voided urine 95% of the time. Increasing insulin doses based on the results obtained in the first situation (i.e., heavier glucosuria in the second sample) poses the potential risk of hypoglycemia during the several-hour period preceding the urine collection. On the other hand, in the second situation (i.e., less glucosuria in the second sample), insulin dose increases are less likely to be made even though they would be warranted to treat the higher glucose levels present during the several-hour period preceding the urine collection. Thus, overtreatment might occur only 5% of the time, but this theoretic figure is probably grossly exaggerated because as long as any glucosuria is present, circulating glucose concentrations are exceeding the T_m for glucose and are far from hypoglycemic levels. Therefore, to simplify management, the results of first-voided urine samples can be used to adjust insulin doses.

Before relying on urine test results, however, a physician must obtain a general idea of the patient's T_m for glucose. Simultaneous blood and second-voided urine tests for glucose must be performed under circumstances that allow such a judgment to be made. For instance, if all tests are conducted when plasma glucose concentrations are >300 mg/dl and urine tests show heavy glucosuria, it is impossible to determine the T_m. On the other hand, if the results of urine tests are negative or show minimal glucosuria while plasma glucose concentrations are markedly elevated, the T_m is high. At plasma glucose levels <200 mg/dl, negative urine test results are appropriate, and again, no decision about the approximate T_m for glucose is possible. However, if glucosuria is present with glucose concentrations much below 200 mg/dl, the patient has a low T_m.

Therefore, simultaneous blood and *double-voided urine* tests must be performed under both fasting and postprandial conditions until appropriate data for determining the T_m are in hand. Only then should the results of first-voided urine tests be relied on exclusively as a basis for insulin dose adjustments. A more detailed rationale for using first-voided urine samples rather than double-voided ones is discussed in Chapter 7. In practical terms, results of blood and urine tests must be matched frequently from the time a patient starts to take insulin until the fasting or late afternoon plasma glucose concentrations fall to the point at which urine tests reveal no glucosuria. If a patient has either a high T_m (often associated with kidney disease or aging) or a low T_m (usually noted in pregnant women and in the occasional diabetic patient who also has an independent renal tubular abnormality), repeated determinations of plasma glucose concentrations at the appropriate times are necessary for proper adjustment of insulin doses.

PATIENT 3

CASE STUDY

A 43-year-old man has had diabetes for 4 years. He is 5 feet 9 inches tall, with a stable weight of 158 pounds. He currently follows an appropriate diet and takes 750 mg of chlorpropamide per day. However, his fasting plasma glucose concentrations have consistently been measured at 220 to 265 mg/dl for the past 4 months. At present, the patient has 0.1% to 0.5% glucosuria before breakfast and excretes glucose in the urine throughout the day and evening. Office records indicate,

however, that he did not have fasting glucosuria before 4 months ago, when his glucose concentrations before breakfast ranged between 130 and 187 mg/dl. Because of the patient's normal T_m, his busy schedule, and his motivation and intelligence, insulin therapy is initiated in an office setting. The patient is obviously not overweight, so the 10 U–5 U split NPH regimen is initially prescribed. A nurse shows him how to inject insulin the first afternoon. He returns the following morning to inject it himself under her supervision. In addition to the technique of insulin injection, instruction is given on the care of insulin and syringes, on urine testing, and on the signs, symptoms, and treatment of hypoglycemia. (The patient has a pathologic aversion to blood and refuses to perform SMBG.) The patient's response to insulin therapy is summarized on the flow sheet in Table 4–9.

COMMENT

The patient, who kept faithful records, was contacted every second day. On 11/11, both the morning and evening doses of NPH insulin were increased because the urine tests before breakfast and before supper showed 0.5% glucosuria. (Because the conversation

Table 4–9. Flow Sheet Showing Response of Patient 3 Using Results of Urine Testing for Initiation of Insulin Therapy

| | Insulin Dose (U) Before | | | | Urine Test Result Before | | | |
| | *Breakfast* | | *Supper* | | | | | |
Date	NPH	Regular	NPH	Regular	*Breakfast*	*Lunch*	*Supper*	*Bedtime*[a]
11/8			5				2%	1%
11/9	10		5		0.5%	2%	1%	0.5%
11/10	10		5		0.5%	1%	0.5%	1%
11/11	10		10		0.5%	1%	0.5%	1%
11/12	15		10		0.1%	1%	0.25%	1%
11/13	15		10		Negative	1%	0.25%	0.5%
11/14	20		10		Negative	0.5%	Negative	0.25%
11/15	20		10		Negative	0.5%	0.1%	0.25%
11/16	20	5	10		Negative	0.1%	Negative	0.1%
11/17	20	5	10		Negative	Negative	Negative	Negative

NPH, neutral protamine Hagedorn.
[a]Urine glucose should be measured before snack (if eaten).

with the patient occurred in the late afternoon, the increase in the morning dose was not implemented until the next morning.) The fasting urine test gave negative results secondary to the increased amount of evening insulin, but the patient continued to excrete some glucose in the urine specimen tested before supper. Therefore, after consultation on 11/13, the morning dose of NPH insulin was raised further, with subsequent clearing of glucosuria in the late afternoon urine test. However, the results of tests done before lunch remained positive, and on the morning of 11/16 the patient was taught how to add a small amount of regular insulin to the NPH insulin in the same syringe. On this insulin regimen (20 U of NPH and 5 U of regular insulin before breakfast, 10 U of NPH insulin before supper), the patient's urine tests consistently yielded negative results except at times of a dietary indiscretion.

This patient had a smooth transition from oral hypoglycemic agents to insulin therapy. The dose of insulin could be adjusted every second day because the pattern of results of urine tests was consistent. In many cases, however, these results are not consistent, and changes in the insulin dose must proceed more slowly until a definite pattern emerges.

PATIENT 4

CASE STUDY

This 42-year-old woman has had diabetes for 8 years. She is 5 feet 7 inches tall, has a large frame, and currently weighs 202 pounds. Despite a 1,300-calorie diet (which is poorly followed) and maximal amounts of a sulfonylurea agent, her urine tests (when done) consistently reveal 1% to 2% glucosuria; these results correspond to her recent plasma glucose concentrations of 320 to 415 mg/dl, as determined at office visits. She has had a problem with alcohol, and therefore metformin (see Chapter 5) is contraindi-

cated. Her sulfonylurea agent is discontinued, and the 20 U-10 U split regimen of NPH insulin is prescribed because of the patient's obesity. She refused to perform SMBG but was willing to test her urine. Her response is summarized on the flow sheet in Table 4-10.

COMMENT

It was convenient for this patient to come to the office before breakfast for glucose determinations. She took her insulin, ate breakfast at a nearby coffee shop, and was contacted later that day about appropriate insulin dose adjustments, which she implemented that evening and the following morning. Fasting glucose concentrations were initially measured and compared with the results of testing a double-voided urine in order to establish her T_m. On 4/5, both insulin doses were increased by 10 U because of persistent heavy glucosuria. On 4/7, the evening dose of NPH insulin was increased by only 5 U because the patient's fasting urine test results and glucose levels had shown some improvement. (This decision is in keeping with the policy of *gradually* increasing insulin doses to avoid hypoglycemia and its attendant disruption of metabolism.) The morning dose of NPH insulin was increased by 10 U because the tests conducted before supper gave consistently poor results. No change in either dose of insulin was made on 4/9 because the fasting tests showed definite improvement and the results of the late afternoon urine tests suggested some improvement. (This decision is in keeping with the principle that changes in insulin therapy should be predicated on a consistent pattern of test results rather than on a group of test results that vary considerably.)

On 4/11, increases were made in both insulin doses because of unacceptable fasting and before supper urine test results. On 4/13, the morning dose of NPH insulin was increased by only 5 U because late afternoon

Table 4–10. Flow Sheet Showing Response of Patient 4 to Initiation of Insulin Therapy

| | Insulin Dose (U) Before | | | | Urine Test Result (Plasma Glucose, mg/dl) Before | | | |
| | *Breakfast* | | *Supper* | | | | | |
Date	*NPH*	*Regular*	*NPH*	*Regular*	*Breakfast*	*Lunch*	*Supper*	*Bedtime*[a]
4/3	20		10		2%	2%	2%	2%
4/4	20		10		2%	2%	2%	2%
4/5	20		20		1% (352)	2%	2%	2%
4/6	30		20		0.5%	2%	1%	1%
4/7	30		25		1% (301)	2%	1%	1%
4/8	40		25		0.5%	1%	0.5%	0.5%
4/9	40		25		0.25% (227)	1%	0.25%	0.5%
4/10	40		25		0.5%	1%	0.5%	1%
4/11	40		30		0.5% (253)	1%	0.5%	0.5%
4/12	50		30		0.25%	1%	0.25%	0.5%
4/13	50		30		0.1% (198)	1%	0.5%	0.5%
4/14	55		30		Negative	0.5%	0.1%	0.25%
4/15	55		35		0.1% (203)	1%	0.25%	0.5%
4/16	60		35		Negative	0.5%	0.1%	0.25%
4/17	60		35	5	Negative (178)	0.5%	Negative	0.1%
4/18	60	5	35	5	0.1%	0.5%	0.25%	0.1%
4/19	60	5	35	5	Negative	0.25%	Negative	Negative
4/20	60	10	35	5	0.25%	0.1%	0.1%	0.25%
4/21	60	10	35	5	0.1%	Negative	0.25%	0.25%
4/22	60	10	35	5	0.1%	0.1%	0.1%	Negative
4/23	60	10	40	5	0.25%	0.25%	Negative	0.1%
4/24	60	10	40	5	Negative	Negative	Negative	Negative
4/25	60	10	40	5	1% (reaction)	0.5%	0.25%	0.1%
4/26	60	10	40	5	Negative	0.25%	0.1%	Negative
4/27	60	10	35	5	0.5% (reaction)	0.5%	0.25%	0.1%
4/28	60	10	35	5	0.1%	0.1%	Negative	0.1%

NPH, neutral protamine Hagedorn.

[a]Urine glucose should be measured before snack (if eaten).

results, although showing definite improvement, still consistently showed 0.25% to 0.5% glucosuria. The evening dose of NPH insulin was not changed because the fasting glucose concentration and urine test results were continually improving. On 4/15, both doses of insulin were again increased; the evening injection was increased in an attempt to lower the fasting plasma glucose concentration below approximately 200 mg/dl, and the morning dose was increased because the tests before supper still showed some spillage.

On 4/17, the T_m was established as normal, and further determinations of plasma glucose levels were made only at routine office visits (see Chapter 7). The amounts of intermediate-acting insulin being administered were deemed appropriate; therefore, small amounts of regular insulin were added to each injection because of persistent glucosuria before lunch and before bed. Two days later (4/19), the urine tests showed some response to the addition of the short-acting component. Five more units of regular insulin were added to the morning dose because of persistent glucosuria before lunch. Arrangements were made to lengthen the period between consultations because the urine tests gave fairly consistent and almost acceptable results. On 4/23, the evening dose of NPH insulin was increased by 5 U in an attempt to eradicate intermittent fasting glucosuria. However, the patient experienced hypoglycemia in the early morning hours of 4/25 and 4/27; she woke up perspiring and had feelings of tremulousness, hunger, and palpitations, all of which were relieved within 10 to 15 minutes by food. As expected, her urine test results deteriorated during that period, and the insulin prescription was returned to 60 U of NPH plus 10 U of regular insulin before breakfast and 35 U of NPH plus 5 U of regular insulin before supper. The fact that the morning and evening doses of insulin were changed independently of each other on 4/7, 4/13, 4/19, 4/23, and 4/27 attests to the efficacy of this approach.

If this obese patient had been able to adhere to her hypocaloric diet, the resulting weight loss would no doubt have obviated her need for insulin and possibly even sulfonylurea agents. Even though an appropriate diet would have been the most effective therapy for this patient, she was unable to benefit from this approach despite continued emphasis by persons involved in her medical care. In my view, the *theoretic* possibility of

a simple, more effective treatment does not justify withholding other forms of therapy that will probably improve diabetic control. Without insulin, this patient's tissues would be exposed to chronic, moderate to marked hyperglyecmia. Although insulin therapy may not be fully effective because of the insulin resistance associated with obesity and her dietary noncompliance, lowering the patient's glucose concentrations should prove helpful in retarding the development of microangiopathic and neuropathic complications.

PATIENT 3 REVISITED

As described earlier, many patients learn to perform SMBG when insulin therapy is started. The physician (or appropriately trained nurse practitioner or diabetes nurse educator) can use these results to adjust the initial insulin doses. Let us assume that patient 3 was taught SMBG by a diabetes nurse educator on his initial visit on 11/8 and his technique proves to be accurate when checked on his return visit the next morning. The results of his SMBG are shown in Table 4-11 in parentheses next to the urine test results discussed previously (see Table

Table 4–11. Comparison of Urine Testing and SMBG in Patient 3 After Initiation of Insulin Therapy

	Insulin Dose (U) Before				Urine (and SMBG) Test Results Before			
	Breakfast		*Supper*					
Date	*NPH*	*Regular*	*NPH*	*Regular*	*Breakfast*	*Lunch*	*Supper*	*Bedtime*[a]
11/8			5				2% (280)[b]	1% (257)
11/9	10		5		0.5% (248)	2% (362)	1% (243)	0.5% (227)
11/10	10		5		0.5% (218)	1% (310)	0.5% (210)	1% (232)
11/11	10		10		0.5% (242)	1% (290)	0.5% (205)	1% (218)
11/12	15		10		0.1% (195)	1% (263)	0.25% (195)	1% (242)
11/13	15		10		Negative (178)	1% (243)	0.25% (189)	0.5% (192)
11/14	20		10		Negative (185)	0.5% (238)	Negative (162)	0.25% (178)
11/15	20		10		Negative (163)	0.5% (189)	0.1% (172)	0.25% (183)
11/16	20	5	10		Negative (172)	0.1% (168)	Negative (165)	0.1% (192)
11/17	20	5	10		Negative (168)	Negative (164)	Negative (149)	Negative (156)

NPH, neutral protamine Hagedorn; SMBG, self-monitoring of blood glucose.

[a]Glucose measurements taken before snack (if eaten).

[b]mg/dl.

4-9). The insulin doses based on the results of the urine tests are maintained in Table 4-11 to point out how the blood glucose results would have changed the dose adjustments. For instance, on 11/13 the evening dose of NPH insulin would have been increased if blood glucose values had been available. A negative urine test result on the morning of 11/13 could have reflected a fasting glucose concentration appropriately low. Because there is simply no way to discern, the negative urine test result has to be the end point. By the same token, the morning dose of NPH insulin would have been increased on 11/17 if the patient were using SMBG; the negative urine test result before supper on 11/16 prevented this adjustment. Finally, regular insulin would have been introduced before breakfast on 11/14 (after talking with the patient on 11/13) instead of on 11/16 and before supper on 11/13 instead of not added at all if only urine tests are used. The value of SMBG goes far beyond speeding up the process of attaining a stable insulin dose when insulin therapy is initiated. It is clear from the information contained in Table 4-11 that near euglycemia cannot be achieved if urine tests for glucose are used to monitor diabetic control. SMBG is necessary to accomplish this.

INITIAL INSULIN THERAPY INVOLVING ONE MORNING INJECTION

Although I routinely start patients on at least two injections of insulin per day, a patient occasionally refuses this approach but agrees to take a single injection. One morning dose of insulin is still being used (unfortunately, in my view) by many physicians. Therefore, a brief discussion using this approach is in order. The principles delineated in the previous section on the initiation of insulin therapy with two daily injections also apply, for the most part, to therapy with a single daily injection. The appropriate dose of intermedi-

ate-acting insulin is established first. If short-acting insulin is necessary, only small amounts are used. If the patient is hospitalized, final adjustments are made after discharge. The initial doses of 10 to 15 U of NPH insulin in lean patients and 25 to 30 U in obese patients are equivalent to the total amount used in the two-injection approach. The rates of increase of 5 U per day in lean patients and 10 U per day in obese and extremely hyperglycemic patients are also similar.

There are some important differences, however. First, in elderly patients—the most likely candidates for single-injection therapy—less stringent control may be acceptable because of decreased life expectancy and the greater risks of hypoglycemia. Second, results of the urine tests or SMBG performed in the evening before supper *and* the following morning before breakfast help determine any changes in the dose of NPH insulin—that is, if either test yields an unacceptable result, the morning dose of NPH should be increased. As discussed previously, when the dose of intermediate-acting insulin is gradually increased, the test performed before supper usually shows a quicker and more sensitive response than the next day's fasting test. Attempts are made to find a dose that controls both daytime and nighttime glucose levels. However, when the dose of NPH insulin is continually increased in an attempt to control the next morning's fasting glucose concentration or urine test result, hypoglycemia is often noted in the late afternoon. In such cases, switching some breakfast or lunch calories to a midafternoon snack may alleviate the problem and even allow further increases in the morning dose of NPH insulin. If this tactic should fail, two choices are left: Either the patient can continue to take one daily injection of a dose that controls glucose levels during the day but allows significant fasting hyperglycemia, or the patient can switch to two injections per day.

Another pattern of response is (fortunately) infrequent. In this situation, intermediate-acting insulins act much more slowly than usual,[15] and nighttime or early morning hypoglycemia occurs at insulin doses that fail to control the daytime hyperglycemia. Use of two daily injections of intermediate-acting insulin would not seem helpful in this instance. Because the dose that precipitated nighttime hypoglycemia was inadequate for daytime needs, addition of a second dose in the evening would only make matters worse unless the morning dose of NPH was reduced—a course that would cause further problems with daytime control. Several other approaches, may be tried: (1) injecting the morning dose of NPH insulin earlier; (2) eating supper later; and (3) delaying and/or increasing the bedtime snack. In my experience, patients with a delayed response to intermediate-acting insulin usually have a normal response to short-acting insulin. Therefore, if a patient is willing to take additional injections, the before breakfast NPH insulin dose is adjusted on the basis of the fasting blood glucose level, and preprandial regular insulin is used as necessary to control the blood glucose levels during the day.

SWITCHING FROM ONE INJECTION OF INTERMEDIATE-ACTING INSULIN IN THE MORNING TO TWO INJECTIONS PER DAY

The main reason to convert a single morning injection regimen to one requiring a second injection of intermediate-acting insulin is because of unacceptable fasting hyperglycemia in the presence of before supper glucose values that are not high enough to allow an increase in the dose of NPH insulin in the morning. The most effective way to accomplish this is simply to add 4 to 5 U of intermediate-acting insulin before supper. It makes little sense to decrease the morning dose, because this is already an effective amount and lowering it would result in poorer control during the day. The patient simply needs more of an effect during the

night, and this is now being supplied by the second injection. It is slowly increased as needed, depending on the results of the fasting test.

PREMIXED INSULINS

Premixed insulin preparations, either commercially available containing either 70% NPH insulin and 30% regular insulin (70/30) or 50% NPH insulin and 50% regular insulin (50/50) or mixed by family members or nurses in syringes (or bottles) with various proportions of intermediate- and short-acting insulins, are increasingly being used, especially for older patients who have difficulty mixing insulins. They are often given as a single daily injection, although they can be used twice a day. The relationship between each test and the individual component of the insulin prescription for both two injections (see Table 4–2) and one injection per day (discussed earlier) applies to premixed insulins as well. However, there are certain constraints on adjusting doses because the amounts of both NPH and regular insulins are being changed concomitantly.

The general rule to follow is that the lowest glucose value limits the dose. For instance, in a patient taking two injections of premixed insulin, the morning dose can be increased as long as neither the before lunch nor before supper glucose level is too low. If either of these declines below the target range or the patient experiences unexplained hypoglycemia between breakfast and lunch or between lunch and supper, the dose cannot be increased any further and indeed will probably need to be decreased slightly. This should occur even if one of the test results (before lunch or before supper) is too high. Similarly, the before supper injection of premixed insulin can be increased as long as the before bed and fasting test results are not too low and unexplained hypoglycemia does not occur between supper and breakfast. If either too low test results or unexplained hypoglycemia occurs during this period, the dose of the premixed insulin must be adjusted downward accordingly. The situation is a little more complex in a patient taking a single daily injection of premixed insulin. Any test result that is too low or unexplained hypoglycemia at any time necessitates decreasing the dose even if three of the four test values are too high. Thus, although using premixed insulins may be easier for patients, their use usually leads to higher glucose levels than if the doses of NPH and regular insulin could be adjusted separately.

DRAWBACKS TO THE SLIDING-SCALE METHOD OF INITIATING INSULIN THERAPY

Two principles guide a physician in initiating insulin therapy. First, insulin should be administered in anticipation of subsequent events so that it is available to *prevent* inordinate hyperglycemia. To reiterate: In a mixed/split insulin regimen, a morning dose of NPH insulin exerts a gradual influence on plasma glucose levels throughout the day, with a maximal effect on the calories ingested during supper, which (in the United States) is usually the patient's largest meal. By the same token, morning and evening doses of regular insulin are given in anticipation of the acute influx of breakfast and supper carbohydrate calories. Finally, the smaller dose of NPH insulin in the evening prevents significant fasting hyperglycemia by making gradually increasing amounts of insulin available throughout the night (as the effect of the larger morning dose of NPH insulin wanes) to restrain hepatic glucose production.

Second, the kind of insulin used (intermediate acting) and the gradually increasing amounts initially prescribed should make for a relatively smooth transition from higher to lower plasma glucose levels. Large fluctuations in glucose concentrations, with the at-

tendant disruption of carbohydrate homeostasis through secretion of counterregulatory hormones, should be avoided.

These two principles are violated when the sliding-scale method of prescribing insulin is used. In this approach, different amounts of short-acting insulin are given (usually every 4 to 6 hours), depending on the outcome of blood glucose levels or urine tests for glucose and ketone bodies. First, treatment is given only after hyperglycemia is marked enough to result in glucosuria. Because the smallest amount of regular insulin is usually given for 0.5% glucosuria, treatment is withheld until relatively high plasma glucose concentrations (approximately 220 to 250 mg/dl or even higher) are attained. This is often the case when blood glucose concentrations are used instead of urine results. Thus, the principle of prescribing insulin to *prevent* significant hyperglycemia is certainly violated. Second, not only is the plasma glucose response to regular insulin fairly rapid, but the majority of the effectiveness of regular insulin is dissipated within 3 to 4 hours. In addition, the hormonal response to the rapid lowering of plasma glucose levels may cause subsequently administered insulin to be less effective. This effect leads to more hyperglycemia, and thus larger amounts of insulin are required than if glucose concentrations had been lowered more gradually. The result is relatively large and rapid fluctuations of glucose levels treated with increasing amounts of short-acting insulin.

The sliding-scale method using urine testing is critically dependent on the accuracy of the results, which involves at least three factors: the timing of collection, a consistent relation between the amount of urinary glucose actually present and that measured, and the T_m for glucose.

The collection and testing of the urine sample in hospitals where it is still done is almost always the responsibility of the nursing staff. Unless a patient is on a diabetic ward where urine collection and testing may be part of the daily nursing routine, this activity may be overlooked when other problems on the ward become pressing. Permanent insulin orders are followed much more dependably, even though they may need frequent modification. Dispensing of medication is such an integral part of the nursing routine that failure to give insulin that has already been ordered is most unusual.

Although both diabetic patients and the medical personnel caring for them may rely on the semiquantitative tests for urinary glucose, a number of factors (often beyond a patient's control) profoundly disrupt the relation between the amount of glucose present and the amount measured. Both falsely high and falsely low results are obtained frequently (see Chapter 7). Thus, the dose of regular insulin administered may not correspond closely to the actual amount of urinary glucose.

Finally, if the T_m is abnormal, the patient can be seriously under- or overtreated. Two personal examples illustrate this problem. An endocrinologic consultation was requested 5 days after prostate surgery for a 76-year-old diabetic man who was feeling lethargic, anorectic, and weak. The patient had been taking small amounts of NPH insulin before surgery. The sliding-scale method of insulin therapy had been ordered after surgery, but the patient had received no insulin in view of consistently negative results in urine tests for glucose. A determination of the plasma glucose concentration, as ordered by the endocrinology consultant, gave a result of 448 mg/dl. Obviously, the very high T_m in this elderly diabetic patient and the failure to measure plasma glucose levels conspired to deprive this patient of needed insulin.

The second patient was a pregnant diabetic woman who was admitted to the hospital several weeks before delivery. The sliding-scale method was prescribed to provide her with any additional insulin she might require during the last part of her third trimester. Her urine tests consistently revealed 2% glucosuria and gave moderate to large results

for ketones. The patient received many extra units of regular insulin each day. The endocrinology consultant requested a random determination of the plasma glucose level, which was measured at 167 mg/dl. A 24-hour urine test for glucose revealed that this patient excreted 174 g/day. Because she was ingesting a 200-g carbohydrate diet, very little of her carbohydrate intake was being used. This loss resulted in starvation (or low-carbohydrate) ketosis (see Chapter 7). Thus, neither the marked glucosuria nor the ketosis was due to uncontrolled diabetes. When the carbohydrate content of the patient's diet was increased to 250 g, the ketosis disappeared. Obviously, the lowered T_m associated with pregnancy was responsible for the administration of unnecessary insulin to this patient.

The sliding-scale method of prescribing insulin is usually used in two situations: either for the initiation of insulin therapy or for the treatment of a patient with insulin during a temporary situation in which the usual relations between eating and insulin therapy are disrupted (e.g., during and after surgery or in critically ill hospitalized patients). In the first instance, the sliding-scale method is chosen in the hope that the amount of short-acting insulin required over several days will help determine the appropriate dose of intermediate-acting insulin. For the reasons just stated, this is a false hope, and the use of this approach simply lengthens the patient's hospital stay. Indeed, the proponents of this approach must recognize that it requires the use of disproportionately large amounts of regular insulin because they recommend that the total dose of short-acting insulin given during the preceding 24 hours be reduced by one third to one half in calculating the dose of NPH insulin for the next day. In my experience, also, there is a large discrepancy between the amount of regular insulin initially given to a recently diagnosed diabetic patient and the amount of intermediate-acting insulin prescribed on discharge from the hospital.

The use of the sliding-scale method in the second situation should also be actively discouraged. It is easy to provide patients in these unusual circumstances with insulin in anticipation of their needs rather than after hyperglycemia has developed (see Chapter 7). The other arguments against using this method (as just summarized) would certainly apply to postoperative and/or critically ill patients.

It should be pointed out that although using blood glucose levels obtained every 4 to 6 hours to regulate repeated doses of regular insulin avoids the problems associated with semiquantitative urine tests for glucose, two important drawbacks remain. First, this approach does not *anticipate* increases in glucose concentrations but delays treatment until hyperglycemia occurs. Second, the caveats concerning the more rapid lowering of glucose levels in response to regular insulin still apply when glucose levels are measured in the blood rather than in the urine.

Finally, the use of sliding-scale insulin in these situations must be differentiated from using it acutely to lower the blood glucose level in ambulatory patients under intensive management (see Chapter 7). In that case, it is appropriate to change the dose of regular insulin on an ad hoc basis to compensate for too high or too low preprandial glucose levels. These adjustments are often necessary to allow a patient to achieve near euglycemia without an inordinate risk of hypoglycemia.

SIDE EFFECTS OF INSULIN THERAPY

The side effects of insulin therapy include delayed *local* skin reactions to injected insulin, true or *systemic* insulin allergy, insulin resistance, insulin-induced lipoatrophy, and insulin-induced lipohypertrophy. Three other possible sequelae of insulin administration are considered *therapeutic* effects, not side effects. The most obvious one, of course, is hypoglycemia. The other two are associated with weight gain in patients whose diabetes was uncontrolled before the initiation or intensification of insulin therapy. These patients commonly gain weight, usually because the glucose calories that were lost in the urine in the markedly hyperglycemic state are now being stored under the influence of insulin. These formerly lost but now retained calories can account for 70% to 100% of the weight gained.[10, 16] An occasional patient accumulates enough extra fluid so that localized or even generalized edema may occur.[17, 18] This *insulin edema* is reversible over time (up to a month) but may be helped by a mild diuretic or in refractory cases by low-dose ephedrine.[19] Insulin normally causes sodium reabsorption in the proximal tubules of the kidneys, and it is believed that insulin edema is a very unusual manifestation of this action. It is more likely to occur in those patients whose diabetes had been markedly out of control for a long time.

Some information about the structure, biosynthesis, and purification of insulin is necessary for an understanding of the pathogenesis of these complications of insulin therapy. Insulin is a polypeptide hormone with a molecular weight of approximately 6,000. As illustrated in the dark area of Figure 4–4, the insulin molecule consists of A and B chains joined by two disulfide bridges. In addition, a disulfide linkage connects amino acids 6 and 11 within the A chain. The steps by which insulin is synthesized in the pancreatic β-cells include (1) the formation of a single long-chain polypeptide; (2) the curving of this string of amino acids back on itself in a configuration that aligns the future A and B chains of insulin opposite each other; (3) the closing of the two disulfide bridges to form a larger polypeptide (molecular weight, ~9,000) called *proinsulin*, which is illustrated by the entire structure in Figure 4–4; and (4) the breaking of this curvilinear molecule at two points, yielding insulin (see Fig. 4–4, solid circles) and the

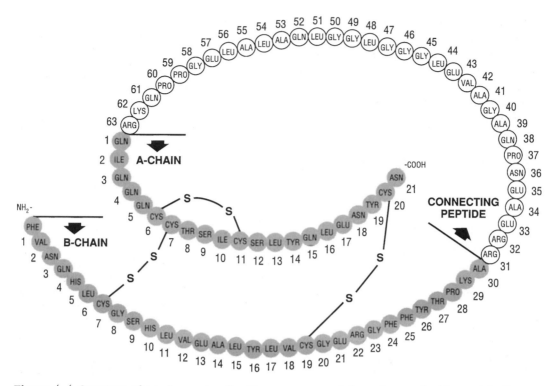

Figure 4-4. Structure of porcine proinsulin. Cleavage occurs at the points marked by straight lines, yielding equimolar amounts of connecting peptide and insulin. The letter *S* connected to the heavy bars represents disulfide linkages between the amino acids indicated. (From Chance RE: Amino acid sequences of proinsulins and intermediates. Diabetes 21 [suppl 2]:461, 1972)

connecting peptide (see Fig. 4-4, open circles).

Insulin and connecting peptide (C-peptide) are packaged in equimolar amounts in the granules of the β-cells and released into the circulation together. C-peptide has no known biologic function but does serve as an important marker of insulin secretion in patients whose insulin levels cannot be measured directly (e.g., because of insulin-binding antibodies).

The conventional way to monitor the purity of insulin preparations is to measure the amount of proinsulin contained in them, which is expressed as parts per million (ppm). In the past 25 years, the purification of insulin preparations has improved dramatically so that now there is <10 ppm in the *impure* preparations used. The pure ones

contain <1 ppm of proinsulin. The preparation and purity of the three general classes of insulin preparations available (i.e., human insulins, purified pork or beef insulins, and standard insulins) are discussed later.

Both IgG and IgE antibodies to insulin are found in patients treated with insulin. Only rarely, however, do these antibodies cause clinical problems in diabetic patients. The IgE antibody seems to be directed specifically against insulin, and high titers are associated with systemic insulin allergy. The situation with regard to IgG antibodies is less clear. It was initially believed that insulin itself stimulated the formation of IgG antibodies. This antigenic response was later thought to be mainly (if not entirely) due to the impurities (proinsulin and other larger-molecular-weight compounds) in the preparation. Although purified insulins were once thought not to be antigenic, studies clearly indicate that IgG antibodies are formed against these purer preparations.[20] Thus, although impurities enhance the IgG antibody response to insulin, insulin itself is probably mildly antigenic.

DELAYED LOCAL REACTION AT THE SITE OF INJECTION

With the earlier, more impure preparations of insulin, local skin reactions at the site of injection were common, occurring in as many as 50% of patients receiving injections for the first time. In patients who have these reactions, symptoms start within 1 month of institution of insulin therapy. A 3- to 6-hour lag period passes before the appearance of the lesions, which are characterized by pruritic, erythematous, indurated areas from 1 to 5 cm in diameter. The lesions become maximal 18 to 24 hours later and last for several days. They are often heralded by a stinging or burning sensation at the time of injection. These reactions are self-limited, invariably disappearing within 1 to 3 months. Because the prevalence and severity of these lesions had been markedly diminished by recrystallization of the older insulin preparations to rid them of contaminants, it is likely that the impurities cause these local reactions. The mechanism may involve a delayed hypersensitivity reaction.[21] In any event, use of the new, more pure preparations has alleviated this problem to a large extent.

Treatment of local delayed reactions to insulin injections should be conservative. If the symptoms are not too troublesome to a patient, no therapy is indicated because the lesions will resolve spontaneously within several months. Skin reactions to the intermediate-acting insulins seem more common than those to the short-acting insulins. Delayed local reactions may occasionally be due to the zinc in the insulin preparations; such

reactions can be successfully treated with zinc-free insulin.[22] Antibodies to protamine in patients taking NPH insulin are common.[23] However, the clinical manifestation of protamine allergy is not a delayed local reaction but either an extremely rare generalized urticarial reaction occurring spontaneously[24] or an anaphylactoid reaction. The latter occurs when protamine is given to reverse heparinization after cardiac catheterization[25] or cardiac surgery[26] in approximately 1% of diabetic patients taking NPH insulin.

Except for switching to a purer preparation, using an insulin of another species has usually not been helpful in treating delayed local reactions. Other therapeutic approaches that have been suggested include systemic use of antihistamines or local injections of antihistamines or glucocorticoids. The adverse effects of these medications must be weighed against the possible benefits in this benign situation. If local injections of an antihistamine are tried, 1 mg of diphenhydramine (Benadryl) for each 10 U of insulin can be added to the same syringe, although antihistamines may be effective only in true or systemic insulin allergy[27] (see below). As long as small doses of steroids are used, adrenal suppression, insulin resistance, and other adverse effects of glucocorticoid therapy should not be a problem. Two glucocorticoid preparations, hydrocortisone and dexamethasone, have been used in the same syringe with insulin. The initial doses of hydrocortisone and dexamethasone are 2 mg and 0.1 mg per injection, respectively. These amounts are gradually increased until the desired effect is achieved. The replacement doses of hydrocortisone and dexamethasone (i.e., the amounts that will suppress the hypothalamic-pituitary-adrenal axis) are 20 mg and 0.75 mg, respectively. It is important to use the smallest possible effective dose—one that preferably is considerably smaller than a full replacement dose. Another important point is that the effect of dexamethasone lasts for more than 24 hours whereas the effect of hydrocortisone lasts for about 8 hours. This shorter-lived effect of hydrocortisone is a theoretic argument for its use, because adrenal suppression may be less likely. On the other hand, if the local reaction flares up after the effect of the glucocorticoid wears off, dexamethasone may be the better agent.

TRUE OR SYSTEMIC INSULIN ALLERGY

Nature of Insulin Allergy

True allergy to insulin, also called *systemic insulin allergy*, is (fortunately) rare, occurring in approximately 0.1% of diabetic patients receiving insulin. It is much more common in patients with a history of interrupted insulin therapy than in those whose therapy has been continuous. The manifestations of insulin allergy are usually seen within 1 or 2 weeks of the resumption of interrupted insulin therapy. The hallmark of true insulin allergy is an *immediate* local reaction (within 30 to 60 minutes) that gradually increases until large areas surrounding the injection site are involved. In approximately one half of the patients, the reaction soon spreads into a generalized urticarial pattern and is occasionally associated with angioneurotic edema or even anaphylactic shock.[28] These systemic reactions are often preceded by gradual increases in the severity of the immediate local reaction, which may serve as a warning that serious difficulties lie ahead unless appropriate therapy (desensitization) is instituted.

These immediate reactions (both local and systemic) seem to be allergic responses to the insulin molecule itself. They are rarely alleviated by the use of extremely pure insulin preparations. The clinical similarity to penicillin allergy is striking, and indeed, the immunologic characteristics of true insulin allergy are almost identical to those of penicillin allergy. Both types of allergy involve (1) exquisite sensitivity to minute amounts of the antigen on conjunctival or intradermal testing; (2) passive transfer of an antibody (identified as IgE) that is capable of sensitizing normal skin to a subsequent challenge by the antigen (i.e., a positive result of Prausnitz-Küstner test); (3) high titers (as measured by direct assays) of IgE antibodies to the particular antigen in question; and (4) successful treatment by desensitization in almost all cases. Although true insulin allergy is mediated by the same antibody (IgE) that causes atopic disease (asthma, allergic rhinitis, urticaria), patients allergic to insulin apparently have no greater predisposition to atopy than do other patients. On the other hand, one third of patients with true insulin allergy had a history of penicillin allergy.[29]

Patients with systemic insulin allergy have high titers of IgE antibodies; these levels decline rapidly (within days) after desensitization but only gradually (over months) after discontinuation of insulin.[30-32] These antibodies also characterize the immunologic response of patients who develop persistent, immediate local reactions without systemic symptoms.[33] The IgE antibodies fix to tissue mast cells (and circulating basophils). When the IgE–mast cell combination is exposed to insulin, a complicated reaction causes the degranulation of the mast cells. The material released by the mast cells is composed of chemical inflammatory mediators, including large amounts of histamine, and is responsible for the urticaria and anaphylactic symptoms exhibited by patients with true insulin allergy.

Treatment of Insulin Allergy

Because pork, beef, and human insulin differ slightly in their amino acid composition (as discussed later in this section), it is theoretically possible that IgE antibodies may be directed against insulin from only one of these species and that switching insulin preparations may be of value. Although such a switch from animal to human insulin is occasionally helpful,[32, 34] true or systemic insulin allergy to human insulin has also been reported.[35-37] Despite the latter, substituting human insulin for pork or beef insulin in a patient with an immediate local skin reaction, with or without generalized urticaria, should probably be attempted before desensitization is carried out. Desensitization is the treatment of choice in a patient with anaphylactoid symptoms.

To desensitize a patient, very small but gradually increasing amounts of insulin are injected after relatively short periods. These minute doses of the antigen bind to IgE, but the amount of histamine and other chemical mediators of inflammation released by the IgE–mast cell combination is too small to cause clinical symptoms. As the dose of injected insulin is gradually increased, the amount of insulin bound to IgE is thought to increase at a slow enough pace that the resultant mast cell degranulation causes no symptoms. Eventually, little or no free (unbound to insulin) IgE remains in the circulation, and the patient can tolerate the usual therapeutic dose of insulin.

Desensitization can be achieved by either of two methods. If the patient has received insulin within the preceding 24 hours, the dose is first decreased by 80% and then increased by 3 to 5 U per injection at daily or twice-daily intervals. In this manner, many patients can be successfully desensitized. If administration of 20% of the usual insulin dose still leads to symptoms of insulin allergy or if the patient has not received insulin within the preceding 24 hours, enough unbound IgE antibodies are probably present to cause difficulties. Under these conditions, injection of more than very small amounts of insulin is extremely uncomfortable for the patient and possibly dangerous; therefore, a complete desensitization program is advisable.

A reasonable schedule for complete desensitization is presented in Table 4–12. The footnote to the table describes the four diluted insulin solutions used, and the table gives details of administration. All injections may be given subcutaneously. If rapid desen-

Table 4–12. Desensitization Schedule for Patients with True (Systemic) Insulin Allergy

Order of Doses	Solution[a]	Volume Injected (ml)	Amount of Insulin Injected (U)
1	D	0.1	0.001
2	D	0.2	0.002
3	D	0.4	0.004
4	C	0.1	0.01
5	C	0.2	0.02
6	C	0.4	0.04
7	B	0.1	0.1
8	B	0.2	0.2
9	B	0.5	0.5
10	A	0.1	1
11	A	0.2	2
12	A	0.5	5[b]

[a]Solutions are designed as follows: A, 1 ml of U-100 (regular insulin) + 9 ml of normal saline (final concentration, 10.0 U/ml); B, 1 ml of solution A + 9 ml of normal saline (final concentration, 1.0 U/ml); C, 1 ml of solution B + 9 ml of normal saline (final concentration, 0.1 U/ml); and D, 1 ml of solution C + 9 ml of normal saline (final concentration, 0.01 U/ml).

[b]Required therapeutic dose may be tried after this point.

sitization is required (i.e., if the patient's glucose levels are markedly out of control or diabetic ketoacidosis is an imminent problem and substantial amounts of insulin are needed soon), insulin is given every 30 minutes. If subtherapeutic amounts of insulin can be tolerated for a day or two, insulin is administered every 2 hours. Regular insulin is given for the first 12 injections (until a dose of 5 U is reached). After that, the required therapeutic dose of either intermediate-acting or fast-acting insulin (depending on the circumstances) may be tried.

Because human insulin will probably be the only species of insulin available in the near future, desensitization to human regular insulin should be carried out.

If a severe local or systemic reaction occurs during the gradual increase of the amount of insulin administered, the dose should be reduced by one dilution and the schedule resumed. If the weakest dilution (0.001 U) listed in Table 4–12 elicits a positive reaction, then even weaker dilutions injected *intradermally* must be tried. Whatever dilution causes no reaction, tests with gradually increasing amounts above that dilution should be continued.

During the course of desensitization, adequate anaphylactic precautions must be taken. Epinephrine, diphenhydramine, methylprednisolone (Solu-Medrol), and intubation equipment must be immediately available. A physician should be immediately available for at least 30 minutes after the administration of each increasing amount of insulin. If this restriction should prove difficult (during the night, for example), the continued administration of the last dilution that was well tolerated by the patient should be performed by an experienced nurse. In this case, injections should be given at 2-hour intervals. The presence of a physician and anaphylactic precautions are mandatory when insulin-allergic patients are receiving increasing amounts of insulin because anaphylactoid reactions can occur suddenly, even when previous smaller doses of insulin administered at 30-minute intervals have not elicited any local reactions.[38]

Desensitization is successful in approximately 95% of patients manifesting systemic insulin allergy.[29] Approximately 50% of patients with persistent local reactions of the immediate type also seem to be helped by desensitization.[29] Once desensitized, these patients should not have their insulin therapy interrupted. Because a schedule calling for at least two injections a day has the theoretic advantage of supplying insulin more constantly to the circulation (as well as usually improving diabetic control), such a regimen should probably be used for all patients who have been successfully desensitized. Indeed, treatment by continuous subcutaneous insulin infusion via an insulin pump has been successful in a patient who was not helped by desensitization to highly purified pork or human insulin.[39] However, some patients may require repeated desensitization despite continuous insulin administration.

Treatment of true insulin allergy with glucocorticoids should be avoided if possible because of the effectiveness of desensitization and the long-term adverse effects of steroid therapy. However, if repeated desensitizations are ineffective, prednisone may bring relief, probably by blocking IgE production. An initial dose of 30 to 40 mg/day should be tapered as rapidly as possible to the lowest amounts feasible, with the patient's allergic manifestations serving as the endpoint. If discontinuation of prednisone is not possible within several weeks, alternate-day therapy may be tried to minimize the adverse effects of the glucocorticoid. Alternatively, injection of dexamethasone[40] or methylprednisolone[41] via the insulin syringe has also been advocated. Because so little experience with glucocorticoid therapy for patients with true insulin allergy has been reported, it is difficult to offer firm recommendations. Fortunately, the need for glucocorticoid therapy in this situation is unusual.

Some patients develop both a delayed local reaction and a true insulin allergy (immediate reaction) concurrently.[27, 42] Taking a detailed history to differentiate the symptoms and signs of this biphasic insulin allergy is important because the treatment for each component may be different.[27]

Occasionally, these patients with systemic signs of allergy are not allergic to the insulin molecule but are reacting to the zinc,[24, 43-45] protamine,[24, 44] and/or the diluting medium[43-45] of the insulin preparation. Insulin desensitization kits obtained from two pharmaceutical companies that manufacture insulin (Lilly and Novo Nordisk) contain appropriate solutions for intradermal testing that allow one to make this diagnosis.

INSULIN RESISTANCE

Insulin resistance is defined clinically as a situation in which a patient requires more than 200 U of insulin daily for more than 2 days. This definition was coined more than 40 years ago, when it was erroneously believed that the human pancreas secreted approximately 200 U of insulin per day. Although it is now known that the normal pancreas secretes only 20 to 40 U of insulin per day, this clinical definition is helpful because it delineates a very small group of patients with a number of unusual underlying problems.

Use of the term *insulin resistance* in this context must be clearly differentiated from its more general use (usually in research areas) to describe situations in which any impairment of insulin action is noted. The broad spectrum of insulin resistance includes (1) situations in which the pancreas hypersecretes a quantity of insulin that maintains carbohydrate metabolism within normal limits; (2) mild glucose intolerance; (3) definite diabetes controlled by diet alone, by oral antidiabetes medications, or by the usual amounts of injected insulin; and (4) cases in which the insulin requirement of a patient clearly falls outside the doses required by the great majority of diabetic patients. The situations to be discussed under the clinical definition of the term *insulin resistance* represent the far end of this spectrum at which the action of insulin is markedly inhibited. For instance, although every acromegalic patient with or without diabetes mellitus manifests insulin resistance in the general sense, only those few requiring the large amounts of insulin specified in the clinical definition of this term need special therapeutic considerations.

Conditions Associated with Insulin Resistance

The conditions associated with the clinical definition of insulin resistance are listed in Table 4–13. Infection, regardless of the causative organism, clearly is a state in which insulin resistance exists, but the mechanisms involved are unknown. The insulin requirements of most diabetic patients with infections rise, but the requirement reaches 200 U per day in only a small minority of patients.

Table 4–13. Conditions Associated with Insulin Resistance

Infection
Gross obesity
Cushing's syndrome
Acromegaly
Hemochromatosis
Lipodystrophic diabetes
Acanthosis nigricans
Werner's syndrome (adult form of progeria)
Insulin degradation at injection site
Idiopathic or immune-mediated (mediated by IgG antibody)

Because the host's defenses against infections caused by bacteria and certain fungi are impaired in the setting of uncontrolled diabetes, it is important to increase the insulin dose appropriately in a vigorous attempt to lower glucose concentrations.

Although obese diabetic patients require significantly more insulin than their non-obese counterparts, relatively few obese patients could be termed insulin resistant in the clinical sense of the term. There seems to be a rough correlation between a patient's degree of obesity and the insulin requirement. The clinical approach to obese diabetic patients is considered in Chapter 7.

Glucocorticoids are potent insulin antagonists that increase hepatic gluconeogenesis (see Chapter 2) and interfere with the ability of insulin to enhance glucose use by the peripheral tissues. Most cases of insulin resistance secondary to Cushing's syndrome are iatrogenic—that is, glucocorticoid therapy is prescribed for treatment of other severe problems (asthma, lupus erythematosus, myasthenia gravis, rejection of transplanted organs, and so on). In general, the increase in the insulin requirement is proportional to the amount of glucocorticoids given. Thus, most patients classified as clinically insulin resistant are taking at least 50 mg of prednisone or its equivalent. (That is not to say that most patients taking 50 mg or more of prednisone are clinically insulin resistant.) Noniatrogenic cases of insulin resistance caused by excessive secretion of glucocorticoids are very unusual.

Acromegaly is the clinical syndrome caused by excessive secretion of growth hormone, usually from a pituitary tumor. One metabolic aspect of this syndrome is insulin resistance induced by growth hormone, the mechanism of which is unknown. Like obese patients and those affected by excessive doses of glucocorticoids, acromegalic patients may manifest a spectrum of conditions ranging from normal carbohydrate metabolism to diabetes of varying severity. Effective therapy exists for most patients with acromegaly, and those whose condition falls under the clinical definition of insulin resistance are few.

Although the great majority of patients whose diabetes is secondary to hemochromatosis do not develop clinical insulin resistance, the number of patients with clinical insulin resistance and hemochromatosis is certainly higher than would be expected. Insulin resistance has also been reported in isolated cases of acute and chronic hepatic degeneration, hepatic infarcts, common-duct stones, fatty liver, Laënnec's cirrhosis, and hepatic failure. The mechanism involved in insulin resistance associated with hemochromatosis and other liver diseases is unknown. Although most reports of such cases originated before IgG antibodies were routinely measured, the production of such antibodies clearly cannot explain many of these cases.

Patients with lipodystrophic diabetes[46] are often unresponsive to large amounts of insulin. Total lipodystrophy, often called *lipoatrophy*, is a syndrome characterized by a complete loss of adipose tissue associated with some or all of the following: ketosis-resistant diabetes, hyperlipidemia, hepatomegaly, increased basal metabolic rates (but normal thyroid test results), and acanthosis nigricans. Partial lipodystrophy, in which loss of adipose tissue occurs in only parts of the body, is more common and is also associated with some or all of the features just listed. Partial lipodystrophy takes two general forms. In the cephalothoracic form, the loss of fat occurs in the upper part of the body, with normal or even excessive amounts of adipose tissue remaining in the lower half. In the second form, the loss of fat occurs in the lower half of the body and sometimes in the upper extremities, but adipose tissue remains over the face and trunk.[47] Patients with total lipodystrophy must also constitute different syndromes. Studies have revealed prereceptor[48] (i.e., increased insulin clearance from the circulation), receptor[49] (i.e., decreased binding of insulin to its receptor), and postbinding defects[50] in various patients with total lipodystrophy. The postbinding defect could be due to a decreased function of the activated receptor once insulin is bound.[51] These rare lipoatrophic syndromes with marked systemic effects should not be confused with insulin-induced (local) lipoatrophy, one of the side effects of insulin (described later).

Insulin resistance is occasionally seen in patients who have acanthosis nigricans without lipoatrophy. Almost all such individuals studied have been females in whom obesity, hirsutism, amenorrhea, and/or polycystic ovaries were also noted. These individuals may tolerate thousands of units of insulin. Insulin resistance in these patients is caused by a marked defect in the binding of insulin to its receptor.[52] There are two clinical subtypes. In some patients (type A), both decreased binding of insulin to its receptor and decreased functioning of the activated receptor have been demonstrated. These abnormalities have been due to various genetic alterations of the insulin receptor in different patients.[53] Type A patients manifest no immunologic features. In contrast, other patients with this syndrome (type B) have antibodies to the insulin receptor itself.[52, 54] These antibodies do not affect the number of receptors available but interfere with the affinity of insulin for its receptor. Some type B patients have intermittent hypoglycemia,[55, 56] which is occasionally life threatening. The hypoglycemia is thought to be due to an insulin-like effect caused by the binding of the antireceptor antibody to the receptor. Why binding of the antireceptor antibody to the receptor only intermittently triggers postreceptor events mimicking the action of insulin is unclear. Type B patients also manifest other immunologic features, such as very high erythrocyte sedimentation rates; elevated levels of antinuclear and anti-DNA antibodies; decreased complement levels; proteinuria; elevated IgG, IgM, and IgA levels; leukopenia; alopecia; and vitiligo. The type B syndrome is one of the autoimmune diseases and has been associated with lupus erythematosus,[57, 58] scleroderma,[59] myositis,[57, 60] and both thrombocytopenia and primary biliary cirrhosis in the same patient.[61]

Werner's syndrome, the adult form of progeria,[62] is a rare familial condition that appears in adults and is characterized by diabetes, short stature, slender extremities but a stocky trunk, premature graying of the hair, baldness, cataracts, skin ulcers, early appearance of atherosclerosis, and premature death. Although diabetes is usually mild, these patients are often unresponsive to large amounts of insulin for unknown reasons.

Destruction of subcutaneously injected insulin in a 16-year-old diabetic girl has been reported.[63] This patient's condition could not be controlled by even as much as 3,000 U of injected insulin per day. Control was achieved by continuous intravenous infusion of approximately 50 to 60 U over a 24-hour period. Although a few more patients with this kind of problem have been described since the original one, this kind of insulin resistance fortunately is very rare.[64] If this cause of clinical insulin resistance can be documented, these patients respond best to continuous intravenous[65] or intraperitoneal[66] insulin.

All of the conditions listed in Table 4–13 and discussed so far can usually be easily excluded in the differential diagnosis. A patient's insulin resistance most often falls into the category described by the term *idiopathic*. In actuality, this designation is not entirely accurate because the basis for the high insulin requirement is known. Many patients receiving insulin injections develop IgG insulin-binding antibodies during the ensuing weeks or months. These antibodies are produced whether or not the patient has diabetes (e.g., they were found to be present in mentally ill patients undergoing insulin shock treatment 40 to 50 years ago). Although IgG antibody production to insulin is much less with the more pure insulin preparations used today, detectable amounts are still found in many patients. In the vast majority of diabetic patients, modest levels of IgG antibodies to insulin (<10 mU of insulin bound per milliliter) cause no difficulty. In approximately 0.1% of insulin-requiring patients, the concentration increases to very high levels (ranging from 50 to many thousands of milliunits of insulin bound per milliliter). The reason for this markedly enhanced response and the subsequent decline to normal levels is completely unknown. As with true insulin allergy, intermittent insulin therapy seems to predispose patients to insulin resistance. Indeed, both insulin allergy (IgE mediated) and insulin resistance (IgG mediated) can be found in the same patient. Although this cause of insulin resistance is an immunogenic one, nitrogen mustard, 6-mercaptopurine, and azathioprine all have been ineffective in alleviating the condition.

Treatment of Insulin Resistance

Several approaches can be effective in patients with immune-mediated (idiopathic) insulin resistance. Theoretically, it may be possible for patients to switch to another insulin preparation that the IgG antibodies either do not recognize or bind to much more weakly. Mammalian insulins differ in their primary amino acid structure only in positions 8, 9, and 10 on the A chain and position 30 on the B chain (Table 4–14). As already discussed, the less pure the insulin preparation,

Table 4–14. Species Differences in Amino Acid Sequence of Mammalian Insulins

Type of Insulin	Position			
	A Chain			B Chain
	8	9	10	30
Beef	Alanine	Serine	Valine	Alaine
Pork	Threonine	Serine	Isoleucine	Alanine
Human	Threonine	Serine	Isoleucine	Threonine
Other				
Dog	Threonine	Serine	Isoleucine	Alanine
Sperm whale	Threonine	Serine	Isoleucine	Alanine
Rabbit	Threonine	Serine	Isoleucine	Serine
Horse	Threonine	Glycine	Isoleucine	Alanine
Sheep	Alanine	Glycine	Valine	Alanine
Sei whale	Alanine	Serine	Threonine	Alanine

the greater is the potential for antibody production. On the other hand, the primary amino acid structure must also have a role because, with preparations of comparable purity, beef insulin is more antigenic than pork or human[67] insulin and pork insulin is more antigenic than human insulin of recombinant DNA origin.[68]

From a clinical point of view, switching insulin preparations is not usually an effective way to treat insulin resistance. First, although the IgG antibodies in non–insulin-resistant patients usually bind more avidly to beef insulin than to pork and human insulin, cross-reactivity does occur. Thus, although a patient's IgG may be directed primarily against beef insulin, the titers are so high that the antibodies also neutralize virtually all of the pork or human insulin. Second, because impure preparations enhance the immune response to insulin, it was hoped that purified insulin preparations would be effective in treating insulin resistance. However, this therapy has often been ineffective.[29, 69]

Finally, although two insulin preparations have been extremely effective in treating insulin resistance, neither is readily available to physicians in this country at present. If insulin is treated with sulfuric acid under the appropriate chemical conditions, the modified insulin molecule that emerges retains

some biologic activity but shows a markedly reduced affinity for binding to IgG antibodies and very little antigenicity in patients never before treated with insulin. It is not surprising, then, that sulfated beef insulin has been used effectively in therapy of insulin resistance.[70] However, although sulfated insulin was first prepared and tested by a Canadian laboratory approximately 30 years ago, it is still not available in the United States except by direct petitioning to the Food and Drug Administration.

The (nonmammalian) fish insulins differ markedly from mammalian insulins in structure. For instance, cod and beef insulins differ in 24 positions on the A chain and 9 positions on the B chain. As might be anticipated, antibodies directed against beef insulin do not bind cod insulin. However, cod insulin retains its biologic activity in mammals and therefore is effective in treating insulin resistance.[71] Unfortunately, nonmammalian insulins are not available in this country.

A third insulin preparation, which is actually an analogue of insulin,[72] has been successfully used to treat a patient with immune-mediated insulin resistance.[73] Lispro insulin (Humalog) is an insulin analogue in which the amino acids at positions 28 and 29 have been switched. The normal insulin molecule dimerizes (i.e., two molecules attach to each other), and thus absorption from the subcutaneous space is delayed somewhat. Lispro insulin is a monomer (i.e., it does not dimerize), and its absorption is much more rapid. Apparently, the monomeric analogue is much less avidly bound to insulin antibodies, thus accounting for its success in this patient. The principle here is the same as for sulfated beef and fish insulins—that is, all three are insulin preparations whose structural changes mask recognition by insulin antibodies but retain biologic activity. If further experience with lispro insulin in immune-mediated insulin resistance confirms this case report, use of this human insulin analogue will probably become the treatment of choice in this unusual situation.

If one of these three insulins is not available, switching to a more purified insulin preparation should be tried. If this is unsuccessful or if the patient developed immune-mediated insulin resistance on one of the pure preparations, other avenues of therapy are usually necessary. Some physicians treat insulin resistance with high doses of glucocorticoids. Although the mechanism by which these agents decrease insulin requirements is not known with certainty, inhibition of IgG antibody production has been postulated. Even if antibody formation were immediately curtailed, however (and this is probably not the case), high insulin requirements would persist for a while because the half-life of IgG is approximately 3 to 4 weeks. Thus, the clinical response to glucocorticoids is often delayed for 1 or 2 weeks, with initial responses occasionally occurring as late as a month after commencement of therapy. During the initial period of treatment, deterioration in diabetic control and even higher insulin requirements are common secondary to the insulin resistance caused by high doses of glucocorticoids. If this therapeutic approach is tried, doses equivalent to approximately 60 mg of prednisone should be used initially and maintained for at least several weeks or until insulin requirements

are definitely lowered. The amount of steroid administered is then decreased rapidly, until either the patient can be taken off the medication entirely or a level is reached below which insulin requirements definitely increase again. Patients frequently require 5 to 10 mg of prednisone for maintenance therapy. Some individuals who are in remission and either are taking low doses of steroids or have discontinued therapy completely may suffer relapse and need subsequent courses. In view of the adverse effects of long-term glucocorticoid administration, complete discontinuation of therapy should be attempted repeatedly. If it is not possible to discontinue treatment, alternate-day therapy should be tried, although there are no published results concerning its efficacy.

Immune-mediated insulin resistance is self-limited, with antibody titers and insulin requirements returning to the usual levels within several months to a year. Because of the potential hazards of long-term glucocorticoid administration, the relatively long lag period before this type of therapy becomes effective, the frequent deterioration in diabetic control after initiation of steroid therapy, and the temporary nature of the clinical course of insulin resistance, I avoid administering glucocorticoid therapy altogether and simply use enough insulin to keep patients asymptomatic (relatively) and to prevent the development of ketosis.

A special preparation of highly concentrated regular pork insulin (U-500) is available for this purpose. The high concentration of insulin in this preparation (500 U/ml) is very convenient for these patients because the usual U-100 insulin would have to be injected in large volumes. Even though the U-500 preparation contains regular insulin, the action is prolonged because of the extremely high antibody titers. After absorption from the subcutaneous injection site, the insulin is quickly bound by the enlarged pool of circulating IgG antibodies before it can act on the insulin-sensitive tissues. Free insulin is subsequently released at a rate that clinically approximates a time course of action between those of short- and intermediate-acting insulins. Thus, one or two injections per day of U-500 regular pork insulin in appropriate amounts usually control diabetes in a patient with immune-mediated insulin resistance. Patients seem to require much less (50% to 75%) of the U-500 preparation than the amounts of U-100 insulin for which it is substituted.[74, 75] Obviously, in this temporary situation, good control is difficult to achieve and should probably not be sought. The goals should be to keep patients from developing ketosis and to lower glucose concentrations to a degree such that the symptoms of hyperglycemia (polyuria, polydipsia, nocturia, and increased susceptibility to infection) are avoided.

Several important considerations must be kept in mind during the treatment of immune-mediated insulin resistance with U-500 regular pork insulin. Small increments in insulin dose are usually ineffective when more insulin is needed. The increase per dose should be at least 10 U and probably close to 20 U, depending on the clinical picture. That is, if a patient's glucose levels are clearly out of control and have shown little or no response to the current insulin regimen, increases of 20 to 25 U should be prescribed. If a patient has begun to respond to increased amounts of insulin, the additional increases in dose should be smaller, that is, 10 to 15 U each time. However, it must be emphasized again that responses to these large amounts of insulin are usually not consistent and predictable in patients with insulin resistance. The dose of insulin may be varied considerably with little change in glucose levels, or conversely, glucose concentrations may vary considerably despite administration of a fixed amount of insulin. Thus, simply keeping patients free of ketosis and symptomatic hyperglycemia is a realistic goal but can often be quite a therapeutic challenge.

Return of Insulin Sensitivity

Insulin sensitivity can return relatively quickly. The reason for a marked decrease in

IgG production is unknown. At this point in the clinical course, hypoglycemia can become a serious problem as the large amounts of already bound insulin are released and act on the tissues. Furthermore, the number of available binding sites for the recently injected insulin on the circulating anti-insulin IgG pool is not large. For this reason, the dose of insulin must be decreased in large decrements (20 to 40 U) once symptoms of hypoglycemia are detected. The reversal of insulin resistance is one of the few situations in which I lower the insulin dose in *anticipation* of hypoglycemia. If the fasting and/or before supper glucose concentrations are <200 mg/dl or if a patient with an appropriate T_m for glucose has negative results of tests for glucosuria at these times, the dose of insulin should be decreased. If the degree of diabetic control remains the same, further decreases in the dose of insulin should be tried until control deteriorates. If the insulin-resistant state has finally been reversed, the decrease stops when the usual therapeutic dose of insulin is reached. If not, continued administration of larger amounts of insulin and continued close follow-up are required.

A smooth transition from insulin resistance to insulin sensitivity often does not occur, and insulin requirements may have to be juggled from day to day, depending on a patient's responses. However, at some point in the clinical course, excessive production of IgG antibodies to insulin ceases, and the return of insulin sensitivity becomes obvious. This change usually takes place over several weeks, an interval consistent with the half-life of IgG antibodies. Although the timing of the decision to return to therapy with intermediate-acting insulins varies from patient to patient, once <100 U of regular insulin is being given at each injection, NPH or lente insulin generally may be tried again. A short interval (2 to 4 hours) between the injection of U-500 regular pork insulin and a clear metabolic response (marked lowering of glucose concentrations) and/or clinical symptoms of hypoglycemia suggests that the high titers of IgG antibodies have diminished; thus, a short interval of action of U-500 insulin may serve as a clue about when to resume therapy with intermediate-acting insulins.

INSULIN-INDUCED LIPOATROPHY

Insulin-induced lipoatrophy (Fig. 4-5) is a loss of subcutaneous fat at the sites of insulin injections. Although this condition seems to be more common in young females than in other patients, it certainly is not limited to this group of insulin-requiring diabetic patients. Even though this form of local lipoatrophy is a benign condition, the cosmetic effect can be disturbing, especially to adolescent girls and young women. Although the cause of this reaction is not known for certain, an immune response to contaminants in the administered insulin preparation may be involved. First, lipoatrophy was found to be two to three times more common in patients who had received the more impure preparations compared with the purified ones.[67, 76] Second, patients with lipoatrophy often describe a local delayed reaction at the site of injection,[29] a response that may be associated with delayed hypersensitivity to impurities in the insulin preparation.[21] Third, the condition of some patients improves in response to local injections of dexamethasone.[77] Fourth, abnormal deposition of immunologic components was found in the dermal vessel walls in biopsy specimens taken from lipoatrophic sites.[78, 78a] In addition, these patients had much higher serum insulin-binding capacities (IgG titers) than insulin-requiring patients without lipoatrophy.[78] Finally, cytokine (tumor necrosis factor-α and interleukin-6) production was markedly increased by macrophages of a patient with lipoatrophy.[78a]

An effective treatment is available for insulin-induced local lipoatrophy. This treatment simply (and perhaps paradoxically) involves injection of pure insulin preparations directly into the involved areas. The response is probably due to a local lipogenic effect of insulin. The technique for injection in these atrophic areas is shown in Figure 4-6, and the results 6 months later are shown in Figure 4-7. In a series of more than 300 patients,[29] more than 80% were successfully treated by injection of standard mixed beef-pork insulin, a preparation more pure than

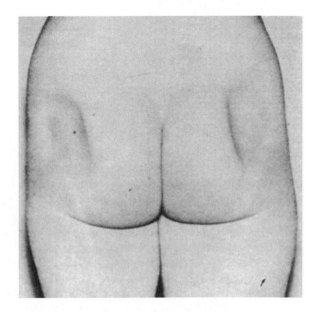

Figure 4–5. Insulin-induced lipoatrophy in a young woman. (From Mazzaferi EL: Endocrinology Case Studies. Medical Examination Publishing Co, Flushing, NY, 1975, p. 161)

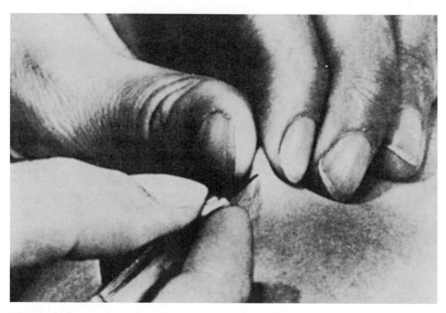

Figure 4–6. Injection of insulin into the affected area of a patient with lipoatrophy. Note the thin skin fold. (From Hulst SGTh: Treatment of insulin-induced lipoatrophy. Diabetes 25:1052, 1976)

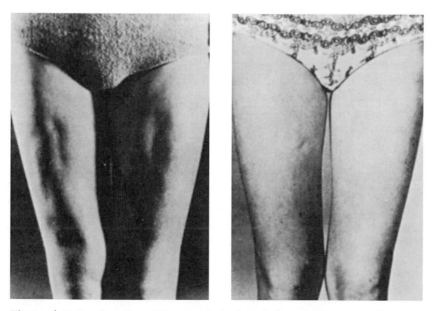

Figure 4–7. Insulin-induced lipoatrophy before (left) and after (right) 6 months of treatment with a purified insulin preparation. (From Hulst SGTh: Treatment of insulin-induced lipoatrophy. Diabetes 25:1052, 1976)

the ones used in the early 1970s. Approximately one quarter of those in whom this approach was not helpful responded to injection of a standard pork preparation. The remainder were successfully treated when a purified preparation of pork insulin was used. Human insulin was successful in a few patients in whom purified pork insulin was ineffective.[79] Thus, in keeping with an allergic basis for lipoatrophy, using the least immunogenic insulin to treat it is the most effective therapy.

Several other considerations need to be kept in mind. First, patients who may still be experiencing delayed local reactions to insulin are often refractory to treatment for lipoatrophy until the skin reaction abates. Second, local injections must be given for 2 to 4 weeks before normal subcutaneous fat tissue even begins to reaccumulate. Third, areas that have filled in may lose their fatty tissue again unless they are reinjected periodically (every 2 to 4 weeks). Fourth, although the evidence implicating an immunogenic basis for lipoatrophy is substantial and injection of pure preparations of insulin into the affected sites is "virtually 100% effective,"[29] an occasional patient develops lipoatrophy in response to subcutaneous injections of purified pork[80] or human[81-82a] insulin, even though the latter was a recombinant DNA–derived preparation.[82, 82a] I have also seen several such patients. Finally, once insulin lipoatrophy is successfully treated, use of the insulin preparation that was effective should be continued. Return to a more immunogenic preparation can be associated with recurrence of lipoatrophy both at new injection sites and in areas previously afflicted but no longer being injected after reaccumulation of fat.[29, 83]

INSULIN-INDUCED LIPOHYPERTROPHY

Some diabetic patients receiving insulin manifest lipohypertrophy of subcutaneous fat tissue at the site of injection (Fig. 4-8). This condition is no doubt due to a local lipo-

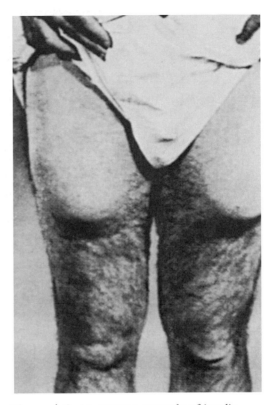

Figure 4–8. An extreme example of insulin-induced lipohypertrophy. (From Krall LP, Zorilla E: Disorders of the skin in diabetes. In Marble A, White P, Bradley RF, Krall LP [eds]: Joslin's Diabetes Mellitus. Lea & Febiger, Philadelphia, 1971, p. 654A)

genic effect of insulin. Although patients are less likely to comment on lipohypertrophy than on atrophy, an older careful study of almost 600 patients[84] revealed some increases in subcutaneous fat at the sites of insulin injection in approximately 40% of males and 18% of females less than 20 years old and in 20% of males and 12% of females older than 20 years. The use of more pure insulin preparations has not changed the approximately 20% prevalence of lipohypertrophy.[29, 85] In my experience, lipohypertrophy is also common at the abdominal sites of needle placement in patients using insulin pumps. One factor that predisposes to this reaction is repeated injections in the same

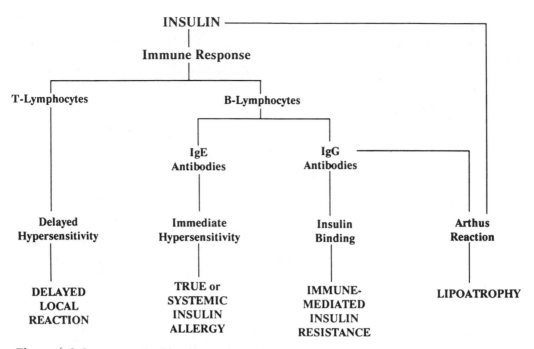

Figure 4–9. Immunogenic side effects of insulin therapy.

place.[85] Once lipohypertrophy develops, patients may tend to continue injecting at this site because many report less pain than at other sites. In addition to cosmetic considerations, continued injection into these areas is probably not wise because absorption of insulin from such sites is delayed[86, 87] and erratic.[87] Avoidance of these lipohypertrophic areas for future insulin injection sometimes results in a gradual disappearance of this extra tissue. Severe insulin-induced lipohypertrophy has been successfully treated with liposuction.[88]

Thus, except for lipohypertrophy, the pathogenesis of the other four side effects of insulin therapy seems to be immunogenic (Fig. 4-9). Stimulation of the T-lymphocyte arm of the immune system leads to delayed hypersensitivity manifested by a *delayed local reaction*. Activation of B lymphocytes leads to formation of IgE and IgG antibodies, causing *true* or *systemic insulin allergy* and *immune-mediated insulin resistance*, respectively. Finally, *lipoatrophy* may be the

result of an Arthus type of reaction in which immune complexes are formed between the antigen (insulin) and circulating (IgG insulin-binding) antibodies, causing activation of complement and infiltration of inflammatory cells.[78]

REFERENCES

1. Waife SE (ed): Diabetes Mellitus, 8th ed. Eli Lilly and Co, Indianapolis, 1980, p. 42
2. Bhaskar R, Chou MCY, Field JB: Time-action characteristics of regular and NPH insulin in insulin-treated diabetics. J Clin Endocrinol Metab 50:475, 1980
3. Galloway JA, Root MA, Bergstrom R et al: Clinical pharmacologic studies with human insulin (recombinant DNA). Diabetes Care 5(suppl 2):13, 1982
4. Ziel FH, Davidson MB, Harris MD et al: The variability in the action of unmodified insulin is more dependent on changes in tissue insulin sensitivity than on insulin absorption. Diabetic Med 5:662, 1988

5. Olsson P-O, Hans A, Henning VS: Miscibility of human semisynthetic regular and lente insulin and human biosynthetic, regular and NPH insulin. Diabetes Care 10:473, 1987

6. Robert JJ, Chevenne D, Debray M: The contribution of intermediate-acting insulin preparations to daytime insulin treatment. Diabetic Med 6:531, 1989

7. Yki-Jarvinin H, Kauppila M, Kujansuu E et al: Comparison of insulin regimens in patients with non-insulin-dependent diabetes mellitus. N Engl J Med 327:1426, 1992

8. Peters AL, Davidson MB: BIDS therapy for treatment of NIDDM: effectiveness and predictors (if any) of success. Diabetes Spectrum 7:152, 1994

9. Chow C-C, Tsang LWW, Sorensen JP et al: Comparison of insulin with or without continuation of oral hypoglycemic agents in the treatment of secondary failure in NIDDM patients. Diabetes Care 18:307, 1995

10. Shank ML, Del Prato S, DeFronzo RA: Bedtime insulin/daytime glipizide: effective therapy for sulfonylurea failures in NIDDM. Diabetes 44:165, 1995

11. Worth R, Home PD, Johnston DG et al: Intensive attention improves glycaemic control in insulin-dependent diabetes without further advantage from home blood glucose monitoring: results of a controlled trial. BMJ 285:1233, 1982

12. Starostina EG, Antsiferov M, Galstyan GR et al: Effectiveness and cost-benefit analysis of intensive treatment and teaching programmes for Type 1 (insulin-dependent) diabetes in Moscow—blood glucose versus urine glucose self-monitoring. Diabetologia 37:170, 1994

13. Muhlhauser I, Bruckner I, Berger M et al: Evaluation of an intensified insulin treatment and teaching programme as routine management of Type 1 (insulin-dependent) diabetes: the Bucharest-Dusseldorf study. Diabetologia 30:681, 1987

14. Davidson MB: The case for routinely testing the first-voided urine specimen. Diabetes Care 4:443, 1981

15. Hallas-Moller K: The lente insulins. Diabetes 5:7, 1956

16. Carlson MG, Campbell PJ: Intensive insulin therapy and weight gain in IDDM. Diabetes 42:1700, 1993

17. Saudek CD, Boulter PR, Knopp RH et al: So-dium retention accompanying insulin treatment of diabetes mellitus. Diabetes 23:240, 1974

18. Wheatley T, Edwards OM: Insulin oedema and its clinical significance: metabolic studies in three cases. Diabetic Med 2:400, 1985

19. Hopkins DFC, Cotton SJ, Williams G: Effective treatment of insulin-induced edema using ephedrine. Diabetes Care 16:1026, 1993

20. Fineberg SE, Galloway JA, Fineberg NS et al: Immunogenicity of recombinant DNA human insulin. Diabetologia 25:465, 1983

21. Ross JM: Allergy to insulin. Pediatr Clin North Am 31:675, 1984

22. Feinglos MN, Jegasothy BV: "Insulin" allergy due to zinc. Lancet 1:122, 1979

23. Nell JL, Thomas JW: Frequency and specificity of protamine antibodies in diabetic and control subjects. Diabetes 37:172, 1988

24. Shore NR, Shelley WB, Kyle CC: Chronic urticaria from isophane insulin therapy. Arch Dermatol 111:94, 1975

25. Levy JH, Ziadan JR, Faraj B: Prospective evaluation of risk of protamine reactions in patients with NPH insulin-dependent diabetes. Anesth Analg 65:739, 1986

26. Levy JH, Schwieger IM, Zaidan JR et al: Evaluation of patients at risk for protamine reactions. J Thorac Cardiovasc Surg 98:200, 1989

27. Loeb JA, Herold KC, Barton KP et al: Systematic approach to diagnosis and management of biphasic insulin allergy with local anti-inflammatory agents. Diabetes Care 12:421, 1989

28. Hanauer L, Batson JM: Anaphylactic shock following insulin injection: case report and review of the literature. Diabetes 10:105, 1961

29. Galloway JA, Bressler R: Insulin treatment in diabetes. Med Clin North Am 62:663, 1978

30. Patterson R, Mellies CJ, Roberts M: Immunologic reactions against insulin. II. IgE anti-insulin, insulin allergy and combined IgE and IgG immunologic insulin resistance. J Immunol 110:1135, 1973

31. Mattson JR, Patterson R, Roberts M: Insulin therapy in patients with systemic insulin allergy. Arch Intern Med 135:818, 1975

32. Bruni B, Barolo P, Blatto A et al: Treatment of allergy to heterologous monocomponent insulin with human semisynthetic insulin. Long-term study. Diabetes Care 11:59, 1988

33. deShazo RD, Mather P, Grant W et al: Evaluation of patients with local reactions to insulin with skin tests and in vitro techniques. Diabetes Care 10:330, 1987

34. Kristensen JS, Falholt K, Jensen I: Sensitisation to human insulin. BMJ 289:1382, 1984

35. Grammer LC, Metzger BE, Patterson R: Cutaneous allergy to human (recombinant DNA) insulin. JAMA 251:1459, 1984

36. Child DF, Johansson GO: IgE antibody studies in a case of generalized allergic reaction to human insulin. Allergy 39:630, 1984

37. Berke L, Owen JA, Atkinson RL: Allergies to human insulin. Diabetes Care 7:402, 1984

38. Goldman RA, Lewis AE, Rose LI: Anaphylactoid reaction to single-component pork insulin. JAMA 236:1148, 1976

39. Valentini U, Cimino A, Rocca L et al: CSII in management of insulin allergy. Diabetes Care 11:97, 1988

40. Wiles PG, Guy R, Watkins SM et al: Allergy to purified bovine, porcine, and human insulins. BMJ 287:531, 1983

41. Grant W, deShazo RD, Frentz J: Use of low-dose continuous corticosteroid infusion to facilitate insulin pump use in local insulin hypersensitivity. Diabetes Care 9:318, 1986

42. deShazo RD, Boehm TM, Kumar D et al: Dermal hypersensitivity reactions to insulin: correlations of three patterns to their histopathology. Allergy Clin Immunol 69:229, 1982

43. Bruni B, Campana M, Gamba S et al: A generalized allergic reaction due to zinc in insulin preparation. Diabetes Care 8:201, 1985

44. Bruni B, Barolo P, Gamba S et al: Case of generalized allergy due to zinc and protamine in insulin preparation. Diabetes Care 9:552, 1986

45. Gin H, Aubertin J: Generalized allergy due to zinc and protamine in insulin preparation treated with insulin pump. Diabetes Care 10:789, 1987

46. Senior B, Gellis SS: The syndromes of total lipodystrophy and of partial lipodystrophy. Pediatrics 33:593, 1964

47. Davidson MB, Young RT: Metabolic studies in familial partial lipodystrophy of the lower trunk and extremities. Diabetologia 11:561, 1975

48. Golden MP, Charles MA, Arquilla ER et al: Insulin resistance in total lipodystrophy: evidence for a pre-receptor defect in insulin action. Metabolism 34:330, 1985

49. Kriauciunas KM, Kahn CR, Muller-Wieland D et al: Altered expression and function of the insulin receptor in a family with lipoatrophic diabetes. J Clin Endocrinol Metab 67:1284, 1988

50. Magre J, Reynet C, Capeau J et al: In vitro studies of insulin resistance in patients with lipoatrophic diabetes. Evidence of heterogeneous postbinding defects. Diabetes 37:421, 1988

51. Magre J, Grigorescu F, Reynet C et al: Tyrosine-kinase defect of the insulin receptor in cultured fibroblasts from patients with lipoatrophic diabetes. J Clin Endocrinol Metab 69:142, 1989

52. Kahn CR, Flier JS, Bar RS et al: The syndromes of insulin resistance and acanthosis nigricans. Insulin-receptor disorders in man. N Engl J Med 294:739, 1976

53. Taylor SI: Molecular mechanisms of insulin resistance: lessons from patients with mutations in the insulin-receptor gene. Diabetes 41:1473, 1992

54. Rodriguez O, Collier E, Arakaki et al: Characterization of purified autoantibodies to the insulin receptor from six patients with type B insulin resistance. Metabolism 41:325, 1992

55. Flier JS, Bar RS, Muggeo M et al: The evolving clinical course of patients with receptor autoantibodies: spontaneous remission or receptor proliferation with hypoglycemia. J Clin Endocrinol Metab 47:985, 1978

56. Taylor SI, Barbetti F, Accili D et al: Syndromes of autoimnmunity and hypoglycemia: autoantibodies directed against insulin and its receptor. Endocrinol Metab Clin North Am 18:123, 1989

57. Tsokos GC, Gorden P, Antonovych T et al: Lupus nephritis and other autoimmune features in patients with diabetes mellitus due to autoantibody to insulin receptors. Ann Intern Med 102:176, 1985

58. Di Paolo S, Giorgino R: Insulin resistance and hypoglycemia in a patient with systemic lupus erythematosus: description of antiinsulin receptor antibodies that enhance insulin binding and inhibit insulin action. J Clin Endocrinol Metab 73:650, 1991

59. Bloise W, Wajchenberg BL, Moncada VY et al: Atypical antiinsulin receptor antibodies in a patient with type B insulin resistance and scleroderma. J Clin Endocrinol Metab 68:227, 1989

60. Fonseca V, Khokher MA, Dandona P: Insulin receptor antibodies causing steroid responsive diabetes mellitus in a patient with myositis. BMJ 288:1578, 1984

61. Selinger S, Tsai J, Pulini M et al: Autoimmune thrombocytopenia and primary biliary cirrhosis with hypoglycemia and insulin receptor autoantibodies. A case report. Ann Intern Med 107:686, 1987

62. Epstein CJ, Martini GM, Schultz AL, Motulsky AG: Werner's syndrome: a review of its symptomatology, natural history, pathological features, genetics, and relationship to the natural aging process. Medicine 45:177, 1966

63. Paulsen EP, Courtney JW III, Duckworth WC: Insulin resistance caused by massive degradation of subcutaneous insulin. Diabetes 28:640, 1979

64. Shade DS, Duckworth WC: In search of the subcutaneous-insulin-resistance syndrome. N Engl J Med 315:147, 1986

65. Paterson KR, Campbell IW, MacRury SM et al: Management of diabetes resistant to subcutaneous insulin with intravenous insulin via an implanted infusion pump. Scot Med J 33:239, 1988

66. Fonseca VA, Menon RK, Shaghn O'Brien PM et al: Successful pregnancy in diabetic controlled with intraperitoneal insulin. Diabetes Care 10:541, 1987

67. Wilson RM, Douglas CA, Tattersall RB et al: Immunogenicity of highly purified bovine insulin: a comparison with conventional bovine and highly purified human insulins. Diabetologia 28:667, 1985

68. Fineberg SE, Galloway JA, Fineberg NS et al: Immunogenicity of recombinant DNA human insulin. Diabetologia 25:465, 1983

69. Yue DK, Turtle JR: New forms of insulin and their use in the treatment of diabetes. Diabetes 26:341, 1977

70. Davidson JK, DeBra DW: Immunologic insulin resistance. Diabetes 27:307, 1978

71. Yalow RS, Berson SA: Reaction of fish insulins with human insulin antiserums. Potential value in the treatment of insulin resistance. N Engl J Med 270:1171, 1964

72. Howey DC, Bowsher RR, Brunelle RL et al: [Lys(B28), Pro(B29)]-human insulin: a rapidly absorbed analogue of human insulin. Diabetes 43:396, 1994

73. Lahtela JT, Knip M, Paul R et al: Severe anti- body-mediated human insulin resistance: successful treatment with the insulin analog lispro. Diabetes Care 20:71, 1997

74. Nathan SM, Axelrod L, Flier JS et al: U-500 insulin in the treatment of antibody-mediated insulin resistance. Ann Intern Med 94:653, 1981

75. Baumann G, Drobny EC: Enhanced efficacy of U-500 insulin in the treatment of insulin resistance caused by target tissue insensitivity. Am J Med 76:529, 1984

76. Deckert T, Andersen OO, Poulsen JE: The clinical significance of highly purified pig-insulin preparations. Diabetologia 10:703, 1974

77. Kumar D, Miller LV, Mehtalia SD: Use of dexamethasone in treatment of insulin lipoatrophy. Diabetes 26:296, 1977

78. Reeves WG, Allen BR, Tattersall RB: Insulin-induced lipoatrophy: evidence for an immune pathogenesis. BMJ 1:1500, 1980

78a. Altan-Gepner C, Bongrand P, Farnarier C et al: Insulin-induced lipoatrophy in type 1 diabetes: a possible tumor necrosis factor-α-mediated dedifferentiation of adipocytes. Diabetes Care 19:1283, 1996

79. Valenta LJ, Elias AN: Insulin-induced lipodystrophy in diabetic patients resolved by treatment with human insulin. Ann Intern Med 102:790, 1985

80. Ramachandran A, Mohan V, Snehalatha C et al: Lipoatrophy with monocomponent insulins: two case reports. Diabetes Care 10:133, 1987

81. Rosman MS: Fat atrophy in human insulin therapy. Diabetes Care 9:436, 1986

82. Page MD, Bodansky HJ: Human insulin and lipoatrophy. Diabetic Med 9:779, 1992

82a. Jaap AJ, Horn HM, Tidman MJ et al: Lipoatrophy with human insulin. Diabetes Care 19:1289, 1996

83. Teuscher A: Treatment of insulin lipoatrophy with monocomponent insulin. Diabetologia 10:211, 1974

84. Marble A, Renold AE: Atrophy of subcutaneous fat following injections of insulin. Proc Am Diabetes Assoc 2:171, 1942

85. Young RJ, Steel JM, Frier BM et al: Insulin injection sites in diabetes—a neglected area? BMJ 283:349, 1981

86. Kolendorf K, Bojsen J, Deckert T: Clinical factors influencing the absorption of ^{125}I-NPH insulin in diabetic patients. Horm Metab Res 15:274, 1982

87. Young RJ, Hannan WJ, Frier BM et al: Diabetic lipohypertrophy delays insulin absorption. Diabetes Care 7:479, 1984

88. Hardy KJ, Gill GV, Bryson JR: Severe insulin-induced lipohypertrophy successfully treated by liposuction. Diabetes Care 16:929, 1993

CHAPTER 5

ORAL ANTIDIABETES AGENTS

SULFONYLUREA AGENTS

BACKGROUND

During World War II, French scientists studying the antibiotic potential of modified sulfonamides noted that the patients (especially those who were malnourished) used in their experiments were unexpectedly dying. Further investigation revealed that hypoglycemia was the cause of death. Because of the overwhelming need for and interest in the antibiotic properties of the sulfonamides, this serendipitous discovery was not considered further until after the war. The first sulfonylurea agent, carbutamide, was introduced into clinical practice for the treatment of diabetes mellitus in 1955 in Germany. (Its use was subsequently discontinued in the United States because of adverse reactions.) Tolbutamide (Orinase) was introduced in the United States the following year, and chlorpropamide (Diabinese) became available a year later. In the 1960s, two more sulfonylurea agents, acetohexamide (Dymelor) and tolazamide (Tolinase), were introduced into clinical practice in the United States. Thus, four sulfonylurea compounds, whose chemical structures are shown in Figure 5–1, have been available in the United States for the treatment of diabetes mellitus for more than 30 years and therefore are known as *first-generation agents*. The sulfonylurea component of these compounds, which is responsible for their hypoglycemic effects, is enclosed by dashed lines in the figure. The different groups attached to the common sul-

fonylurea structure give each compound unique pharmacokinetic properties.

In 1984, two sulfonylurea compounds that had been used in Europe for many years were introduced into the United States. These second-generation agents are glyburide (Micronase, DiaBeta, Glynase) and glipizide (Glucotrol, Glucotrol XL) (Fig. 5–2). In 1996, another sulfonylurea agent, glimepiride (Amaryl), was approved by the Federal Drug Administration for use in this country.

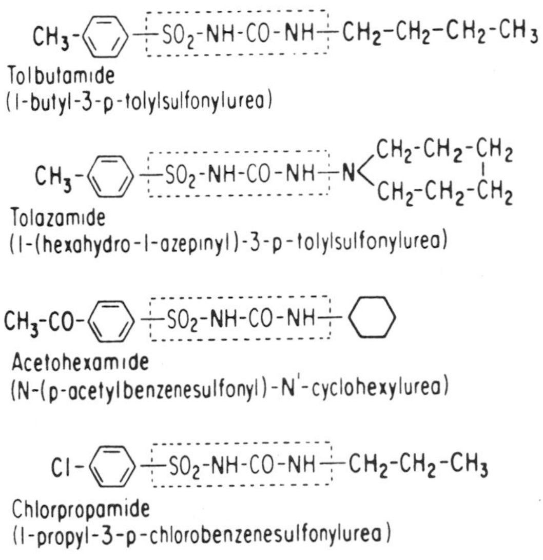

Figure 5–1. Chemical structure of the four first-generation sulfonylurea agents. The common sulfonylurea structure, enclosed by dotted lines, is the active component of each molecule. The attached groups are responsible for the various metabolic fates of each drug. (From Williams RH, Porte D Jr: The pancreas. In Williams RH, ed, Textbook of Endocrinology, 5th ed. WB Saunders, Philadelphia, 1974, p. 502)

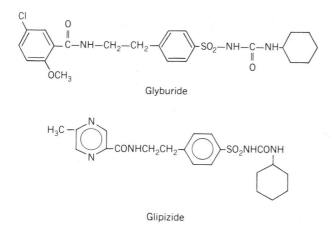

Glyburide

Glipizide

Figure 5–2. Chemical structure of the two second-generation sulfonylurea agents available for use in the United States.

MECHANISM OF ACTION

Sulfonylurea agents are ineffective in animals whose β-cells have been removed by pancreatectomy or destroyed by chemicals. These compounds do not work in diabetic patients who are ketosis prone—the biochemical manifestation of marked insulin deficiency (see Chapter 2). With the advent of a radioimmunoassay that could measure insulin concentrations in the physiologic range, these levels were found to be increased in both peripheral and portal veins after the *acute* administration of these compounds. These data strongly suggested that the hypoglycemic effect of the sulfonylurea agents is due to stimulation of insulin secretion. However, the situation after long-term administration of sulfonylurea agents is more complex. Glucose concentrations are lower, and insulin levels are either unchanged[1-3] or, more likely, increased.[3] A number of studies have demonstrated that sulfonylurea agents sensitize the pancreatic β-cells to glucose and other secretagogues.[4, 5] The β-cell response, however, is dependent on the prevailing glucose levels, and thus interpretation of the insulin response is complicated. This phenomenon is illustrated by the following observation. The insulin response to intravenous administration of the β-adrenergic agonist isoproterenol and the amino acid arginine is similar in type 2 diabetic patients

before and after sulfonylurea agent therapy.[6] However, as just stated, the response to these non–glucose-secretagogues is dependent on the prevailing glucose concentrations, which are obviously lower after treatment. If the glucose concentrations are artificially raised to the value before treatment, insulin secretion in patients on therapy is markedly enhanced compared with their initial responses.[6] These relationships are depicted in Figure 5-3.

The mechanism by which sulfonylurea agents enhance the β-cell response has been delineated in recent years.[4, 5] Insulin secretion follows depolarization of the β-cell membrane, which leads to opening of voltage-dependent calcium channels and an influx of calcium ions. The increase in intracellular calcium triggers the release of insulin by a mechanism that is not clearly understood. Glucose-stimulated insulin secretion occurs after the entry and subsequent metabolism of glucose by the β-cells. This leads to increased adenosine triphosphate (ATP) synthesis, which in turn blocks an ATP-sensitive potassium channel (Fig. 5–4). The closure of these ATP-sensitive potassium channels depolarizes the β-cell membrane, and the pathways of insulin secretion are stimulated as just described. Sulfonylurea agents bind to a receptor that is either closely linked to or possibly part of this ATP-sensitive potassium channel and in this manner

Figure 5–3. The acute insulin response (AIR) to arginine before (U) and during chronic chlorpropamide therapy (Rx). The responses during treatment were measured both at the new lowered basal glucose concentration and after the glucose level was artificially raised to values noted before therapy. (From Judewitsch RG, Pfeifer MA, Best JD, et al: Chronic chlorpropamide therapy of noninsulin-dependent diabetes augments basal and stimulated insulin secretion by increasing islet sensitivity to glucose. J Clin Endocrinol Metab 55:321, 1982)

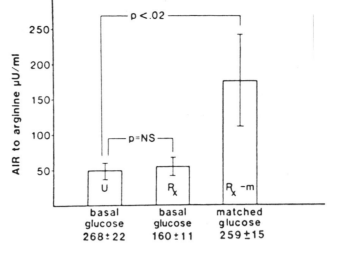

enhance both glucose-induced insulin secretion and the insulin response to nonglucose stimuli.

Four other potential mechanisms by which sulfonylurea agents may help reduce glucose concentrations have been proposed.[4, 5] Strong evidence shows that these drugs potentiate the action of insulin on peripheral tissues (i.e., adipose tissue, muscle, and liver). This effect occurs at a step of hormone action that is distal to insulin binding to its receptor. Second, they may reduce the hepatic extraction of insulin, 50% of which is normally cleared on each passage

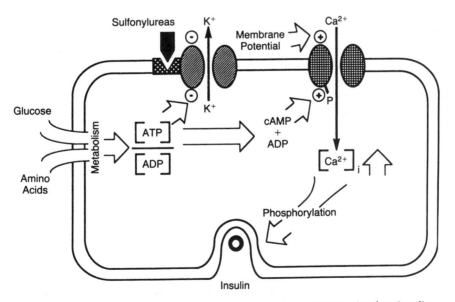

Figure 5–4. Proposed mechanism by which sulfonylurea agents stimulate insulin secretion. ATP, adenosine triphosphate; ADP, adenosine diphosphate; cAMP, cyclic adenosine monophosphate; P, phosphate; K^+, potassium ion; Ca^{2+}, calcium ion. (From Gerich JE: Oral hypoglycemic agents. N Engl J Med 321:1231, 1989)

through the liver, thus leading to higher hormone concentrations in the peripheral circulation. Third, sulfonylurea agents may directly (in the absence of insulin) suppress hepatic glucose production. Finally, these drugs reduce glucagon levels. It must be emphasized, however, that these non–β-cell effects of sulfonylurea agents cannot be clinically important because they are ineffective in type 1 diabetic patients and animal models of diabetes in which insulin secretion has been abolished.

PHARMACOLOGY

Sulfonylurea agents are rapidly absorbed from the gastrointestinal tract. The time course of their absorption does not vary with age[7] but may be reduced by hyperglycemia in both normal[8] and diabetic[9] subjects, possibly secondary to decreased gastric motility. Appreciable concentrations in plasma can be measured by 1 hour after ingestion. The compounds are transported in the blood bound to serum proteins, mostly albumin. Plasma levels of drug vary widely for reasons that are not entirely clear. In the case of tolbutamide, rates of disappearance vary over a 10-fold range among individuals. This variation is due to genetic differences in the enzyme of the rate-limiting degradative step.[10] Thus, although generalizations are made about the pharmacology of these drugs, the data cited may not strictly apply to individual patients.

Tolbutamide is oxidized in the liver, and its metabolites, which are inactive, are excreted by the kidneys. The approximate half-life of the parent compound is 4 to 5 hours, and the duration of action is from 6 to 12 hours. Therefore, this drug should be taken 2 or 3 times a day.

Early investigators originally concluded that chlorpropamide was not metabolized in humans but rather was simply bound to serum proteins and excreted in the urine. This metabolic fate would account for its long half-life of about 36 hours and its prolonged duration of action of up to 60 hours. However, subsequent experiments showed that most of the drug administered was recovered in the form of urinary metabolites.[4] From a clinical viewpoint, the prolonged duration of action not only suggests that the metabolites must have hypoglycemic activity[4] but allows administration of the drug only once a day. Because of its long half-life, however, steady-state levels are not reached for 7 to 10 days.

Acetohexamide is degraded by the liver and kidneys. Its metabolites, however, have hypoglycemic activity, and one of them, hydroxyhexamide, is 2.5 times as active as the parent compound. The metabolites are excreted by the kidneys. The fact that hydroxyhexamide is actively secreted by the renal tubules probably accounts for its uricosuric effect, mediated via inhibition of tubular reabsorption of uric acid. (In type 2 diabetes with hyperuricemia, an additional benefit of acetohexamide is a mild decrease in serum concentrations of uric acid.[11]) Therefore, although the half-life of acetohexamide is 1 to 2 hours, its duration of action ranges from 12 to 24 hours mainly because of the activity of hydroxyhexamide, whose half-life is 4 to 5 hours. The drug is given once or twice per day, depending on the dose.

Tolazamide is metabolized to six major byproducts, one of which has some hypoglycemic activity. However, the effect of the metabolite is weaker than that of the parent compound. The degradative products are excreted by the kidneys. The serum half-life of tolazamide and its active metabolite is about 7 hours. The duration of action ranges from 12 to 24 hours, and the drug is given once or twice a day, depending on the dose.

Glyburide is metabolized in the liver. Two of its degradative products have been shown to have considerable hypoglycemic activity.[12] The metabolites are excreted roughly equally by the kidneys, appearing in the urine, and by the biliary tract, appearing in the feces. The serum half-life is approximately 10 hours, and the drug has a duration of action up to 24 hours. It is given once or twice a day, depending on the dose. A micronized formulation (Glynase) that is available is absorbed more completely than DiaBeta or Micronase. This increased bioavailability simply means that lower doses are used. Otherwise, there is no difference between the micronized and nonmicronized preparations of glyburide.

Glipizide is almost completely inactivated in the liver, and the degradative products are excreted in the urine. The serum half-life of the parent compound is approximately 3 to 4 hours. Its therapeutic effect has been reported to range between 10 and 24 hours. Glucotrol is given once or twice a day, depending on the dose. A long-acting form of glipizide (Glucotrol XL) is now available. Once-a-day dosing is appropriate for this formulation.

Glimepiride is metabolized in the liver to products that have no more than one third of the biologic activity of the parent compound. Like the metabolites of glyburide, they are excreted about equally by the liver and kidneys.

SIDE EFFECTS (Table 5-1)

Sulfonylurea agents have been taken by millions of people with diabetes for a number of years and are well tolerated by most patients. The prevalence of side effects is <5%; use of the drugs must be discontinued in only 1% to 2%. Hypoglycemia, although considered to be an adverse effect, is actually an extension of the pharmacologic effect of the sulfonylurea agents.

The most common side effects of the sulfonylurea agents are gastrointestinal and cutaneous. The gastrointestinal effects are dose related and may disappear when the dose is reduced. These reactions often abate within several weeks even if the dose is not reduced. The gastrointestinal symptoms include anorexia, heartburn, nausea with occasional vomiting, feelings of abdominal fullness, and flatulence. The common adverse cutaneous effects are morbilliform, maculopapular, or urticarial rashes, which are often characterized by erythema and pruritus. Some cross-reactivity may occur among the sulfonylurea agents.

Disulfiram-like reactions have been reported to occur with chlorpropamide therapy. Disulfiram (Antabuse) is a drug used in the treatment of alcoholism. The first degradative product of ethanol is acetaldehyde, which is further metabolized to acetyl coen-

Table 5–1. Side Effects of Sulfonylurea Agents

More Common	Rare
Gastrointestinal	*Skin Lesions*
Anorexia	Photosensitivity
Heartburn	Lichenoid eruptions
Nausea with occasional vomiting	Erythema multiforme
Abdominal distention	Exfoliative dermatitis
Flatulence	
	Hematologic Disorders
Rash	Leukopenia
Morbilliform	Agranulocytosis
Maculopapular	Aplastic anemia
Urticarial	Hemolytic anemia
Other (Chlorpropamide Only)	*Hepatic Disorders*
Alcohol flushing syndrome	Intrahepatic cholestasis (chlorpropamide usually, but
Hyponatremia (syndrome of inappropriate antidiuretic hormone secretion)	others also)
	Hepatitis (glyburide)

zyme A. Disulfiram inhibits the enzyme for the latter reaction, which causes an accumulation of acetaldehyde. The build up of acetaldehyde causes some or all of the following reactions within 5 to 10 minutes of alcohol ingestion: feelings of warmth, flushing, headache, nausea, vomiting, sweating, and thirst. More severe reactions occur occasionally, including respiratory difficulty, chest pain, hypotension, orthostatic syncope, confusion, and vertigo. Reactions can last from 30 minutes to several hours. Chlorpropamide also inhibits this enzyme, but much less completely. Only relatively mild symptoms usually develop in the disulfiram-like reactions precipitated by chlorpropamide. The prevalence of these reactions is unclear; various reports have cited prevalences from <1% to 33% among patients taking chlorpropamide. This discrepancy is obviously related to the amount of alcohol consumed by patients and the perseverance of the physician in questioning patients.

The other side effects of the sulfonylurea agents are uncommon (<1%) or rare (isolated case reports). Other skin reactions include photosensitivity, lichenoid eruptions, erythema multiforme, and exfoliative dermatitis. Adverse hematologic effects include leukopenia, agranulocytosis, thrombocytopenia, hemolytic or aplastic anemia, or pancytopenia. Intrahepatic cholestatic jaundice, most commonly with chlorpropamide therapy, has been reported; this condition is usually reversed by discontinuation of the drug. Three patients with possible glyburide-induced hepatitis have been reported.[13, 14] Fevers, eosinophilia, nonspecific proctocolitis, hepatic porphyria, and porphyria cutanea tarda have also been reported. Sulfonylurea agents may decrease the thyroidal uptake of radioactive iodine to some extent, but they have not been shown to cause goiters or hypothyroidism.

Chlorpropamide[15, 16] and rarely tolbutamide may cause the syndrome of inappropriate secretion of antidiuretic hormone (SIADH). The drugs cause this condition not only by stimulating the release of the hormone by the hypothalamus but also by potentiating its inhibitory effect on free water excretion by the distal renal tubule. Therefore, serum sodium concentrations decline to abnormally low levels, and patients can present with headache and lethargy that may progress to stupor, coma, and seizures. Elderly patients are much more susceptible to this effect, especially if they are also taking a diuretic. The other sulfonylurea agents do not cause SIADH. Some of them even appear to have a mild diuretic effect, which is not of any clinical significance.

A number of years ago, the University Group Diabetes Program (UGDP) reported that patients taking the sulfonylurea agent tolbutamide had higher cardiovascular mortality than those treated with diet alone or insulin.[17, 18] Specifically, 823 patients were randomized into one of four treatment groups as follows: (1) a fixed dose (1.5 g) of tolbutamide; (2) lactose placebo; (3) intermediate-acting insulin given in a conventional manner to lower glucose concentrations to near euglycemia if possible; and (4) a standard dose of intermediate-acting insulin (10 to 16 U, depending on body size) to determine if insulin had any effects independent of its glucose-lowering capabilities. Eight years after recruitment of patients began, the use of tolbutamide was discontinued. The UGDP investigators concluded that tolbutamide therapy was associated with a significant increase in mortality due to cardiovascular causes compared with patients receiving the placebo medication. If true, these results would have an important bearing on the treatment of type 2 diabetic patients.

However, in my view, at least three major defects in the UGDP study invalidate its conclusions. First, although patients were randomized into the treatment groups, unfortunately and inexplicably, patients receiving tolbutamide had more baseline cardiovascular risk factors than the placebo group. In fact, the differences in two very important risk factors, total cholesterol levels and one or more major electrocardiographic abnormalities, reached statistical significance. Second, the cardiovascular mortality in the placebo group was inexplicably low compared with the tolbutamide group during the period in which the sulfonylurea agent was being used in the study.

The third drawback to the UGDP study was the manner in which data for patients who dropped out of the study or whose medication was changed were handled statistically. The usual procedure in therapeutic trials is to exclude data for such patients from statistical analysis and not to ascribe subsequent events to the patients' original treatment.[19] The UGDP investigators chose to ascribe all subsequent events to the original treatment, regardless of whether the patient had discontinued the treatment or had been switched to another form of therapy. Approximately 25% of patients in both the tolbutamide groups and the placebo group had either dropped out (i.e., were unavailable for follow-up for ≥1 year) or changed medications by the time the use of tolbutamide was discontinued.[20] Thus, the deaths of some patients were attributed to a form of treatment to which they had not been exposed for a number of years before their demise.

Thus, serious questions can be raised about the validity of the conclusion reached by the UGDP study that tolbutamide therapy is associated with a significant increase in mortality due to cardiovascular causes. These and related arguments caused the American Diabetes Association, which initially supported the UGDP study, to reassess its position and withdraw its endorsement.[21]

In addition to these arguments against the UGDP study, five other prospective studies have investigated the cardiovascular events in patients taking sulfonylurea agents, usually tolbutamide.[22-26] None of these reported a deleterious effect of these drugs on the cardiovascular system. Although the design of each of these prospective studies was some-

what different from that of the UGDP study, the number of patients treated with tolbutamide was more than twice the number in the UGDP study,[17] and they were observed for similar periods. Second, in none of the studies (including the UGDP study) was the incidence of nonfatal cardiovascular events increased in patients taking tolbutamide. This fact speaks against a generalized toxic effect of tolbutamide on the vasculature, because if such an effect were exerted, more morbidity (in addition to higher mortality) would be expected. If the conclusions of the UGDP study are valid at all, tolbutamide must affect a patient's ability to survive such an event instead of causing conditions that are more likely to precipitate the event. Finally, a retrospective analysis of 239 diabetic patients monitored for 16 years in the well-known Framingham Study also failed to link sulfonylurea agents with excessive cardiovascular mortality.[27]

Therefore, in view of all of these data (described in much greater detail in the second edition of this book), I do not hesitate to prescribe sulfonylurea agents to type 2 diabetic patients under the appropriate conditions. This conclusion is based on what I perceive to be serious flaws in the UGDP study and the lack of supporting evidence in the six studies briefly mentioned.

DRUG INTERACTIONS

Other drugs can affect the hypoglycemic action of sulfonylurea agents in two general ways. First, drugs that either impair glucose tolerance or cause hypoglycemia would be expected to influence the effect of sulfonylurea agents in diabetic patients. This interaction would be *indirect*, because the interfering drugs would act by the same mechanisms as in nondiabetic subjects. Potassium-losing diuretics, glucocorticoids, estrogen compounds, and phenytoin (Dilantin) can impair the action of sulfonylurea agents. Conversely, salicylates, propranolol, monoamine oxidase inhibitors (of the hydrazine type), disopyramide, pentamidine, quinine, and ethanol (although not a prescribed drug) might indirectly potentiate the hypoglycemic effect of sulfonylurea agents.

Second, drugs may have a *direct* effect on the action of the sulfonylurea agents—that is, an interaction occurs in which the interfering drug affects the absorption, distribution, metabolism, or excretion of the sulfonylurea agents themselves. For instance, phenylbutazone enhances the hypoglycemic effect of acetohexamide by interfering with the renal excretion of hydroxyhexamide, its major degradative product, which is more potent than the parent compound. A moderate number of drugs displace the sulfonylurea agents from their albumin binding sites, interfere with the enzymes responsible for their degradation, and/or alter their half-lives in the circulation.[28, 29] However, some of these effects are contradictory; for example, although displacement of sulfonylurea agents from albumin binding sites should decrease their half-lives, a number of drugs have been found to displace these agents and to increase their half-lives. Furthermore, most of these interfering drugs have not been shown to have a clinical effect on the action of sulfonylurea agents. Therefore, only the relatively few drugs that have actually caused hypoglycemia by potentiating the effects of the sulfonylurea agents are considered here.

Sulfonamides are the most important class of drugs that potentiate the effect of sulfonylurea agents by displacing them from their albumin binding sites.[28, 29] Older drugs that have also caused hypoglycemia in patients taking sulfonylurea agents, probably by the same mechanism, are phenylbutazone (Butazolidin) and clofibrate (Atromid-S).[28, 29] Chloramphenicol (Chloromycetin) and *bis*-hydroxycoumarin (dicumarol) have also caused hypoglycemia in patients taking sulfonylurea agents, probably by inhibiting hepatic microsomal enzymes involved in drug degradation.

One final point should be made about drug interactions involving sulfonylurea

agents. The nonpolar character of the side chains of the second-generation agents causes them to bind to serum proteins (primarily albumin) by nonionic forces. This is in contrast to the ionic binding of the first-generation compounds. This difference in binding plus the much smaller doses of the second-generation sulfonylurea agents could theoretically lead to fewer drug interactions with glyburide and glipizide than the first-generation ones. However, to my knowledge and that of another reviewer,[28] no clinical evidence supports this supposition. I have seen sulfonamide-induced hypoglycemia in several patients taking second-generation sulfonylurea agents.[29a]

GENERAL GUIDELINES FOR CLINICAL USE

Patients with diabetes present with one of three general levels of symptoms: (1) asymptomatic; (2) mildly symptomatic (slight increase in urination with compensatory increased fluid ingestion); or (3) markedly symptomatic (marked polyuria, polydipsia, nocturia, polyphagia with weight loss). Glucose concentrations in the latter group often exceed 400 mg/dl. Young (<30 years old), lean patients in the third group, especially if significant ketosis is present, most likely have type 1 diabetes and require insulin. Although all of the others have type 2 diabetes, the initial treatment differs. All patients require nutritional (and exercise—see Chapter 7) counseling, but diet therapy alone should be used in asymptomatic patients. There is no justification for exposing patients to potential side effects of drugs if diet alone is effective. Diet alone may also be appropriate for obese patients with only mild, easily tolerated symptoms. Therapeutic decisions after the first month of diet treatment are shown in Table 5-2.

Patients failing to respond to diet alone or those whose mild symptoms are deemed severe enough to require pharmacologic therapy are started on small amounts of an oral drug (Table 5-3). Because it takes ap-

Table 5–2. Guidelines for Therapeutic Decision After 1 Month of Initial Treatment with Diet Alone in Asymptomatic or Mildly Symptomatic Type 2 Diabetic Patients

Fasting Plasma Glucose Concentration (mg/dl)

Initial	*After First Month*	*Decision*
>300[a]	>300	Start oral drug
>300	<300; <50 decrease	Start oral drug
>300	<300; >50 decrease	Continue diet alone[b]
200–300	≥200; <50 decrease	Start oral drug
200–300	≥200; >50 decrease	Continue diet alone[b]
200–300	<200	Continue diet alone[b]
<200	≥200	Start oral drug
<200	<200	Continue diet alone[b]

[a] Unlikely to be asymptomatic or to have only mild symptoms unless the renal threshold for glucose is very high.

[b] Fasting plasma glucose concentration and glycated hemoglobin level should be measured at the end of the second month, and further therapeutic decisions based on goals and principles used to treat patients on long-term therapy (see text).

proximately five half-lives for a newly administered drug to reach equilibrium concentrations, the response to the drug should be evaluated 1 to 2 weeks later by measuring a fasting plasma glucose (FPG) level. The goal is to reduce the FPG concentration to <140 mg/dl. To achieve this, the dose of the oral agent should be increased in small incremental steps every 2 weeks or so until the FPG level is <140 mg/dl or the maximal dose for that drug is reached. The ultimate goal is to achieve a glycated hemoglobin level of <1.5% above the upper limit of normal for the assay used. This test, however, requires 2 to 3 months to reflect the new levels of glycemia and cannot be used to judge the initial response to changes in therapy. (How to proceed when the maximal dose of a sulfonylurea agent is reached and control is unsatisfactory as reflected in glycated hemoglobin levels measured at least 2 to 3 months after initiating therapy or on a more chronic basis is addressed later.)

A third (overriding) factor that drives therapeutic decisions about sulfonylurea agents, in addition to FPG and glycated hemoglobin levels, is hypoglycemia. Hypoglycemia in the late afternoon or late morning, if lunch is delayed, is not uncommon in patients taking

Table 5–3. Recommended Initial Doses of Sulfonylurea Agents for Type 2 Diabetic Patients

	Initial Dose (mg)		
	Asymptomatic Diet Failures*[a] *or Patients with Mild* *Symptoms with Indicated FPG		
Agent	*<180 mg/dl*	*>180 mg/dl*[b]	***Markedly Symptomatic Patients*[c]**
Tolbutamide (Orinase)	500[d]	1,000[d]	—
Acetohexamide (Dymelor)	250	500	—
Tolazamide (Tolinase)	100	250	1,000 (500)
Chlorpropamide[e] (Diabinese)	100	250	750 (250)
Glyburide (DiaBeta, Micronase)	1.25	2.5	20 (7.5)
Glipizide (Glucotrol)	2.5	5.0	40 (15)
Glyburide (Glynase)	0.075	1.5	12 (6)
Glipizide (Glucotrol XL)	2.5	5.0	20 (10)
Glimepiride (Amaryl)	1.0	2.0	8 (4)

FPG, fasting plasma glucose concentration.

[a] Relatively asymptomatic patients should be treated with diet alone initially (see text for full discussion).

[b] For patients >65 years old, use dose for younger patient with FPG <180 mg/dl.

[c] Dose in parentheses indicates starting dose for patients >65 years of age. Increase quickly after 1 week if no response seen.

[d] Total dose given twice per day.

[e] Chlorpropamide should not be a first-line agent in patients >65 years of age.

sulfonylurea agents, even when the FPG concentration is >140 mg/dl.[30, 31] If documented, either by measurement or by a compelling description (signs and/or symptoms promptly relieved by ingestion of simple carbohydrate), the presence of hypoglycemia dictates a change in therapy regardless of FPG and glycated hemoglobin levels (Table 5-4). Thus, FPG concentrations measured approximately 2 weeks after a dose change reflect the response to that change, and glycated hemoglobin levels measured every 2 to 3 months reflect the average glycemia during the preceding period and drive therapeutic decisions regardless of the FPG concentrations. Hypoglycemia takes precedence over the other two.

Although in the past I used 1- to 2-hour postprandial glucose concentrations to monitor patients in whom FPG levels were <140 mg/dl,[32] I rarely do so at present for three reasons. First, postprandial values are dependent on the carbohydrate content of the meal and the time elapsed between eating and blood sampling. Some patients manipulate these variables to "look good" to their health care provider. Second, it is difficult for some working people to arrange their schedules to go to a laboratory or their doctor's office at the appropriate time to have a postprandial glucose concentration measured. Third, in my experience, postprandial glucose levels do not seem to correlate as well with glycated hemoglobin values

as do FPG concentrations. This is perhaps not surprising because FPG levels are fairly stable in type 2 diabetic patients not taking insulin and are obviously independent of meal content and timing of sampling. Measuring postprandial glucose concentrations is helpful, however, in one situation—that is, in those patients in whom the FPG level is <100 mg/dl but the glycated hemoglobin level is >1.5% above the upper limit of normal for the assay used when measured at least 2 months after the last change of oral drug therapy. It is possible that these are the unusual patients whose postprandial rise of glucose concentrations are high enough to yield such a glycated hemoglobin level. If this should prove to be the case when postprandial glucose concentrations are measured, either a cautious increase in the dose of the sulfonylurea agent or introducing metformin or acarbose is indicated.

Although many physicians start markedly symptomatic type 2 diabetic patients on insulin, this is most often not necessary. The vast majority of them respond quickly and satisfactorily to a maximal dose of a sulfonylurea agent. Because older patients are more sensitive to these drugs, a half-maximal dose is used initially in those older than 65 years. If they have not responded in a week, the dose is increased to a maximal one. These patients have usually been markedly symptomatic for weeks to months. Hence, the few weeks it takes to determine whether

Table 5–4. General Guidelines for Adjusting the Dose of Sulfonylurea Agents

FPG	Hypoglycemia	Glycated Hemoglobin	Decision
≥140	No	≥1.5% above the ULN	Increase dose
≥140	No	<1.5% above the ULN	No change
<140	No	≥1.5% above the ULN	Increase dose
<140	No	<1.5% above the ULN	No change
Regardless	Yes	≥1.5% above the ULN	Decrease dose *and* add metformin
Regardless	Yes	<1.5% above the ULN	Decrease dose *or* change drug[a]

FPG, Fasting plasma glucose concentration (mg/dl); ULN, upper limit of normal.

[a] If a patient is taking one of the five more effective drugs (i.e., chlorpropamide, glipizide, glyburide, glimepiride, or tolazamide), change to a comparable dose of either acetohexamide (preferred) or tolbutamide.

they will respond to sulfonylurea agents pose little additional risk as long as they are closely monitored.

My approach to a markedly symptomatic type 2 diabetic patient, depicted in Figure 5–5, is based on responses in more than 100 such individuals. After the drug is started, the patient should be telephoned in several days and seen in a week. The decision to start insulin in obese patients at this time is based on the prevailing symptoms, whereas in lean patients, the FPG concentration drives the decision. This seeming discrepancy stems from the observation that regardless of the FPG level 1 week after starting

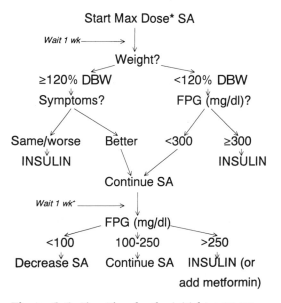

Figure 5–5. Algorithm for the initial treatment of markedly symptomatic type 2 diabetic patients with a maximal dose of one of the four most effective sulfonylurea agents (chlorpropamide, glipizide, glyburide, or tolazamide). *Start with half of the maximal dose in patients ≥65 years old and increase to maximal dose at 1 week if symptoms do not improve. +After the first week, measure FPG concentration every 2 to 4 weeks until it plateaus. DBW, desirable body weight; FPG, fasting plasma glucose; max, maximal; SA, sulfonylurea agent.

the sulfonylurea agent, almost all obese patients had fewer symptoms and did not require insulin subsequently (even when it had been started in the first few because of their very high FPG concentrations). In contrast, regardless of any change in symptoms in lean patients, if FPG concentrations remained very high after 1 week, insulin was soon necessary. The fact that obese patients have much more β-cell reserve than lean ones may explain this difference. The decision in the first several weeks is more likely to involve reduction of the sulfonylurea agent dose than choosing whether to start insulin.

The initial responses[33] of 55 carefully monitored, markedly symptomatic type 2 diabetic patients to maximal doses (or half-maximal for those >65 years of age) of one of the four most effective sulfonylurea agents (see Table 5–3) is shown in Figure 5–6. After 4 months, six patients remained on a maximal dose, 29 were taking a submaximal dose, 11 were being treated with diet alone, and only 3 needed insulin. Six patients were unavailable for follow-up. Many of these 55 patients were ketotic, and some even had mildly lowered serum bicarbonate levels (indicating a compensated ketoacidosis). Neither of these metabolic abnormalities predicted a lack of response. Thus, treating markedly symptomatic type 2 patients with high doses of sulfonylurea agents is successful in most cases and avoids not only the very labor-intensive process of starting patients on insulin (which occurs in the hospital in many practice settings) but also the significant alterations in the life styles of these patients. The few who do require insulin often need it weeks to months later because of an unsatisfactory response. At that time, they are not so symptomatic and may even be asymptomatic, and insulin adjustments can be made more gradually than in markedly hyperglycemic, symptomatic patients. Moreover, insulin therapy can be initiated in an office or outpatient setting rather than in the hospital.

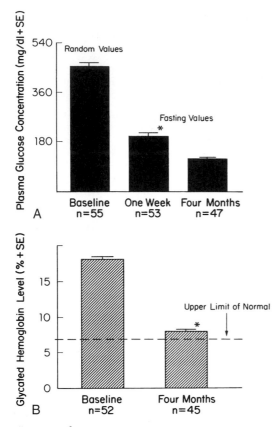

Figure 5–6. Response of markedly symptomatic type 2 diabetic patients to maximal dose of sulfonylurea agents (or half of maximal dose in patients ≥65 years old). SE, standard error of the mean. *A*: Glucose concentrations. *, P < 0.001 versus baseline and 4 months. *B*: Glycated hemoglobin levels. *, P < 0.001 versus baseline.

SELECTING A REGIMEN

The oral antidiabetes drugs available in the United States are listed in Table 5-5. The pharmacology of the sulfonylurea agents was discussed earlier (and that of metformin and acarbose is described later). The choice of agent is based on differences in effectiveness, side effects, compliance, and cost.

Obviously, potency (i.e., response per milligram of the drug) is clinically irrelevant. The relative effectiveness of the preparations can be determined in two ways. First, the proportion of newly diagnosed, ketosis-resistant diabetic patients whose disease is controlled by each drug can be compared. (Theoretically, these patients should have failed to respond satisfactorily to dietary therapy alone.) The second and more rigorous method is to evaluate how many patients who fail to respond appropriately to maximal doses of one drug will respond to another one. Only tolbutamide and chlorpropamide, the first two sulfonylurea agents released, have been compared in this manner. By both criteria, chlorpropamide is clearly more effective than tolbutamide.[34]

Despite numerous reports in the literature comparing two or more sulfonylurea agents, few evaluations use either of the criteria mentioned earlier. In most studies, patients are switched from a submaximal dose of one agent and started on another one. In a few, small numbers of untreated patients have been given glyburide, glipizide, and/or chlorpropamide, and the percentage adequately controlled has not differed. In terms of successfully treating a patient who has failed to respond to one of the sulfonylurea agents, no comparisons have been made in large numbers of patients, with the exception of tolbutamide versus chlorpropamide,[34] already mentioned. I have had extensive experience with acetohexamide and believe that it is more effective than tolbutamide but less so than chlorpropamide (i.e., failures on maximal doses of acetohexamide can often be rescued by chlorpropamide). In regard to choosing among glyburide, glipizide, tolazamide, and chlorpropamide, my impression of the literature is that few patients who have not responded to one of these agents respond satisfactorily to another, and no one of these drugs is clearly superior to any other.

The side effects of these drugs have already been discussed. Chlorpropamide is associated with two (hyponatremia, alcohol flushing) not shared by the others. Although all of them can cause intrahepatic cholesta-

Table 5–5. Selected Characteristics of Oral Antidiabetes Medications

Generic Name	Trade Name	Tablet Size (mg)	Usual Daily Dose Range (mg)	Maximal Dose (mg)	Duration of Action (h)
Tolbutamide	Orinase[a]	250, 500	500–2,000 (divided)	3,000	6–12
Chlorpropamide	Diabinese[b]	100, 250	100–500 (single)	750	60
Acetohexamide	Dymelor[c]	250, 500	250–1,500 (single or divided)	1,500	12–24
Tolazamide	Tolinase[a]	100, 250, 500	100–750 (single or divided)	1,000	12–24
Glyburide	Micronase[a] DiaBeta[d]	1.25, 2.5, 5.0	2.5–10 (single or divided)	20	12–24
	Glynase[a] (micronized glyburide)	1.5, 3.0, 6.0	1.5–6.0 (single or divided)	12	12–24
Glipizide	Glucotrol[c]	5, 10	5–20 (single or divided)	40	10–24
	Glucotrol XL (long-acting glipizide)[c]	5, 10	5–10 (single)	20	24–48
Glimepiride	Amaryl[d]	1, 2, 4	1–4	8	≈24
Metformin	Glucophage[f]	500, 850	1,000–2,000 (divided)	2,500 (2,550)	6–12
Acarbose	Precose[g]	50, 100	75–150 (divided)	300	Not absorbed

[a] Upjohn Co., Kalamazoo, MI.
[b] Pfizer Inc., New York, NY.
[c] Eli Lilly and Co., Indianapolis, IN.
[d] Hoechst-Roussel Pharmaceuticals, Somerville, NJ.
[e] Pratt Pharmaceuticals, New York, NY.
[f] Bristol-Myers Squibb Company, Princeton, NJ.
[g] Bayer Corporation, West Haven, CT.

sis, it is more likely with chlorpropamide. In terms of compliance, tolbutamide would be the most difficult because the drug must be taken two or three times a day. Chlorpropamide, the long-acting formulation of glipizide, and glimepiride are the least difficult because they need be taken only once a day. With the others, the first half (tolazamide, glyburide, glipizide) or two thirds (acetohexamide) of the maximal dose is taken with breakfast and the remainder (if necessary) before supper. When considering cost, not only the price per tablet but the number of pills a patient may take per day must be considered. Generic preparations are currently available for all sulfonylurea agents except Glynase, Glucotrol XL, and Amaryl. Costs, however, depend on local market conditions, which now include negotiated prices in managed care settings.

In regard to the four factors involved in selecting a particular sulfonylurea agent (effectiveness, side effects, compliance, and cost), the following would seem a fair summary. Tolbutamide is the least effective and acetohexamide is next but less so than the five remaining, chlorpropamide, tolazamide, glyburide, glipizide, and glimepiride, all of which seem clinically equivalent. Chlorpropamide is least desirable in regard to side effects but, along with Glucotrol XL and Amaryl, easiest to use in terms of compliance. There is little to distinguish among the other four with regard to side effects and compliance. One factor, in addition to costs, that now influences which sulfonylurea agent to use includes which drugs are on the formularies of health maintenance organizations.

The recommended initial doses of the sulfonylurea agents are listed in Table 5-3. A markedly symptomatic patient is given maximal doses of one of the five most effective agents, tolazamide, chlorpropamide, glyburide, glipizide, or glimepiride. The initial dose of a sulfonylurea agent in either asymptomatic type 2 diabetic patients for whom dietary therapy has failed or for mildly symptomatic patients depends on the prevailing FPG concentration. If this value is <180 mg/dl, the lowest-strength tablet or one half of that in the case of glipizide and glynase, is used (see Table 5-3). If the value exceeds 180 mg/dl, the next highest tablet strength is chosen. The patient should be monitored every 1 to 4 weeks while the initial dosage adjustments are being made. An exception to the suggestions offered in Table 5-3 is patients over 65 years of age. I recommend starting all these asymptomatic or mildly symptomatic individuals on the lowest dose listed regardless of their FPG concentration. For older markedly symptomatic patients, the initial dose is approximately one third to one half of the maximal dose (see Table 5-3). The dose can be quickly increased up to maximal amounts if little or no response occurs within a week. Other than these changes in initial doses, there is no difference in the way in which older and younger patients are monitored.

The therapeutic goals are summarized in Table 5-4 and have already been discussed. The dose of the sulfonylurea agent is gradually increased until either the goals are achieved or the maximal dose is being given. Chlorpropamide, Glucotrol XL, and Amaryl are always given once a day because of their long durations of action. Up to 1 g of acetohexamide is taken in the morning, with the final 500 mg taken in the evening. For tolazamide, doses of up to 500 mg are taken in the morning and any additional amounts necessary are given in the evening. Tolbutamide should be given two or three times a day because of its short duration of action. In the case of glyburide, the first 10 mg is taken in the morning and the remainder in the evening. With glipizide, the initial 20 mg is given before breakfast and any additional amount before the evening meal.

If therapy with tolbutamide or acetohexamide fails, a switch to maximal doses of one of the other five agents improves diabetic control in a significant number of patients. If control is unsatisfactory on one half to two thirds of the maximal dose of a drug, increasing it to the maximum should be tried. Although this often results in some improvement,[34a] it may not yield a glycated hemoglobin level <1.5% above the upper limit of normal for the assay used. In this situation, further therapy is usually necessary (either adding metformin or BIDS therapy—discussed later). Adding a second sulfonylurea agent to the first one is ineffective.[35]

Type 2 diabetic patients with renal insufficiency present a special problem. Although none of the sulfonylurea agents are recommended for these patients, insulin therapy is sometimes not feasible. No comparative studies have investigated the use of sulfonylurea agents in these patients. However, on the basis of the metabolic characteristics of these drugs, the following approach seems reasonable. Tolbutamide is preferred because its degradative products are inactive. If it is ineffective, glipizide would be my next choice, followed by tolazamide, because their degradative products, although excreted by the kidneys, have only weak hypoglycemic activity. Chlorpropamide, glyburide, acetohexamide, and glimepiride should be avoided because their degradative products have significant hypoglycemic activity and are also excreted by the kidneys. The lowest dose of the selected agent should be used initially and increased cautiously. I usually attempt to control glucose levels in these patients with sulfonylurea agents before using insulin therapy. Patients experiencing renal failure are often unusually sensitive to insulin, presumably because degradation of insulin by the kidneys is impaired and its half-life is prolonged. Therefore, hypoglycemia is always a potential problem for these patients, regardless of the therapeutic approach. In addition, chronic renal failure itself is sometimes associated with fasting hypoglycemia.[36]

Discussions of the sulfonylurea agents usually include comments on the percentage of patients who experience primary and secondary failure with this form of therapy and refer to the number of patients who did just as well when drug treatment was discontinued. The percentage of primary failure (i.e., patients who never respond satisfactorily to the drug) ranges from 5% to 40%, and secondary failure (i.e., patients who initially respond but later become refractory) ranges from 3% to 30%. Many of these data were generated before the proper criteria for selection of appropriate patients to receive sulfonylurea agents were established. Therefore, they have little bearing on the decision about whether to use these drugs in an individual patient. If the criteria outlined earlier for selecting candidates for treatment with sulfonylurea agents are used, patients who will certainly be unresponsive (i.e., young, lean ketosis-prone patients) and those whose diabetes can be controlled by dietary therapy alone will be eliminated from consideration. Thus, the risk of primary failure will be minimized, and unnecessary exposure to the sulfonylurea agents is avoided. A persistent incidence of secondary failure does not, in my view, invalidate the use of the sulfonylurea agents. For whatever period type 2 diabetic patients can experience satisfactory control with sulfonylurea agents, they will be able to avoid the inconvenience, discomfort, and relative inflexibility of meal and activity patterns required by insulin therapy. If the guidelines discussed earlier are followed, patients in whom these drugs fail will have glucose levels that are out of control for only a short period before either insulin is started or metformin is added. The efficacy of this approach is supported by the fact that after diet failure, those patients who respond to sulfonylurea agents show the same degree of improvement in diabetic control as those patients treated with insulin instead of a sulfonylurea agent.[37-39]

METFORMIN[40, 41]

BACKGROUND

Metformin is a biguanide, a derivative of guanidine. The history of these compounds can be traced to medieval times, when the plant *Galega officinalis*, also known as goat's rue or French lilac, was used to treat diabetes in southern and eastern Europe. The active ingredient in this plant was isoamylene guanidine. In 1918, guanidine was shown to possess hypoglycemic activity. Guanidine was too toxic for clinical use, and although a series of guanidine derivatives were synthesized and tested in the 1920s, interest waned after insulin became available. Interest was rekindled after the successful experience with sulfonylurea agents in the 1950s and in 1957 phenformin was introduced into the United States and metformin in France, and in 1958 buformin in Germany (Fig. 5-7). Buformin never gained wide acceptance, but phenformin in this country and metformin in Europe and Canada were used more and more frequently for treating type 2 diabetes.

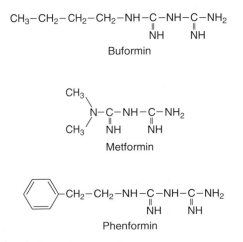

Figure 5-7. Structural formulae of the biguanide drugs.

Phenformin was discontinued in the United States in 1976 because of an association with lactic acidosis. Metformin has continued to be used because careful monitoring revealed at least a 10-fold less risk of lactic acidosis, which occurred primarily in patients with contraindications to its use. The drug was approved by the Federal Drug Administration after two large multicenter studies[42] were carried out in the United States and was released for clinical use here in 1995.

CHEMISTRY

Two chemical properties of biguanides are thought to account for their metabolic effects. First, their nonpolar side chains determine the degree to which they are lipophilic, a characteristic that allows them to bind to the hydrophobic phospholipids of biologic membranes. Phenformin is more lipophilic than metformin and therefore has a stronger affinity for mitochondrial membranes. This property probably explains its much greater propensity to cause lactic acidosis. Second, under physiologic conditions, biguanides exist in protonated (polar) forms. Once bound to biologic membranes, this hydrophilic part of the molecule is thought to change the surface potential, possibly accounting for the myriad metabolic effects of the drug (discussed later).

PHARMACOLOGY

Metformin is absorbed mainly from the small intestine. Its bioavailability is 50% to 60%. Peak levels are achieved approximately 2 hours after ingestion. Metformin does not bind to plasma proteins, and 90% is excreted unchanged in the urine within 12 hours. The plasma half-life ranges from 1.5 to 4.5 hours but is prolonged, not unsurprisingly, in the presence of renal insufficiency. Renal clearance of metformin is greater than creatinine clearance, indicating active tubular secretion of the drug. Cimetidine competes with metformin at the renal tubule inhibiting its clear-

ance and thereby increasing its availability.[43] This is the only drug interaction reported. Guar gum decreases the absorption of metformin in normal subjects.[44] Finally, the accumulation of the drug in the walls of the gastrointestinal tract is 10- to 100-fold that in the plasma, consistent with its major side effects and one possible mechanism of action to lower glucose levels in hyperglycemic patients (discussed later).

MECHANISM OF ACTION

In diabetic patients, metformin lowers elevated glucose concentrations toward normal but does not cause hypoglycemia. The drug does not lower glucose concentrations in normal subjects. Therefore, it is an antihyperglycemic agent rather than a hypoglycemic one. It does not increase insulin secretion. How it decreases hyperglycemia is not clear.[40, 41, 45, 46] Possible mechanisms are listed in Table 5–6. Although each of these is supported by one or more studies, many of them are not found in others. A few generalizations can be made. In regard to the gastrointestinal tract, anorexia per se would not

Table 5–6. Possible Sites and Mechanisms of Action of Metformin

Gastrointestinal

Decreased or delayed absorption of glucose
Increased conversion of glucose to lactate by intestinal cells
Inducing anorexia

Hepatic (Decreased Glucose Output Secondary to Inhibition of Gluconeogenesis)

Direct effect
Potentiating insulin effect

Peripheral Tissues (Muscle and Fat)

Direct effect[a]
Potentiating insulin effect
  Increased insulin receptor binding
  Postbinding mechanism(s)[a]

[a] One of the mechanisms may be increased translocation of glucose transporters to the plasma membrane.

seem to be primarily important. Diminished hepatic glucose output is probably a factor, but the decrease is less than the reduction in the FPG concentration, suggesting that other mechanisms may be important. In general, postprandial glucose levels are lowered more than fasting ones, implicating an important effect on peripheral tissues. Although increased insulin binding has been found in a number of studies, especially in vitro ones, little correlation is noted between this effect and lowering of glucose concentrations. Therefore, an effect on insulin binding by metformin is not thought to be important. The lack of hypoglycemia may be explained by failure of insulin secretion to increase and/or by the increased production of lactate, an important precursor for gluconeogenesis. Thus, increased hepatic glucose production via lactate conversion to glucose may protect against hypoglycemia. Although the literature concerning how metformin lowers elevated glucose concentrations is inconsistent, the effects on all three tissues are probably important. In summary, metformin may work by limiting glucose entry from the gastrointestinal tract, decreasing hepatic glucose production, and enhancing insulin action in the peripheral tissues (i.e., as an insulin sensitizer). The precise mechanisms by which these are accomplished are unknown.

ADVERSE SIDE EFFECTS

The major side effect of metformin therapy is gastrointestinal. As many as 20% of patients (a few studies record even higher percentages) experience one or more of the following: anorexia, metallic taste, abdominal discomfort, nausea, vomiting, and diarrhea. These side effects are often transient and can be minimized if the drug is taken with meals and if the initial dose is low and gradually increased every week or two. Published studies claim that only approximately 5% of patients discontinue the drug because of gastrointestinal side effects, although anecdotal experience would suggest that this may be an underestimate. Higher doses of the drug are often limited by one or several of these gastrointestinal symptoms.

Lactic acidosis is a rare but often fatal (mortality rates approximate 50%) side effect. It almost always occurs in patients in whom the drug is contraindicated (Table 5–7). Renal insufficiency is an obvious contraindication because the drug is excreted unchanged in the urine and accumulates if kidney function is impaired. The vast majority of metformin-associated lactic acidosis occurs in patients with decreased renal function. The pharmaceutical company marketing metformin states that it should not be given to males whose serum creatinine concentration is ≥1.5 mg/dl and to females whose value is ≥1.4 mg/dl. Hepatic dysfunction is also a contraindication, presumably because lactate might not be metabolized normally in patients with liver disease. No published guidelines describe the level of hepatic impairment at which metformin should be avoided. I arbitrarily use levels of transaminases that are twice normal to exclude the drug. Alcohol abuse or binge drinking is a contraindication because the

Table 5–7. Contraindications to the Use of Metformin

Drug Should Not Be Started	Drug Should Be Temporarily Withheld
Renal impairment (serum creatinine level ≥1.5 mg/dl in males or ≥1.4 mg/dl in females)	Cardiovascular collapse
Hepatic disease	Acute myocardial infarction
History of alcohol abuse/binge drinking	Acute congestive heart failure
Acute or chronic acidosis	Severe infection
	Use of iodinated contrast material
	Major surgical procedure

metabolism of ethanol generates reducing equivalents (NADH) that push the equilibrium between lactate and pyruvate toward lactate (i.e., lactate tends to accumulate). Finally, use of metformin should probably be avoided in the unusual patient who already has an acute or chronic acidosis due to another cause because any accumulation of lactate could worsen his or her metabolic status.

In several conditions, patients taking metformin should have the drug temporarily withheld (see Table 5-7). Because lack of oxygenation is an important cause of lactic acidosis, metformin would certainly be contraindicated in patients at risk for hypoxia. These situations include acute cardiovascular collapse, acute myocardial infarction, and acute congestive heart failure. Because severe infections can lead to lactic acidosis, metformin should be discontinued in these cases as well. The drug should also be stopped several days before the use of iodinated contrast material because renal function often decreases for a short time after its administration. Finally, metformin should not be used in patients undergoing major surgical procedures. The drug can be restarted after the foregoing situations are reversed.

As stated earlier, the incidence of lactic acidosis associated with metformin is 10-fold less than that associated with phenformin because of their chemical and pharmacologic differences. Approximately 100 cases of lactic acidosis have been associated with metformin, and almost all of these have occurred in patients in whom the drug was contraindicated and in a few who attempted suicide with it.[47] In Canada, no reported episodes of lactic acidosis were associated with metformin use during a 12-year period (covering approximately 56,000 patient-years), during which intensive monitoring was carried out for the final 6 years. Therefore, if used properly, metformin presents very little risk of lactic acidosis. In fact, the incidence of sulfonylurea agent–induced severe hypoglycemia is 5.5-fold higher than metformin-

associated lactic acidosis (0.22 vs. 0.04 total cases per 1000 patient-years), although their mortality rates are similar (0.02 vs. 0.01 fatal cases per 1000 patient-years).[48] Appropriate observation of patients taking metformin should include routine monitoring of renal and hepatic function every 6 months or so to identify any risk for the development of lactic acidosis.

Metformin may decrease intestinal absorption of vitamin B_{12} and folate, especially the former. However, there are only a few isolated case reports of a megaloblastic anemia attributed to vitamin B_{12} deficiency associated with metformin therapy.[40, 49] In view of the widespread use of the drug during the past nearly 40 years, one must question whether metformin was wholly responsible for the anemia. Certainly, it would not appear to be cost-effective to routinely screen patients taking metformin for vitamin B_{12} malabsorption or deficiency. A simple test for anemia carried out periodically should suffice.

FAVORABLE SIDE EFFECTS

In this discussion, effects of metformin not directly related to lowering elevated glucose concentrations are considered side effects. Certain of these have favorable clinical outcomes. As already mentioned, the drug does not cause hypoglycemia when used as monotherapy. (Hypoglycemia may occur when metformin is added to a sulfonylurea agent, but this is due to the latter.) Metformin is also a weight stabilizer. Patients whose diabetic control is improved by sulfonylurea agents typically gain 5 to 10 pounds, whereas those using insulin may add even more. A small initial weight loss of several pounds is often noted with metformin, and this levels out after 3 to 6 months at 1% to 3% below the pretreatment weight. No correlation between the amount of weight lost and the improvement of diabetic control has been found.

Metformin also has favorable effects on

circulating lipids. Triglyceride levels are lowered most consistently, with decrements of 10% to 20% in normotriglyceridemic patients and up to 50% in hypertriglyceridemic ones. It is difficult, however, to determine exactly how much of this improvement in type 2 diabetic patients is due to an action of the drug independent of its glucose-lowering effect. Some of it must be a direct effect on lipids because metformin lowers triglyceride levels in nondiabetic individuals as well. Total and low-density lipoprotein (LDL) cholesterol concentrations are lowered more modestly (5% to 10%) in some, but not all, studies. Although a few studies have also noted a small but significant rise in high-density lipoprotein (HDL) cholesterol levels, the majority have not. The results of the large multicenter study carried out in the United States[42] are consistent with these observations. Statistically significant decrements in triglyceride (16%), total cholesterol (5%), and LDL cholesterol (7%) levels and an insignificant increase (3%) in HDL cholesterol levels were noted in patients who responded to metformin therapy.

CLINICAL USE

Metformin can be used either as monotherapy as the first drug given should diet and exercise fail to achieve satisfactory control, or it can be added to sulfonylurea agents should they be inadequate when pushed to the maximal dose. When used as monotherapy, metformin and sulfonylurea agents produce similar responses in both obese and nonobese patients, approximately a 20% to 25% fall in FPG concentrations. Metformin is available in two tablet sizes, 500 and 850 mg. To minimize the gastrointestinal side effects, a small dose should be started with a meal, either one 850-mg or 500-mg tablet with breakfast and supper. Gastrointestinal symptoms seem to be less in some patients if the drug is taken with some food already in the stomach. If the twice-a-day initial dose causes intolerable side effects, one 500-mg

tablet can be tried. As with sulfonylurea agents, the FPG concentration is measured a week or two later to determine if a satisfactory response (<140 mg/dl) has been achieved. This is unlikely with the smaller doses, especially if the initial FPG concentration was >180 mg/dl. The dose of metformin should be increased gradually every week or two until one of three events occurs: (1) The FPG concentration decreases to <140 mg/dl, at which time the dose is maintained until a glycated hemoglobin level obtained 2 months hence determines whether satisfactory control (a value <1.5% above the upper limit of normal for the assay used) has been achieved; if not, the dose is increased one step and the patient is reevaluated in several weeks for gastrointestinal symptoms and measurement of an FPG concentration. If that remains <140 mg/dl, glycated hemoglobin is measured in 2 months and the process repeated if necessary (unlike with sulfonylurea agent therapy, there is no danger of hypoglycemia as the metformin dose is increased as long as the drug is used as monotherapy). (2) A maximal dose of the drug has been reached (five 500-mg tablets [2500 mg] or three 850-mg tablets [2550 mg]) (see later discussion for next decision). (3) A dose causes intolerable gastrointestinal side effects; in this case, a sulfonylurea agent should be substituted for metformin because the results of monotherapy with both drugs are similar and one would wish to determine if satisfactory control could be achieved with one agent before considering combined therapy.

If the 850-mg tablets are used, the progression is simple: one pill before breakfast, then supper, and finally lunch. Some patients have fewer gastrointestinal side effects with the initial tablet before supper rather than breakfast. The progression with the 500-mg tablets is as follows: 500 mg with supper; 500 mg with breakfast and 500 mg with supper; 500 mg with breakfast, 500 mg with lunch, and 500 mg with supper; 1000 mg with breakfast, 500 mg with lunch, and 500 mg with supper; and finally, 1000 mg with breakfast, 500 mg with lunch, and 1000 mg with supper. The use of the 850-mg tablets is simpler, but if gastrointestinal side effects are a problem, the more gradual increase using the 500-mg tablets may be helpful. In my experience, intolerable gastrointestinal symptoms, if they occur, usually become manifested at doses of metformin ≥1500 mg.

The results of the large multicenter study carried out in the United States[42] are representative of the reported worldwide experience. Two groups of mildly to moderately obese (120% to 170% of desirable body weight) type 2 diabetic patients who had failed to experience improvement (FPG concentrations >140 mg/dl) with diet alone (protocol 1) or maximal doses (20 mg) of glyburide (protocol 2) were studied. In protocol 1, the patients were given either placebo or metformin in gradually increasing doses. In protocol 2, the patients were either maintained on the maximal dose of glyburide (with placebo added), switched to gradually increasing doses of metformin (plus placebo), or had gradually increasing doses of metformin added to their maximal dose of glyburide. Their glycemic responses are shown in Figures 5–8 and 5–9. The initial FPG concentration was approximately 250 mg/dl in all of the groups. The initial deterioration in control in the patients switched to metformin in protocol 2 was because glyburide was stopped and the initial dose of metformin was low and increased gradually.

Metformin should not be used as monotherapy in patients with type 1 diabetes. When added to insulin therapy in these patients, insulin doses decrease somewhat but improvement in control is not impressive. Therefore, this combination in type 1 patients is not recommended. Too few studies have evaluated the results of adding metformin to the regimen of insulin-requiring type 2 diabetic patients to make any recommendations at present. However, should future experience with this approach show that it is not very effective, simply giving enough

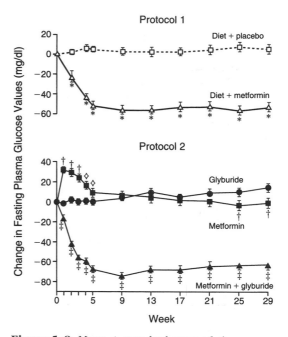

Figure 5–8. Mean ± standard error of changes in fasting plasma glucose concentrations in type 2 diabetic patients enrolled in two large multicenter studies in the United States. See text for description of protocols 1 and 2. *P < 0.001 between the placebo and metformin groups in protocol 1; †P < 0.001 between metformin and glyburide groups in protocol 2; ◇P < 0.01 between metformin and glyburide groups in protocol 2; ‡P < 0.001 between combination therapy (metformin + glyburide) and glyburide groups in protocol 2. (From DeFronzo RA, Goodman AM, and the Multicenter Metformin Study Group: Efficacy of metformin in patients with non-insulin-dependent diabetes mellitus. N Engl J Med 333:541, 1995)

insulin yields excellent control, even in very obese patients.[50, 51] Finally, although no teratogenic effects due to metformin have been reported, it is recommended that the drug not be used in pregnancy.

SULFONYLUREA AGENTS VERSUS METFORMIN

Because the efficacy of sulfonylurea agents and metformin is similar as monotherapy in

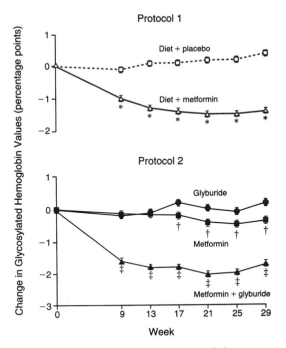

Figure 5–9. Mean ± standard error of changes in glycated hemoglobin levels in type 2 diabetic patients enrolled in two large multicenter studies in the United States. See text for description of protocols 1 and 2. *P < 0.001 between the placebo and metformin groups in protocol 1; †P < 0.01 between metformin and glyburide groups in protocol 2; ‡P < 0.001 between the combination therapy (metformin + glyburide) and glyburide groups in protocol 2. (From DeFronzo RA, Goodman AM, and the Multicenter Metformin Study Group: Efficacy of metformin in patients with non-insulin-dependent diabetes mellitus. N Engl J Med 333:541, 1995)

both lean and obese type 2 diabetic patients, the choice of which one to start with rests with their other effects rather than their glycemic ones (Table 5–8). Nonglycemic factors favoring sulfonylurea agents are their few side effects, their ease of use, and the fact that most of them are available in a generic form, which should mean lower costs to patients. Potential hypoglycemia and weight gain as control is improved are unfavorable factors, as is an allergy to sulfa drugs in the

few patients who have it. The nonglycemic factors favoring metformin are the absence of hypoglycemia, a favorable effect on the dyslipidemia associated with type 2 diabetes, and the weight-stabilizing effect of the drug. The unfavorable factors are the high prevalence of gastrointestinal side effects, which require careful gradual dose increases and can be dose limiting in some patients, and the fact that the drug is contraindicated in certain circumstances (renal and hepatic dysfunction, alcohol abuse, and acute or chronic acidosis), which necessitates ongoing monitoring and the need to discontinue it temporarily in patients with acute cardiovascular collapse, myocardial infarction or congestive heart failure, or severe infections, as well as in those undergoing major surgery or studies with iodinated contrast media. In addition, it probably is more expensive than generic sulfonylurea agents.

Whichever one is selected, the dose should be gradually increased until either satisfactory control is achieved or the maximum dose is reached without attaining it. (With metformin, intolerable gastrointestinal side effects may be the limiting factor.) If control is unsatisfactory when the maximum (tolerated) dose is reached, the other drug should be added (if there are no contraindications). If the tolerated dose of metformin is 1 g or less at this point, it can be discontinued and the patient treated with a sulfonylurea agent alone. In the unusual situation in which hypoglycemia limits the sulfonylurea agent dose and the glycated hemoglobin level reflects inadequate control, metformin should be added (if there are no contraindications) if the dose of the sulfonylurea agent is one half of the maximal dose or greater. If the sulfonylurea agent dose is less than one half of the maximal dose, metformin can be substituted. The principle here is that if the patient is on a low dose of one of the drugs that cannot be increased, monotherapy with the other should be tried before combining the two. At higher doses, it is unlikely that monotherapy with the other one would lead

Table 5–8. Metformin Versus Sulfonylurea Agents as Monotherapy: Nonglycemic Factors

Drug	Pro	Con
Metformin	No weight gain	Gastrointestinal side effects common
	No hypoglycemia	Potential for lactic acidosis (if contraindications exist)
	Favorable effect on lipids	Possible slower dose titration
		More frequent dosing
		More expensive
Sulfonylurea agents	Few side effects	Hypoglycemia
	More rapid dose titration usually possible	Weight gain possible
	Often less frequent dosing	Sulfa allergy (rare)
	Available as cheaper generic	

to satisfactory control because the two drugs are equally effective.

When the second drug is added, the same principles underlying the dose increases of each one used as monotherapy apply in this circumstance, as well as the same precautions for their use. One should be especially alert to the possibility of hypoglycemia when metformin is added to a maximal dose of a sulfonylurea agent. In many cases, monitoring (especially in the late afternoon) has documented the need to reduce the dose of the sulfonylurea agent to avoid hypoglycemia.

COMBINATION THERAPY

As mentioned earlier, patients failing to experience improvement with maximal doses of sulfonylurea agents could improve their diabetic control if metformin were added to their regimen. Similarly, in patients not responding to maximal (tolerated) doses of metformin, adding a sulfonylurea agent improves diabetic control as well. If metformin were contraindicated (see Table 5–7) or intolerable gastrointestinal side effects limited its use, evening NPH insulin could be added to the maximal dose of the sulfonylurea agent. (This approach, bedtime insulin, daytime sulfonylurea, is termed BIDS.) BIDS therapy is preferred to discontinuing the oral drugs and starting two or more injections of insulin because not only is it simpler, but

BIDS has been shown to be as effective as split/mixed and preprandial regular/evening NPH insulin regimens in studies lasting up to 12 months.[52–54a] There is no reported experience of adding evening NPH insulin to maximal (tolerated) doses of metformin, which is perhaps not surprising because only an allergy to sulfa drugs is an absolute contraindication to sulfonylurea agent therapy. Therefore, unless metformin is contraindicated or not tolerated, most patients are treated with a combination of the two oral drugs. If metformin is not used, most patients undergo BIDS therapy (see Chapter 4 for description of implementation).

If diabetic control is unsatisfactory on maximal (tolerated) doses of the two oral drugs, there are three alternatives: (1) adding evening NPH insulin to the combination; (2) stopping the sulfonylurea agent and adding evening NPH insulin; or (3) stopping metformin and adding evening NPH insulin. My personal preference is to discontinue metformin and convert to BIDS therapy for the following reasons. First, some patients have gastrointestinal side effects with metformin, and stopping the drug obviously alleviates them in these individuals. Second, it is preferable to treat patients with the simplest possible regimen that achieves satisfactory control, and two drugs rather than three meet this criterion. Finally, sulfonylurea agents are easier to use than metformin because the latter requires ongoing monitoring to ascertain that contraindications to its use have not developed, and withholding it temporarily is necessary under certain circumstances (see Table 5–7). Finally, at least some sulfonylurea agents (the long-acting preparation of glipizide, glimepiride, and chlorpropamide) are once-a-day medications, whereas metformin must be taken two or three times a day.

If satisfactory control (in most patients, glycated hemoglobin levels <1.5% above the upper limit of normal for the assay used) is not achieved on a combination of a maximal dose of one of the five most effective sulfonylurea agents and a dose of evening NPH insulin that maintains the fasting blood glucose concentration between 80 and 120 mg/dl, metformin is added back and gradually increased until either satisfactory control is achieved or a maximal (tolerated) dose of the second oral drug is reached. (If the patient has not been taking metformin for more than a week, the drug usually needs to be started again at a low dose and gradually increased to minimize the gastrointestinal side effects.) As mentioned already, because split/mixed and preprandial regular/evening NPH insulin regimens do not yield better control than BIDS therapy,[52–54a] I do not change from evening NPH insulin plus daytime oral drugs to one of the insulin-alone regimens unless the glycated hemoglobin level is >3.0% above the upper limit of normal for the assay used. My reasoning is that at this high level of glycated hemoglobin, an insulin-alone regimen, even if the patient is not compliant enough to take full advantage of it, has a better chance of improving diabetic control than if the glycated hemoglobin level is between 1.5% and 3.0% above the upper limit of normal for the assay used.

ADDING A SULFONYLUREA AGENT TO INSULIN

Adding a sulfonylurea agent to the regimen of patients with poor control on insulin has been advocated by some. (This approach should not be confused with BIDS therapy, in which evening intermediate-acting insulin is added for patients with poor control on oral drugs.) To date, at least 22 English-language studies[55] have been conducted to investigate the efficacy of this mode of combination therapy. The types of studies fall into essentially two groups: concurrent studies and crossover studies. In a concurrent study, patients receiving a sulfonylurea agent (most commonly glyburide) combined with insulin are compared with other patients receiving a placebo plus insulin. In a crossover study, patients act as their own controls—patients' response to a sulfonylurea agent plus insulin is compared with their response to a placebo plus insulin or, in a few studies, to their response to insulin alone. At some point in the trial, they are changed from one mode of therapy to the other, hence the term *crossover*. In most studies (both concurrent and crossover), the patients were poorly controlled on insulin before the trial was initiated and the effect of adding a sulfonylurea agent evaluated.

At least eight concurrent studies (Table 5–9) have been reported, involving a total of 162 patients monitored for a mean of 27 weeks (range, 6 to 52). The group receiving placebo showed no changed in their FPG concentrations, glycated hemoglobin levels, or insulin dose. The group receiving a sulfonylurea agent plus insulin had a modest reduction in their FPG concentrations and glycated hemoglobin levels. In those studies in which insulin doses were allowed to vary, a decrease was also observed in the final amount of insulin used by the patients also taking a sulfonylurea agent.

At least 14 crossover studies involved 185 patients receiving each treatment an average of 12 weeks. The comparisons were made at the end of each treatment period (see Table 5–9). The results were very similar to concurrent studies, with almost the same difference in FPG concentrations and glycated hemoglobin levels. Insulin doses, when

Table 5–9. Insulin Versus Insulin Plus Sulfonylurea Agent Treatment in Type 2 Diabetic Patients

	FPG (mg/dl)		Glycated Hemoglobin (%)		Insulin (U/day)	
	Before	*After*	*Before*	*After*	*Before*	*After*
Concurrent studies[a]						
Number of studies	6[b]	6[b]	7[b]	7[b]	5[c]	5[c]
Placebo (80 patients)	209	193	10.8	11.1	63	62
Sulfonylurea agent (82 patients)	203	170	10.7	10.0	66	48
Crossover studies[a, d]						
Number of studies		13[b]		13[b]		8[c]
Placebo		198		10.6		48
Sulfonylurea agent	185 patients	162		9.8		41

FPG, Fasting plasma glucose concentration.

[a] See text for discussion.

[b] Number of studies in which this variable was measured.

[c] Number of studies in which insulin dose was allowed to vary; in the others, insulin dose was either kept fixed or reported in U/kg.

[d] Measurement made at the end of the study period in which patients had been treated with placebo plus insulin or sulfonylurea agent plus insulin.

allowed to vary, fell but to a lesser extent than in the concurrent studies.

Several observations can be made from these results. The patients taking a sulfonylurea agent plus insulin did have a modest lowering of their FPG concentrations and slightly less than a 1% reduction in their glycated hemoglobin values. They also had an overall decrease in the number of units of insulin they were taking per day. It should be noted, however, that diabetic control remained fairly poor. Because the goal of diabetes treatment is to achieve near euglycemia, and this goal can usually be reached with the use of appropriate (although often large) amounts of insulin,[50, 51] it seems that adding sulfonylurea agents to patients poorly controlled on insulin offers no advantage. Adding sulfonylurea agents also increases the risk of both potential side effects and the costs of therapy.

Some have argued that high insulin levels may accelerate progression of atherosclerosis.[56] If that were the case, a possible benefit of adding a sulfonylurea agent for patients with diabetes poorly controlled on insulin might include reduced circulating levels of

insulin (if the insulin dose could legitimately be reduced). However, the argument that insulin *causes* atherosclerosis is becoming much less tenable.[57] Furthermore, many of the studies summarized in Table 5–8 showed that the patients who responded to the addition of sulfonylurea agents were those who were capable of increasing their endogenous insulin secretion. Therefore, after a sulfonylurea agent is added, circulating insulin levels would either be higher if the insulin dose were kept constant or unchanged if the insulin dose were lowered. In neither situation would insulin levels be decreased.

ACARBOSE*

MECHANISM OF ACTION AND PHARMACOLOGY

Acarbose, marketed in the United States in 1996 as Precose, is a complex oligosaccha-

---

* I wish to thank John Amatruda, M.D., of Bayer Corporation, Pharmaceutical Division, for providing me with a preprint of a postmarketing survey[61] and unpublished data obtained from clinical trials.

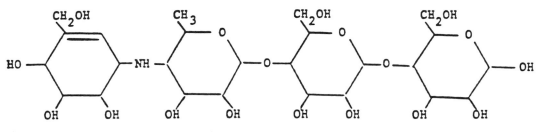

Figure 5–10. Structural formula of acarbose.

ride (Fig. 5-10) that competitively inhibits intestinal brush border α-glucosidases, which hydrolyze sucrose and intermediate starches. The drug binds reversibly and with high affinity to the carbohydrate attachment site of the α-glucosidases. Acarbose also has a moderately inhibitory effect on pancreatic α-amylase, which hydrolyzes starches in the lumen of the small intestine (Fig. 5-11). Therefore, by delaying digestion of carbohydrates in the small intestine, acarbose reduces the rate of glucose absorption, causing a blunting of the postprandial rise in glucose concentrations.

Acarbose has a relatively long half-life in the gastrointestinal tract because it is not metabolized until reaching the large intestine. There it is broken down principally by bacterial enzymes. Less than 2% of an oral dose of acarbose is absorbed into the circulation, where it is excreted as an intact drug by the kidneys.

EFFICACY

Acarbose has been studied in a large number of type 2 diabetic patients in randomized, double-blind, placebo-controlled studies,[58-60] mostly as either monotherapy or added to sulfonylurea agents after this modality of treatment had failed. It was added to either metformin or insulin in a smaller number of

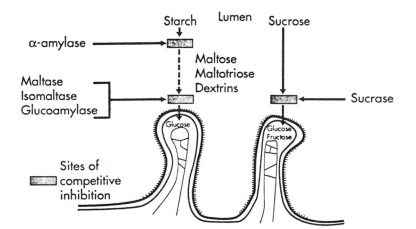

Figure 5–11. Sites of action of acarbose in the gastrointestinal tract. In normal digestion, pancreatic α-amylase hydrolyzes complex starches into oligosaccharides, which are further hydrolyzed by α-glucosidases located in the intestinal brush border to glucose and other monosaccharides, which are then absorbed. Acarbose competitively inhibits both of these enzymatic steps.

type 2 diabetic patients.[59] The results were similar in all groups in these studies. In general, glycated hemoglobin levels fell 0.5% to 0.75%, FPG concentrations 5 to 25 mg/dl, and 1-hour postprandial glucose concentrations 20 to 50 mg/dl, depending on the dose. The results were more impressive in a postmarketing survey of 10,462 patients cared for by 2,375 German physicians.[61] Eight percent of these patients had type 1 diabetes, 90% had type 2 diabetes, and in 2% the type was not stated. Of the type 2 patients, 29% were taking acarbose as monotherapy, 58% had it combined with a sulfonylurea agent, 9% with insulin, and 4% with both a sulfonylurea agent plus insulin. After 12 weeks of acarbose therapy in the type 2 diabetic patients, glycated hemoglobin levels had fallen 1.5%, FPG concentrations 52 mg/dl, 1-hour postprandial glucose concentrations 63 mg/dl, and 2-hour postprandial glucose concentrations 58 mg/dl. The results were remarkably similar in the much smaller number of type 1 diabetic patients: 1.5%, 51 mg/dl, 55 mg/dl, and 51 mg/dl, respectively. The more robust responses in the postmarketing survey can perhaps be attributed to the fact that these patients were in poorer control when acarbose was started than in the more carefully selected study patients. It is well known that the higher the initial values, the larger is the reduction when appropriate diabetic therapy is initiated. Another possible factor is that in the controlled studies, dietary intervention was carried out in the run-in period before the drug was introduced. In this instance, the effect of acarbose is superimposed on any dietary effect. In a postmarketing survey, there is no diet run-in and it is likely that acarbose has a greater effect if a strict diet is not being followed.

SIDE EFFECTS

The major side effect of acarbose is gastrointestinal distress. Because digestion of ingested carbohydrates is delayed by the drug, polysaccharides and disaccharides reach the large intestine, where they are hydrolyzed by bacterial enzymes. This results in an osmotic effect with secretion of water into the colon and metabolism of the breakdown products, yielding a number of metabolites such as short-chain fatty acids, hydrogen gas, carbon dioxide, and methane. The formation of these products can cause flatulence (the most common gastrointestinal side effect), abdominal pain, and diarrhea. Abdominal pain and diarrhea tend to return to pretreatment levels over time. Flatulence may persist but usually declines in frequency and intensity with time. These symptoms are more likely to occur early after initiating acarbose therapy but can be minimized if a low dose is used initially and increased gradually (see the later discussion of dosing).

Elevations of hepatic transaminase values were twice as common in acarbose-treated patients compared with placebo-treated patients in the controlled studies. These elevated levels returned to normal after discontinuation of the drug, as well as in the majority of episodes in which treatment was continued. When drug dose was taken into account, the prevalence of transaminase elevations was similar in placebo-treated patients and those receiving 300 mg/day or less of acarbose. Thus, the increased risk occurred in patients receiving larger amounts of the drug. However, in the international postmarketing experience involving more than a half million patients, 19 Japanese patients developed markedly elevated transaminase levels (>500 IU/L), and 12 of them also had jaundice. The dose of acarbose in 15 of the 19 was 300 mg/day or greater, and 13 of the 16 for whom weights were available weighed <60 kg (132 pounds). In the 18 cases for which follow-up was available, hepatic function improved or resolved completely when acarbose was discontinued.

Acarbose as monotherapy does not cause hypoglycemia. If added to a sulfonylurea agent or insulin, hypoglycemia may occur because these agents are working on a lowered glycemia caused by acarbose. *If hypoglycemia does occur in a patient taking acarbose, it must be treated with glucose (e.g., dextrose tablets) rather than sucrose or other carbohydrate-containing preparations because acarbose does not inhibit the absorption of the former as it does the latter.* Small reductions in hematocrit were noted in study patients receiving acarbose compared with placebo controls, but no changes occurred in total hemoglobin levels. There is no effect on lipid levels. When used as monotherapy, acarbose does not cause weight gain as control is improved, nor does it increase insulin concentrations. When acarbose is used in combination with a sulfonylurea agent, the weight gain and increased insulin concentrations often noted with this class of drugs are diminished. Although only very small amounts of acarbose are absorbed, plasma concentrations of the drug in volunteers with renal impairment were increased in proportion to renal dysfunction. Because no clinical studies have been carried out on diabetic patients with creatinine levels >2.0 mg/dl or in pregnancy, use of the drug in these patients is not recommended. Acarbose should not be used by patients with cirrhosis, inflammatory bowel disease, colonic ulcerations, or partial bowel obstruction or by those predisposed to bowel obstruction. Digestive enzyme preparations that hydrolyze carbohydrates (e.g., pancreatin, amylase) and intestinal adsorbents (e.g., charcoal) may reduce the effect of acarbose and should not be taken at the same time.

CLINICAL USE

Acarbose is currently supplied in 50-mg and 100-mg tablets, but a 25-mg tablet will be available soon. The 50-mg tablet is scored on one side so that it can easily be broken in half. The recommended starting dose is 25 mg tid to be taken with the first bite of each main meal. This starting dose has led many patients in this country to discontinue the drug because of flatulence. Although it takes

longer to reach a clinically effective level, starting with 25 mg with a single meal and gradually adding the drug with a second and then a third meal leads to better patient acceptance. The drug apparently is less effective if taken as little as 30 minutes before eating. The dose is increased to 50 mg tid and then to 100 mg tid if necessary at 4- to 8-week intervals. Doses >300 mg/day are not recommended because at higher doses there occur, (1) only slightly improved glycemic control, (2) more gastrointestinal side effects, and (3) a much greater risk of elevated transaminase levels. Although type 2 diabetic patients weighing <60 kg (132 pounds) are very uncommon in this country, the maximal dose of acarbose in these patients should be 50 mg tid. It is recommended that serum transaminase levels be measured every 3 months during the first year of treatment with acarbose and periodically thereafter. If elevated values are noted, a reduction in the dose or discontinuation of the drug may be indicated, especially if the elevations persist.

It is recommended that the response be monitored by 1-hour postprandial glucose concentrations and that the minimum dose be used to give the maximum benefit—that is, if the last dose tried does not improve the response, the amount of the drug should be lowered to the amount that gave a comparable response to the higher dose. Because very few physicians in this country have prescribed acarbose, little first-hand experience or reported literature is available to evaluate this recommended approach. However, I would be concerned that the timing of the blood sample and, more importantly, the carbohydrate content of the meal might be variable enough to limit the usefulness of a single 1-hour postprandial glucose concentration to evaluate the effect of each dose. Certainly, after the appropriate dose is determined, glycated hemoglobin levels could guide therapy. Given this situation, I would suggest that, once a dose is taken before each main meal, it should be maintained for

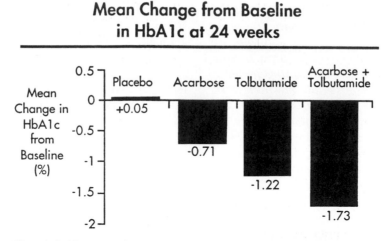

Figure 5–12. Mean changes in glycated hemoglobin levels in type 2 diabetic patients receiving either placebo, acarbose, tolbutamide, or acarbose + tolbutamide. (From Coniff RF, Shapiro JA, Seaton TB: Multicenter, placebo-controlled trial comparing acarbose [BAY g 5421] with placebo, tolbutamide, and tolbutamide-plus-acarbose in non-insulin-dependent diabetes mellitus. Am J Med 98:443, 1995)

8 weeks, at which time a glycated hemoglobin level be measured and used to decide if the dose should be increased. (After rapidly lowering glucose concentrations in poorly controlled type 2 diabetic patients and maintaining near euglycemia for 4 months, 75% of the new steady-state glycated hemoglobin level is achieved in the first 2 months.[62]) In this manner, overall glycemia (and possibly gastrointestinal tolerance) would determine the eventual dose of acarbose. Only actual experience will tell us which approach is better.

When acarbose should be used in the overall therapeutic approach to type 2 diabetic patients is not settled at present. Because of its inability to cause hypoglycemia, a cogent argument could be made to use it as monotherapy in patients who have not responded to dietary changes especially in those whose glycated hemoglobin levels are only several percent above the upper limit of normal. On the other hand, a therapeutic response to sulfonylurea agents may be observed in a shorter period because the dose can be increased more rapidly, the response to a sulfonylurea agent was greater than to acarbose when both were used as monotherapy[60] (Fig. 5–12), and gastrointestinal side effects rarely limit using sulfonylurea agents. Acarbose should also be useful when given to patients whose disease is not well controlled on sulfonylurea agents, metformin, or insulin.[59] The real world postmarketing survey[61] would suggest a greater response to acarbose than found in the controlled studies.[56, 59, 60] The niche for acarbose may be as adjunct therapy in type 2 diabetes for cases not satisfactorily controlled by the other modalities of treatment. It might also be very useful in older patients, in whom hypoglycemia may be a greater risk and metformin may more likely be contraindicated because of the lowered glomerular filtration rate in this population.

REFERENCES

1. Chu PC, Conway MJ, Krouse HA, Goodner CJ: The pattern of response of plasma insulin

and glucose to meals and fasting during chlorpropamide therapy. Ann Intern Med 68:757, 1968

2. Reaven G, Dray J: Effect of chlorpropamide on serum glucose and immunoreactive insulin concentrations in patients with ketosis-resistant diabetes mellitus. Diabetes 16:487, 1967

3. Peters AL, Davidson MB: Reduction of hyperinsulinemia by glyburide—scientific fact or advertising fiction? Diabetes Care 15:719, 1992

4. Gerich JE: Oral hypoglycemic agents. N Engl J Med 321:1231, 1989

5. Groop LC: Sulfonylureas in NIDDM. Diabetes Care 15:737, 1992

6. Judzewitsch RG, Pfeifer MA, Best JD et al: Chronic chlorpropamide therapy of noninsulin-dependent diabetes augments basal and stimulated insulin secretion by increasing islet sensitivity to glucose. J Clin Endocrinol Metab 55:321, 1982

7. Sartor G, Melander A, Schersten B et al: Influence of food and age on the single-dose kinetics and effects of tolbutamide and chlorpropamide. Eur J Clin Pharmol 17:285, 1980

8. Groop LC, Luzi L, DeFronzo RA et al: Hyperglycaemia and absorption of sulphonylurea drugs. Lancet 2:129, 1989

9. Esmatjes E, Vinuesa P, Navarro P et al: The effect of hyperglycemia on glipizide absorption in NIDDM patients. Diabetes Care 18:1075, 1995

10. Scott J, Poffenbarger PL: Pharmacogenetics of tolbutamide metabolism in humans. Diabetes 28:41, 1979

11. Yu TF, Berger L, Gutman AB: Hypoglycemic and uricosuric properties of acetohexamide and hydroxyhexamide. Metabolism 17:309, 1968

12. Rydberg T, Roder M, Jonsson A et al: Hypoglycemic activity of glyburide (glibenclamide) metabolites in humans. Diabetes Care 17:1026, 1994

13. Goodman RC, Dean PJ, Radparvar A, Kitabchi AE: Glyburide-induced hepatitis. Ann Intern Med 106:837, 1987

14. Meadow P, Tullio CJ: Glyburide-induced hepatitis. Clin Pharmacol 8:470, 1989

15. Garcia M, Miller M, Moses AM: Chlorpropamide-induced water retention in patients with diabetes mellitus. Ann Intern Med 75:549, 1971

16. Kadowaki T, Hagura R, Kajinuma H et al: Chlorpropamide-induced hyponatremia: incidence and risk factors. Diabetes Care 6:468, 1983

17. University Group Diabetes Program: A study of the effects of hypoglycemic agents on vascular complications in patients with adult-onset diabetes I. Design, methods and baseline results. Diabetes 19(suppl 2):747, 1970

18. University Group Diabetes Program: A study of the effects of hypoglycemic agents on vascular complications in patients with adult-onset diabetes. II. Mortality results. Diabetes 19(suppl 2):789, 1970

19. Feinstein AR: Clinical biostatistics. XXXV. The persistent clinical failures and fallacies of the UGDP study. Clin Pharmacol Ther 19:78, 1976

20. Kilo C, Miller JP, Williamson JR: The Achilles heel of the University Group Diabetes Program. JAMA 243:450, 1980

21. Whitehouse FW, Arky RA, Bell DI et al: The UGDP controversy (policy statement). Diabetes 28:168, 1979

22. Keen H, Jarrett RJ, Fuller JH: Tolbutamide and arterial disease in borderline diabetics. In Malaisse WJ, Pirart J (eds): Proceedings of the Ninth Congress of the International Diabetes Federation. Excerpta Medica, Amsterdam, 1974, p. 558

23. Paasikivi J, Wahlberg F: Preventive tolbutamide treatment and arterial disease in mild hyperglycemia. Diabetologia 7:323, 1971

24. Feldman R, Crawford D, Elashoff R, Glass A: Oral hypoglycemic drug prophylaxis in asymptomatic diabetes. In Malaisse WJ, Pirart J (eds): Proceedings of the Ninth Congress of the International Diabetes Federation. Excerpta Medica, Amsterdam, 1974, p. 574

25. Persson G: Cardiovascular complications in diabetics and subjects with reduced glucose tolerance. Acta Med Scand Suppl 605:25, 1977

26. Ohneda A, Maruhama Y, Itabashi H et al: Vascular complications and long-term administration of oral hypoglycemic agents in patients with diabetes mellitus. Tohoku J Exp Med 124:205, 1978

27. Garcia MJ, McNamara PM, Gordon T, Kannell WB: Morbidity and mortality in diabetics in the Framingham population. Sixteen year follow-up study. Diabetes 23:105, 1974

28. Jackson JE, Bressler R: Clinical pharmacology of sulphonylurea hypoglycemic agents. Drugs 22:211;295, 1981

29. Hansen JM, Christensen LK: Drug interactions with oral sulphonylurea hypoglycaemic drugs. Drugs 13:24, 1977

29a. Edwards TH, Braunstein GD, Davidson MB: Glyburide-induced hypoglycemia in an elderly patient: similarity of first-generation and second-generation sulfonylurea agents. Mt Sinai J Med 52:644, 1985

30. Trovati M, Burzacca S, Mularoni E et al: Occurrence of low blood glucose concentrations during the afternoon in type 2 (non-insulin-dependent) diabetic patients on oral hypoglycaemic agents: importance of blood glucose monitoring. Diabetologia 34:662, 1991

31. Pedersen O, Hother-Nielsen O, Bak J et al: Effects of sulfonylureas on adipocyte and skeletal muscle insulin action in patients with non-insulin-dependent diabetes mellitus. Am J Med 90(suppl 6A):22S, 1991

32. Davidson MB: Rational use of sulfonylureas. Postgrad Med 92:69, 1992

33. Peters AL, Davidson MB: Maximal dose glyburide therapy in markedly symptomatic patients with type 2 diabetes: a new use for an old friend. J Clin Endocrinol Metab 81:2423, 1996

34. Katz HM, Bissel G: Blood sugar lowering effects of chlorpropamide and tolbutamide. A double blind cooperative study. Diabetes 14:650, 1965

34a. Davidson MB, Ficks LG, Peter AL: There is benefit to increasing the sulfonylurea dose. Diabetes Spectrum 10:91, 1997

35. Salo S, Groop L: Combination of two sulfonylureas. Does it make sense? Diabetes Care 11:751, 1988

36. Uraemic hypoglycaemia (editorial). Lancet I:660, 1986

37. Multi-centre study: UK prospective study of therapies of maturity-onset diabetes. I. Effect of diet, sulphonylurea, insulin or biguanide therapy on fasting plasma glucose and body weight over one year. Diabetologia 24:404, 1983

38. Firth RG, Bell PM, Rizza RA: Effects of tolazamide and exogenous insulin on insulin action in patients with non-insulin-dependent diabetes mellitus. N Engl J Med 314:1280, 1986

39. Nathan DM, Russell A, Godine JE: Glyburide or insulin for metabolic control in non-insulin-dependent diabetes mellitus. A randomized, double-blind study. Ann Intern Med 108:334, 1988

40. Bailey CJ, Turner RC: Metformin. N Engl J Med 334:574, 1996

41. Davidson MB, Peters AL: An overview of metformin in the treament of type 2 diabetes mellitus. Am J Med 102:99, 1997

42. DeFronzo RA, Goodman AM, Multicenter Metformin Study Group: Efficacy of metformin in patients with non-insulin-dependent diabetes mellitus. N Engl J Med 333:541, 1995

43. Somogyi A, Stockley C, Keal J et al: Reduction of metformin renal tubular secretion by cimetidine in man. Br J Clin Pharmacol 23:44, 1987

44. Gin H, Orgerie MB, Aubertin J: The influence of guar gum on absorption of metformin from the gut in healthy volunteers. Horm Metab Res 21:81, 1989

45. Klip A, Leiter LA: Cellular mechanism of action of metformin. Diabetes Care 13:696, 1990

46. Bailey CJ: Metformin—an update. Gen Pharmacol 24:1299, 1993

47. Lucis OJ: The status of metformin in Canada. Can Med Assoc J 128:24, 1983

48. Bailey CJ, Nattrass M: Treatment—metformin. Baillieres Clin Endocrinol Metab 2:455, 1988

49. Callaghan TS, Hadden DR, Tomkin GH: Megaloblastic anaemia due to vitamin B_{12} malabsorption associated with long-term metformin treatment. BMJ 280:1214, 1980

50. Andrews WJ, Vasquez B, Nagulesparan M et al: Insulin therapy in obese, non-insulin-dependent diabetes induces improvements in insulin action and secretion that are maintained for two weeks after insulin withdrawal. Diabetes 33:634, 1984

51. Henry RR, Wallace P, Gumbiner B et al: Intensive conventional insulin therapy for type 2 diabetes: metabolic effects during a 6-month outpatient trial. Diabetes Care 16:21, 1993

52. Yki-Jarvinin H, Kauppila M, Kujansuu E et al: Comparison of insulin regimens in patients with non-insulin-dependent diabetes mellitus. N Engl J Med 327:1426, 1992

53. Peters AL, Davidson MB: BIDS therapy for treatment of NIDDM: effectiveness and pre-

dictors (if any) of success. Diabetes Spectrum 7:152, 1994

54. Chow C-C, Tsang LWW, Sorenson JP et al: Comparison of insulin with or without continuation of oral hypoglycemic agents in the treatment of secondary failure in NIDDM patients. Diabetes Care 18:307, 1995

54a. Shank ML, Del Prato S, DeFronzo RA: Bedtime insulin/daytime glipizide: effective therapy for sulfonylurea failures in NIDDM. Diabetes 44:165, 1995

55. Peters AL, Davidson MB: Insulin plus sulfonylurea agent for treating type 2 diabetes. Ann Intern Med 115:45, 1991

56. Stout RW: Overview of the association between insulin and atherosclerosis. Metabolism 34:7, 1985

57. Davidson MB: Clinical implications of insulin resistance syndromes. Am J Med 99:420, 1995

58. Coniff RF, Shapiro JA, Seaton TB: Long-term efficacy and safety of acarbose in the treatment of obese subjects with non-insulin-dependent diabetes mellitus. Arch Intern Med 154:2442, 1994

59. Chaisson J-L, Josse RG, Hunt JA et al: The efficacy of acarbose in the treatment of patients with non-insulin-dependent diabetes mellitus: a multicenter controlled clinical trial. Ann Intern Med 121:928, 1994

60. Coniff RF, Shapiro JA, Seaton TB: Multicenter, placebo-controlled trial comparing acarbose (BAY g 5421) with placebo, tolbutamide, and tolbutamide-plus-acarbose in non-insulin-dependent diabetes mellitus. Am J Med 98:443, 1995

61. Spengler M, Cagatay M: The use of acarbose in the primary-care setting: evaluation of efficacy and tolerability of acarbose by postmarketing surveillance study. Clin Invest Med 18:325, 1995

62. Tahara Y, Shima K: The response of GHb to stepwise plasma glucose change over time in diabetic patients. Diabetes Care 16:1313, 1993

DIABETIC KETOACIDOSIS AND HYPEROSMOLAR NONKETOTIC SYNDROME

CHAPTER

6

DIABETIC KETOACIDOSIS

PATHOPHYSIOLOGY

Diabetic ketoacidosis (DKA) is caused by a profound lack of effective insulin. Published studies routinely report some measurable insulin concentrations, but these low levels (usually <10 μU/ml) are clearly inadequate in the metabolic milieu of marked hyperglycemia, ketosis, and acidosis. Although levels of the counterregulatory hormones (catecholamines, glucagon, growth hormone, and cortisol) are elevated as the result of stress,[1] such elevations do not *cause* the metabolic derangements that lead to DKA. Elevated levels of these hormones simply potentiate the effect of a lack of insulin; patients can become at least mildly ketoacidotic in the absence of high levels of these hormones.

The clinical hallmarks of DKA are acidosis, dehydration, and electrolyte depletion. The mechanisms behind these conditions are outlined in Figure 6-1. The effect of a lack of insulin on all three general areas of metabolism—carbohydrate, protein, and fat—figures prominently in the pathophysiology of DKA. In the absence of effective insulin, ingested carbohydrate is not utilized by the three insulin-sensitive tissues (liver, muscle, and adipose tissues). This impairment of glucose uptake causes hyperglycemia. Furthermore, in the late postprandial state, after the carbohydrate content of the diet has been stored, insulin is critically important in the modulation of glucose production by the liver. In the absence of effective insulin, enhanced hepatic glucose production further increases the already elevated glucose concentrations. In fact, more than half of the reduction in plasma glucose concentrations secondary to insulin administration in the treatment of DKA is due to decreased hepatic glucose production.[1] Hyperglycemia, in turn, causes an osmotic diuresis that results in water and electrolyte depletion. The water and electrolyte losses cause dehydration, which is clinically manifested as intravascular volume depletion. The fluid losses are hypotonic to plasma, and a hyperosmolar state therefore develops.

In protein metabolism, a lack of insulin reinforces fluid and electrolyte depletion. In the absence of effective insulin, the transport of amino acids into cells and the incorporation of these intracellular amino acids into protein are decreased. In addition, the inhibition of protein degradation by insulin is lost. Therefore, the effects of a lack of insulin on amino acid transport, protein synthesis, and protein degradation all cause protein catabolism, which results in increased release of amino acids from muscle tissue. Some of these amino acids are gluconeogenic precursors and are converted to glucose by the liver. The rate of gluconeogenesis is controlled by the amount of appropriate substrates delivered to the liver. Therefore, the increased flux of amino acids from muscle contributes significantly to hyperglycemia, with its attendant fluid and electrolyte losses. The amino acids not utilized for gluconeogenesis are metabolized by the liver to fulfill energy demands. This increased nitrogen loss leads to a depletion of lean body mass, which is an important component of the weight loss suffered by the affected patients.

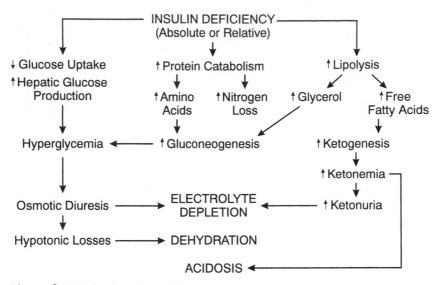

Figure 6–1. Pathophysiology of diabetic ketoacidosis.

In the case of fat metabolism, the lack of effective insulin also contributes to fluid and electrolyte depletion. However, ketosis and eventual acidosis are solely attributable to the lack of an insulin effect on adipose tissue. A critical aspect of insulin action on this tissue is an inhibition of the breakdown of triglycerides, a pathway termed lipolysis (see Chapter 2). Increased lipolysis results in elevated concentrations of glycerol and free fatty acids (FFA) in plasma. Because glycerol is a gluconeogenic precursor, its increased flux from adipose tissue enhances gluconeogenesis even further. This enhancement, of course, leads to more pronounced hyperglycemia and greater fluid and electrolyte losses. Some of the FFA can be utilized by tissues for energy purposes or reconstituted as hepatic triglycerides. However, as discussed in Chapter 2, the most important determinant of ketone body formation (ketogenesis) is the amount of FFA delivered to the liver. The ketogenic pathway is further activated by the presence of the low insulin and high glucagon concentrations that characterize DKA. The ketone bodies (acetoacetate and β-hydroxybutyrate) are weak acids that must be buffered on release by the liver into the circulation (ketonemia). As more and more ketone bodies are produced, the body bases become depleted and acidosis ensues. In addition to causing acidosis, the ketone bodies also contribute to the loss of electrolytes. Although they can be utilized to some extent by various body tissues, the capacity to metabolize ketone bodies is soon exceeded, and they are excreted into the urine (ketonuria). This event exacerbates electrolyte depletion because cations must be excreted with the ketone bodies. These are the mechanisms, then, by which a lack of insulin affects carbohydrate, protein, and fat metabolism and leads to the dehydration, electrolyte depletion, and acidosis that characterize DKA.

LOSSES

The usual fluid and electrolyte losses sustained by patients experiencing DKA are marked, as shown in Figure 6-2. The values in this figure are derived from two kinds of studies. In one type of study, the use of insulin was discontinued in ketosis-prone diabetic patients, and the amounts of fluid and electrolytes lost over a 24-hour period were

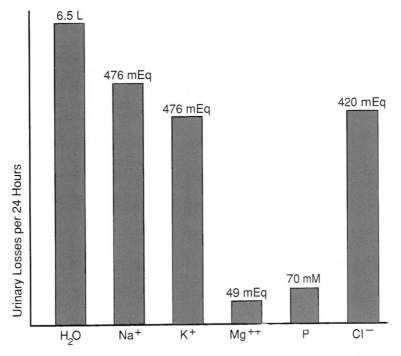

Figure 6–2. Urinary losses of water and electrolytes in patients with diabetic ketoacidosis.

measured. In the other type, the amounts of fluid and electrolytes needed to treat patients experiencing DKA in the first 24-hour period were carefully tabulated. In a "typical" 70-kg individual, the fluid, sodium, potassium, and chloride losses depicted in Figure 6-2 are indeed impressive. Extracellular water represents 17% of body weight, or ~12 L in our reference subject. Therefore, more than one half of the extracellular fluid compartment was lost. The amount of exchangeable sodium in a normal individual is 41 mEq/kg. The sodium loss in these diabetic subjects represented >15% of this total exchangeable pool. Similarly, the chloride loss was between 15% and 20% of the normal chloride pool (33 mEq/kg). Approximately 10% of total body potassium (50 to 54 mEq/kg) was excreted by these subjects. Of the total exchangeable magnesium pool (10 mEq/kg), 7% was lost under these circumstances.

The situation with regard to phosphorus is more complicated. The body of a 70-kg man, for example, contains ~712 g, or 23,000 mmol, of phosphorus. Of this amount, 80% is in bone and 9% in muscle. However, the bulk of the intracellular phosphorus is in organic form, and only a small fraction is inorganic. Thus, although the amount of phosphorus lost in the urine of these diabetic subjects during a 24-hour period is a minuscule percentage of total body phosphorus, it represents a relatively substantial part of the available inorganic phosphorus pool. Balance studies performed during several weeks after recovery from DKA have demonstrated substantial retention of phosphorus (up to 400 mmol). These studies probably underestimate net phosphorus losses because they were completed before the pre-DKA weight had been regained. The problems of phosphorus homeostasis in the treatment of DKA is discussed in greater detail later.

Table 6–1. Precipitating Causes of Diabetic Ketoacidosis

Cause	Percent
Infection	30–40
Cessation of insulin	15–20
New-onset diabetes	20–25
Myocardial infarction	
Pancreatitis	
Shock and hypovolemia	10–15
Stroke	
Other medical diseases	
No precipitating event	20–25

From DeFronzo RA, Matsuda M, Barrett EJ: Diabetic ketoacidosis: a combined metabolic-nephrologic approach to therapy. Diabetes Rev 2:209, 1994.

CAUSES

The precipitating causes of DKA are listed in Table 6-1. The most common cause is infection. New onset of type 1 diabetes is the second most common cause, followed closely by omission or reduction of the current insulin dose. Various medical conditions account for the remainder of the identifiable causes. No precipitating event can be identified in approximately one quarter of patients admitted to the hospital with DKA. It should be emphasized, however, that DKA is potentially preventable in the approximately 50% of patients in whom the precipitating cause is infection or reduced insulin doses (often a combination of the two).

SYMPTOMS

The symptoms of DKA are listed in Table 6-2. Polyuria and polydipsia are simply mani-

Table 6–2. Symptoms of Diabetic Ketoacidosis

Polyuria	Anorexia
Polydipsia	Nausea
Weakness	Vomiting
Lethargy	Abdominal pain
Myalgia	"Dyspnea"
Headache	

festations of osmotic diuresis secondary to hyperglycemia. Weakness, lethargy, headache, and myalgia are relatively nonspecific symptoms. The gastrointestinal and respiratory symptoms, however, are specifically related to DKA.

Although documentation is difficult, ketosis is probably responsible for many of the gastrointestinal symptoms. (Ketosis secondary to low carbohydrate intake—i.e., starvation ketosis—is associated with anorexia, nausea, and occasionally vomiting.) In any event, nausea, vomiting, and abdominal pain are often noted in patients with DKA. The abdominal pain can be quite severe and may even suggest an intraabdominal process requiring surgery.

When questioned more closely, patients who complain of dyspnea (shortness of breath on exertion) are found actually to be having difficulty in catching their breath even while sitting or lying quietly. This symptom, of course, represents hyperventilation, which is the ventilatory response to metabolic acidosis originally described by Kussmaul.

SIGNS

The signs of DKA are listed in Table 6-3. Low body temperatures are not generally recognized as characteristic of patients experiencing DKA. The depth of respiration, not the rate, characterizes Kussmaul respirations. Patients often have a normal respiratory rate

Table 6–3. Signs of Diabetic Ketoacidosis

Hypothermia
Hyperpnea (Kussmaul respirations)
Acetone breath
"Dehydration" (intravascular volume depletion)
Hyporeflexia
Acute abdomen
Stupor (→ coma)
Hypotonia
Uncoordinated ocular movements
Fixed, dilated pupils

but on closer inspection are noted to be breathing very deeply. The signal for this hyperventilation is acidosis, which stimulates the respiratory center in the brain. The resulting respiratory alkalosis offsets the metabolic acidosis to some extent but cannot compensate for it entirely in the absence of treatment.

The structures and relations among the ketone bodies are depicted in Figure 6-3. Acetoacetate is irreversibly converted to acetone, some of which is excreted by the lungs. Acetone has a fruity odor that is often apparent on a patient's breath, although not all observers can distinguish this odor.

Although the term *dehydration* is often used to describe patients experiencing DKA, the signs really result from intravascular volume depletion. In adults, the most sensitive sign of intravascular volume depletion is a change in the way in which the neck veins fill. When normally hydrated subjects lie entirely horizontally (i.e., without a pillow), the neck veins fill from below up to one half to two thirds of the way to the angle of the jaw. This sign is essentially a clinical measurement of venous pressure, which is normally ~7 cm H_2O. To ascertain whether the jugular veins are filling from below, the vein near the clavicle should first be occluded just above the clavicle so that its course can be delineated as it fills from above. Next, the vein should be occluded near the angle of the jaw to determine how far over the clavicle it fills from below. It is helpful to empty the vein by "milking" it while it is occluded from above so that the advancing column of blood can be seen as the vein subsequently fills from below the clavicle. If the vein is not filled from below or is filled to less than

one half of the distance to the angle of the mandible, the intravascular volume is significantly reduced.

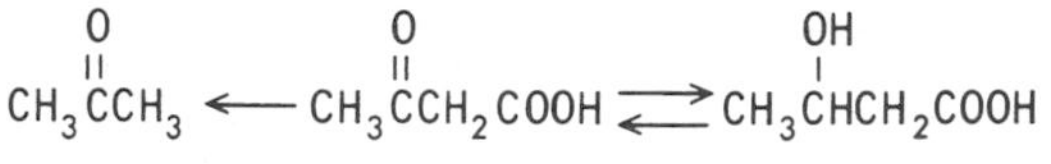

The only other reliable sign of intravascular depletion in adults is supine hypotension or a fall of systolic blood pressure by 20 mm Hg or greater when the patient moves from a lying to a sitting or standing position. So that equilibrium is ensured, at least 1 minute should elapse before the semivertical or vertical blood pressure is recorded. This orthostatic change in systolic blood pressure is a less sensitive measurement than decreased filling of the neck veins and thus represents a more marked deficit in intravascular volume. (It must be kept in mind, however, that diabetic patients with dysfunction of the autonomic nervous system may manifest orthostatic changes in blood pressure in the absence of any fluid loss.)

The other signs often considered in the determination of dehydration are really not very helpful. Dry mucous membranes are noted in patients who breathe with their mouth open. Soft eyeballs and poor skin turgor are seen, at least in adults, only with profound dehydration.

Hyporeflexia may be noted in patients experiencing DKA. If not present initially, it often develops during treatment as the potassium concentration ([K]) falls. (The response of potassium to therapy is discussed later.)

The abdominal examination of patients experiencing DKA can yield striking results. Abdominal tenderness to palpation and muscle guarding are usual. Bowel sounds may be diminished or even absent. Rebound tenderness is often noted. In an occasional patient, a boardlike abdomen with no bowel sounds and rebound tenderness may suggest a catastrophic intraabdominal process requiring immediate surgery. However, these signs are caused by DKA, although the mechanism underlying them is unknown. Except for the unusual patient in whom DKA may be precipitated by such an event, these signs resolve as the patient's biochemical status improves. In any event, because surgery is

$$CH_3\overset{\overset{\textstyle O}{\|}}{C}CH_3 \longleftarrow CH_3\overset{\overset{\textstyle O}{\|}}{C}CH_2COOH \rightleftarrows CH_3\overset{\overset{\textstyle OH}{|}}{C}HCH_2COOH$$

| Acetone | Acetoacetate | β-hydroxybutyrate |

Figure 6-3. Structure of and relation among the ketone bodies.

contraindicated in patients with DKA because of the extremely high related mortality, treatment of DKA must precede surgical intervention, and signs suggesting the need for surgery almost invariably disappear with treatment.

The mental status of patients experiencing DKA ranges from completely alert to comatose and is not related to the degree of ketosis or acidosis. In fact, a patient's mental status seems best correlated with plasma osmolarity (Fig. 6-4). Various degrees of lethargy, stupor, and coma are observed in most patients, and altered mental status is an important sign of DKA.

Hypotonia, uncoordinated ocular movements, and fixed, dilated pupils are (fortunately) unusual symptoms that are associated with a poor prognosis (as is very deep coma).

DIFFERENTIAL DIAGNOSIS

The diagnosis of DKA is simple if it is considered in the differential. A urine sample showing marked glucosuria and ketonuria or an undiluted plasma sample giving a strongly positive result in the nitroprusside test for acetoacetate is sufficient for the diagnosis. However, too often, these tests are not performed and the diagnosis is regrettably delayed.

Other conditions that may mimic DKA to various degrees and the clinical similarities between these conditions and DKA are listed in Table 6-4. Although coma is certainly encountered in DKA, most diabetic patients who present in coma are found to have suffered cerebral vascular accidents, simply because many more diabetic patients have strokes than have episodes of DKA.

A brainstem hemorrhage may be confused with DKA because both conditions may be associated with glucosuria and hyperventilation. The hyperventilation in brainstem hemorrhage is explained by the fact that the respiratory center is located in the brainstem. In the 19th century, Claude Bernard

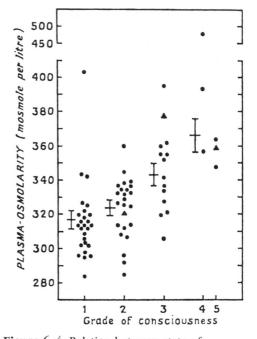

Figure 6–4. Relation between state of consciousness and calculated plasma osmolarity in 70 episodes of diabetic ketoacidosis. The means (horizontal line) are shown, and ± 1 SEM is enclosed in brackets. The three triangles refer to three values reported as exceeding those shown. States of consciousness were defined as follows: (1) awake or mildly drowsy (26 episodes); (2) moderately drowsy but easily arousable and fully oriented (24 episodes); (3) very drowsy but arousable by loud questioning and then partially oriented (14 episodes); (4) stuporous, barely responsive, and then not oriented (3 episodes); and (5) comatose (4 episodes). (From Fulop M, Tannenbaum H, Dreyer N: Hyperosmolar coma. Lancet 2:635, 1973)

showed that stimulation of an area in the brainstem resulted in glucosuria, or "piqûre" diabetes.

The many features that distinguish DKA from hypoglycemia are listed in Table 6-5. In hypoglycemia, the onset is rapid (within minutes), gastrointestinal symptoms are lacking, signs of intravascular volume depletion are absent, and respiration is normal. In DKA, in contrast, the onset is slow (over a

Table 6–4. Differential Diagnosis of Diabetic Ketoacidosis (DKA)

Cerebrovascular accident (altered mental status)[a]
Brainstem hemorrhage (hyperventilation, glucosuria)
Hypoglycemia (altered mental status, tachycardia)
Metabolic acidosis (hyperventilation, anion gap
    acidosis)
　Uremia
　Salicylates
　Methanol
　Ethylene glycol
Gastroenteritis (nausea, vomiting, abdominal pain)
Pneumonia (hyperventilation)

[a]Clinical similarities to DKA are listed in parentheses.

period of hours), gastrointestinal symptoms and signs of intravascular volume depletion are prominent, and Kussmaul respirations are noted. In DKA, tachycardia is present secondary to intravascular volume depletion. In hypoglycemia, the sympathetic nervous system is fully activated, and in addition to tachycardia, the patient may exhibit tremors, anxiety, hunger, tingling of the fingers and around the mouth, palpitations, and sweating. Sweating leads to cool, wet skin that contrasts with the dry, flushed skin of patients in DKA. Although glucosuria is usually minimal or absent in hypoglycemia, the test result can be positive if the bladder contains

Table 6–5. Features Distinguishing Diabetic Ketoacidosis from Hypoglycemia

	Condition	
Feature	*DKA*	*Hypoglycemia*
Onset	Slow	Fast
Gastrointestinal symptoms	Yes	No
Intravascular volume depletion	Yes	No
Respiration	Deep	Normal
Sympathetic nervous system signs and symptoms	Tachycardia only	Yes
Glucosuria	≥2%	±
Ketonuria	Strong	Negative

DKA, diabetic ketoacidosis.

urine formed during a hyperglycemic period preceding the onset of hypoglycemia. The presence of ketonuria establishes the diagnosis of DKA, whereas its absence indicates a diagnosis of hypoglycemia. The diagnosis of DKA is clearly untenable in the absence of ketonuria.

The other conditions listed—metabolic acidosis, gastroenteritis, and pneumonia—all can be ruled out by the absence of significant ketosis. Although ketonuria may be present if carbohydrate intake has been poor, a less than strongly positive result in the nitroprusside test for ketone bodies in undiluted plasma essentially rules out DKA.

INITIAL LABORATORY VALUES

The results of pertinent laboratory tests in patients presenting with DKA are listed in Table 6-6. Glucose concentrations obviously can vary considerably, and a substantial number of patients experiencing DKA have initial glucose values of <300 mg/dl.[2] In a series of 211 episodes of DKA, 37 patients had severe acidosis—that is, [HCO_3] <10 mEq/L—and "euglycemia." Glucose concentrations were between 200 and 300 mg/dl in 21 patients, between 100 and 200 mg/dl in 9, and <100 mg/dl in 7! Thus, 17.5% of patients in this report presented with glucose levels of <300 mg/dl although they were experiencing severe DKA.[2] Others have also found that glucose concentrations are unrelated to the severity of the acidosis.[3]

The nitroprusside test for ketone bodies yields strongly positive results in undiluted plasma, and these results most often remain strongly positive through several dilutions. The result of this test does not represent the full extent of the ketosis, however, because the nitroprusside reagent measures only acetoacetate and not β-hydroxybutyrate. (Actually, acetone is also measured, but it is only 5% as active as acetoacetate on a molar basis and occurs in patients with DKA at levels that are only two to four times higher than those of acetoacetate.) The ratio of β-hy-

Table 6–6. Initial Laboratory Values for Patients Experiencing Diabetic Ketoacidosis

Test	Result	Remarks
Glucose	300–800 mg/dl	Concentrations not related to severity of DKA
Ketone bodies	Strong at least in undiluted plasma	Measures only acetoacetate, not β-hydroxybutyrate
[HCO$_3$]	0–15 mEq/L	
pH	6.8–7.3	
[Na]	Low, normal, or high	Total body depletion; concentration dependent on relative H$_2$O loss and amount shifted from intracellular to extracellular space
[K]	Low, normal, or high	Total body depletion; heart responsive to extracellular concentration
Phosphate	Usually normal or slightly elevated; occasionally slightly low	Associated with phosphaturia; marked decrease with treatment in levels of both serum and urine phosphates
Creatinine/BUN	Usually mildly increased	May be prerenal; spurious increases in creatinine by acetoacetate in some automated methods
WBC count	Usually increased	Possibility of leukemoid reaction (even in absence of infection)
Amylase	Often increased	Predominant form of salivary gland origin
Lipase	Sometimes increased	Even markedly elevated values do not necessarily mean acute pancreatitis present
Hemoglobin, hematocrit, total protein	Often increased	Secondary to contracted plasma volume
AST, ALT, LDH	Can be mildly elevated	Spurious increases in transaminases due to acetoacetate interference in older colorimetric methods

[HCO$_3$], concentration of bicarbonate; [Na], concentration of sodium; [K], concentration of potassium; BUN, blood urea nitrogen; WBC, white blood cell; AST, aspartate aminotransferase; ALT, alanine aminotransferase; LDH, lactic dehydrogenase; DKA, diabetic ketoacidosis.

droxybutyrate to acetoacetate varies greatly in DKA but may be as high as 3:1 to 5:1.[4-6] A rapid and specific assay for β-hydroxybutyrate that can be carried out on a drop of blood or plasma (e.g., KetoSite-ketone test card, GDS Diagnostics, Elkhart, IN) has become available. However, at present, this test is not widely used and there is little reported experience with it.

The decreases in [HCO$_3$] and pH do reflect the severity of metabolic derangement. However, if a patient is vomiting much, the tendency for a metabolic alkalosis blunts the decline in [HCO$_3$] and pH.[1] In fact, patients have been reported with marked hyperglyce-mia and ketosis and such severe vomiting that the resulting metabolic alkalosis has more than compensated for the ketoacidosis causing initial elevations of [HCO$_3$] and pH.[7] Severe intravascular volume depletion causes a contraction alkalosis, further limiting the reduction of [HCO$_3$] and pH.

Although total body depletion of sodium stores occurs in DKA, the serum concentration of sodium ([Na]) may be low, normal, or high and depends on water balance. If hyperlipidemia is present, the serum [Na] measured is falsely low. If hyperlipidemia is absent, the serum [Na] is simply a measure of the relative amounts of the cation and body water. Because urinary fluid losses are hypotonic, plasma osmolality becomes elevated, and a high serum [Na] would be expected. However, polyuria leads to polydipsia and the amount of water ingested affects the [Na]. If an appropriate amount of water is consumed, the [Na] may be normal. If an excess amount is ingested, the [Na] decreases. Vomiting further complicates the relation between sodium and water. In addition, the osmolar contribution of the hyperglycemia tends to decrease [Na] by drawing water from the intracellular to the extracellular space. Finally, if intravascular volume depletion is profound, antidiuretic hormone is secreted in an attempt to restore the vascular volume, even at the expense of decreasing serum osmolality and [Na].[8] (Hypertriglyceridemia can cause a pseudohyponatremia by displacing plasma water with lipid, and elevated triglyceride levels commonly occur in patients with markedly uncontrolled diabetes. The [Na] is decreased by 1.6 mEq/L for each 1000 mg/dl triglyceride concentration.) At presentation, the [Na] is normal in half of the patients, low in one quarter, and elevated in one quarter.[1] Although correcting the [Na] to take into account the effect of hyperglycemia (i.e., by raising the value by 1.6 mg/dl for each 100 mg/dl of glucose above 100 mg/dl[9]) has been advocated to give a truer picture of water balance,[1] the corrected value does not alter the clinical dictum that patients in DKA need saline repletion to restore their vascular volume, regardless of the [Na]. (The rate and osmolality of the replacement solutions are discussed later in the treatment section.)

Similar considerations pertain to the initial [K], which may be low, normal, or high. There is a profound total body depletion of potassium regardless of the serum concentration, and affected patients must have their stores replenished with potassium salts. The clinical situation with regard to potassium homeostasis in DKA is somewhat complicated and is also discussed in greater detail later in the treatment section.

Serum phosphorus concentrations are usually normal or even slightly elevated in untreated DKA. This finding is associated with marked phosphaturia (which accompanies all forms of metabolic acidosis). The explanation given is that acidosis leads to the breakdown of intracellular organic compounds and that inorganic phosphate is thus liberated, transferred into the plasma, and subsequently excreted in the urine. Treatment of DKA results in a gradual reduction of phosphaturia (over 8 to 10 hours) and a marked decrement of serum phosphorus concentrations, which may not reach their nadir for several days. The hypophosphatemia is presumably the result of the uptake of inorganic phosphorus by cells that had been phosphorus deficient.

Creatinine and blood urea nitrogen (BUN) levels are usually increased in DKA. This increase often represents prerenal azotemia caused by diminished perfusion of the kidneys secondary to intravascular volume depletion. An additional reason for elevated creatinine concentrations (but not BUN values) is interference by acetoacetate in some automated assays.[10] Therefore, a valid assessment of renal function must await resolution of DKA. In many cases, however, BUN and creatinine values do not return to normal, a result reflecting underlying diabetic nephropathy.

Not only is leukocytosis common in DKA, but leukemoid reactions with white blood cell (WBC) counts of 20,000 to 40,000/mm³ are occasionally seen. The high WBC counts are associated with lymphopenia and eosinopenia. This leukocyte response to DKA is thought to reflect increased adrenocortical activity and dehydration. Therefore, leukocytosis itself is not a reliable sign of infection in this setting. However, the WBC differential may provide an important clue. Patients with a higher percent of band neutrophils (bands) and a lower percent of segmented ones (segs) are much more likely to have a major infection.[11] In this study, 153 patients admitted with a diagnosis of DKA were divided into four groups. Group one (n = 111) manifested no infection during the first 48 hours. Group two (n = 11) had minor infections (upper respiratory, candidiasis, periodontal disease, viral pharyngitis) developing within the first 48 hours; these did not require antibiotics. Group three (n = 19) had a major infection (sepsis, abscess, meningitis, cellulitis, exudative pharyngitis, mucormycosis) that was not clinically apparent initially but became so within the first 48 hours. Group 4 (n = 12) had a major infection (pneumonia, pulmonary tuberculosis, wet gangrene) that was clinically evident on admission. All four groups had elevated WBC counts (per mm^3) of 13,890, 12,273, 16,258, and 20,358, respectively. The percent of band forms in the differential was higher in patients with a major infection (6.3, 4.7, 23.5, and 21.1, respectively), with a corresponding decrease in the percent of segmented polys (72.7, 72.5, 58.1, and 60.1, respectively). Using an admission band neutrophil count of ≥10% as diagnostic of a major infection, the sensitivity was 100% and the specificity was 80%. That is, all patients with a major infection had ≥10% band neutrophils (sensitivity) whereas 80% of patients with ≥10% band neutrophils had a major infection (specificity).

Amylase values are elevated in >50% of patients with DKA.[12] However, the increase in the majority of instances is in amylase of salivary origin rather than in that of pancreatic origin.[13, 14] Furthermore, the levels and origin of amylase do not correlate with signs and symptoms suggestive of pancreatitis.[13, 14] Thus, hyperamylasemia probably represents transient nonspecific leakage of this enzyme from its two tissues of origin and does not support a diagnosis of pancreatitis in DKA.

Lipase levels, which are considered more specific for pancreatic damage than amylase, can also be elevated in DKA, although not as frequently as amylase.[12] Although it is stated in textbooks that hyperlipasemia in DKA diagnoses pancreatitis, the published data do not substantiate that claim. Nsien and colleagues[12] reported that three patients with DKA, no abdominal symptoms, and marked elevations of lipase had negative results of computed tomography (CT) scans of the pancreas. In my own experience with six patients in DKA who had elevated lipase levels (three with mild increases and three with marked increases), all of the patients with mild increases had negative results of CT scans of the pancreas whereas two of the three with marked increases had changes consistent with acute pancreatitis. The third had mild changes in the head of the pancreas, but the radiologist was reluctant to make that diagnosis. Two of the three with marked elevations of lipase (including the one with the mild changes on the CT scan) had a positive history of alcohol abuse. All three of the patients with marked elevations of lipase had abdominal signs and symptoms consistent with acute pancreatitis. Thus, very high levels of lipase (increases over 10-fold) in patients with DKA and abdominal signs and symptoms may indicate acute pancreatitis (especially in patients with an alcoholic history), but in many instances this is not the case. Clinical judgment is required here. If a patient with marked hyperlipasemia can resume oral intake within a day or two, this would seem to be inconsistent with the diagnosis of acute pancreatitis. If the biochemical changes of DKA have been reversed and the patient remains unable to tolerate oral feedings for several more days, the patient may have acute pancreatitis.

The frequent increases in hemoglobin, hematocrit, and total proteins in DKA simply reflect the decreased volume of plasma. Therefore, a low normal or slightly decreased hematocrit or hemoglobin value on admission indicates a probable anemia that will require further evaluation after DKA is treated.

In the recent past, tests for the enzymes serum aspartate aminotransferase (AST), alanine aminotransferase (ALT), and lactic dehydrogenase (LDH) often gave falsely elevated results because of interference by acetoacetate in the colorimetric methods used. Many laboratories are now using kinetic procedures for the measurement of these enzymes; in these procedures, false-positive results are not a problem. If the level of any of these enzymes is found to be elevated in patients who are ketotic, the physician should ascertain that the method used involves direct measurements of reduced nucleotides via changes in ultraviolet absorption rather than coupling with a diazonium salt (the colorimetric method). However, levels of serum enzymes such as AST, ALT, creatine phosphokinase (CPK), and 5'-nucleotidase are truly elevated in many patients with DKA. Severe abnormalities are usually explained by readily apparent clinical disease. Elevated levels are not related to the degree of abdominal symptoms, nor are they caused by acidosis per se. When no cause can be found, the enzyme levels usually return to normal after treatment for DKA.

Discerning readers have probably noticed that the anion gap ($[Na]-[Cl]-[HCO_3]$) has not been discussed. Because of the impact of vomiting and contraction alkalosis discussed earlier, as well as other limitations in its interpretation,[15] uncritical reliance on the anion gap in the diagnosis and treatment of DKA can be misleading.

TREATMENT

The treatment of DKA can be conveniently discussed under six separate categories: general therapeutic approaches, fluid replacement, insulin therapy, potassium replacement, phosphate replacement, and bicarbonate therapy. Obviously, all six areas must be considered in clinical decisions, but if each area is considered separately, the decisions are usually straightforward and a coherent treatment plan emerges. Some of these areas of treatment are controversial, and valid arguments can be made on both sides of the issues. Indeed, in many cases, it is difficult to be certain that one course of action is distinctly better for a given patient.

General Considerations

The use of all deliberate speed is appropriate in the treatment of DKA. Therapy within minutes is not necessary, but a delay of treatment for several hours can be detrimental to patients. Certain general principles should be followed. First, only one physician should be in charge of the patient's care and should assume full responsibility for therapeutic decisions. Second, a diabetic ketoacidosis progress record (Fig. 6-5) should be started *as soon as therapy is initiated.* Too often, this record is constructed from memory many hours after treatment has begun. An accurate and updated progress record enables any health professional involved in the care of the patient to become quickly familiar with the treatment given and the response to therapy. This progress record is extremely important in situations in which responsibility for the patient's care is transferred (e.g., when house staff coverage in teaching hospitals or evening and weekend coverage in the private sector causes a transfer of responsibility to personnel not familiar with the patient). At that juncture, it is wise for the two physicians involved to discuss the patient's progress record, what has transpired, and what is planned. Unfortunately, the physician taking over the patient's care is often unaware of important information because it is not on the progress record and has not been communicated by the doctor going off duty.

Third, and most obvious, an appropriate site for intravenous fluid administration is necessary. Because many hours of fluid administration will be necessary, a small needle tenuously placed in a peripheral vein should not be relied on.

Fourth, urine samples are necessary not only in making the diagnosis of DKA but in monitoring a patient's response to therapy. In addition, it must be ascertained that a patient is not experiencing renal shutdown before potassium replacement is started. Therefore, if a patient does not urinate spontaneously, bladder catheterization, which

(a) Enter as applicable: 1 = ALERT   2 = LETHARGIC (easily aroused)
   3 = STUPOR (aroused with difficulty)   4 = COMA (unresponsive)

DATE	SIGNS			SERUM						URINE	TREATMENT						
											INSULIN		FLUIDS				
TIME	BP (↑ or→)	RESP	(a) CNS	GLUCOSE	HCO₃	K	Na	Cl	Cr / BUN	GLUCOSE / KETONES	TIME START	AMT (U/hr)	TIME START	TYPE	AMT (L)	K (mEq)	HCO₃ (mEq)

Figure 6–5. Sample diabetic ketoacidosis progress record. BP, blood pressure; ↑, sitting or standing; →, lying; RESP, respiratory; CNS, central nervous system; Cr, creatinine; BUN, blood urea nitrogen; Amt, amount; K, potassium; HCO₃, bicarbonate.

rarely should be undertaken in diabetic patients, is indicated. In this instance, the initial bladder specimen should be cultured to ascertain whether the DKA is associated with (precipitated by?) a urinary tract infection. Once the catheter is placed, the resulting pyuria makes such an assessment difficult.

Fifth, because the possibility of pulmonary aspiration is enhanced considerably in comatose patients, a nasogastric tube should be put in place and continuous suction applied until patients become more responsive. In more alert patients, this maneuver is restricted to those with signs of gastric distention.

The sixth general principle concerns the ordering of laboratory tests and the timing of samples. This discussion is limited to those tests that are concerned specifically with the diagnosis and treatment of DKA. I routinely order measurements of glucose, electrolytes, phosphate, and creatinine or BUN values. Although measuring the initial pH and degree of ketosis is not necessary for either diagnosis or monitoring the response to therapy, these values will document the severity of the DKA. If an arterial puncture cannot be done, measurement of venous or nonarterialized capillary blood pH is still useful as long as it is recognized that this value may be slightly lower than that obtained with a concomitant arterial sample. Indeed, some maintain that these sampling sites (i.e., nonarterial) should be used routinely.[16] I often do not obtain a blood pH in a straightforward case of DKA.

The degree of ketosis is best reflected in the last dilution in which the nitroprusside test for acetoacetate yields a *strongly* positive result. Determination of the last dilution in which any reaction is noted is not helpful. The advantage of measuring plasma ketone bodies by this semiquantitative technique is that the results are available immediately. If possible, the nitroprusside test should be performed near the patient's bedside by the physician or an appropriately trained person. If the sample is sent to the laboratory, by the time the results are returned they are not helpful in many instances. Although the rapidity with which the results of the nitroprusside test are known would seem to make them very useful in therapeutic decisions, monitoring of the patient's response by using this test may be misleading during the first 4 to 6 hours for reasons discussed later. On the other hand, rapid determination of β-hydroxybutyrate could be useful in establishing the diagnosis. The initial value was 8.3 mmol/L (normal, <0.20 to 0.25 mmol/L) in a small series of patients with DKA.[17] There was no indication in this report, however, of how to use subsequent values to determine therapy.

After treatment is started, glucose and electrolyte concentrations should be measured every 2 hours until the [HCO_3] reaches ~12 mEq/L; at this time, sampling every 4 hours becomes appropriate. Phosphate concentrations should be measured initially and every 4 to 6 hours. If phosphate levels are elevated, calcium and magnesium concentrations in serum should also be measured. The BUN or creatinine test is repeated after the patient is adequately rehydrated.

Fluid Administration

Solutions containing dextrose should not be used initially (unless the glucose concentration is <200 mg/dl) because the additional glucose could not be utilized and would simply increase the degree of hyperglycemia. Because an occasional patient with DKA also has lactic acidosis (as described later), most diabetologists also avoid the use of solutions containing lactate. The controversy surrounding fluid administration involves the osmolality of the saline solution that should be used.

A patient experiencing DKA has two separate problems that are specifically treated by fluid administration. One is the hyperosmolal state of the circulation (secondary to hypotonic fluid losses), and the other is intravascular volume depletion. The first problem should be treated with hypo-osmolal solutions, and the second requires saline to replenish the plasma volume. The argument against using a hypo-osmolal solution (usually one-half normal or 0.45% saline) as the initial fluid replacement in DKA is that it does not reverse intravascular volume depletion as rapidly as does normal saline, and vital organs may continue to be underperfused for a longer period. On the other hand, the argument against the use of normal or isotonic (0.9%) saline as the initial fluid is its hyperosmolality (308 mOsm/kg) compared with normal plasma osmolality (285 mOsm/kg). Proponents of the use of normal saline point out that plasma osmolality in DKA is most often >310 mOsm/kg, and therefore a hyperosmolal solution is not really being infused. However, potassium and its anion (20 to 40 mEq of each) are often added to the first bottle (as described later) so that the osmolality is increased to 348 or 388 mOsm/kg. The need to reduce the plasma osmolality in DKA (and the possible danger of increasing it) is represented by the inverse relation between the patient's level of consciousness and plasma osmolality, as depicted in Figure 6–4.

Given these considerations, I use normal saline when intravascular volume depletion is profound and 0.45% saline when plasma volume contraction is more moderate. The two clinical signs of intravascular volume depletion (an orthostatic decline in systolic pressure of 20 mm Hg or greater and decreased neck vein filling from below) are very helpful in making this clinical distinction. (Supine hypotension reflects an even greater degree of intravascular volume depletion than a normal supine systolic blood pressure with orthostatic changes on sitting or standing.) As long as a patient has supine hypotension or orthostatic changes, reflecting more profound dehydration, normal saline is the preferred solution. When the blood pressure can be maintained while the patient is sitting or standing but neck vein filling is still low, the administration of 0.45%

saline can be begun. Regardless of the degree of dehydration, 0.9% saline is used if the serum [Na] is <130 mEq/L, and 0.45% saline is used if the serum [Na] is >150 mEq/L. These recommendations are summarized in Table 6–7. When the neck veins fill appropriately, the patient is rehydrated, and further administration of intravenous (IV) fluid is unnecessary (unless, for some reason, oral intake is not feasible, in which case maintenance fluids are required). Patients with known orthostatic changes in blood pressure secondary to dysfunction of the autonomic nervous system present a problem. For these patients, I first use 1 L of 0.9% saline and then switch to 0.45% saline unless the serum [Na] dictates otherwise.

The rate of fluid administration is important. A common cause of an apparent lack of response to insulin treatment is too slow a rate of fluid replacement. (A typical situation might involve an infusion rate of 200 ml/h and glucose concentrations that remain within 50 mg/dl of their initial level for several hours.) It has even been suggested that initially insulin has little, if any, effect on hyperglycemia and that the reduced glucose concentrations are secondary to rehydration, which results in urinary disposal of the excess glucose.[18, 19] One liter of fluid per hour should be given for at least the first 2 hours and even longer if orthostatic changes are noted. (The amount of fluid deficit shown in Figure 6–2 should be kept in mind.) As the signs of intravascular volume depletion abate, the rate of fluid administration can be decreased appropriately, usually to 500 ml/h. Intravenous administration of saline is usually continued until the intravascular volume has been fully restored (signified by normal filling of the neck veins from below) or when the patient can easily tolerate oral fluids.

Because it takes longer to correct acidosis than to correct hyperglycemia, it is almost always necessary to add dextrose to the fluids being administered at some point during treatment. When glucose concentrations

Table 6–7. A Guide to Choosing Normal or Half-Normal Saline to Treat Diabetic Ketoacidosis

Factors in Choosing Saline Type			
Serum Sodium (mEq/L)	*Supine or Orthostatic Hypotension*	*Neck Vein Filling*	Type of Saline
130–150	Present	Decreased	Normal
130–150	Absent	Decreased	Half-normal
<130	Immaterial	Immaterial	Normal
>150	Immaterial	Immaterial	Half-normal

have declined to ~250 mg/dl, 5% dextrose should be added to the infusion. (The reason for preventing glucose levels from falling rapidly to <250 mg/dl is discussed later). The average decrement in glucose concentrations is 75 to 100 mg/dl/h. Therefore, the time at which dextrose is needed can often be estimated if this rate of reduction in glucose level can be documented during the early phase of treatment. Because the osmolality of 5% dextrose in water is 277 mOsm/kg, the appropriate fluid for infusion is 5% dextrose-0.45% saline. By the time dextrose is needed, most patients have been rehydrated to the point at which 0.45% saline is appropriate. However, if intravascular volume depletion is still severe, a 5% dextrose-0.9% saline solution should be used. The hyperosmolality of the infusate decreases appreciably as glucose is metabolized or excreted and leaves the vascular space.

Insulin Treatment

In the past, most authorities recommended administration of high doses of insulin at frequent intervals for the treatment of DKA. Several studies have directly compared the efficacy and side effects of using much lower doses of insulin (2 to 10 U/h) instead of the previously recommended approach.[20-23] The reversal of the DKA state was similar regardless of the dose of insulin given. However, patients treated with lower doses of insulin had less hypoglycemia and hypokalemia than those given the higher "conventional" amounts.

These reports, however, were not universally accepted, and doubts were raised about the effectiveness of lower-dose insulin treatment in patients with severe DKA (i.e., those presenting in coma).[24] A subsequent report, however, compared the response to lower-dose insulin therapy and that to high-dose therapy in comatose or stuporous patients.[25] No differences were found in the rate of decrement of glucose concentrations, the control of acidosis, or the time elapsed before the patient became mentally alert. Finally, mortality in DKA was similar in 113 episodes treated with infrequent large amounts of insulin (4.4%) and in 237 episodes treated with frequent or continuous small doses of insulin (4.6%).[26]

Additional comparisons have demonstrated that the route of administration of lower doses of insulin (IV, subcutaneous, or intramuscular) has little influence on a patient's response.[27] Using a loading dose of insulin also makes no difference, not a surprising finding because the initial glucose response may be largely dependent on rehydration, as was discussed earlier.

Therefore, I treat all patients who are experiencing DKA with a low-dose IV infusion of regular insulin. To simplify the protocol, I do not use a loading dose because no clinical evidence shows that it is necessary. I use the IV route of administration to minimize the trauma of repeated injections for patients. The initial dose is 5 U/h. A solution of 0.2 U/ml is prepared by addition of 100 U (1.0 ml of U-100 regular insulin) to 500 ml of 0.9% saline. Although insulin is adsorbed to the glass bottle and plastic tubing, it is not necessary to add albumin to this solution. Rather, to avoid the expense and time wasted in waiting for albumin to arrive from the pharmacy, 50 to 100 ml of the insulin solution may simply be discarded into the sink (through the tubing after it is attached to the bottle). This procedure saturates the adsorption sites, and the appropriate amount of insulin is delivered to the patient.[28] The insulin solution is then administered via an IV infusion pump at a rate of 25 ml/h (0.2 U/ml × 25 ml/h = 5 U/h). The insulin is either piggy-backed onto the IV line delivering the rehydration fluid or administered via a separate vein. I avoid adding the insulin to the fluids used for rehydration because as the rate of administration of these fluids changes, either the amount of insulin delivered also changes or new solutions with different insulin concentrations have to be prepared. It is much simpler to control the rate of insulin delivery separately.

In most patients, this rate of insulin administration (5 U/h) is effective. However, if the glucose concentration does not decrease by 10% from its initial level after 2 hours of administration at this rate (and if fluid replacement is adequate, as described earlier), the infusion rate of insulin should be doubled to 10 U/h. This step is necessary in only a very small minority of cases and seems to be more commonly required (as expected) in obese and infected patients. When an occasional patient still does not respond and the glucose level again fails to decrease by 10% from the initial level within 2 more hours, the infusion rate should be doubled once more (to 20 U/h) at 4 hours. In fact, the infusion rate should be doubled every 2 hours until the patient starts to respond with a persistent lowering of the glucose concentration. Although infusion rates above 10 U/h are necessary in only an occasional patient, this approach serves to identify early those few patients with DKA who are truly insulin resistant; thus, they are provided with increasing amounts of insulin. The highest in-

fusion rate in my experience was 80 U/h; this rate was used in an obese patient with severe DKA in whom immune-mediated insulin resistance (see Chapter 4) was subsequently diagnosed.

An insulin concentration of 0.2 U/ml is particularly appropriate in this form of treatment of DKA. When 5 or 10 U of insulin per hour is required, the volume of fluid delivered in addition to the rehydration fluid is small enough (25 and 50 ml/h, respectively) to be excluded from calculations of fluid balance. Only at an infusion rate of ≥20 U of insulin per hour (which is rarely necessary) does the amount of additional fluid (100 ml/h) become large enough to require consideration in the overall fluid management. Conversely, after the metabolic derangements of DKA have mostly been reversed, patients often require infusion of insulin at a slower rate (1 to 3 U/h) until the appropriate time for administration of intermediate-acting insulin (as described in the following paragraph). At a concentration of insulin of 0.2 U/ml, infusion rates of 5 to 15 ml/h are required, and such infusions can be accurately delivered by currently available IV infusion pumps.

When the [HCO_3] is >15 mEq/L (see the following discussion of delayed return of [HCO_3] to normal) and the patient is able to drink and to eat light foods, the insulin infusion can be discontinued and administration of intermediate-acting (NPH) insulin started. It is helpful to give the first dose of intermediate-acting insulin in the morning or in the evening (i.e., at a time when the patient normally receives it). In this way, adjustments can be made in the manner described in Chapter 4. Because patients recovering from DKA probably are not eating the usual number of calories initially, the first dose of NPH insulin should be approximately two thirds of the usual amount. If a patient has a documented infection, however, the prehospitalization dose of insulin is given. The decreased caloric intake is probably offset by the insulin resistance associated with infection. Patients in whom this episode of DKA is the initial manifestation of diabetes should be given the usual starting doses of NPH insulin discussed in Chapter 4. Although these patients are not eating normally, these initial doses are usually lower than those that the patients eventually require and thus are not excessive.

A question often arises about the interval between the discontinuation of regular insulin infusions and the administration of NPH insulin. If a patient eats at the time when NPH insulin is first administered, the insulin infusion is continued for 1 or 2 hours (with the interval determined by the size of the meal). This regular insulin helps dispose of the ingested calories during the 2- to 4-hour lag period before intermediate-acting insulin starts to act. On the other hand, if NPH insulin is injected when the patient is not eating, the insulin infusion is stopped at the time of injection. In many patients, the regular insulin seems to exert some tissue effects for 1 or 2 hours after the infusion is discontinued and thereby helps to control the glucose concentration during the lag period before NPH insulin begins to act.

In many instances, a number of hours elapse between the time that acidosis clears and the time appropriate for administration of NPH insulin (morning or evening). In this situation, insulin infusion should be continued, but at a slower rate (1 to 3 U/h). Glucose concentrations should be measured every 4 hours, and the infusion rate should be titrated according to the patient's response. Plasma glucose levels under these circumstances obviously depend on the rate of glucose administration. Once a patient has recovered from DKA, 5% dextrose in water should be infused at the same rate as in any other patient who is not taking oral nourishment (i.e., ~50 g of glucose during every 8-hour period, or 125 ml/h. As just discussed, infusion of regular insulin is either discontinued at the time of injection of NPH insulin (if the patient is not eating) or continued for 1 or 2 hours (if the patient is eating). With these guidelines, the switch from insulin infusion to injection of intermediate-acting insulin after recovery from DKA is a relatively simple process.

Potassium Replacement

In considering potassium therapy, one is faced with a certain dilemma. Although the total body depletion of potassium is profound (see Fig. 6–2), the heart responds to extracellular concentrations, which, as shown in Table 6–6, can be high as well as normal or low. Therefore, potassium replacement may be contraindicated initially. However, because all modes of therapy reduce the serum [K], unless the patient is anuric, potassium replacement is required at some time (usually soon) after treatment is started.

Rehydration lowers the serum [K] in two ways. First, as the plasma volume is expanded, the [K] decreases simply through dilution. Second, an expanding intravascular volume improves renal perfusion. Improved perfusion increases urinary glucose excretion, and the resulting osmotic diuresis enhances urinary potassium losses.

Insulin treatment also lowers the serum [K] by two separate mechanisms. First, insulin directly stimulates the uptake of potassium by adipose tissue, muscle, and liver. Second, the entry of glucose into these tissues further enhances potassium uptake. Although it is commonly held that potassium leaves the cell and enters the extracellular fluid compartment as hydrogen ions enter the cell to be buffered, this probably does not occur in DKA.[29] Therefore, correction of the acidosis (with a postulated subsequent return of potassium into the cell) does not result in lowering of [K]. The major determinants of the serum [K] on admission for DKA are the degree of ketoacidemia and hyperglycemia,[29] both of which are accounted for solely by the insulinopenia.

Although the [K] measured in the laboratory is obviously the ultimate criterion on which clinical decisions must be based, the electrocardiogram (ECG) provides a reasonable alternative in the interval before laboratory results are available. The effect of potassium on the T-wave of the ECG is depicted in Figure 6–6. Hyperkalemia causes a tall, symmetrically peaked T-wave, whereas hypokalemia is associated with low or flat T-waves and the development of U-waves if the [K] is low enough. The relation between the shape of the T-wave and the serum [K] may vary among patients. Therefore, the actual [K] cannot be predicted by the T-wave configuration on the ECG. However, in a given patient, the changes in the T-waves are consistent and predict corresponding changes in [K]. That is, a serum [K] of 6.0 mEq/L may be associated with abnormally tall and peaked T-waves in one patient but with normal-appearing T-waves in another. In both patients, however, the T-wave decreases in

amplitude during treatment. By the same token, a serum [K] of 2.6 mEq/L may be associated with low T-waves in one patient and flat T-waves in another. Treatment (without appropriate potassium replacement) flattens out the T-waves in the first patient and causes the appearance of U-waves in the second. Thus, no matter what the actual configuration of the T-wave at the beginning of treatment, the change from the initial serum [K] can be predicted by a corresponding change in the T-wave.

Because both hyperkalemia and hypokalemia have detrimental effects on the cardiovascular and respiratory systems, the goal of potassium replacement is to maintain the serum [K] within the normal range. If a patient presents with hyperkalemia, potassium replacement should be delayed until the serum [K] has fallen into the normal range. If

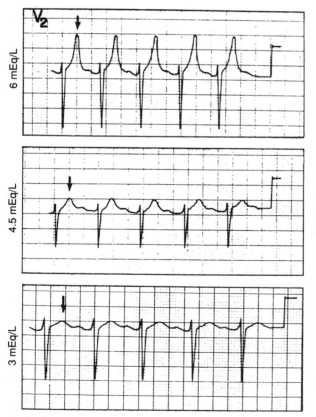

Figure 6–6. Relation between serum concentration of potassium [K] and T-wave configurations.

the initial serum [K] is normal, the goal of potassium replacement should be to maintain this normal level. If hypokalemia is initially noted, potassium replacement should restore the serum [K] to normal relatively quickly; however, the patient's cardiovascular system must not be jeopardized by too rapid administration of potassium. At presentation, the great majority of patients have a normal or elevated [K].[1] A low [K] reflects very severe potassium deficiency. If the [K] is <3.0 mEq/L, insulin should be withheld until potassium repletion raises the [K] above that value. Remember that initial rehydration alone is effective therapy.[18, 19]

To replete potassium in a safe, timely manner, the following approach is recommended. An ECG is performed as soon as is feasible, and the lead II, V_1, or V_2 tracing is either placed in the patient's chart or posted at the bedside for further comparisons. (If one of the V leads is used to monitor T-wave changes and the electrodes are not left on, it is wise to mark the locations of the chest electrodes so that their accurate placement on subsequent ECGs can be ensured. This prevents alterations due to differences in electrode placement.) Potassium replacement is not begun if the patient is anuric or if the T-waves either are abnormally tall and peaked or have a high normal configuration. If the T-waves are normal, 20 mEq of potassium (with an appropriate anion, which is discussed later) is added to the first liter of replacement fluid. If the T-waves are low or flat, 40 mEq of potassium is added. An ECG tracing of the same lead is taken every 1 or 2 hours, and appropriate changes in the potassium replacement regimen are made as necessary. For instance, when the abnormally tall or high normal T-wave falls into a normal configuration, 20 mEq of potassium is added to the infused fluids. If the patient had a normal T-wave on the previous ECG and was receiving 20 mEq of potassium per liter and the current tracing shows a low or flat T-wave, the potassium content of the replacement fluid should be increased to 40

mEq/L. Increases above this concentration should not be based on ECG changes alone. However, if the serum [K] is <2.5 mEq/L, the potassium content of the replacement fluid should be increased to 60 mEq/L (and the insulin withheld as mentioned earlier). In the rare instance when the serum [K] is <2.0 mEq/L, 80 mEq of potassium per liter can be given. These larger amounts, however, should be administered only with ECG monitoring. Furthermore, because administration of these high concentrations of potassium may be extremely irritating to the peripheral vein, use of more than one access route may be necessary or (if more than one route is impractical) a central line may need to be established.

As treatment continues, it may be possible to decrease the rate of potassium administration as the low T-waves return to normal and the serum [K] rises. There is no need to replace the entire potassium deficit by the IV route. After the patient is able to eat, potassium should be supplied by the oral route, either via food intake or, if the serum [K] remains low, by potassium supplementation (12 to 15 mEq three times a day with meals).

Phosphate Replacement

Serum phosphate concentrations are usually slightly elevated or in the high normal range in patients admitted in DKA, and they decline, often to very low levels, during the first 24 hours of treatment without phosphate replacement.[21, 30-34] Some earlier evidence showed that these low levels of phosphate might impair tissue oxygenation by inhibiting the production of red blood cell 2,3-diphosphoglycerate.[35] This compound decreases the affinity of hemoglobin for oxygen, thereby enhancing oxygen delivery to peripheral tissue. Hence, lower levels would theoretically cause oxygen to be more tightly bound to hemoglobin and less available to the tissues. However, impairment of tissue oxygenation could not be corroborated in subsequent studies.[31, 33] Furthermore, phosphate replacement had no effect on the rates of (1) glucose decrement[32-34]; (2) pH rise[31, 33, 34]; (3) increase in bicarbonate levels[33]; (4) fall in ketone bodies[33]; (5) recovery of mental status[32, 33]; (6) requirements for insulin[32, 33]; or (7) mortality.[32-34] In addition to the lack of demonstrable clinical efficacy for phosphate treatment in DKA, there are two other reasons to be wary of its use. First, phosphate infusions are contraindicated for patients with renal insufficiency, and initially it is difficult to ascertain whether the increased creatinine and BUN levels represent prerenal azotemia, spurious increases in creatinine values secondary to high acetoacetate concentrations, or true renal failure. Second, overly zealous administration of phosphate has been reported to cause symptomatic hypocalcemia,[36, 37] although in general the reduction in calcium levels during phosphate replacement in DKA is modest.[31-33] On the other hand, serum phosphate concentrations can fall to extremely low levels (even to <1 mg/dl) during therapy for DKA, and the potential hazards of severe hypophosphatemia (muscle weakness, respiratory failure, hemolytic anemia, hemorrhage, rhabdomyolysis, and neurologic dysfunction) must be kept in mind.[38]

On the basis of all these considerations, I use the following approach. Potassium is replaced with the chloride anion unless the serum phosphate concentrations are initially low or in the low normal range. In that case, half of the potassium is given as the chloride and half as the phosphate salt. In addition, I use phosphate for one half of the potassium replacement as soon as an initially high serum level declines into the normal range because of the likelihood of a continued decrease unless phosphate is given. In any event, continued monitoring of serum phosphate and calcium levels is important to prevent unexpected hyperphosphatemia or hypocalcemia.

Inorganic phosphate exists in serum in two valence states, HPO_4^{2-} and $H_2PO_4^-$ the proportions vary with the pH. Therefore, the number of millequivalents in 1 mmol of phosphate is not constant. In contrast, because the amount of phosphate as expressed in millimoles does not vary, phosphate replacement should be calculated in millimoles.[39] Although potassium phosphate for injection is a mixture of two salts, KH_2PO_4 and K_2HPO_4, the important consideration is the total amount of phosphate being administered. Most potassium phosphate preparations for IV use contain 4.4 mEq/ml of potassium and 3 mmol/ml of phosphate.

Bicarbonate Therapy

The use of bicarbonate is another controversial area in the treatment of DKA. In my view, most patients experiencing DKA do not require and therefore should not receive bicarbonate therapy. Although some standard texts state that a pH of <7.0 is incompatible with life (or words to that effect), two important caveats must be issued. First, this assertion applies to a chronic situation, whereas DKA is an acute acidosis. Second, and probably more important, the acid-base status of the cerebrospinal fluid (CSF), not the pH of the systemic circulation, determines brain function.[40] In contrast to respiratory acidosis, in which systemic pH and that of CSF diminish in parallel,[40] the pH of CSF is much higher than the systemic pH in DKA,[40, 41] for reasons discussed later.

There are many cogent arguments against the administration of bicarbonate to patients with DKA. First, endogenous bicarbonate is generated during insulin treatment.

Second, not only is intracellular pH normally much lower than extracellular pH, it is relatively uninfluenced by the acid-base status of the surrounding interstitial fluid. Rather, the partial pressure of carbon dioxide (Pco_2) has a much greater effect. The lowered Pco_2 of DKA raises the intracellular pH.[42] Thus, the intracellular pH may be normal or close to it even though a patient has a systemic acidosis.

Third, because bicarbonate administration usually reverses systemic acidosis relatively quickly, hypokalemia becomes a much greater problem. Indeed, before the relation between bicarbonate therapy and hypokalemia was recognized, a number of patients treated with alkali died of cardiac arrhythmias. More recently, hypokalemic respiratory arrest occurring during bicarbonate administration in DKA has been rediscovered.[43]

Fourth, administration of bicarbonate enhances the paradoxic acidosis of the CSF that develops during the treatment of DKA. The mechanism of enhancement can be understood by means of the following rearrangement of the Henderson-Hasselbalch equation, which expresses the relation among pH, $[HCO_3]$, and P_{CO_2}.

$$pH \propto \frac{[HCO_3]}{P_{CO_2}} \qquad (1)$$

Because CO_2 crosses freely from blood to CSF and vice versa, it quickly equilibrates between the two. Bicarbonate, on the other hand, diffuses much more slowly across the blood-brain barrier.[40] The difference between the rate of diffusion of CO_2 and that of bicarbonate explains both the higher pH of the CSF in DKA and the paradoxic fall of the pH of CSF during treatment. In the untreated state, as the $[HCO_3]$ falls, it is lower in the systemic circulation than in the CSF because of the delayed attainment of equilibrium. Because CO_2, on the other hand, equilibrates rapidly between the blood and CSF, CO_2 tension is the same on both sides of the blood-brain barrier. As can be appreciated from the equation just cited, the pH is higher in the CSF than in the plasma. As treatment progresses, both the P_{CO_2} and the $[HCO_3]$ increase in the plasma. In the CSF, the increase in the $[HCO_3]$ is delayed compared with that in the P_{CO_2}, so that the pH actually falls. Bicarbonate therapy enhances this decrease in the pH of CSF.[41, 44] Because mental status correlates with the pH of CSF rather than with systemic pH,[40] bicarbonate therapy could be deleterious.

Fifth, fatal cerebral edema is a rare cause of death in DKA that is discussed in more detail later. The histologic changes in the brain resemble those of anoxia.[42] Treatment of experimentally induced DKA in dogs with systemic bicarbonate caused a marked reduction in the partial pressure of oxygen in the CSF compared with that in dogs whose regimen did not include bicarbonate.[45]

Sixth, bicarbonate administration in patients with DKA increased hepatic ketogenesis, resulting in an initial rise in acetoacetate concentrations followed by a rebound increase in β-hydroxybutyrate levels after the alkali was discontinued.[46] There was a 6-hour delay in the improvement of ketosis compared with the control group in DKA not receiving bicarbonate.[46]

Seventh, a retrospective analysis[47] of 73 cases of severe DKA treated with bicarbonate compared with 22 episodes of DKA treated without bicarbonate revealed no differences between the two groups in rates of (1) decrease in plasma glucose levels; (2) increase in plasma bicarbonate concentrations; (3) arterial pH; and (4) neurologic recovery. This study is representative of several other retrospective ones that could document no improved outcome in patients treated with bicarbonate.

Eighth, a prospective study[48] of patients with severe DKA (pH 6.9 to 7.14), half of whom received bicarbonate, also showed no difference in the rates of (1) decrease in plasma glucose levels; (2) decrease in concentrations of plasma ketone bodies; (3) increase in arterial pH; (4) increase in plasma bicarbonate levels; and (5) increase in CSF pH and bicarbonate concentrations. Thus, in the absence of any advantages to bicarbonate therapy in DKA, why expose patients routinely to the potential hazards of this treatment?

In several situations, however, bicarbonate therapy should be considered. First, patients with life-threatening hyperkalemia should be given bicarbonate. A second circumstance in which bicarbonate therapy might be considered is in severe acidosis (pH <7.2) with shock that is unresponsive to intravascular volume repletion. If rehydration with saline (which is distributed throughout the entire extracellular fluid compartment) is initially ineffective, the intravascular volume should be expanded with plasma, albumin, or even whole blood (all of which are contained within the vascular volume). If these measures do not restore the blood pressure, bicarbonate therapy is indicated. The rationale for the use of alkali under these circumstances is that severe, prolonged acidosis may impair left ventricular contractility, whereas a more rapid reversal of acidosis may improve cardiac output.

Finally, a patient with a maximal ventilatory response (P_{CO_2} = 10 mm Hg) and a [HCO_3] ≤ 5 mEq/L has a very small buffer reserve. Any further reduction in [HCO_3] would theoretically have a profound effect on the pH. Although in my experience patients with these values have been successfully treated without bicarbonate administration, alkali treatment is often used under these circumstances. To avoid alkalosis overshoot (i.e., posttreatment alkalosis), it is recommended to infuse only that amount of bicarbonate that raises the [HCO_3] to 10 to 12 mEq/L.[1] Other sources of an alkalosis overshoot are bicarbonate generated from the metabolism of ketone bodies and the 24- to 36-hour persistence of hyperventilation after the acidosis is corrected.[49] Because these two are beyond the control of the physician, it makes sense to limit the amount of exogenous bicarbonate to minimize the possibility of an alkalosis overshoot.

If bicarbonate therapy is to be used to treat DKA, it should *never* be given in the form of an IV bolus. Death secondary to hypokalemia has occurred under these circumstances, even when the [K] was elevated at the time of administration. Bicarbonate should be added to 0.45% saline and infused into the patient over at least a 1-hour period. An ampule of $NaHCO_3$ contains 44 mEq of Na and HCO_3 each, or a total of 88 mEq.

Therefore, the osmolality of a solution containing 1 ampule of $NaHCO_3$ in 1 L of 0.45% saline is 242 mOsm/kg. Addition of 20 mEq of potassium plus 20 mEq of an appropriate anion yields a true isotonic solution (282 mOsm/kg). If more potassium replacement is indicated (and potassium administration should be generous when bicarbonate is infused), 40 mEq of potassium plus 40 mEq of appropriate anions should be added. The addition of these amounts of $NaHCO_3$ and potassium plus its anion to 0.45% saline gives a solution with an osmolality of 322 mOsm/kg (which is lower than that of isotonic saline plus potassium replacement). In the unusual situation in which more alkali therapy is appropriate (for instance, if a patient is in shock with a profound acidosis), addition of two ampules of $NaHCO_3$ plus 40 mEq of potassium and 40 mEq of its anion to 1 L of *distilled water* gives a solution containing 256 mOsm/kg. Finally, in the rare instance in which potassium replacement is not indicated (because of hyperkalemia and/or anuria), addition of two ampules of $NaHCO_3$ to 1 L of 0.45% saline yields a solution containing 330 mOsm/kg.

Thus, various combinations of saline, bicarbonate, and potassium can be given, with the choice depending on the clinical situation. The following points should be emphasized: (1) do not give boluses of bicarbonate; (2) infuse $NaHCO_3$ over a period of hours; (3) include generous amounts of potassium; and (4) use solutions with osmolalities of ~250 to 330 mOsm/kg. I do not attempt to calculate the amount of alkali that should be given to replenish the bicarbonate pool. Instead, I simply monitor the serum [HCO_3] and usually discontinue bicarbonate therapy when the pH exceeds 7.30 or the [HCO_3] reaches 10 to 12 mEq/L.

RESPONSE TO THERAPY

Glucose concentrations decline at a rate of 75 to 100 mg/dl/h in patients receiving low-dose insulin infusions for the treatment of DKA. In general, glucose levels reach 200 to 300 mg/dl within 4 to 5 hours. At this time, because of the continued need for insulin to treat the still uncorrected ketosis and acidosis, dextrose must be added to the infusion to avoid hypoglycemia. The insulin infusion rate can be decreased to 2 to 3 U/h unless the addition of dextrose to the rehydration fluid (usually as 5% dextrose in one-half normal saline) increases plasma glucose concentrations.

Ketosis is reversed in ~12 to 24 hours, although some patients may have detectable ketone bodies for several days. This may be due to the generation of acetone by the spontaneous decarboxylation of acetoacetate. As mentioned earlier, acetone is weakly reactive to nitroprusside. Its concentration in DKA exceeds that of acetoacetate.[50] Because of its solubility in fat and slow excretion via the lungs and kidneys, the half-life of plasma acetone in treated patients with DKA ranged from 8 to 15 hours.[50] These factors probably account for the persistence of ketonuria and the smell of acetone on the breath 24 to 48 hours after the correction of acidosis. As shown in Figure 6-7, levels of β-hydroxybutyrate and acetoacetate (which initially favors the former by a ratio of 3:1 to 5:1) shifts so that the concentration of the latter falls less rapidly (and may even increase early in treatment) than that of the former. This has important clinical ramifications if the patient's course is being monitored by the nitroprusside test for plasma ketone bodies. Because only acetoacetate is measured by this method, it may appear that the ketosis is not responding to treatment or even that it is worsening, although the total amount of ketone bodies is actually decreasing (hours 2 through 8 in Fig. 6-7).

Direct measurement of β-hydroxybutyrate concentrations would avoid the uncertainties of interpretation surrounding the assessment of ketosis by nitroprusside. One study of 15 patients evaluated the clinical utility of rapid determinations of β-hydroxybutyrate in

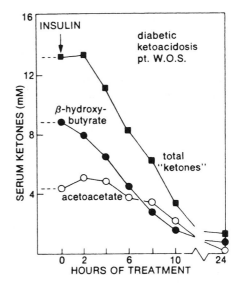

Figure 6–7. Response of serum ketone bodies to treatment in diabetic ketoacidosis. (See text for discussion.) (From Upjohn Co: Current Concepts. Coma in the Diabetic. The Upjohn Co, Kalamazoo, MI, 1974, p. 16)

the management of DKA.[17] The initial concentration was 8.5 mmol/L. DKA was considered resolved when two of the following three criteria were met: (1) [HCO_3] ≥18 mEq/L; (2) venous pH ≥7.32; and (3) calculated anion gap ≤14 mEq/L. At resolution, β-hydroxybutyrate concentrations were 0.52 mmol/L (range 0.1 to 0.8 mmol/L). The researchers concluded that rapid determinations of β-hydroxybutyrate levels were "useful in establishing the diagnosis of DKA and in the management of selected patients, i.e., those with prolonged metabolic acidosis, combined diabetic and lactic acidosis, and other mixed acid-base disorders." This statement implies that this measurement, although helpful in making the diagnosis, may not be particularly necessary in the management of routine cases of DKA.

Monitoring of the reversal of acidosis strictly on the basis of changes in the [HCO_3] may also be somewhat misleading. Frequently, the [HCO_3] seems to remain low (between 12 and 18 mEq/L) after most other signs, symptoms, and biochemical abnormalities associated with DKA have markedly improved. If the pH is measured at this time, it is frequently >7.3, while both the [HCO$_3$] and the P$_{CO_2}$ are low.[51, 52] Thus, the metabolic acidosis has been almost compensated at this point by a respiratory alkalosis (see Equation 1). Indeed, if patients are observed closely, deep respirations are noted even though tachypnea is frequently absent. This explains the discrepancy between the time when the pH returns to >7.3 (~8 to 9 hours) and that when the [HCO$_3$] returns to normal (14 to 24 hours).

During this period of recovery from DKA, the acid-base status is labeled as a hyperchloremic acidosis. The anion gap has returned to normal, and increased chloride levels replace the ketone bodies. The mechanism of these changes is thought to be the following. The conversion of ketone bodies to bicarbonate is the major source of the regenerated alkali. However, ketone bodies are lost in the urine before treatment and during rehydration, and therefore, an insufficient amount of bicarbonate is formed to replace totally the acidic ketone bodies in the extracellular space.[53, 54] The chloride ion makes up the deficit during this period until more bicarbonate ion is generated from other sources. The important clinical lesson to keep in mind is that decreased [HCO$_3$] after approximately 8 hours of treatment probably does not mean that the patient's pH is still low and requires further therapy for an acidosis. The increase in [HCO$_3$] and decline in serum chloride levels to normal values should occur spontaneously in the next 12 to 24 hours.

Full replacement of total body water may require 1 or 2 days and obviously can be completed by the oral route. Full repletion of intracellular electrolytes can take up to 10 days. Nitrogen balance may require several weeks to return to normal.

Life-threatening complications associated with DKA are listed in Table 6–8. Mortality in DKA has been reported to be between 3% and 30% although the more recent figures have been between 5% and 10%. No single factor seems to predict which patients will fare poorly. The presence of a complicating condition is often associated with a poor outcome. Age and the duration and degree of unconsciousness have also been cited as relevant factors. For instance, in 317 episodes of DKA in adults admitted to a hospital in England, 43% of those of over 50 years of age died, whereas the mortality rate was only 3.4% in patients younger than 50 years.[55] In 128 episodes of DKA in adults admitted to a hospital in the United States, 18% of those over 50 years of age died, compared with 6% of those younger than 50.[56] The severity of hyperglycemia or acidosis does not seem to be of prognostic importance. Deaths are usually a result of infections, arterial thrombosis, or unrelenting shock.[19] Because infection leads to death in only 2% of patients with DKA, routine antibiotic coverage is not indicated. On the other hand, a thorough evaluation for a source of infection is mandatory in every patient with DKA. Adult respiratory distress syndrome (almost always in smokers) is as an important cause of death in DKA.[57]

Death secondary to arterial thrombosis has been reported to be relatively common in all published studies of patients with DKA. The site may be ubiquitous and can involve any of the following arteries: coronary, carotid, mesenteric, iliac, renal, splenic, or pancreaticoduodenal. The clinical manifestations usually become apparent late in the course of treatment or even after recovery from DKA. It has been suggested that the treatment itself may trigger a number of phenomena that increase the propensity of patients with DKA to develop vascular thromboses.

Hypotension, azotemia, and oliguria leading to anuria as a result of severe intravascular volume depletion in combination with hyperosmolality are often associated with a poor prognosis.[58] Like vascular thrombosis, irreversible shock may develop during the course of treatment. Thus, vigorous rehydration at the beginning of treatment may be helpful. Decreased cardiac output secondary

Table 6–8. Life-Threatening Complications Associated with Diabetic Ketoacidosis

Cerebral edema	Disseminated intravascular coagulation
Serious infection	Adult respiratory distress syndrome (smokers)
Unrelenting shock	Aspiration
Cardiac arrest (hyperkalemia)	Pulmonary embolus
Respiratory arrest (hypokalemia)	Rhabdomyolysis
Arterial thrombosis	Pneumomediastinum and subcutaneous emphysema

to severe prolonged acidosis may also contribute to a poor outcome through impairment of left ventricular function. If acidosis does not improve in this situation, treatment with bicarbonate may be helpful. However, preexisting heart disease may also be a major and untreatable factor.

Rhabdomyolysis is a common complication of DKA and is related to the degree of hyperosmolality.[59, 60] Pneumomediastinal emphysema secondary to the 20 to 30 mm Hg increase in alveolar pressure caused by Kussmaul respirations is probably much more common than realized.[61] Fortunately, neither of these seems to make a major contribution to mortality.

Although cerebral edema is an unusual cause of death in the entire population of patients with DKA, 95% of cases occur in patients <20 years of age and 33% in children <5 years old.[62] The usual clinical setting is one in which the patient is showing marked clinical and biochemical improvement but then lapses back into a fatal coma while the metabolic abnormalities return completely to normal. At autopsy, cerebral edema is found. Although clinically evident cerebral edema is often fatal, rapid recognition and treatment with mannitol is helpful. If treatment is administered soon after signs of neurologic deterioration, approximately half of patients (most often children) are left with mild or no disability.[63, 64]

It was once thought that cerebral edema was solely a manifestation of treatment. In fact, several studies documented that most patients undergoing treatment for DKA probably go through a stage of mild cerebral edema. In one study,[65] CSF pressures were monitored continuously in five (adult) patients during the first 10 hours of therapy. In four of the five patients, the CSF pressure was normal before initiation of treatment but became elevated during the course of therapy. In the fifth patient, the CSF pressure was elevated initially and increased even further during treatment. The highest pressure recorded was 600 mm H_2O, and four of the five patients had sustained elevations in pressure for at least 2 hours. All of these patients were alert on admission but became drowsy during the interval when CSF pressure was greater than normal. One patient developed slurred speech and became semistuporous 3 hours after treatment was begun. Another patient became incoherent and agitated at 4 hours and semistuporous at 6 hours.

Cerebral edema during the treatment of DKA with low-dose insulin infusions was evaluated by means of serial repeat echoencephalograms.[66] A decrease in the width of the lateral ventricles was taken as an indication of cerebral edema. Nine of 11 patients showed significant decreases in lateral ventricle size at some time during the 15-hour period after treatment was started. Seven of the nine patients who had diminished lateral ventricle width also showed "hash marks," which are characteristic of cerebral edema by this technique. By 20 hours, the size of the lateral ventricle had returned to normal in all patients. In this study, no patient exhibited clinical evidence of cerebral edema. More recently, cerebral edema was evaluated by performing cranial CT scans in six children being treated for DKA.[67] The scans were performed as soon as possible after the blood glucose level had fallen to <250 mg/dl and 3 to 6 days after admission, just before discharge from the hospital. Two patients were lethargic at the time of the first scan, but no patient had any other abnormal neurologic sign during treatment. All of the initial scans showed a statistically significant narrowing of the third and lateral ventricles compared with the subsequent one. Although the results on the early scan did not permit an unequivocal diagnosis of cerebral edema, comparison of the two scans showed an alteration in brain volume compatible with mild brain swelling during treatment for DKA in these children who showed no clinical signs of abnormal neurologic function (except for lethargy).

It now seems clear that cerebral edema is also present before treatment. Not only is it evident on CT scans before therapy is initiated,[68, 69] but fatal cerebral edema has been reported either before treatment was begun[70] or 1.5 hours after it was started, with only minimal changes in pH, glucose, and electrolytes values.[71] The degree of cerebral edema before therapy was proportional to the glucose concentration and inversely proportional to the bicarbonate level.[69] The recognition that cerebral edema is present before treatment may help lessen the emotional and legal consequences that can attend this unfortunate outcome.

Why an occasional, usually young patient develops fatal cerebral edema and how this devastating outcome can be prevented are unknown. Three observations, however, suggest a therapeutic approach that may limit the possibility of developing clinical cerebral edema during therapy. First, changes of cerebral edema on CT scan during treatment correlated very highly with changes in calculated plasma osmolality[69]—that is, the more rapid the fall, the more brain swelling. Second, although Rosenbloom[63] could find no correlation between clinical cerebral edema and rates of hydration, tonicity of administered fluid, or rates of correction of glucose (or bicarbonate) concentrations, others have noted that clinical cerebral edema occurred

in patients whose [Na] failed to rise as glucose concentrations fell[72] and did not if [Na] remained stable or increased.[72, 73] Because [Na] would be expected to increase as glucose levels declined (all other things being equal),[9] the failure to rise implies overhydration with free water.

Third, experiments in animals have demonstrated that a rapid decline of the plasma glucose concentration after a 4-hour period of marked hyperglycemia causes cerebral edema. The mechanism involved may be the delay in attainment of equilibrium between glucose levels in CSF and those in plasma. Glucose concentrations decrease more rapidly in the blood than in the CSF during treatment. This discrepancy results in a less marked decrease in CSF osmolality than in plasma osmolality, so that fluid enters the CSF compartment. Because expansion of this compartment is limited by the cranium, increased pressure and cerebral edema develop. Greater decrements in glucose concentrations and osmolalities in plasma than in CSF have been documented in patients undergoing treatment with high-dose insulin regimens.[41, 44]

These observations suggest that the development of clinical cerebral edema during treatment may be associated with a rapid decline in plasma osmolality. This could occur if glucose concentrations are lowered too quickly and/or hypotonic solutions are given too rapidly. Thus, it seems wise to lower glucose levels gradually (75 to 100 mg/dl/h) and to support the glucose concentration by adding dextrose to the infusate when it reaches ~250 mg/dl. In children, avoiding rapid rates of rehydration to ≤4 L/m² during the first 24 hours[74] and ensuring that [Na] does not decline during treatment by adjusting the tonicity of the infusate[72, 73] may also be beneficial.

HYPEROSMOLAR NONKETOTIC SYNDROME

Although hyperosmolar nonketotic syndrome (HNKS) was first described before

1900 and sporadic cases were reported in the first half of this century, this syndrome has received ever-increasing attention since 1957. The "pure" syndrome has been defined[75] variously as glucose concentrations of 500 to 800 mg/dl, hyperosmolality >320 to 350 mOsm/kg, and profound intravascular volume depletion in the absence of "significant" ketosis (usually defined as a nitroprusside reaction of ≤2+ in a 1:1 dilution of plasma). The serum bicarbonate concentration is >15 mEq/L, and by definition, the serum pH is >7.3. The plasma glucose values often are even higher (ranging to >2000 mg/dl), as is the hyperosmolality (sometimes >400 mOsm/kg). A depressed sensorium is frequently encountered, especially if the plasma osmolality is >350 mOsm/kg. Affected patients are usually older than those presenting with DKA. In practice, patients who have these characteristics of HNKS are often also mildly ketotic and acidotic. Indeed, DKA and HNKS represent two ends of a continuous spectrum, and many patients have various aspects of each syndrome.[76] As might be expected, the pathogenesis, clinical presentation, and treatment of HNKS are similar to those of DKA in most respects. Several exceptions are important, however. The following discussion briefly mentions the similarities between the two conditions but emphasizes the differences.

PATHOPHYSIOLOGY

As outlined in Figure 6-1, a lack of effective insulin in carbohydrate and protein metabolism leads to intravascular volume depletion ("dehydration") and electrolyte depletion. The unregulated lipolysis that results from a lack of effective insulin on fat metabolism causes ketosis and the resultant acidosis. If lipolysis were not increased, ketosis and acidosis would not ensue and patients would manifest only depletion of intravascular volume and electrolytes. Because, in fact, only the latter two manifestations characterize pa-

tients in HNKS, the relatively normal lipolysis in this setting must be explained.

Two explanations have been offered. Because the regulation of lipolysis is so sensitive to insulin (see Chapter 2), the levels of insulin in patients in HNKS may be sufficient to control this pathway but not to prevent catabolism in the carbohydrate and protein pathways. In general, however, plasma insulin concentrations have been similar in DKA and in HNKS when measured. On the other hand, FFA levels are generally lower in HNKS than in DKA, a finding that reinforces the view that lipolysis is better controlled in HNKS. In vitro data suggest that hyperosmolality itself inhibits lipolysis.[77] Thus, the combination of some effective insulin acting in an environment of greatly increased osmolality may account for the lack of ketosis and subsequent acidosis. This is not an entirely satisfactory explanation, however, because the marked increase in serum osmolality occurs later in the evolution of HNKS and would not account for the restrained lipolysis early on.

LOSSES

The losses sustained in DKA and depicted in Figure 6-2 are often exceeded in patients in HNKS (Table 6-9). In the absence of ketosis and acidosis, which cause severe gastrointestinal symptoms in patients with DKA and force them to seek medical attention within 1 or 2 days, many patients tolerate polyuria and polydipsia for weeks, thus losing great quantities of fluid and electrolytes.

CAUSES

Conditions associated with the onset of HNKS are listed in Table 6-10. The mechanism by which these conditions induce HNKS is evident in most but not all cases. HNKS can be the initial manifestation of diabetes mellitus in older patients. In most other cases, the onset of HNKS is associated with a condition that is known to impair

Table 6–9. Comparison of Deficits of Water and Electrolytes in Hyperosmolar Nonketotic Syndrome and Diabetic Ketoacidosis

	HNKS	DKA
Water (L)	9	6
Water (ml/kg)[a]	100–200	100
Na (mEq/kg)	5–13	7–10
Cl (mEq/kg)	5–15	3–5
PO$_4$ (mmol/kg)	3–7	5–7
Mg (mEq/kg)	1–2[b]	1–2
Ca (mEq/kg)	1–2[b]	1–2

HNKS, hyperosmolar nonketotic syndrome; DKA, diabetic ketoacidosis.

From DeFronzo RA, Matsuda M, Barrett EJ: Diabetic ketoacidosis: a combined metabolic-nephrologic approach to therapy. Diabetes Rev 2:209, 1994

[a] Per kilogram of body weight.

[b] Assumed to be equal to deficits occurring in DKA.

insulin action or insulin secretion or both, especially if ready access to fluids is not available. The patient usually is ill, although the mechanistic relationship to HNKS is not always clear. *The important point to keep in mind, however, is that patients with HNKS are very likely to have a precipitating cause that requires a diligent search unless it is obvious.* Even patients in whom HNKS is the initial manifestation of diabetes may have an underlying condition that precipitated it.

Infection, occurring commonly in patients with HNKS, is well known to cause insulin resistance. Inflammation or tumors of the pancreas probably reduce insulin secretion. The potent insulin resistance of growth hormone and glucocorticoids explains the association of HNKS with acromegaly and Cushing's syndrome, respectively.

Several of the miscellaneous conditions listed in Table 6–10 would be expected to cause stress-related secretion of growth hormone, catecholamines, cortisol, and glucagon. These conditions include extensive burns, hypothermia, and heat stroke. HNKS in burned patients is often associated with high carbohydrate intake, either orally or IV. It may also develop in hospitalized patients given large amounts of carbohydrate in tube

feedings or via total parenteral nutrition without enough free water and/or insulin. Dialysis patients have usually received hypertonic solutions in the dialysate. Secretion of the stress hormones would also be expected if a patient were ill enough with any of the other conditions listed in Table 6–10.

The mechanisms by which the drugs listed in Table 6–10 cause HNKS are clear. Diazoxide and phenytoin (Dilantin) directly inhibit insulin secretion, as does hypokalemia. Propranolol, a β-adrenergic blocker, inhibits lipolysis. As was just mentioned, glucocorticoids cause insulin resistance. Finally, HNKS was found to occur in patients treated for cardiac arrest with 7.5% NaHCO$_3$ (although it is no longer routinely used). The injection of a hypertonic solution in a situation of overwhelming stress (in which levels of all of the counterregulatory hormones were no doubt extremely elevated) would explain this association. Because older patients take

Table 6–10. Predisposing or Precipitating Factors of Hyperosmolar Nonketotic Syndrome

Acute Illness	Drugs/Therapy
Previously undiagnosed diabetes mellitus	Calcium channel blockers
	Chlorpromazine
Acute infection	Chlorthalidone
(32% to 60%)	Cimetidine
Pneumonia	Diazoxide
Urinary tract infection	Encainide
Sepsis	Ethacrynic acid
Cerebrovascular accident	Immunosuppressive agents
Myocardial infarction	L-Asparaginase
Acute pancreatitis	Loxapine
Acute pulmonary embolus	Phenytoin
Intestinal obstruction	Propranolol
Dialysis, peritoneal	Steroids
Mesenteric thrombosis	Thiazide diuretics
Renal failure	Total parenteral nutrition
Heat stroke	
Hypothermia	
Subdural hematoma	
Severe burns	
Endocrine	
Acromegaly	
Thyrotoxicosis	
Cushing's syndrome	

many drugs, it is possible that some of the ones listed in Table 6-10 are not related to the onset of HNKS despite the fact that in some cases a clear temporal relationship was found between starting the drug and the onset of the syndrome.

SYMPTOMS

Except for dyspnea, all of the symptoms of DKA listed in Table 6-2 also apply to HNKS. Polyuria and polydipsia are very intense for 3 to 7 days before treatment and have often been present for several weeks. Although less prevalent than in DKA, abdominal pain, nausea, and vomiting do occur in HNKS. However, rather than the gastrointestinal symptoms that often motivate patients with DKA to seek medical attention, the usual reason for which patients in HNKS are brought to a medical facility is their lack of normal responsiveness. Many also present with focal neurologic symptoms, which are discussed in more detail in the next section.

SIGNS

Many of the signs of DKA (see Table 6-3) do not apply to HNKS. Patients in HNKS often have an elevated temperature, which is usually caused by an infection.[78] Because marked ketosis and acidosis are not present, hyperpnea, acetone breath, and signs of an acute abdomen are lacking. Intravascular volume depletion is usually profound, and the related signs are therefore uniformly present.

The neurologic picture in HNKS differs dramatically from that in DKA in many patients. Coma due to the altered metabolic conditions per se is not noted when the serum osmolality is <340 to $350 \, mOsm/kg$.[75] Thus, it is more likely in patients with HNKS, occurring in 10% to 20% of episodes.[75, 78, 79] Although a depressed sensorium (albeit not coma) is common to both syndromes, focal neurologic signs and symptoms are frequently noted in patients in HNKS.[80-82] Seizures, often resistant to anticonvulsant ther-

apy, are frequent (occurring in 10% to 15% of patients), and hallucinations and psychic disturbances are not uncommon. Focal dysfunctions include aphasia, homonymous hemianopsia, hemiparesis, hemisensory defects, unilateral hyperreflexia, and unilateral Babinski signs; all of these focal dysfunctions may be postictal but may also occur independently of seizures. Abnormal muscle tone, tonic eye deviations, and nystagmus are less frequent. Hyperpnea (in the absence of acidosis) is common and probably reflects stimulation of the medullary centers by non–acid-base parameters. In contrast to the Kussmaul respirations of DKA, in which both inspiratory and expiratory phases are increased, the hyperpnea of HNKS is reported to affect the expiratory phase only. Hyperthermia is a terminal event. Signs of nuchal rigidity have been reported in patients in HNKS, even though meningitis was found to be absent by means of appropriate tests. Abnormalities in electroencephalograms are seen and are unaffected by treatment with anticonvulsant agents. These abnormalities disappear when hypotonic fluids are given, although it may take several days for a complete return to normal.

DIFFERENTIAL DIAGNOSIS

As with DKA, the diagnosis of HNKS is easily made once it is considered. The usual difficulty is that only various neurologic possibilities are considered initially. Patients in HNKS are commonly admitted to the neurology or neurosurgical service, and the diagnosis of HNKS is made only when the results of routine urine and blood tests are known. This delay in the institution of appropriate treatment is partially responsible for the much poorer prognosis in HNKS than in DKA.

INITIAL LABORATORY VALUES

The similarities and differences between the initial laboratory values in DKA (see Table 6-6) and those in HNKS should be apparent from the foregoing discussion. Glucose concentrations are generally higher in HNKS. Although the [Na] and [K] can be low, normal, or high in both syndromes, the [Na] in HNKS is more likely to be higher than in DKA. As discussed earlier, an artificial reduction of the [Na] due to hypertriglyceridemia must be kept in mind, especially because patients in HNKS have a longer prodrome than those in DKA and consequently are more likely to develop elevated triglyceride levels. (During therapy, as glycemia is lowered and serum osmolality decreases, the [Na] rises because water is drawn back into the intracellular space, the reverse of what occurred as HNKS developed.) Serum osmolality is also higher in HNKS than in DKA. The *total* serum osmolality can be calculated as follows:

$$Osmolality = 2 \ [Na + K] \\ + \frac{[glucose]}{18} + \frac{[BUN]}{2.8} \quad (2)$$

In order to determine the *effective* serum osmolality, the final term is dropped from Equation 2 because urea is freely distributed between the extracellular and intracellular compartments. However, the calculated *total* osmolality corresponds better with the measured serum osmolality values. Changes in serum phosphate levels are similar to those in DKA. Both [HCO$_3$] and pH values are normal in the pure syndrome of HNKS. The biochemical indices of plasma volume contraction (BUN, creatinine, hematocrit, hemoglobin, and total protein) are generally higher in HNKS because intravascular volume depletion is usually greater. Phosphate concentration, amylase levels, WBC counts, and serum enzyme changes have not been systematically reported in HNKS. The latter two values, of course, would depend on the presence of associated conditions. CPK levels may be elevated, sometimes to extremely high values, secondary to the rhabdomyolysis caused by the marked hyperosmolality.[78]

TREATMENT

The points discussed in the earlier section on general considerations in the treatment of DKA apply for the most part in HNKS, with several modifications. With regard to laboratory tests, if significant ketosis is absent, an initial measurement of pH is unnecessary. In the unusual event that the [HCO$_3$] is low (<15 mEq/L), pH can be measured. Because most patients in HNKS are older and many have preexisting heart disease, monitoring of their cardiovascular status during fluid replacement is critically important. For this reason, placement of a central venous pressure line or, if possible, a right heart catheter that measures pulmonary capillary wedge pressure should be considered in patients with a history of congestive heart failure.

The same controversy surrounding fluid administration in DKA exists in relation to HNKS. Because the correlation between plasma osmolarity and depression of sensorium is even higher in HNKS (Fig. 6-8) than in DKA (see Fig. 6-4), some investigators argue that hypotonic solutions should be used and plasma osmolality reduced fairly rapidly. Others point out that patients in HNKS are even more vulnerable to the effects of intravascular volume depletion than are those with DKA and thus that rehydration with 0.9% saline should take precedence. Because there are few scientific data on which to base a choice between these two philosophies, I use the same approach in both HNKS and DKA with regard to fluid administration (see Table 6-7). If supine hypotension or orthostatic changes were present initially and normal saline given, fluid administration is switched to 0.45% saline as soon as the orthostatic changes have been reversed. As was just mentioned, precipitation of congestive heart failure during saline administration is all too common in patients in HNKS. Frequent monitoring of their cardiovascular status by physical examination and hemodynamic methods (if available) is

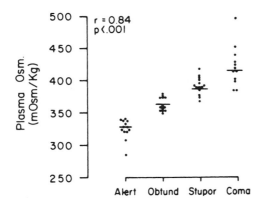

Figure 6–8. Relation between state of consciousness and measured plasma osmolarity in 53 patients in hyperosmolar nonketotic coma. States of consciousness were defined as follows: (1) alert—the patient responds immediately and appropriately to normal stimuli; (2) obtundation—the patient is in a state of dull indifference in which increased stimulation is required to evoke a response; (3) stupor—the patient can be aroused only by vigorous and continuous stimulation; and (4) coma—the patient exhibits little or no response to stimulation. For calculation of the correlation coefficient (r), scores of 1 through 4 were given for each state of consciousness, respectively. For each group, plasma osmolarity was significantly different ($P < 0.01$) from that of the adjacent group(s). (From Arieff AI, Carrol H: Cerebral edema and depression of sensorium in nonketotic hyperosmolar coma. Diabetes 23:525, 1974).

extremely important to a successful outcome. The one exception to the previous discussion on fluid replacement involves patients who have advanced renal failure and who develop HNKS. Under these conditions, glucosuria leading to an osmotic diuresis may be markedly impaired[83] so that the hyperglycemia-induced shift of water from the intracellular to the extracellular space is retained. These patients differ from the typical presentation of HNKS in that the prodrome of polyuria and polydipsia is absent and the initial [Na] is low. In this situation, little or no fluid may be required—only insulin to

lower glucose concentrations so that water shifts back from the extracellular to the intracellular space. Dialysis may be necessary in some instances.

Insulin is given to patients in HNKS in the same manner as to those with DKA. When the glucose concentration declines to ~250 mg/dl, the rate of insulin infusion is decreased to 2 to 3 U/h and dextrose is added to the administered fluid. Cerebral edema is much less common in HNKS than in DKA. In the few reported cases, the symptoms began when the glucose concentration was well below 250 mg/dl,[81, 84] and almost all occurred in children,[84] similar to the situation in DKA.

Because patients in HNKS are not experiencing ketosis or acidosis, the glucose level is the sole biochemical endpoint. However, it often is many hours or even a few days before these patients are able to tolerate oral intake because of their mental status and/or associated conditions. Under these circumstances, 50 g of dextrose should be administered every 8 hours, and the dose of insulin infused should be decreased appropriately (1 to 3 U/h) on the basis of plasma glucose determinations every 4 hours. The transition from insulin infusion to subcutaneous administration of insulin is made as described for DKA.

The same considerations for potassium replacement that apply to patients with DKA are pertinent to those in HNKS, with two caveats. Because more patients in HNKS may have underlying renal disease, urinary potassium losses may be lower. Bicarbonate therapy is obviously inappropriate for patients in HNKS. These two factors lessen the possibility of hypokalemia. However, because patients with preexisting heart disease may be more susceptible to the effects of potassium, potassium replacement must still be monitored carefully.

In my experience, phosphate homeostasis follows a pattern similar to that in DKA. Because many of these patients also have underlying renal disease, close monitoring of phosphate concentrations is required before administering phosphate. The same general approach for phosphate replacement in HNKS as in DKA should be used.

PROGNOSIS

The prognosis for patients in HNKS is worse than that for those with DKA. Older mortality reports ranged from 15% to 60%, with most values between 30% and 50%. More recent reports have suggested a lower mortality, between 10% and 20%.[56, 85, 86] This improvement may be related to earlier recognition of HNKS and more aggressive fluid administration.[78] Early mortality (<72 hours) is usually due to sepsis, progressive shock, or an underlying illness, whereas later mortality is usually caused by thromboembolic events or the effects of treatment.[79] An unfavorable outcome is more likely in older patients, with higher degrees of dehydration (as evidenced by the BUN level), higher [Na], higher serum osmolality (which reflects the length of the prodromal period), and lower level of consciousness.[75] Although

elevated levels of CPK reflecting rhabdomyolysis are common, especially in those patients with very high serum osmolalities, myoglobinuric acute tubular necrosis is rare, usually occurring in the presence of shock or preexisting renal disease.[79]

The causes of death are usually related to associated conditions rather than to the metabolic derangements per se. Gram-negative sepsis and pneumonia are particularly lethal to patients in HNKS. In addition to infections, vascular events (e.g., thrombosis) are frequent causes of death. Renal failure is often present in these patients. As mentioned earlier, the presenting neurologic symptoms may take 3 to 5 days to resolve completely, even though the metabolic parameters may long since have returned to normal.

Finally, in contrast to patients with DKA, all of whom eventually require insulin therapy after recovery, many patients who recover from HNKS can be treated with oral antidiabetic medications and/or dietary therapy alone. These approaches are particularly effective in patients whose initial manifestation of diabetes was HNKS.

Table 6–11. Comparisons of Some Salient Features of Diabetic Keotacidosis and Hyperosmolar Nonketotic Syndrome

| Feature | Conditions | |
	Diabetic Ketoacidosis	*Hyperosmolar Nonketotic Syndrome*
Age of patient	Usually <40 years	Usually >40 years
Duration of symptoms	Usually <2 days	Usually >5 days
[Glucose]	Usually <800 mg/dl	Usually >800 mg/dl
[Na]	More likely to be normal or low	More likely to be normal or high
[K]	High, normal, or low	High, normal, or low
[HCO₃]	Low	Normal
Ketone bodies	At least 4+ in 1:1 dilution	<2+ in 1:1 dilution
pH	Low	Normal
Serum osmolality	Usually <350 mOsm/kg	Usually >350 mOsm/kg
Cerebral edema	Often subclinical; occasionally clinical	Not evaluated if subclinical; rarely clinical
Prognosis	3% to 10% mortality	10% to 20% mortality
Subsequent course	Insulin therapy required in virtually all cases	Insulin therapy not required in many cases

[Glucose], serum concentration of glucose; [Na], serum concentration of sodium; [HCO₃], serum concentration of bicarbonate; [K], serum concentration of potassium.

DIABETIC KETOACIDOSIS VERSUS HYPEROSMOLAR NONKETOTIC SYNDROME

Some of the salient features of DKA and "pure" HNKS are compared in Table 6–11. In clinical practice, however, a patient often presents with some features of each syndrome. In some patients (usually those who are relatively young), acidosis is predominant, with a more moderate rise in serum osmolality. In others (usually older patients), serum osmolality is markedly increased in combination with either fully compensated acidosis (i.e., a slight decrease in [HCO_3] and a normal pH) or mild acidosis (i.e., a slight decrease in pH with a moderate reduction in [HCO_3]). Whatever the balance between acidosis and hyperosmolality, the approach to treatment is similar for DKA and HNKS.

REFERENCES

1. DeFronzo RA, Matsuda M, Barrett EJ: Diabetic ketoacidosis: a combined metabolic-nephrologic approach to therapy. Diabetes Rev 2:209, 1994
2. Munro JF, Campbell IW, McCuish AC, Duncan LJP: Euglycaemic diabetic ketoacidosis. BMJ 2:578, 1973
3. Brandt KR, Miles JM: Relationship between severity of hyperglycemia and metabolic acidosis in diabetic ketoacidosis. Mayo Clin Proc 63:1071, 1988
4. Stephens JM, Sulway MJ, Watkins PJ: Relationship of blood acetoacetate and 3-hydroxybutyrate in diabetes. Diabetes 20:485, 1971
5. Owen OE, Block BS, Patel M et al: Human splanchnic metabolism during diabetic ketoacidosis. Metabolism 26:381, 1977
6. Reichard GA, Skutches CL, Hoeldtke RD et al: Acetone metabolism in humans during diabetic ketoacidosis. Diabetes 35:668, 1986
7. Sanders G, Boyle G, Hunter S et al: Mixed acid-base abnormalities in diabetes. Diabetes Care 1:362, 1978
8. Walsh CH, Baylis PH, Malins JM: Plasma arginine vasopressin in diabetic ketoacidosis. Diabetologia 16:93, 1979
9. Katz MA: Hyperglycemia-induced hyponatremia calculation of expected serum sodium depression. N Engl J Med 289:843, 1973
10. Molitch ME, Rodman E, Hirsch CA, Dubinsky E: Spurious serum creatinine elevations in ketoacidosis. Ann Intern Med 93:280, 1980
11. Slovis CM, Mork VGC, Randall JS et al: Diabetic ketoacidosis and infection: leukocyte count and differential as early predictors of serious infection. Am J Emerg Med 5:1, 1987
12. Nsien EE, Steinberg WM, Borum M et al: Marked hyperlipasemia in diabetic ketoacidosis: a report of three cases. J Clin Gastroenterol 15:117, 1992
13. Warshaw A, Feller ER, Lee KH: On the cause of raised serum-amylase in diabetic ketoacidosis. Lancet 1:929, 1977
14. Vinicor F, Lehrner LM, Karn RC, Merritt AD: Hyperamylasemia in diabetic ketoacidosis: sources and significance. Ann Intern Med 91:200, 1979
15. Salem MM, Mujais SK: Gaps in the anion gap. Arch Intern Med 153:1625, 1992
16. Hale PJ, Nattrass M: A comparison of arterial and non-arterialized capillary blood gases in diabetic ketoacidosis. Diabetic Med 5:76, 1988
17. Umpierrez GE, Watts NB, Phillips LS: Clinical utility of β-hydroxybutyrate determined by reflectance meter in the management of diabetic ketoacidosis. Diabetes Care 18:137, 1995
18. Wäldhausl W, Kleinberger G, Korn A et al: Severe hyperglycemia: effects of rehydration on endocrine derangements and blood glucose concentration. Diabetes 28:577, 1979
19. Clements RS Jr, Vourganti B: Fatal diabetic ketoacidosis: major causes and approaches to their prevention. Diabetes Care 1:314, 1978
20. Kitabchi AE, Ayyagari V, Guerra SMO, Medical House Staff: The efficacy of low-dose versus conventional therapy of insulin for treatment of diabetic ketoacidosis. Ann Intern Med 84:633, 1976
21. Piters KM, Kumar D, Pei E, Bessman AN: Comparison of continuous and intermittent intravenous insulin therapies for diabetic ketoacidosis. Diabetologia 13:317, 1977
22. Pfeifer MA, Samols E, Wolter CF, Winkler CF: Low-dose versus high-dose insulin therapy for diabetic ketoacidosis. South Med J 72:149, 1979

23. Soler NG, Wright AD, FitzGerald MG, Malins JM: Comparative study of different insulin regimens in management of diabetic ketoacidosis. Lancet 2:1221, 1975

24. Madison LL: Low-dose insulin: a plea for caution. N Engl J Med 294:393, 1976

25. Morris LR, Kitabchi AE: Efficacy of low-dose insulin therapy for severely obtunded patients in diabetic ketoacidosis. Diabetes Care 3:53, 1980

26. Sheppard MC, Wright AD: The effect on mortality of low-dose insulin therapy for diabetic ketoacidosis. Diabetes Care 5:111, 1982

27. Fisher JN, Shahshahani MN, Kitabchi AE: Diabetic ketoacidosis: low-dose insulin therapy by various routes. N Engl J Med 297:238, 1977

28. Peterson L, Caldwell J, Hoffman J: Insulin adsorbance to polyvinylchloride surfaces with implications for constant-infusion therapy. Diabetes 25:72, 1976

29. Adrogue HJ, Lederer ED, Suki WN et al: Determinants of plasma potassium levels in diabetic ketoacidosis. Medicine 65:163, 1986

30. Kanter Y, Gerson JR, Bessman AN: 2,3-Diphosphoglycerate, nucleotide phosphate, and organic and inorganic phosphate levels during the early phases of diabetic ketoacidosis. Diabetes 26:429, 1977

31. Gibby OM, Veale KEA, Hayes TM et al: Oxygen availability from the blood and the effect of phosphate replacement on erythrocyte 2,3-diphosphoglycerate and haemoglobin-oxygen affinity in diabetic ketoacidosis. Diabetologia 15:381, 1978

32. Keller U, Berger W: Prevention of hypophosphatemia by phosphate infusion during treatment of diabetic ketoacidosis and hyperosmolar coma. Diabetes 29:87, 1980

33. Fisher JN, Kitabchi AE: A randomized study of phosphate therapy in the treatment of diabetic ketoacidosis. J Clin Endocrinol Metab 57:177, 1983

34. Wilson HK, Keuer SP, Lea AS et al: Phosphate therapy in diabetic ketoacidosis. Arch Intern Med 142:517, 1982

35. Ditzel J, Standl E: The problem of tissue oxygenation in diabetes mellitus. Acta Med Scand 578(suppl):49, 1975

36. Zipf WB, Bacon GE, Spencer ML et al: Hypocalcemia, hypomagnesemia, and transient hypoparathyroidism during therapy with potassium phosphate in diabetic ketoacidosis. Diabetes Care 2:265, 1979

37. Lavis VR: Treatment of diabetic ketoacidosis (letter). Diabetes Care 2:385, 1979

38. Knochel JP: The pathophysiology and clinical characteristics of severe hypophosphatemia. Arch Intern Med 137:203, 1977

39. Lentz RD, Brown DM, Kjellstrand CM: Treatment of severe hypophosphatemia. Ann Intern Med 89:941, 1978

40. Posner JB, Plum F: Spinal-fluid pH and neurologic symptoms in systemic acidosis. N Engl J Med 297:605, 1967

41. Ohman JL Jr, Marliss EB, Aoki TT, et al: The cerebrospinal fluid in diabetic ketoacidosis. N Engl J Med 284:283, 1971

42. Matz R: Diabetic acidosis, rationale for not using bicarbonate. N Y State J Med 76:1299, 1976

43. Dorin RI, Crapo LM: Hypokalemic respiratory arrest in diabetic ketoacidosis. JAMA 257:1517, 1987

44. Assal J-Ph, Aoki TT, Manzano FM, Kozak GP: Metabolic effects of sodium bicarbonate in management of diabetic ketoacidosis. Diabetes 23:405, 1974

45. Bureau MA, Begin R, Berthiaume Y et al: Cerebral hypoxia from bicarbonate infusion in diabetic acidosis. J Pediatr 96:968, 1980

46. Okuda Y, Adrogue HJ, Field JB et al: Counterproductive effects of sodium bicarbonate in diabetic ketoacidosis. J Clin Endocrinol Metab 81:314, 1996

47. Lever E, Jaspan JB: Sodium bicarbonate therapy in severe diabetic ketoacidosis. Am J Med 75:263, 1983

48. Morris LR, Murphy MB, Kitabchi AE: Bicarbonate therapy in severe diabetic ketoacidosis. Ann Intern Med 105:836, 1986

49. Narins R: Acid-base disorders: definitions and introductory concepts. In Narins R (ed): Clinical Disorders of Fluid and Electrolyte Metabolism. McGraw-Hill, New York, 1994, pp. 755–767

50. Sulway MJ, Malins JM: Acetone in diabetic ketoacidosis. Lancet 2:736, 1970

51. Oh MS, Carroll HJ, Goldstein DA, Fein IA: Hyperchloremic acidosis during the recovery phase of diabetic ketosis. Ann Intern Med 89:925, 1978

52. Oh MS, Banerji MA, Carroll HJ: The mechanism of hyperchloremic acidosis during the

recovery phase of diabetic ketoacidosis. Diabetes 30:310, 1981

53. Halperin ML, Bear RA, Hannaford MC, Goldstein MB: Selected aspects of the pathophysiology of metabolic acidosis in diabetes mellitus. Diabetes 30:781, 1981

54. Adrogué HJ, Wilson H, Boyd AE III et al: Plasma acid-base patterns in diabetic ketoacidosis. N Engl J Med 307:1603, 1982

55. Gale EAM, Dornan TL, Tattersall RB: Severely uncontrolled diabetes in the over-fifties. Diabetologia 21:25, 1981

56. Carroll P, Matz R: Uncontrolled diabetes mellitus in adults: experience in treating diabetic ketoacidosis and hyperosmolar nonketotic coma with low-dose insulin and a uniform treatment regimen. Diabetes Care 6:579, 1983

57. Carroll P, Matz R: Adult respiratory distress syndrome complicating severely uncontrolled diabetes mellitus: report of 9 cases and a review of the literature. Diabetes Care 5:574, 1982

58. Beigelman PM: Severe diabetic ketoacidosis (diabetic "coma"): 482 episodes in 257 patients; experience of three years. Diabetes 20:490, 1971

59. Singhal PC, Abramovici M, Venkatesan J: Rhabdomyolysis in the hyperosmolal state. Am J Med 88:9, 1990

60. Wang L-M, Tsai S-T, Ho L-T et al: Rhabdomyolysis in diabetic emergencies. Diabetes Res Clin Pract 26:209, 1994

61. Caramori MLA, Gross JL, Friedman R et al: Pneumomediastinum and subcutaneous emphysema in diabetic ketoacidosis. Diabetes Care 18:1311, 1995

62. Hammond P, Wallis S: Cerebral oedema in diabetic ketoacidosis: still puzzling—and often fatal. BMJ 305:203, 1992

63. Rosenbloom AL: Intracerebral crises during treatment of diabetic ketoacidosis. Diabetes 13:22, 1990

64. Bello FA, Stone JF: Cerebral edema in diabetic ketoacidosis in children. Lancet 336:64, 1990

65. Clements RS Jr, Blumenthal SA, Morrison AD, Winegrad AI: Increased cerebrospinal-fluid pressure during treatment of diabetic ketosis. Lancet 2:671, 1971

66. Fein IA, Rackow EC, Sprung CL, Grodman R: Relation of colloid osmotic pressure to arterial hypoxemia and cerebral edema during crystalloid volume loading of patients with diabetic ketoacidosis. Ann Intern Med 96:570, 1982

67. Krane EJ, Rockoff MA, Wallman JK et al: Subclinical brain swelling in children during treatment of diabetic ketoacidosis. N Engl J Med 312:1147, 1985

68. Hoffman WH, Steinhart CM, El Gammal T et al: Cranial computed tomography in children and adolescents with diabetic ketoacidosis. J Neuroradiol 9:733, 1988

69. Durr JA, Hoffman WH, Sklar AH et al: Correlates of brain edema in uncontrolled IDDM. Diabetes 41:627, 1992

70. Glasgow AM: Devastating cerebral edema in diabetic ketoacidosis before therapy. Diabetes Care 14:77, 1991

71. Couch RM, Acott PD, Wong GWK: Early onset fatal cerebral edema in diabetic ketoacidosis. Diabetes Care 14:78, 1991

72. Harris GD, Fiordalisi I, Harris WL et al: Minimizing the risk of brain herniation during treatment of diabetic ketoacidemia: a retrospective and prospective study. J Pediatr 117:22, 1990

73. Harris GD, Fiordalisi I: Physiologic management of diabetic ketoacidemia: a 5-year prospective pediatric experience in 231 episodes. Arch Pediatr Adolesc Med 148:1046, 1994

74. Duck SC, Wyatt DT: Factors associated with brain herniation in the treatment of diabetic ketoacidosis. J Pediatr 113:10, 1988

75. Ennis ED, Stahl EJvB, Kreisberg RA: The hyperosmolar hyperglycemic syndrome. Diabetes Rev 2:115, 1994

76. Wachtel TJ, Tetu-Mouradjian LM, Goldman DL et al: Hyperosmolarity and acidosis in diabetes melliitius: a three-year experience. J Gen Intern Med 6:495, 1991

77. Turpin BP, Duckworth WC, Solomon SS: Stimulated hyperglycemic hyperosmolar syndrome. Impaired insulin and epinephrine effects upon lipolysis in the isolated rat fat cell. J Clin Invest 63:403, 1979

78. Matz R: Hyperosmolar nonacidotic uncontrolled diabetes: not a rare event. Clin Diabetes 6:25, 1988

79. Lorber D: Non-ketotic hypertonicity in diabetes. Endocrinologist 3:29, 1993

80. Maccario M: Neurological dysfunction associated with nonketotic hyperglycemia. Arch Neurol 19:525, 1968

81. Guisado R, Arieff AI: Neurologic manifesta-

tions of diabetic comas: correlation with biochemical alterations in the brain. Metabolism 24:665, 1975

82. Morres CA, Dire DJ: Movement disorders as a manifestation of nonketotic hyperglycemia. J Emerg Med 7:359, 1989

83. Gerich JE, Martin MM, Recant L: Clinical and metabolic characteristics of hyperosmolar nonketotic coma. Diabetes 20:228, 1971

84. Arieff AI: Cerebral edema complicating nonketotic hyperosmolar coma. Miner Electrolyte Metab 12:383, 1986

85. Khardori R, Soler NG: Hyperosmolar hyperglycemic nonketotic syndrome. Am J Med 77:899, 1984

86. Wachtel TJ, Silliman RA, Lamberton P: Predisposing factors for the diabetic hyperosmolar state. Arch Intern Med 147:499, 1987

OFFICE MANAGEMENT OF THE DIABETIC PATIENT

It is unfortunate that most of a physician's training in the care of diabetic patients occurs in a hospital. The treatment of these patients belongs in an office setting. The weekly diabetes clinic experience or the exposure to diabetes in the primary care clinics, which may last from 1 to several months and serves as the house officer's experience in office management, is woefully inadequate. More than with most diseases, diabetes care requires an ongoing dialogue between patient and physician, and unlike individuals with other diseases, diabetic patients themselves make many important decisions about their care. They need appropriate education and guidance by their physician and other health professionals. With the proper interaction between patient and physician, many hospitalizations can be avoided. As discussed in Chapters 4 and 6, insulin therapy can be initiated and stabilized and mild diabetic ketoacidosis (DKA) can even be treated outside of the hospital in motivated patients if an office routine is established for this purpose.

No matter how experienced and dedicated a physician is, both patients' knowledge of diabetes and their appropriate judgments in soliciting help from a physician are usually the critical factors that prevent minor problems from becoming major ones. The education of diabetic patients is considered in detail in Chapter 10, which was written for patients as well as for the personnel (often nurses) carrying out the teaching. Although most physicians have neither the time nor the inclination to teach patients themselves, it is crucial that diabetic patients

understand the material appropriate to their disease, as summarized in Chapter 10. If other professionals are not available to teach the diabetic patients, I urge physicians to read Chapter 10 before carrying out the instructions. Too often, medical jargon prevents effective communication between patient and physician, and patients often are too overwhelmed to ask questions. Appropriate dietary information for patients is described in Chapter 3.

INITIAL EVALUATION AND GENERAL FOLLOW-UP

The recommendations[1] of the American Diabetes Association regarding history, physical examination, and laboratory evaluation during the initial visit are summarized in Tables 7-1 to 7-3. A few comments about some of these elements are in order. For patients taking insulin, it is important to ascertain the frequency, timing (i.e., whether they commonly occur at a specific time of the day), and possible causes of hypoglycemic episodes. Information about unexplained hypoglycemia and especially about severe hypoglycemia (i.e., initiation of treatment by another person is necessary) is critically important to elicit. It is also very helpful to determine a patient's typical schedule (i.e., time [and dose] of insulin injections, meals, snacks, and exercise) to give more appropriate advice about insulin therapy.

Blood pressure should be monitored closely and treated vigorously if elevated (see Chapter 8). In addition to the well-known

Table 7–1. Recommended Elements of the History on the Initial Visit

- Symptoms, results of laboratory tests, and special examination results related to the diagnosis of diabetes
- Prior glycohemoglobin records
- Eating patterns, nutritional status, and weight history; growth and development of children and adolescents
- Details of previous treatment programs, including nutrition and diabetes self-management training
- Current treatment of diabetes, including medications, meal plan, and results of glucose monitoring and patient's use of the data
- Exercise history
- Frequency, severity, and cause of acute complications such as ketoacidosis and hypoglycemia
- Prior or current infections, particularly skin, foot, dental, and genitourinary
- Symptoms and treatment of chronic complications associated with diabetes: eye; kidney; nerve; genitourinary (including sexual), bladder, and gastrointestinal function; heart; peripheral vascular; foot; and cerebrovascular
- Other medications that may affect blood glucose levels
- Risk factors for atherosclerosis: smoking, hypertension, obesity, dyslipidemia, and family history
- History and treatment of other conditions including endocrine and eating disorders
- Family history of diabetes and other endocrine disorders
- Gestational history: hyperglycemia, delivery of an infant weighing >9 pounds, toxemia, stillbirth, polyhydramnios, or other complications of pregnancy
- Life style, cultural, psychosocial, educational, and economic factors that might influence the management of diabetes

Adapted from American Diabetes Association. Clinical practice recommendation. Diabetes Care 20(suppl 1):S5, 1997

detrimental effects of hypertension— macrovascular diseases of the heart and central nervous system—hypertension is also associated with accelerated microvascular damage to the eyes[2–4] and kidneys.[5, 6] Because periodontal disease is more common in people with diabetes,[7] the oral examination should include an evaluation of the gums. Examination of the thyroid gland is important in patients with type 1 diabetes because of the association with Hashimoto's thyroiditis, another autoimmune disease.

Because diabetic patients have an increased susceptibility to macrovascular disease, it is important to carry out baseline recording of pulses and to check for the presence or absence of bruits. These pulses include the carotid, femoral, popliteal (more easily palpated if the leg is slightly bent), posterior tibialis, and dorsalis pedis. The arteries to be examined for bruits are those of the neck (carotid), abdomen (aorta), flanks (renal), and groin (iliac). Because diabetic patients are at risk for neuropathy, a baseline evaluation of the functioning of at least two components of the peripheral nervous sys-

tem should be performed. Such an evaluation assesses the threshold for vibratory sensation (especially in the lower extremities) and the reflexes. Impairment of one or both of these components is the initial sign of peripheral neuropathy.

Examination of the feet should also determine whether patients can feel the 5.07 (10-g) monofilament. This simple device, developed to assess patients with leprosy, has been very helpful in delineating which patients are at increased risk for amputation. Patients who are insensate to the 5.07 monofilament are nearly 20 times more likely to develop a foot ulcer that those who can feel it.[8] (The 5.07 [10-g] monofilament can be ordered from Sensory Testing Systems, 1815 Dallas Dr., Suite 11A, Baton Rouge, LA 70806, phone [504] 927-7923, fax [504] 926-9053.)

The rationale for the laboratory evaluation is straightforward. Evaluation of the glycemic, lipid, and renal status of patients is necessary because, as discussed elsewhere, overwhelming evidence shows that restoring these indices toward normal has a positive

Table 7–2. Recommended Elements of the Physical Examination on the Initial Visit

- Height and weight measurements (and comparison with norms in children and adolescents)
- Sexual maturation (during peripubertal period)
- Blood pressure determination (with orthostatic measurements when indicated) and comparison with age-related norms
- Ophthalmoscopic examination (preferably with dilation)
- Oral examination
- Thyroid palpation
- Cardiac examination
- Abdominal examination (e.g., for hepatomegaly)
- Evaluation of pulses (by palpation and auscultation)
- Hand/finger examination
- Foot examination
- Skin examination (including insulin injection sites)
- Neurologic examination

Adapted from American Diabetes Association: Clinical practice recommendations. Diabetes Care 20(suppl 1):S5, 1997

clinical benefit. The rationale for a baseline electrocardiogram (ECG) is that this information is valuable if patients are ever evaluated for chest pain due to possible coronary artery disease. This supposition has been challenged, however, by two studies[9, 10] of patients with chest pain in an emergency room. Neither was able to document the utility of a baseline ECG in the decision about whether to admit the patient to the hospital. Furthermore, a careful review of the literature did not substantiate that a resting ECG was a useful screen for coronary artery disease or that early detection of ECG abnormalities led to any clinical interventions that improved health outcomes.[11]

Finally, diabetic patients should wear some form of identification. This is especially important for those taking insulin. If a patient is unable to give a history and a family member or friend is unavailable, he or she may accidentally be given inappropriate and perhaps dangerous therapy unless the medical personnel present are aware of the diabetes.

Medic Alert bracelets or necklaces are the best form of identification. The information needed for ordering them is included in the Appendix to Chapter 10.

The elements of the history, physical examination, and management plan on the initial visit recommended by the American Diabetes Association[1] listed in Tables 7–1, 7–2, and 7–4, respectively, are very complete and represent the best possible approach to patients with diabetes. Similar extensive recommendations are suggested for the continuing care of diabetic patients.[1] However, given the current time and financial constraints under which physicians now practice, adhering to these recommendations, in my view, is often not practical or even possible in some circumstances. The following 11 guidelines are suggested for the appropriate care of diabetes-related problems. These are mostly evidence-based outcome or process measures that have been shown to affect the health of patients *directly*. It is important to understand the difference between an outcome and a process measure. An example of

Table 7–3. Recommended Elements of the Laboratory Evaluation on the Initial Visit

- Fasting plasma glucose determination (a random plasma glucose value may be obtained in an undiagnosed symptomatic patient for diagnostic purposes)
- Glycohemoglobin
- Fasting lipid profile: total cholesterol, high-density lipoprotein (HDL) cholesterol, triglycerides, and low-density lipoprotein (LDL) cholesterol
- Serum creatinine in adults; in children if proteinuria is present
- Urinalysis: glucose, ketones, protein, sediment
- Determination for microalbuminuria (e.g., timed specimen or albumin-to-creatinine ratio) in postpubertal patients who have had diabetes at least 5 years and all patients with type 2
- Urine culture, if sediment is abnormal or symptoms are present
- Thyroid function test(s) when indicated
- Electrocardiogram (in adults)

Adapted from American Diabetes Association: Clinical practice recommendations. Diabetes Care 20(suppl 1):S5, 1997

Table 7–4. Recommended Elements of the Management Plan to Be Instituted at the Initial Visit

- Statement of short- and long-term goals
- Medications (insulin, oral glucose-lowering agents, glucagon, antihypertensive and lipid-lowering agents, other endocrine drugs, and other medications)
- Individualized nutrition recommendations and instructions, preferably by a registered dietitian familiar with the components of the dietary management of diabetes
- Recommendations for appropriate life style changes (e.g., exercise, smoking cessation); patient and family education for self-management that is consistent with the National Standards for Diabetes Patient Education Programs, preferably provided by a Certified Diabetes Educator
- Monitoring instructions; self-monitoring of blood glucose (SMBG), urine ketones, and use of a record system; frequency of SMBG should be individualized according to clinical circumstances, the form of treatment used, and the response to treatment; urine glucose may be considered as an alternative only if the patient is unable or unwilling to perform blood glucose testing or if the only goal is avoidance of symptomatic hyperglycemia
- Annual comprehensive dilated eye and visual examinations by an ophthalmologist for all patients age 12 and older who have had diabetes for 5 years, all patients older than 30 years, and any patient with visual symptoms and/or abnormalities
- Consultation for podiatry services as indicated
- Consultation for specialized services as indicated
- Agreement on continuing support and follow-up and return appointments
- Instructions on when and how to contact the physician or other members of the health care team when the patient has not been able to solve problems and for management of acute problems
- For women of childbearing age, discussion of contraception and emphasis on the need for optimal blood glucose control before conception and during pregnancy
- Dental hygiene

Adapted from American Diabetes Association: Clinical practice recommendations. Diabetes Care 20(suppl 1):S5, 1997

a process measure would be a requirement to measure a glycated hemoglobin level four times a year. This *process* measure has not been shown to affect the health of diabetic patients because glycated hemoglobin values remain fairly constant (and usually high) in an individual patient over many years.[11a-15] The outcome measure would be a target value to be achieved. This *outcome* measure is associated with markedly reduced risks for retinopathy, nephropathy, and neuropathy in both type 1[16] and type 2[17] diabetic patients. Those process measures (e.g., foot examinations) that almost assuredly will lead to improved outcomes (e.g., fewer amputations) are included in the guidelines, although no controlled studies have directly proved the connection.

1. *Glycated hemoglobin levels.* The target value for glycated hemoglobin levels should be $\leq 2\%$ above the upper limit of normal for the assay used. This level is se-

lected because the risks of development and progression of both retinopathy[16, 17] and nephropathy[17, 18] markedly increase in diabetic patients who maintain higher glycated hemoglobin values. If the target level is being met, glycated hemoglobin levels should be measured at least every 6 months (although more frequent measurements identify deterioration of diabetic control sooner). If the target level is not met, glycated hemoglobin levels should be measured at least every 3 months.

2. *Low-density lipoprotein (LDL) cholesterol concentrations.* LDL cholesterol concentrations should be measured at least yearly or more often as necessary. The target value for diabetic patients without coronary artery disease should be <160 mg/dl and for those with coronary artery disease <130 mg/dl. These are minimum target values; many experts would argue for levels of <130 mg/dl and <100 mg/dl, respectively, because

coronary artery disease is such a devastating problem for patients with diabetes and regression of coronary artery lesions has been demonstrated in patients whose LDL cholesterol concentrations were lowered to <100 mg/dl. (See Chapter 8 for a thorough discussion of LDL cholesterol concentrations and the evidence for the benefits of lowering them.)

3. *Fasting triglyceride (TG) concentrations*. Fasting TG concentrations should be measured at least yearly or more often as necessary. Target values for diabetic patients without coronary artery disease should be <400 mg/dl and for those with coronary artery disease <200 mg/dl. Some experts recommend that fasting TG concentrations should be kept below 200 mg/dl or even 150 mg/dl in all diabetic patients. Although interventional studies are currently being conducted, no published data delineate the impact of lowering TG levels on coronary artery disease. However, hypertriglyceridemia is associated with coronary artery disease in type 2 diabetic patients. Furthermore, it is also associated with small, dense LDL particles that are more atherogenic than normally constituted LDL particles. Lowering TG concentrations restores LDL particles to normal size and density. For these reasons, which are explained in more detail in Chapter 8, two expert panels[19, 20] have recommended that TG concentrations be lowered in diabetic patients.

4. *Renal evaluation*. A dipstick test for urinary protein should be performed every year. If the results are negative or trace, an evaluation for microalbuminuria should be carried out. If microalbuminuria or clinical proteinuria (defined by a ≥1+ positive dipstick test) is confirmed, the patient should be treated with an angiotensin-converting enzyme (ACE) inhibitor unless contraindicated. The rationale for this guideline and the methods for evaluating microalbuminuria are discussed in detail in Chapter 8.

5. *Blood pressure*. The blood pressure should be measured at every regularly sched-

uled visit for diabetes or more often as necessary. The target value should be ≤130/85 mm Hg for all patients <60 years of age and all patients with any evidence of renal disease. The target value is ≤160/90 mm Hg for patients ≥60 years old without renal disease. The rationale for this guideline is discussed in Chapter 8.

6. *Visits*. A regularly scheduled visit for diabetes should occur at least every 6 months as long as target values for glycated hemoglobin levels, TG, and LDL concentrations and blood pressure are met. Should any of these exceed target values, patients should be seen at least every 3 months (or more often as necessary to achieve these goals). This guideline is based on expert opinion and is consistent with the recommendations of the American Diabetes Association.[1]

7. *Retinal examination*. A funduscopic examination should be performed every year through dilated pupils or retinal photographs taken through either dilated or undilated pupils in all diabetic patients older than 30 years. The examination is not recommended for type 1 diabetic patients younger than 30 years within the first 5 years of diagnosis or for those who have not yet reached puberty, regardless of the duration of the disease. The examination should be carried out or the photographs read by professionals experienced in the evaluation of diabetic retinopathy. This guideline has been recommended by both the American Diabetes Association[1] and the American Academy of Ophthalmology[21] because early detection of diabetic retinopathy leading to laser photocoagulation at the appropriate time can prevent blindness.[22, 23] Detecting and treating diabetic retinopathy is more cost-effective than many other routine health interventions.[24]

8. *Foot examination*. The feet should be examined at every regularly scheduled visit for diabetes because at least half of lower extremity amputations in diabetic patients are preventable by early detection and appropriate treatment.[25] This guideline is con-

sistent with the recommendations of the American Diabetes Association.[1]

9. *Weight*. Patients should be weighed at every regularly scheduled visit for diabetes. Although long-term dietary success occurs in only a minority of the 80% to 90% of type 2 diabetic patients who are obese, documentation of current weight with continued encouragement for weight loss is successful in some patients. Conversely, documentation of unexplained weight loss may identify patients whose diabetic control is poor. This guideline is consistent with the recommendations of the American Diabetes Association.[1]

10. *Smoking*. Smoking assessment should be carried out yearly. Patients who are current smokers should be counseled or referred to a smoking cessation program. The doubling of the risk of myocardial infarctions in smokers and the removal of this increased risk after cessation certainly do not have to be described to readers of this book. Furthermore, not only is the risk for peripheral vascular disease in smokers much more than doubled (see Chapter 8), but smoking also increases the risks for diabetic retinopathy and nephropathy.

11. *Aspirin*. Diabetic patients ≥40 years old should receive low-dose (75 to 325 mg) enteric coated aspirin each day unless contraindicated. The beneficial effect of low-dose aspirin is clear in patients with established coronary artery disease, whether they have diabetes or not.[26] The issue of using aspirin in the general population for primary prevention of coronary artery disease has been debated,[27-29] and a case made for using it "in those with uncontrolled risk factors for the development of coronary events."[28] Diabetic patients certainly fall into that category, given their propensity for developing cardiovascular disease and our present inability to identify the factor(s) involved. Although caution has been raised about the use of aspirin in the presence of diabetic retinopathy,[28] no increased risk of retinal or vitreous bleeding, even with relatively high

doses of aspirin, was found in patients with established retinopathy enrolled in the Early Treatment Diabetic Retinopathy Study for a median period of 5 years.[30]

Other guidelines recommended by the American Diabetes Association[1]—for example, those concerned with education, nutritional counseling, and self-monitoring of blood glucose (SMBG)—have not been included because these are process measures that have not by themselves been directly shown to result in improved outcomes. In fact, substantial data demonstrate that diabetes education per se, although improving knowledge, does not lead to better outcomes unless management of diabetes is also involved.[31] Similarly, SMBG in diabetic patients treated with diet alone or pills, although perhaps improving motivation and knowledge of the effect of various foods on blood glucose levels, is not associated with better diabetes control.[32-34] Although diabetes education, nutritional counseling, and SMBG (especially in insulin-requiring patients) are most often necessary for improved outcomes, they are not sufficient by themselves. Adhering to process measures that do not result in better outcomes matters little. Conversely, as long as the targets in the outcome measures are met, the process by which they are achieved is immaterial.

MONITORING DIABETIC CONTROL

The importance of strict diabetic control was discussed in Chapter 2. The attainment of this goal is critically dependent on the ability to monitor the degree of control achieved. At present, five general methods are used to assess diabetic control, each of which will be discussed in detail: (1) semiquantitative testing of urine for glucose and ketone bodies; (2) quantitative measurements of urine glucose in timed samples; (3) fasting and/or postprandial whole blood or plasma glucose determinations obtained sporadically at a chemistry laboratory or a physician's office;

(4) SMBG; and (5) measurement of glycated hemoglobin (Hgb), Hgb A_{1c}, or Hgb A_1 levels, or other proteins (serum albumin, serum total protein).

SEMIQUANTITATIVE URINE TESTING

Evaluation of the results of urine testing requires an understanding of the concept of the renal threshold for glucose (T_m). Glucose is filtered at the glomerulus and reabsorbed back into the circulation in the proximal tubule. When the capacity of the proximal tubule to reabsorb glucose is exceeded, glucose appears in the urine. The amount of glucose reabsorbed is related to its concentration in the glomerular filtrate and to the rate at which it is presented to the renal tubular cells. It also is linked to sodium reabsorption in the proximal tubule. Therefore, the classic concept that the proximal tubule has an intrinsic maximal capacity to reabsorb glucose is not accurate. However, the concept of a limit to glucose reabsorption in the proximal tubule (even if it depends on other variables) is useful clinically. Under normal conditions, glucose does not appear in the urine until the plasma glucose concentration exceeds ~180 mg/dl—that is, at plasma levels below this value, virtually all of the glucose is reabsorbed and does not reach the urine. Therefore, the normal T_m is ~180 mg/dl. This level is relatively variable among patients. It tends to be lower in younger patients and to increase with age. Pregnancy lowers the T_m considerably for reasons that are not entirely clear. Pregnant women can even manifest glucosuria with normal plasma glucose concentrations (100 to 120 mg/dl). Renal disease, including diabetic nephropathy, raises the T_m. This explains why some (usually older) patients may be aglucosuric at elevated glucose levels (250 to 350 mg/dl).

Four different products are available for urinary testing of glucose: (1) Clinitest tablets, (2) Clinistix, (3) Diastix, and (4) Chemstrip uG. (In two of them, Diastix and Chemstrip uG, a separate area on the strip has been included on which ketone bodies can also be measured. These products are named Keto-Diastix and Chemstrip uGK.) Clinitest tablets use a copper reduction reaction and may also measure substances other than glucose. Either 2 or 5 drops of urine are added to 10 drops of water before testing. With the remaining three methods, a piece of paper or a cellulose strip is simply dipped into the urine. These methods rely on a reaction involving the enzyme glucose oxidase, which is specific for glucose. The product of the reaction, hydrogen peroxide, reacts with another enzyme impregnated on the strip to produce nascent oxygen, which oxidizes a dye and thus causes the color of the strip to change. Each strip is coupled to a different dye. Substances that interfere with the measurement of urinary glucose by methods using glucose oxidase usually inhibit the oxidation of the dye, not the enzyme reactions.[35]

These four methods have different ranges of sensitivity (Table 7-5). Because the relationship between positive reactions expressed as the plus signs and the actual amount of urinary glucose varies considerably among the different tests, the results should be reported only as percentages. Clinistix is not suitable because each color change represents a range of glucose levels. The two-drop Clinitest method extends readings at higher levels of urinary glucose (between 2% and 5%). Diastix and the five-drop Clinitest method are the most comparable, with approximately equal changes in urinary glucose associated with discernible color changes between 0.25% and 2%. Chemstrip uG combines the advantages of high sensitivity, range up to 5%, and discernible color changes as urinary glucose concentrations gradually increase from the lowest to the highest concentration. However, one needs to wait 2 minutes for a final reading, compared with 30 seconds or less with the other strips.

At least three factors contribute to a poor correlation between plasma glucose values and the concomitant results of urine tests for

Table 7–5. Comparison of Results Among Different Methods of Testing for Urinary Glucose

Product	Glucose Concentration (%)							
	0.1	0.25	0.5	0.75	1	2	3	5
Clinitest (5-drop)		Trace	+	+ +	+ + +	+ + + +		
Clinitest (2-drop)[a]		b			b	b	b	b
Diastix	Trace	+	+ +		+ + +	+ + + +		
Clinistix[c]	... Light ... (+)		... Medium ... (+ +)		... Dark ... (+ + +)			
Chemstrip uG	b	b	b		b	b	b	b

Blank spaces indicate that there are no color blocks for those concentrations.

[a]The 2-drop chart provides a "trace" color block without a percentage value; a trace result merely indicates glucosuria of <0.5%.

[b]Measures percentage of glucosuria at these levels, but equivalent + values are not available.

[c]Estimates relative presence of glucose but cannot show percentage value.

From Ames Co.: Home Urine Testing for the Diabetic. Ames Co, Division Miles Laboratories, Elkhart, IN, 1976

glucose: a wide range of renal thresholds,[36] varying glucose reabsorption by the proximal tubule within the same patient,[37] and interference with urinary glucose measurements due to certain constituents[38] in and properties[39] of the urine itself. Both falsely low and falsely high readings are common and differ among the various methods. In a study evaluating the first four methods listed in Table 7–5, 500 urine samples from both diabetic and nondiabetic patients were tested, both as collected and after a precise amount of glucose was added. Approximately 25% of the samples gave falsely low readings, and almost half gave falsely high readings.[39] Only Clinistix and Diastix gave falsely low readings. In half of the urine samples yielding falsely low results, ascorbic acid (vitamin C) and/or a breakdown product of salicylic acid (aspirin) were found. Both of these substances interfere with oxidation of the dye, as mentioned previously. Aspirin and vitamin C are so commonly ingested that patients often do not mention them to physicians. In addition, numerous other, unidentified compounds were found in the urine specimens, probably representing the diverse medications that the patients were taking or the degradative products thereof. Although substances that might interfere with the results of Chemstrip uG have not been evaluated extensively, vitamin C was noted to yield falsely low or even negative results. One would expect that Diastix, Clinistix, and Chemstrip uG all would react similarly.

Almost half of the urine specimens gave falsely high values,[39] and two thirds of these occurred with Clinitest tablets. Low urine osmolalities (usually <100 mOsm/kg) were consistently associated with falsely high readings. The effect of the usual procedure of collecting a second-voided urine specimen 30 minutes after a patient drinks 16 ounces of water was evaluated in nine additional patients.[39] Falsely high readings were found in all nine samples tested with Clinitest tablets, in five of nine tested with Clinistix, and in four of nine tested with Diastix. These results raise a serious question about the accuracy of testing second-voided urine samples (discussed later).

In addition to vitamin C and aspirin derivatives, several other substances have been implicated in interference with the results of urine testing for glucose. Highly colored urine (i.e., due to bilirubin or nitrofurantoin) may prevent accurate readings owing to a masking of the color reaction. Ketone bodies in moderate to large amounts may depress Diastix but not Chemstrip uG readings. Protein in the urine may cause excessive foaming with Clinitest tablets and difficulty in interpreting the final color development, thus leading to artificially low readings. Non–glucose-reducing sugars, aspirin, and β-lactam cephalosporins and penicillins cause false-positive reactions with Clinitest tablets[35, 38] but do not affect the glucose oxidase method used in the other urine-testing products. Although vitamin C added directly to urine samples also may cause a false-positive reaction with Clinitest tablets, this effect was not noted in urine collected from subjects who ingested large oral doses of ascorbic acid.[38] The same pertains to isoniazid and methyldopa (Aldomet). Both of these drugs caused falsely low readings with the glucose oxidase method (by inhibiting dye development) when added directly to urine[35] but had no effect on urine samples from patients taking the medications.[40, 41] On the other hand, urine samples collected from patients taking L-dopa gave falsely high readings with Clinitest tablets and falsely low readings with Clinistix.[32, 38] Presumably, all tests using the oxidation of a dye would show the same effect. Some evidence suggests that nalidixic acid, p-aminosalicylic acid (PAS), and the x-ray contrast medium diatrizoate (Hypaque) interfere with Clinitest tablets, and the glucose oxidase method is invalidated by phenazopyridine (Pyridium) and diatrizoate.[38] Finally, large amounts of urinary 5-hydroxyindoleacetic acid (5-HIAA), often found in patients with the carcinoid syndrome, also block oxidation of the dye and cause false-negative results with tests using the glucose oxidase method.[32] Table 7–6 summarizes the effects of substances that interfere with tests for urinary glucose.

Two chemical reactions measure ketone bodies. The more common one uses nitroprusside (Ketostix, Keto-Diastix, Labstix, Acetest tablets), and the newest strip (Chemstrip uK) uses nitroferricyanide. (Chemstrip uGK measures both glucose and ketone bodies.) Various substances also interfere with the tests for urinary ketones. Urine from patients taking L-dopa gives a false-positive test result for ketone bodies with nitroprusside.[42–44] However, results were negative with Acetest tablets,[43, 44] possibly because this test may be less sensitive. Methyldopa also yields

false-positive results for ketone bodies with nitroprusside.[42] False-positive results with nitroprusside also occur with paraldehyde.[42] Pyridium, on the other hand, may mask slightly positive reactions for ketone bodies with nitroprusside.[42] False-negative results have been reported when these strips have been exposed to air for an extended time or when urine specimens have been highly acidic (e.g., after high intake of ascorbic acid [vitamin C]). Finally, urine from patients taking captopril, the oral angiotensin-converting enzyme inhibitor, yields false-positive results for ketone bodies with both nitroprusside and nitroferricyanide.[45] This last observation suggests that situations in which interference with the nitroprusside method occurs also apply to nitroferricyanide.

The timing of urine collections obviously affects the results, but the reasons for this are mainly physiologic. A specimen obtained before breakfast when a patient is in the fasting state is least likely to show glucosuria simply because the plasma glucose concentration is usually lowest at that time. Thus, the fasting urine test is the least sensitive—that is, it is least likely to show altered metabolism. The next most sensitive urine test is that performed on a sample collected preprandially. In this case, 3 to 6 hours usually has elapsed since the last meal, and the height of the postprandial glucose surge is over. A second-voided urine sample taken at this time measures the efficiency with which the meal-derived carbohydrates have been cleared by 3 to 6 hours and is more likely to show glucosuria than is the fasting specimen. However, the first-voided, preprandial urine sample is even more sensitive because it reflects the entire period after the meal, during which time postprandial glucose concentrations have reached their maximum. A sample collected 1 to 2 hours postprandially is most likely to show glucosuria, because it is not diluted with urine that may be sugar-free after the plasma glucose level has fallen below the T_m.

Although some diabetologists recommend

Table 7–6. Effect of Substances That Interfere with Results of Urine Tests for Glucose

Substance[a]	Method[b]	
	Nonspecific[c]	Specific[d]
Ascorbic acid (vitamin C)	↑ [e]	↓
Salicylic acid (aspirin)	↑	↓
Decreased osmolality	↑	
Ketone bodies		↓ [f]
Protein	↓	
Cephalosporins (β-lactam)	↑	
Penicillins (β-lactam)	↑	
Non–glucose-reducing sugars	↑	
Isoniazid (INH)		↓ [e]
Methyldopa (Aldomet)		↓ [e]
L-Dopa	↑	↓
5-HIAA		↓
Nalidixic acid	↑	
PAS	↑	
Phenazopyridine (Pyridium)		↓
Diatrizoate (Hypaque)	↑	↑

5-HIAA, 5-hydroxyindoleacetic acid; PAS, *p*-aminosalicylic acid.

[a]Effect may be due to degradative product of substance.

[b]↑, falsely high; ↓, falsely low.

[c]Refers to nonspecific reducing method using Clinitest tablets.

[d]Refers to glucose oxidase method using Clinistix or Diastix. Although all of these products were not tested for each interfering substance, it is assumed that all would be affected.

[e]Effect is noted only when the substance is added directly to the urine; no effect is seen when the patient ingests the substance.

[f]Does not interfere with Chemstrip uG or K.

that patients doing urine testing routinely collect and test a second-voided urine specimen and discard the initial one without testing it, this approach has been challenged. The arguments on each side follow.

The results of the second-voided specimen reflect what is happening at the time that the sample is collected. When these results are compared with the prevailing plasma glucose concentration, the T_m is evident. (However, the T_m is not an exact glucose level, and several comparisons that result in a small range and yield an approximate value for the T_m are needed.) Because this sample is not "contaminated" with glucose that may have been excreted several hours before, the results of the second-voided specimen reflect more accurately the effect of exogenous insulin acting at that particular moment. Depending on which preparation has been injected and when (see Chapter 4, Table 4–1), the preprandial urine tests take place at times of peak insulin action. Therefore, the results are helpful in adjusting the insulin dose.

On the other hand, the same facts can be used to support routine testing of first-voided specimens. Overlooking postprandial glucosuria by testing only the second-voided sample may delude both patient and physician into thinking that diabetic control is really better than it is. Because tight control is so important (see Chapter 2), significant postprandial glucosuria must be appreciated and adjustments made to abolish it. A forceful argument against the routine testing of double-voided urine specimens is the impracticality of the method. Many patients do not have or will not take the time to urinate twice before meals. Indeed, a survey of almost 1,200 urine tests on the inpatient diabetic ward at Cedars-Sinai Medical Center during a period when testing of both first- and second-voided urines was allegedly part of the nursing routine revealed that the second-voided urine was not tested 45% of the time!

If second-voided urine were tested routinely, how often would it yield results different from those of the first-voided specimen? Several studies have attempted to answer this question (Table 7–7). The results were the same 60% to 80% of the time. As was expected, only a small number (5%) of second-voided specimens gave higher readings than the initial sample. First-voided urine gave higher readings in only 14% to 33% of the comparisons. For reasons already discussed, more glucosuria might have been anticipated in the first-voided specimen more often than it was found. Perhaps falsely high readings caused by the formation of dilute urine in the process of collecting the second sample were responsible for this discrepancy.

In view of these considerations, I use the following approach to urine testing. For ketosis-resistant (type 2) patients, I prefer Diastix because they are simple to use and the color changes represent gradually increasing amounts of glucose (see Table 7–5). Although the latter feature is also characteristic of Clinitest tablets, testing with them requires so much preparation and time that patient compliance is profoundly limited. Clinistix has too broad a range of glucose concentrations for each color change. Chemstrip uG is accurate and compares favorably with other test strips. However, the 2-minute waiting period for full color development (compared with 30 seconds with Diastix)

may deter many patients from using this product. On the hand, because ketonuria does not interfere with the results for glucosuria, Chemstrip uG may be advantageous for type 1 diabetic patients either for routine use or when patients are ill and more likely to spill ketone bodies (discussed later).

Ketosis-prone (type 1) patients should not test with Diastix because moderate to large amounts of ketone bodies may depress the glucose readings. In this situation, a falsely low reading is not appreciated because patients are not aware of ketonuria. If Keto-Diastix are used, results of <1% urinary glucose in the presence of moderate or large ketone bodies requires retesting with Clinitest tablets or Chemstrip uG. This is important because uncontrolled diabetes with falsely low glucose readings must be distinguished from "starvation" ketosis (described later).

When diabetes is initially diagnosed and the patient is introduced to urine testing, it is important to know the T_m to interpret the results. Measuring the T_m was described in Chapter 4 and requires, of course, routine testing of second-voided urine samples. However, once the T_m has been determined, I do not usually ask patients to test a double-voided urine sample. It should be obvious from this discussion that semiquantitative urine testing for glucose is at best only a crude index of diabetic control. A measure of the imprecise relation between urine tests and prevailing plasma glucose levels is shown in Figure 7–1. Most negative test re-

Table 7–7. Comparison of Test Results for Urine Glucose Using First- and Second-Voided Urine Samples

			Results (%)		
Reference	Method	No. of Comparisons	*Same*	*First-voided higher*	*Second-voided higher*
Guthrie et al[46]	Clinitest (2-drop)	754[a]	62	33	5
McCarthy[47]	Tes-Tape	406	81	14	5
Davidson[48]	Keto-Diastix	646	72	23	5

[a]Three comparisons in the published report were omitted from this table because the patients ate between the first- and second-voided urine collections.

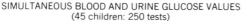

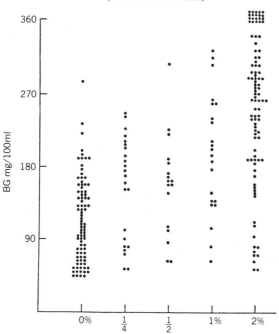

Figure 7–1. Correlation between glucosuria measured by the 5-drop Clinitest method and simultaneous blood glucose concentrations in 45 diabetic children. (From Tattersall R, Gale E: Patient self-monitoring of blood glucose and refinements of conventional insulin treatment. In Skyler JS, Cahill CF [eds]: Diabetes Mellitus. Yorke Medical Books, Stoneham, MA, 1981, p. 101)

sults for glucosuria correspond to blood glucose levels <180 mg/dl, and most test results of 2% or greater are associated with blood glucose concentrations >180 mg/dl. However, there is so much overlap that interpretation of a single test result is extremely difficult. Other studies evaluating plasma glucose values and second-voided urine samples yield distressingly similar results.[49, 50]

In addition to the important effects of the renal threshold, possible interfering substances in the urine, and osmolality, the interpretation of urine test results is also affected by whether or not the bladder is emptied completely. However, many patients do not or cannot consistently perform SMBG, and therefore, in these individuals urine testing is still the most practical and accurate way to judge day-to-day diabetic control. Despite the caveats discussed earlier concerning urine testing, it has been forcefully argued that this method of assessing diabetic control may have advantages over SMBG[51]

because results reflect a period that is physiologically more important than glucose concentrations at a single instance. In fact, in a crossover study of type 1 diabetic patients comparing urine testing with SMBG, both methods of monitoring produced similar levels of glycemic control.[52] In another study of type 1 patients who could not afford SMBG, urine testing resulted in a reduction of DKA episodes and other diabetes-related hospitalization admissions.[53] Therefore, although SMBG is preferred, those patients who either cannot or will not use this method of monitoring should be strongly encouraged to test their urine routinely for glucose.

QUANTITATIVE URINE TESTING

A more accurate assessment of diabetic control by means of testing urine is quantitative measurement by the chemistry laboratory of the amount of glucose excreted. The advantages of this method are as follows: (1) it eliminates the influence of substances that give falsely low or falsely high readings; (2) it eliminates the influence of urinary osmolality; (3) it measures the exact level of glucosuria; and (4) it allows assessment of diabetic control over longer periods.

The quantitative method also has several disadvantages. The major one is the inconvenience of accurate urine collection. The bladder must be emptied at both the beginning and end of the evaluation period, and *all* urine passed during that period must be brought to the laboratory. As with semiquantitative methods, the T_m for glucose has an important effect on the level of glucosuria. In addition, the amount of dietary carbohydrates may influence the interpretation of the results. A commonly accepted criterion for good control is excretion of <10% of the total dietary carbohydrate intake. Therefore, a patient who loses 22 g of urinary glucose in 24 hours would be considered well controlled if he or she ate 250 g of carbohydrates but only fairly well controlled if the diet consisted of only 150 g of carbohydrates. In my view, the disadvantages clearly outweigh any advantages, and therefore I do not use this method of evaluating diabetic control.

PLASMA GLUCOSE MEASUREMENTS

The plasma glucose concentration obviously is the best available index of diabetic control. However, because it reflects the situation only at that particular moment, the results may not represent a patient's usual metabolic state. For instance, if the trip to the laboratory, clinic, or physician's office is stressful for a patient, the resulting glucose value will be higher than usual. Alternatively, some patients (at least some of mine) change their usual pattern of treatment just before testing (e.g., by adhering to their diet or even occasionally by taking extra insulin). Obviously, the glucose concentration will be lower than their usual level. Therefore, although I rely

on plasma glucose concentrations for assessment of control, I usually do not *change* therapy (i.e., add an oral antidiabetic medication for a patient on diet alone or start insulin) on the basis of one (spurious?) value. Comparing the plasma glucose concentration with a glycated hemoglobin level (discussed later) (and/or the pattern of urine test results in the few patients who are performing them) is very helpful in deciding both the validity of the first result and whether to alter the therapeutic regimen.

On the other hand, after starting or changing the dose of a sulfonylurea agent or metformin, I measure the fasting plasma glucose (FPG) concentration approximately 2 weeks later to determine if a dose change is necessary (see Chapter 5 for rationale).

Even if the value were spurious, 2 weeks of a slightly higher or lower amount of the drug is unlikely to lead to dangerous clinical consequences. Although I prefer an FPG concentration measured in the laboratory as a basis for a therapeutic decision to alter the dose, it is difficult for some patients to get to the laboratory before breakfast. For these patients and for those in whom one can vouch for the accuracy of their SMBG values by comparing results measured by them on their meter and in the laboratory on samples obtained at the same time, fasting blood glucose (FBG) concentrations measured at home could serve as a substitute. In that situation, I prefer to base my decision on FBG levels on 3 consecutive days approximately 2 weeks after the dose change. Keep in mind, however, that the results provided by many but not all meters are whole blood values, which are approximately 12% lower than plasma values. Repeated spurious FPG or FBG results would be exposed by the glycated hemoglobin test result obtained every 2 to 3 months. In contrast, a single isolated plasma glucose level is probably not an adequate assessment on which to adjust an insulin dose without other confirmatory information (e.g., symptoms of hypoglycemia or uncontrolled diabetes, glycated value, urine test results, repeated plasma glucose levels).

The timing of plasma glucose measurements also is important in evaluating control. A postprandial sample obtained 1 to 2 hours after a patient has eaten is the most sensitive index, because glucose levels are maximal at this time. The total carbohydrate content of the meal affects this result. The preprandial glucose concentration is the next most sensitive index of how efficiently meal-derived carbohydrates have been cleared from the plasma. Finally, the fasting glucose concentration is the least sensitive index of diabetic control, because it does not reflect a postprandial challenge to the pancreas. In diabetic patients (not receiving insulin), the glucose level is usually at its lowest in the fasting state, and as carbohydrate metabolism deteriorates, this value is the last to rise. Recommendations concerning the timing of samples under different circumstances are discussed later.

GLYCATED (GLYCOSYLATED) HEMOGLOBIN

Measurements of Hgb A_1, Hgb A_{1c}, and, most recently, glycated hemoglobin[54, 55] were introduced into clinical practice approximately 15 years ago as an index of long-term diabetic control and are now widely used.

[The term *glycosylated hemoglobin*, as commonly used, refers not to a glycoside (the product of glycosylation reaction) but rather to a ketoamine that is an Amadori product (discussed later). The Joint Commission on Biochemical Nomenclature recommends that the term *glycation* be used instead of *glycosylation* when the structure referred to is not a glycoside. *Glycation* refers to any carbohydrate–protein linkage, regardless of structure or method of synthesis. Therefore, the term *glycated* hemoglobin or other proteins is used in this book.] Because the terminology can be confusing, some knowledge of the biochemistry of red blood cells (RBCs) is necessary for understanding the rationale for measuring and interpreting levels of these three species of hemoglobin in diabetic patients.

In normal individuals, 90% of hemoglobin consists of two alpha and two beta chains and is called *Hgb A*. Approximately 2% of hemoglobin contains two alpha and two delta chains (Hgb A_2, a normal variant), whereas 1% is fetal hemoglobin (Hgb F), which is composed of two alpha and two gamma chains. The remaining 7% of hemoglobin also consists of two alpha and two beta chains, with either glucose or a derivative of glucose attached to the beta chain. If glucose is attached, the resulting hemoglobin is called *Hgb A_{1c}*. Hgb A_{1c} is the major component of these hemoglobins and constitutes approximately 5% of total hemoglobins in nondiabetic persons. A number of hemoglobins with glucose derivatives attached have also been isolated. Two of these are Hgb A_{1a} and Hgb A_{1b}, each of which makes up approximately 1% of total hemoglobins in nondiabetic individuals. Because all these hemoglobins contain glucose or one of its derivatives, they are known collectively as *Hgb A_1*.

These additions to the end of the beta chain change the charge characteristics of Hgb A so that the molecules travel faster in certain chromatographic separation techniques, such as ion chromatography, electrophoresis, or high-performance liquid chromatography (HPLC). In older terminology, this fraction was called the fast, or minor, hemoglobins. In 1968, diabetic individuals were first noted to have a higher percentage of fast hemoglobins than did control subjects. Because the structure of these hemoglobins was not yet appreciated, investigators thought that the increase in minor hemoglobins was related in some way to the genetic composition of the diabetic population. Subsequent studies of both animals and humans showed clearly that this was not the case.

The reaction between glucose and the beta chain of hemoglobin is (1) slow, (2) mostly irreversible, (3) not mediated by an enzyme, (4) continuous over the life span of the RBC, and (5) proportional to the glucose concentration to which the RBC is exposed. Thus, the amount of Hgb A_1 or its major component, Hgb A_{1c}, is a time-integrated measure of the prevailing glucose concentration to which the RBCs have been exposed. As such (within certain limitations), it should be helpful in monitoring diabetic control. A number of studies have demonstrated that levels of either Hgb A_{1c} or Hgb A_1 (depending on which was measured) are proportional to FPG concentrations, postprandial glucose levels, values obtained during a glucose tolerance test, amount of urinary glucose excreted, and clinical estimates of control. One such correlation is shown in Figure 7-2. In this study, the components of Hgb A_1 were measured in a group of children with a wide spectrum of diabetic control. Biochemical criteria[56] for the different de-

grees of control were as follows: (1) excellent—essentially normal postprandial glucose concentrations on periodic clinic visits, aglycosuria, no ketonuria; (2) good—same as in (1), except for occasional minimal transient glucosuria (trace to 2% in no more than one of three to four daily urine specimens); (3) good to fair—somewhat more frequent transient glucosuria, usually related to dietary indiscretions; (4) fair—varying amounts of glucosuria in approximately half of the samples tested, occasionally transient ketonuria, postprandial glucose concentrations usually between 150 and 300 mg/dl; and (5) poor—various degrees of glucosuria in most urine specimens tested. The relation between the degree of control and levels of Hgb A_{1c} or Hgb A_1 in these cases is striking. The difference between the patients with the best control and the nondiabetic group is minimal. Note that Hgb A_{1a} and Hgb A_{1b} levels are similar in all groups and that the

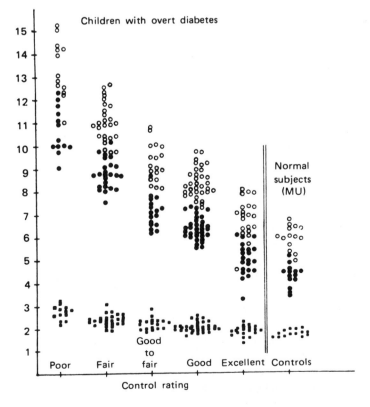

Figure 7–2. Relation between diabetic control in children and the various fractions of glycated hemoglobin. (■) Hgb A_{1a+b}; (●) Hgb A_{1c}; (○) Hgb A_{1a+b+c}. (From Jackson RL, Hess RL, England JD: Hemoglobin A_{1c} values in children with overt diabetes maintained in varying degrees of control. Diabetes care 2:391, 1979)

fraction that changes in diabetic patients is Hgb A_{1c}. Therefore, the differences in the amount of Hgb A_1 among the groups are due to changes in Hgb A_{1c}.

Early longitudinal studies revealed that levels of Hgb A_{1c}[57] and Hgb A_1[58] correlate best with the degree of diabetic control obtained several months earlier.

This would be expected because of the 120-day life span of the RBC and because the glycation reaction of hemoglobin is mostly irreversible. The lag period before an improvement in diabetic control is reflected in changes in Hgb A_{1c} levels as shown in Figure 7–3. Comparison of the relatively rapid decline in urinary glucose level with the gradual decline of Hgb A_{1c} values shows that the latter did not reach a plateau until 6 weeks after tight control was achieved. Similarly, the maximal Hgb A_{1c} value was reached 2 to 3 months after diabetic control was allowed to deteriorate.[59] A more detailed kinetic analysis revealed that 50% of the Hgb A_{1c} level was determined by the glucose concentra-

tions during the preceding month, 25% by the month before that, and 12.5% each in the third and fourth month before the measurement.[60] Clinically, this means that a glycated hemoglobin level obtained 2 months after adjusting therapy reflects 75% of the change in glycemia; a value 3 months later reflects 87.5%.

Glycation of hemoglobin is more complex than what has already been described in at least two respects. The reaction of glucose with the terminal amino acid (valine) on the beta chain of hemoglobin is depicted in Figure 7–4. The first product formed, the aldimine, is not stable and mostly dissociates back to glucose and Hgb A. This compound is called *labile* Hgb A_1 or pre-A_{1c}. A small amount of pre-A_{1c} is slowly converted to Hgb A_{1c}, a ketoamine, by a molecular (Amadori) rearrangement. The formation of Hgb A_{1c} is irreversible and, as described earlier, remains for the duration of the life span of the RBC. Unfortunately, pre-A_{1c} is also measured by both the widely applied ion chromatography

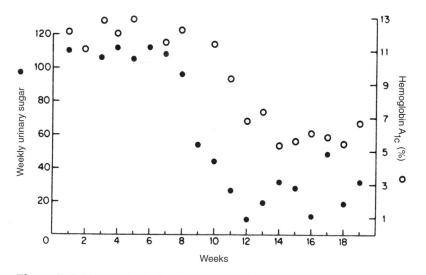

Figure 7–3. Temporal relation between weekly urinary glucose levels and Hgb A_{1c} in one patient. Urinary glucose was measured semiquantitatively with Clinitest tablets (on a scale of 0 to 4+) four times a day. The results were summed every 7 days to obtain a mean weekly index. (From Koenig RJ, Peterson CM, Jones RL et al: Correlation of glucose regulation and hemoglobin A_{1c} in diabetes mellitus. N Engl J Med 295:417, 1976)

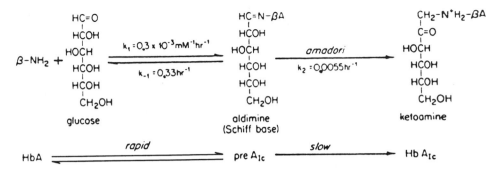

Figure 7–4. Reaction between glucose and the N-terminus of the β-chains of hemoglobin. (From Bunn HF: Evaluation of glycosylated hemoglobin in diabetic patients. Diabetes 30:613, 1981)

used to measure glycated hemoglobin as well as by HPLC and electrophoresis. This explained the findings of older studies in which Hgb A_{1c} levels (1) fell 1% to 2% within a day or two of bringing patients with uncontrolled diabetes into near euglycemia[61, 62]; (2) rose rapidly after control was allowed to deteriorate[61, 63]; and (3) varied day to day by 1% to 4%.[64] Fortunately, most methods used today routinely remove the labile or pre-A_{1c} fraction, although clinicians need to ascertain from the laboratory that this is indeed true before evaluating glycated hemoglobin levels.

Other disadvantages of separation by charge differences are that the results are influenced by the conditions under which the blood is collected, shipped, and stored; the columns are very sensitive to changes in temperature and buffer pH; and falsely high levels may be found in thalassemia (Hgb F coelutes with Hgb A_1), uremia, and lead poisoning, and in patients ingesting large doses of aspirin, and with high blood levels of alcohol, triglycerides, and bilirubin.[58, 61] Some hemoglobinopathies invalidate measurements of Hgb A_{1c} and Hgb A_1. In addition to thalassemia, falsely high values are found in hemoglobinopathies J, K, I, H, Bart's, Raleigh (β_1 ala), Long Island (β_2 pro), and South Florida (β_1 met).[65] Falsely low values are noted in hemoglobinopathies S, D, C, E, G, Lepore, and O-Arab.[65, 66] Interference by

many of the foregoing factors varies, depending on the assay used,[67] and again, physicians should ascertain the performance of the method used in their laboratory.

Hgb A_{1c} or Hgb A_1 is not a true measure of glycated hemoglobin.[68] More refined analyses showed that only 60% to 80% of Hgb A_{1c} is glycated. However, glucose forms ketoamine linkages with another amino acid (lysine). This glycated hemoglobin cannot be separated from Hgb A by charge separation because this reaction does not change the charge properties of hemoglobin. However, ketoamine linkages between glucose and hemoglobin (or any protein, for that matter) form a specific chemical configuration that causes these compounds to bind to phenylboronate resins. This property allows the separation (by affinity chromatography) of glycated hemoglobin (regardless of the site of the glucose reaction) from nonglycated hemoglobin. Fortuitously, the values of Hgb A_{1c} and glycated hemoglobin are similar because the amount of nonglycated hemoglobin in Hgb A_{1c} is approximately the same as the amount of glycated hemoglobin in Hgb A that is not measured by the ion chromatography method of separation. Pre-A_{1c} and aldimine linkages are not bound to the phenylboronate resin, and consequently, measures of total glycated hemoglobin by affinity chromatography are a valid index of long-term diabetic control. Methods based on immuno-

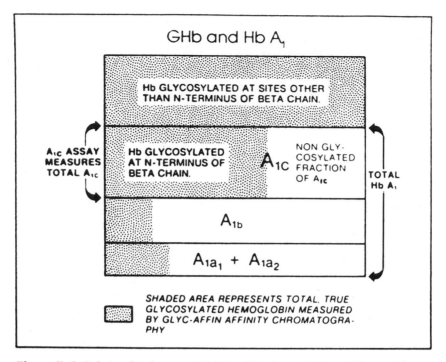

Figure 7–5. Relationship between Hgb A_{1c}, Hgb A_1, and glycated hemoglobin. The latter is measured by affinity chromatography or immunoassay. (From Teupe B: Quantitative determination of glycated hemoglobin using affinity chromatography. In Service FJ, Sheehan J [eds]: Symposium Proceedings. The Role of Glycated Hemoglobin in the Management of Diabetes. Isolab, Akron, OH, 1988, p. 9)

assay that also separate glycated hemoglobin from nonglycated hemoglobin by differences in their chemical structures have now been used.[67] Other advantages of methods based on structural differences are that the results are not influenced by conditions of blood collection, shipping, and storage, and because specific chemical configurations are involved, falsely elevated values are not a problem. The relationship between Hgb A_{1c}, Hgb A_1, and total glycated hemoglobin measured by either affinity chromatography or immunoassay is shown in Figure 7–5.

Regardless of which method is used, two additional important points must be kept in mind in interpreting the results. Because glycation occurs throughout the life span of the RBC, the presence of conditions that shorten RBC survival (hemolytic anemias, bleeding)

produce falsely low values. Conversely, if the life span of the RBC is extended (e.g., by splenectomy), the values are falsely high. Finally, ingestion of large amounts (e.g., ≥ 1.0 g/day) of vitamins C[69] and E[70] may lower glycated hemoglobin levels by blocking glycation of proteins.

There seems to be little doubt that levels of total glycated hemoglogin, stable Hgb A_{1c}, and stable Hgb A_1 are an excellent time-integrated measure of overall diabetic control. They are valuable in assessing control, both in diabetic populations and in individual patients. However, because the lag period before this index reflects changes in diabetic control, it is not as helpful in deciding changes in day-to-day therapy. For instance, a physician would not necessarily know exactly what change to make in the insulin prescription on the basis of a high level of glycated hemoglobin. On the other hand, this measure may be of value in patients whose office test results (or the record they bring to the office) do not coincide with other indices of diabetic control. Glycated hemoglobin levels should be used routinely to monitor diabetic control, because physicians' estimates of control based on historical and laboratory data collected during a routine office visit correlated poorly with the degree of control assessed by Hgb A_{1c} levels.[71]

Many patients attempting to achieve near euglycemia measure glucose levels before meals and bedtime but not postprandially as well. Even though preprandial levels seem satisfactory, glycated hemoglobin values not infrequently are higher than anticipated. This requires further efforts to achieve control, the need for which would not have been evident simply by evaluating the results of SMBG. The relation between fasting and 2-hour postprandial glucose concentrations obtained at clinic visits and stable Hgb A_{1c} values in type 1 diabetic patients is depicted in Figure 7–6. This information furnishes a general context in which to judge diabetic control from a stable Hgb A_{1c} value (upper limit of normal is 6.1%). In general, it is believed that a 1% change in Hgb A_{1c} values

represents a change in the average blood glucose concentration of approximately 30 mg/dl.[58, 72]

Glycation of proteins is a general phenomenon, and enhanced glycation of many proteins occurs in diabetes. Glycated total serum proteins are increased in diabetic patients, and albumin constitutes approximately 80% of the major proteins glycated.[73] Because the half-life of serum albumin is 17 to 20 days, one might expect changes in glycated serum albumin to reflect changes in diabetic control more quickly than changes in glycated hemoglobin (half-life of 56 days). Although this is indeed the case when newly diagnosed diabetic patients were brought under control,[74] glycated albumin and glycated hemoglobin gave the same information in stable insulin-requiring diabetic patients.[75]

Glycated albumin is usually measured by boronate affinity chromatography[76] (similar to the method for glycated hemoglobin) or by a fructosamine assay.[77] The latter method is a colorimetric one that is rapid, precise, and cheap (it can be automated). The correlation between serum fructosamine and glycated hemoglobin levels ranges from 0.17 to 0.80.[78-83] Serum fructosamine results are influenced by serum albumin concentrations[84] (in contrast to the glycated albumin method), and as with Hgb A_{1c} measurements,

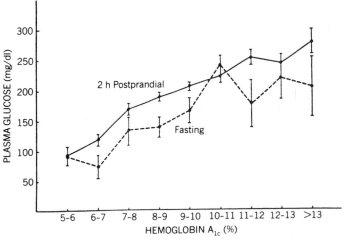

Figure 7–6. Relationship between stable Hgb A_{1c} and both fasting and 2-hour postprandial plasma glucose concentrations in diabetic youths. Points and vertical lines represent means ± SEM of a total of 1,172 values in 187 patients. (From Goldstein DE, Parker KM, England JD et al: Clinical application of glycosylated hemoglobin measurements. Diabetes 31[suppl 3]:70, 1982)

a large percentage of what is measured as serum fructosamine may not be due to protein glycation but to a nonspecific reducing activity of the serum.[85] Serum fructosamine levels are inversely related to body weight and are independent of glycemia.[86] For instance, in a study of 160 type 1 diabetic patients with a body mass index (kg/m^2) of 25.1 and 200 type 2 diabetic patients with a body mass index of 30.6, a Hgb A_{1c} level of approximately 9% correlated with serum fructosamine ranges of 390 to 405 and 325 to 335 μmol/L, respectively. (Robert Thompson, M.D.: Personal communication. Amylin Pharmaceuticals, San Diego, CA.) From a clinical decision-making viewpoint, I see no advantage in measuring glycated products with a shorter half-life and therefore use glycated hemoglobin levels almost exclusively. Others also do not recommend using fructosamine measurements to evaluate diabetic control.[80, 82, 83, 87–89]

SELF-MONITORING OF BLOOD GLUCOSE

SMBG by patients in their usual home environments is widely accepted as important by health care professionals and is performed by millions of diabetic patients.[90, 91] The procedure involves pricking the finger (relatively painlessly) with a lancet, which is almost always inserted into a spring-loaded device, to obtain a drop of blood that is placed on a pad at the end of a strip (see Chapter 10 for a description of accomplishing this). In most systems, the reagents on the pad consist of an enzyme that converts glucose into a substance that reacts with a dye, causing a color change. In older systems (some of which are still in use), the blood is left on the strip for a specific time and then wiped off; another period is allowed to elapse before the color is either visually compared with a chart on the reagent strip vial or inserted into a small meter that displays an exact glucose concentration. More recently developed systems are nonwipe ones—that is, the strip is inserted into the meter before blood is placed on it and the glucose concentration is displayed in less than a minute without further manipulation by the operator. In some of these newer systems, the oxidation of glucose by the enzyme embedded in the strip generates a small electric current that is measured and converted into a glucose concentration that is displayed on the meter. Currently available lancets, spring-loaded devices, strips, and meters are described yearly in the October issue of *Forecast*, published by the American Diabetes Association.

According to a Consensus Statement of the American Diabetes Association,[91] health care professionals should use the results of SMBG to (1) set glycemic goals; (2) develop recommendations for pharmacologic therapy; (3) evaluate the effectiveness of pharmacologic therapy; (4) instruct patients to interpret and respond to blood glucose patterns; (5) evaluate the impact of dietary factors on glycemic control; (6) modify therapy during acute/intercurrent illnesses and when receiving medications that may affect glycemic control; (7) modify the management plan in response to changes in activity; and (8) identify hypoglycemia unawareness and strategies for treatment. These are laudable and, in many patients, achievable goals. Other patients, however, do not perform SMBG. In a national survey of nearly 2,500 diabetic patients older than 18 years,[92] only a third did. In the type 1 diabetic population, 40% of patients monitored once or more a day, 39% monitored less than once a day, and 21% never did. In the type 2 diabetic population using insulin, 26% monitored at least once a day, 27% monitored less than once a day, and 47% did not monitor at all. These disappointing patterns can be improved by educating physicians and patients.[93] Such a community intervention in Michigan resulted in increasing SMBG from 29% to 85% in type 1 diabetic patients, from 6% to 82% in insulin-requiring type 2 diabetic patients, and from 2% to 31% in type 2 diabetic patients not using insulin between 1981 and 1991.

At least four factors limit SMBG—discomfort, inconvenience, cost, and frustration—because health care professionals do not evaluate and discuss the results with patients.[90] The first two factors may be overcome if physicians can convince patients of the importance of the derived information. This implies, of course, that the last reason would not be a barrier.

Unfortunately, SMBG is expensive, largely because of the cost of the strips. If a visual method is used, the strips can be split in half (lengthwise) without sacrificing accuracy.[94] Using strips that can be read visually has two other potential advantages. The first is a visual confirmation of the glucose concentration recorded by the meter when the particular result may be unexpected by the patient. (Of course, this check identifies only problems with the meter, not with a patient's technique, which is the usual reason for discrepant values.) Second, the visually read strips may be kept in a dark, dry environment (e.g., put back into the vial, which contains a desiccant) and read at a later date by another trained individual.[95] Not all investigators agree, however, that the colors are maintained under these conditions.[96, 97] With the introduction of meters with alert signals to identify faulty technique and with the capacity for memory storage of data, there is much less reason now to use a visual method.

A Consensus Development Conference recommended that the results of SMBG systems be within 10% of "true" glucose concentrations between 30 and 400 mg/dl 100% of the time.[90] Although such accuracy may be approached under controlled laboratory conditions,[98, 99] the results are usually much less accurate in the field.[90] Most of this discrepancy is due to patients' technique (including failure to clean and/or calibrate the meter properly) rather than problems with the meter itself.[90] For this reason, I routinely have patients perform SMBG at the time that their blood is drawn and compare their result with a simultaneous venous sample measured in the laboratory. Using a drop of the venous blood only measures the accuracy of their meter. Two important factors must be considered when comparing a patient's (whole blood) glucose value from the meter versus the laboratory-measured (plasma) glucose concentration. Whole blood results are approximately 12% lower than plasma levels because the volume of distribution of glucose in whole blood is decreased owing to the presence of RBCs, yet the results are expressed per total volume. To complicate the issue further, some meters are calibrated to give whole blood results, others are calibrated to give values equivalent to plasma concentrations (even though the sample measured is whole blood), and some are calibrated somewhere in between. Different meters from the same company are calibrated to give either whole blood or plasma equivalent values (e.g., Lifescan). Obviously, both patients and health care providers need to know this characteristic of the meter being used, and it can only be identified (at the time of writing) by contacting the company.

Although the usual goal for SMBG is accuracy within 10% to 15% of the laboratory-derived value, this evaluation ignores the clinical consequences of any differences between the measured and actual value. An error grid analysis (Fig. 7–7) attempts to assess which differences might lead to inappropriate clinical decisions and which ones are clinically benign. This error grid analysis[100] is based on the following assumptions: (1) Target blood glucose values should be between 70 and 180 mg/dl; (2) steps will be taken to bring glucose values outside of this range to within it; (4) treatment resulting in subsequent values outside of this range is inappropriate; and (5) failure to treat blood glucose values <70 mg/dl and >240 mg/dl is also inappropriate.

Five zones are demarcated in the error grid analysis (see Fig. 7–7). Zone A includes

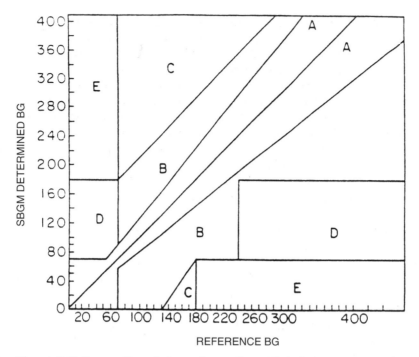

Figure 7–7. Error grid analysis used to evaluate clinical consequences of the results of self-monitoring of blood glucose (SMBG). The reference BG (blood glucose) is a laboratory measured value. See text for description. (From Clarke WL, Cox D, Gonder-Frederick LA et al: Evaluating clinical accuracy of systems for self-monitoring of blood glucose, Diabetes Care 10:622, 1987)

all values either within 20% of the reference (laboratory measured) glucose concentration or <70 mg/dl when the reference value is also <70 mg/dl. These can be considered clinically accurate measurements because the appropriate treatment (or lack of treatment) would occur. The upper and lower zones B contain values that deviate more than 20% from the reference glucose level but that, based on the assumptions enumerated earlier, should lead to either no treatment or appropriate treatment (i.e., the resultant glucose value would be in the target range). Thus, although values in zone B might fall outside of the 10% to 15% goal of accuracy, no adverse clinical consequences would occur. Values in both zones C would lead to mistaken treatment of acceptable glucose levels and result in concentrations out-

side of the target range. Zone D values would lead to no treatment in situations that clearly required treatment. In these situations, patients believe that the glucose concentrations are within the target range, but the actual values lie outside. Failure to treat values that fall within zone D on the left (i.e., near the *y* axis) could have serious hypoglycemic clinical consequences within a relatively short period. Values falling within both zones E would lead to inappropriate treatment—that is, hyperglycemic patients would be treated for hypoglycemia and vice versa. If hypoglycemic patients received treatment for hyperglycemia, the clinical consequences could be dangerous indeed.

The results of evaluating thousands of measurements by error grid analysis are very reassuring.[100] When values are determined by various meters, 74% to 98% fall within zone A, 0% to 20% in zone B, almost none in zone C, 0% to 5% in zone D, and virtually none in zone E. The results of error grid analysis of nearly 1,000 visually derived values were also quite reassuring, with 80% falling within zone A, 17% in zone B, and 3% in zone D.[100] Although a visual assessment of glucose concentrations can be fairly accurate (Fig. 7–8), patients' performance must be verified because a blue-yellow vision deficit (which interferes with a correct visual interpretation) is more common in diabetic patients than in the general population, especially in those patients with retinopathy and even more so in those who have received laser treatment.[101]

Although extensive studies have addressed possible drug interactions affecting the results of urine testing (discussed earlier), little information about possible drug interference with SMBG is available. Glucose concentra-

tions were artificially lowered when a patient receiving a continuous dopamine infusion used an SMBG technique.[102] This was subsequently confirmed by in vitro testing. Concentrations of ascorbic acid (vitamin C), acetaminophen (Tylenol), and salicylic acid (aspirin) that would be found in the medium to high therapeutic range in patients taking these agents on an ongoing basis also depressed glucose concentrations in SMBG systems by 20% or more when studied in vitro.[103] However, unlike the situation with dopamine, I am unaware of any reports attesting to the clinical consequences of these in vitro results. It should be noted, however, that finger-stick glucose concentrations measured in hypotensive patients (systolic blood pressure <80 mm Hg) were falsely low (only two thirds of venous values).[104]

The Consensus Conference[90] recommends SMBG for all insulin-treated patients, especially those who are pregnant, whose diabe-

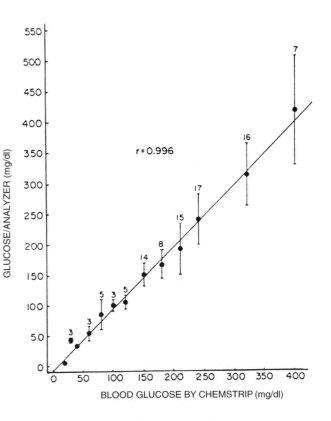

Figure 7–8. Relationship between blood glucose values obtained by visual reading of Chemstrip and laboratory method on the same sample of blood. Results summarize 98 specimens provided by 17 adolescents and adults. (From Kubilis P, Rosenbloom AL: Accurate home glucose monitoring without a meter. Diabetes Care 5:640, 1980)

tes is unstable, who have hypoglycemia un-awareness (discussed later), who are on intensive insulin regimens, and who have abnormal renal thresholds. I urge all insulin-requiring patients to perform SMBG to the extent that their abilities and income allow. As discussed later, my preference is for daily tests up to four times a day. The use of SMBG by patients not taking insulin is more controversial. Theoretically, one might ex-pect that the results of SMBG would enhance patients' motivation and compliance, al-though (as mentioned earlier) when tested this could not be confirmed.[32-34] Motivated individual patients, however, can be helped to determine which carbohydrate-containing foods are more likely to provoke hyperglyce-mia.

Poor compliance may also extend to pa-tients who are ostensibly performing SMBG. A number of studies using meters with mem-ories (unbeknownst to patients) have dem-onstrated fraudulent results written in the logbook by a distressingly large number of patients (up to 40%).[105-107] The discrepancies noted tended to obscure episodes of hyper-glycemia and hypoglycemia. This distortion of the true record underscores the impor-tance of routinely measuring glycated hemo-globin levels as a totally objective criterion of glycemic control. In a large group of pa-tients, SMBG and glycated hemoglobin val-ues correlated quite well (Fig. 7-9).

Three other points should be made about SMBG. First, it has been repeatedly demon-strated that the more frequently SMBG is performed in insulin-requiring patients, the better the diabetic control achieved. One example of this is shown in Figure 7-10 in 14 patients treated with insulin infusion pumps. Second, if a preprandial value is high (and a patient's schedule permits), the meal can be delayed so that the preprandial regu-lar insulin has an opportunity to lower the glucose level before the ingested food raises it again. The postprandial glycemia thus is less than if the meal had been eaten on time. Alternatively, if a patient is not already taking it, lispro insulin (Humalog—see Chapter 4) can be substituted for the regular insulin preparation. Finally, a major problem en-countered by patients using SMBG is that health care professionals often do not review their data.[90] Improved diabetic control does occur when communication between pa-tients and health care professionals addresses the results of SMBG.[108] The frequency of this interaction between patient and professional can be decreased if patients are taught how to interpret SMBG data, a situation that oc-curs only too rarely.[90] The following section deals with this issue.

MONITORING PATIENTS WHO TAKE INSULIN

It is not widely appreciated that sensitivity to exogenous insulin in diabetic patients can vary over time.[109] This can happen in the absence of a recognizable cause (e.g., infec-tion, weight change, emotional stress) and occurs more often in type 1 diabetic pa-tients. For this reason, it is usually inadequate to assign an insulin regimen to a patient and evaluate it only every 3 to 6 months during an office visit. Insulin doses need to be changed much more frequently, either by the physician or by the patient with the physician's guidance. This requires that pa-tients collect ongoing information about their degree of diabetic control.

As just mentioned, the more often insulin-requiring patients perform SMBG (or urine testing), the tighter is their control. Under ideal circumstances, physicians need SMBG results seven or eight times a day: before and after each meal and before the bedtime snack. A 3 AM value occasionally is also nec-essary, especially when insulin doses affect-ing overnight glucose homeostasis are changed. Because this amount of home blood glucose monitoring is unrealistic for most patients, I describe an approach that basically uses four bits of information per day but allows decisions to be made with fewer data as well.

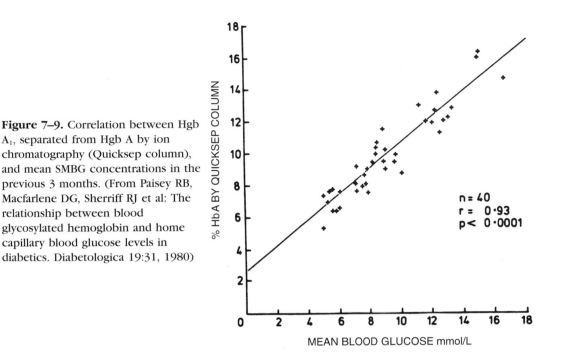

Figure 7–9. Correlation between Hgb A₁, separated from Hgb A by ion chromatography (Quicksep column), and mean SMBG concentrations in the previous 3 months. (From Paisey RB, Macfarlene DG, Sherriff RJ et al: The relationship between blood glycosylated hemoglobin and home capillary blood glucose levels in diabetics. Diabetologica 19:31, 1980)

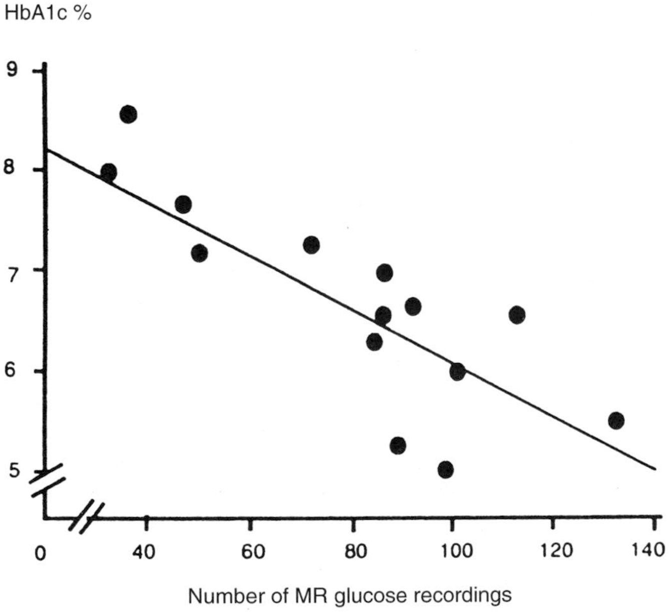

Figure 7–10. Correlation ($r = -0.85$) between number of SMBG measurements recorded in a memory reflectance meter (MR) for 21 days and Hgb A_{1c}. (From Ziegler O, Kolopp M, Got I et al: Reliability of self-monitoring of blood glucose by CSII-treated patients with type I diabetes. Diabetes Care 12:184, 1989)

Table 7–8. Onset and Peak Action of Insulin Preparations Used to Achieve Tight Diabetic Control

Insulin	Description	Action (Hours) Onset	Peak
Lispro	Rapid-acting	~1/4	~1
Regular	Short-acting	½–1	2–4
NPH	Intermediate-acting	3–4	8–14
Ultralente	Long-acting	6–8	14–20

Although it was addressed in Chapter 4 (see Table 4-1), the onset and peak action of the insulin preparations most often used to achieve tight control are presented in Table 7-8. I prefer not to use Lente insulin under these circumstances because both a blunted rise in serum insulin concentrations and a delayed decline in glucose levels occur when regular insulin is added to the Lente preparation as compared with neutral protamine Hagedorn (NPH) insulin.[110, 111] Although Ultralente preparations also retard the absorption of regular insulin,[112] no other choice is available for a suitable long-acting insulin. Mixing lispro insulin with either NPH[113] or Lente[114] preparations, however, does not affect the time course of action of the rapid-acting insulin. The actual times throughout a 24-hour period during which each type of insulin is effective and the timing of the tests reflecting that activity are summarized in Table 7-9. Six different insulin regimens for achieving tight control are summarized in Table 7-10. Regimen F, insulin infusion pump therapy, is included for completeness and for comparison with the other approaches. In my view, only physicians who are experienced with this mode of therapy and who will devote the extra amount of time that it requires should supervise patients on pump therapy.

Five degrees of diabetic control are presented in Table 7-11. Algorithms for adjusting insulin doses are summarized in Tables 7-12 and 7-13. These rules are based on *retrospective* data—that is, insulin doses are changed in response to indices of control occurring in the recent past. Effective use of this approach requires a relatively consistent diet and exercise pattern. Many patients can be taught to adjust their insulin doses *prospectively*—that is, the amount of insulin taken before a meal is a combination of a basic dose, an adjustment based on the blood glucose level at that time, and an adjustment based on the anticipated amount of food to be eaten or exercise to be performed. The prospective approach, which usually yields better control, is discussed later.

Rules for adjusting insulin doses based on results obtained during the previous 3 days

Table 7–9. Period During Which Glucose Is Controlled by Various Components of the Insulin Regimen and Timing of Tests Reflecting That Activity

Insulin	Time Injected	Period of Activity	Test Reflecting Insulin Action
Regular Lispro	Before a meal	Between that meal and either the subsequent one or the bedtime snack (if insulin taken before supper)	Both following meal before which insulin is injected and before subsequent meal or bedtime snack (if insulin taken before supper)
NPH	Before breakfast	Between lunch and supper	Before supper
NPH	Before supper or before bed	Overnight	Before breakfast
Ultralente	Before breakfast *or* before supper *or* half of dose at each time	Mostly overnight because regular insulin overrides its effect during the day	Before breakfast

Table 7–10. Various Insulin Regimens for Achieving Strict Diabetic Control

Regimen	Before breakfast	Before lunch	Before supper	Before bed
		Time Administered[a]		
A	NPH/regular (lispro)	—	NPH/regular (lispro)	—
B	NPH/regular (lispro)	—	Regular (lispro)	NPH
C	Regular (lispro)	Regular (lispro)	NPH/regular (lispro)	—
D	Regular (lispro)	Regular (lispro)	Regular (lispro)	NPH
E[b]	Ultralente/regular (lispro)	Regular (lispro)	Regular (lispro)	—
F	Insulin pump [small amount of regular (lispro) insulin infused throughout 24-hour period (*basal*) with *boluses* of regular (lispro) insulin given before each meal]			

[a]Regular insulin usually injected 30 minutes before designated meal.
[b]Ultralente may also be given either entirely before supper or half of dose before breakfast and half before supper.

are listed in Table 7–12. Many patients, however, fail to show consistent enough changes over a 3-day period to indicate clearly a need to change the insulin dose. However, the trend over a longer time frame demonstrates a need for an adjustment. Therefore, rules for using the data gathered in a week's period are listed in Table 7–13.

An example of using these rules is provided in Table 7–14. This lean type 2 patient is taking NPH and regular insulin 30 minutes before breakfast and before supper (regimen A in Table 7–10) and is using Chemstrips read visually four times a day for home blood glucose monitoring. Her desired level of control is preprandial values ≤120 mg/dl (num-

ber 3 in Table 7–11). During the week of January 21, she made two changes in her insulin dose. She raised the before supper NPH insulin by 2 U on Thursday because her fasting blood glucose concentrations exceeded the target level of 120 mg/dl for three straight mornings. She also increased her morning regular insulin by 2 U at the beginning of the following week because the number of values before lunch that exceeded the target level (four) minus the number below 70 mg/dl (zero) and the number of unexplained hypoglycemic reactions (zero) was 4. The pattern of results before supper was such that neither the 3- nor 7-day rule dictated a change in the morning injection of NPH. The reaction before supper on Wednesday is disregarded, because there was an explanation for it. The reaction between supper and bed on Saturday, for which there was no apparent explanation, is counted as a low value. Therefore, neither the 3- nor 7-day rule would apply here. Although four values were greater than the target level before bedtime, the hypoglycemic reaction has to be subtracted. In addition, the 240 mg/dl value before bed on Wednesday should not be counted because it followed a hypoglycemic reaction and probably represented rebound hyperglycemia. Consequently, the dose of regular insulin before supper is not

Table 7–11. Degrees of Diabetic Control in Order of Increasing Strictness

1. Before meal and bedtime snack glucose concentrations of ≤180 mg/dl
2. Before meal and bedtime snack glucose concentrations of ≤150 mg/dl
3. Before meal and bedtime snack glucose concentrations of ≤120 mg/dl
4. One- to 2-hour postmeal glucose concentrations of ≤200 mg/dl[a]
5. One- to 2-hour postmeal glucose concentrations of ≤150 mg/dl

[a]Concentration used for visual reading of Chemstrip bG would be 210 mg/dl, a value half-way between the colors designating 180 mg/dl and 240 mg/dl.

Table 7–12. Algorithm for Adjusting Insulin Doses Based on Retrospective Data (3-Day Rule)

1. Select one of the first three levels of diabetic control desired.[a]
2. If blood glucose is greater than the upper target level at the same time of day for 3 days in a row, increase the dose of the appropriate insulin by 1 to 2 U[b] as follows:
   (a) If before breakfast test result too high:

Regimen	Insulin
A	NPH—before supper
B	NPH—before bed
C	NPH—before supper
D	NPH—before bed
E	Ultralente
F	Increase basal rate by either 0.1 U/h or 2 U/24-h period

   (b) If before lunch test result too high:

Regimen	Insulin
A through E	Regular (lispro)—before breakfast
F	Bolus—before breakfast

   (c) If before supper test result too high:

Regimen	Insulin
A and B	NPH—before breakfast
C through E	Regular (lispro)—before lunch
F	Bolus—before lunch

   (d) If before bedtime snack[c] test result too high:

Regimen	Insulin
A through E	Regular (lispro)—before supper
F	Bolus—before supper

3. If blood glucose level is <70 mg/dl[d] at the same time of day for 3 days in a row, decrease the dose of the appropriate insulin as shown in 2 above.
4. A mild hypoglycemic reaction (which is easily treated) and for which there is no apparent reason (e.g., delay of meal, less food, increased exercise, error in insulin dose) counts as a <70 mg/dl blood glucose value before the next meal even though the glucose value measured at that time will probably be high. For example:

Time of Reaction	Meal to Which <70 mg/dl Should Be Assigned
Between breakfast and lunch	Lunch
Between lunch and supper	Supper
Between supper and bedtime	Bed
Between going to bed and arising	Breakfast

5. If a severe hypoglycemic reaction for which there is no apparent reason occurs, the appropriate insulin dose should be decreased as shown in 2 above the very *next* time it is to be given.
6. Once the desired level of diabetic control is consistently achieved, consider advancing to the next level of increasing strictness (see Table 7-11).
7. For the 4th and 5th levels, glucose concentrations between 1 and 2 hours after meals must be measured. If these values exceed the upper target level for 3 days in a row (assuming consistency in the size of the meals), increase the dose of the regular or lispro insulin taken before that meal.

[a]See *Goals of Therapy* in text for which level to select initially.

[b]Three to 4 U may be more appropriate in obese patients (>120% of desirable body weight; see the Appendix at the end of this chapter for estimation of desirable body weight).

[c]Bedtime snack not necessary for regimen F; however, a test at this time still needs to be done to evaluate response to before supper bolus dose.

[d]For patients using Chemstrips, color nearer the midrange between 40 and 80 mg/dl is considered <70 mg/dl but color nearer the 80 mg/dl value is not.

Table 7–13. Algorithms for Adjusting Insulin Doses Based on Retrospective Data (7-Day Rule)

1. Use at end of each week *only* if no change had been made using 3-day rule in that particular component of insulin dose.
2. If number of test results greater than desired value *minus* number of test results <70 mg/dl[a] plus unexplained episodes of hypoglycemia is four or greater, increase appropriate component of insulin dose by 1 or 2 U.[b]
3. If number of test results <70 mg/dl[a] plus unexplained episodes of hypoglycemia *minus* number of test results above desired level is 4 or greater, decrease appropriate component of insulin dose by 1 or 2 U.[b]
4. If criteria of number 2 or number 3 not met, no change of insulin dose.

[a]Value may be higher for older patients, those who experience hypoglycemia without symptoms, and those with autonomic neuropathy.

[b]Three to four units may be more appropriate for obese patients.

changed at the beginning of the next week. The results during the week of January 28 led to a 2-U increase in the morning regular insulin dose on Sunday (3-day rule) and a decrease of the morning NPH dose on Monday of the following week (7-day rule).

Many patients, of course, are unwilling to perform SMBG consistently four times a day. Because the minimum information concerning diabetic control should ideally reflect the time between breakfast and lunch, lunch and supper, supper and bed, and overnight (i.e., four times per 24-hour period), a urine test for glucose may be substituted for the blood glucose value before a meal or at bedtime. First-voided urine should be tested because it reflects a large part of the period for which we are interested in ascertaining the degree of control. Any positive result is considered unsatisfactory (i.e., the target level has been exceeded), whereas a negative test result must be considered satisfactory (i.e., the target level has been met). Urine tests for glucose are really not suitable for monitoring patients who are striving for tight control because positive results often appear only when blood glucose values exceed the least

strict target level (number 1 in Table 7–11). However, some information is better than none, and many patients can usually be persuaded to provide the physician with a combination of blood and urine values.

Table 7–15 depicts adjustments of insulin doses based on the results of both kinds of tests. The patient is a 35-year-old salesman who has had type 1 diabetes for 13 years. His desired level of control is also preprandial values ≤120 mg/dl (number 3 in Table 7–11). An insulin regimen consisting of Ultralente insulin in the morning with three injections of regular insulin before each meal (regimen E in Table 7–10) was suitable for him because of his erratic eating patterns related to his job. He also uses Chemstrips read visually for SMBG. When he is with clients, he feels that he cannot perform SMBG before meals but can often test a urine sample before eating. He is more consistent with SMBG at home in the mornings, evenings, and weekends. The results of his before breakfast test dictated an increase in the dose of Ultralente insulin on Friday of the week of February 1 by a slight modification of the 3-day rule. If there is a 1-day hiatus in the test results (which occurred on Wednesday), the patient simply ignores it and considers whether the values surrounding it meet the 3-day criteria. If a 2-day hiatus occurs, the 3-day rule is not applicable (see before dinner results during the same week). Therefore, on Friday morning, after the value of 150 mg/dl was obtained, the dose of Ultralente was raised by 2 U. The results of the before lunch tests did not show any need for a change in the dose of morning regular insulin by the 3-day rule.

I also use a modification of the 7-day rule when patients test intermittently. The results of 2 weeks are pooled with the currently applied criteria that changes should be made if a majority of the results dictate it (at least eight values should be available). By these criteria, the before breakfast regular insulin dose still remains unchanged, because only three of the nine exceeded the target level. However, the modified 7-day rule dictated an

Text continued on page 228

Table 7–14. SMBG Results and Insulin Dose Adjustments in a Patient Testing Four Times a Day

Week beginning Monday 1/21 (Date)

Day of Week	Insulin Injections				Monitoring								
	Break	Lunch	Supper	Bed	Breakfast		Lunch		Supper		Bedtime	Overnight	Remarks
					Before	After	Before	After	Before	After			
Mon	34N 10R		10N 8R		120		120		100		120		
Tues	34N 10R		10N 8R		180		240		150		180		
Wed	34N 10R		10N 8R		150		180		—		240		Dinner delayed, reaction at 6 PM
Thurs	34N 10R		12N[a] 8R		150		120		120		100		Dose change— 3-day rule
Fri	34N 10R		12N 8R		120		180		150		150		
Sat	34N 10R		12N 8R		100		120		180		—		Reaction 4 hours after eating supper, ? reason
Sun	34N 10R		12N 8R		120		150		100		150		

Week beginning Monday <u>1/28</u> (Date)

Day of Week	Insulin Injections				Monitoring								Remarks
	Break	Lunch	Supper	Bed	Breakfast		Lunch		Supper		Bedtime	Overnight	
					Before	After	Before	After	Before	After			
Mon	34N <u>12R</u>		12N 8R		80		150		80		80		Dose change— 7-day rule
Tues	34N 12R		12N 8R		100		120		60		100		
Wed	34N 12R		12N 8R		120		120		40		150		Symptoms of reaction just before supper obtained, ? reason
Thurs	34N 12R		12N 8R		120		150		120		120		
Fri	34N 12R		12N 8R		150		180		60		100		
Sat	34N 12R		12N 8R		100		150		100		120		
Sun	34N <u>14R</u>		12N 8R		80		100		60		100		Dose change— 3-day rule[b]

R, regular insulin; N, NPH insulin.

[a]Changed insulin dose is underlined the first time that it is recorded.

[b]Dose of NPH insulin also decreased to 32 U on Monday, 2/4.

Table 7–15. Insulin Dose Adjustments in a Patient Using Intermittent SMBG and Urine Tests for Glucose

Week beginning Monday 2/1 (Date)

Day of Week	Insulin Injections				Monitoring								
	Break	Lunch	Supper	Bed	Breakfast		Lunch		Supper		Bedtime	Overnight	Remarks
					Before	After	Before	After	Before	After			
Mon	20U 8R	4R	10R		120		—		100		150		
Tues	20U 8R	4R	10R		150		0.5%		—		100		
Wed	20U 8R	4R	10R		—		Neg		0.1%		80		
Thurs	20U 8R	4R	10R		180		120		1%		180		
Fri	22U[a] 8R	4R	10R		150		—		—		150		Dose change—3-day rule
Sat	22U 8R	4R	10R		120		Neg		—		320		Severe reaction in late afternoon several hours after exercise
Sun	22U 8R	4R	10R		100		150		150		180		

Week beginning Monday 2/8 (Date)

Day of Week	Insulin Injections				Monitoring								Remarks
					Breakfast		Lunch		Supper		Bedtime	Overnight	
	Break	Lunch	Supper	Bed	Before	After	Before	After	Before	After			
Mon	22U 8R	4R	<u>12R</u>		120		—		120		120		Dose change—3-day rule
Tues	22R 8R	4R	12R		80		Neg		0.1%		—		
Wed	22U 8R	4R	12R		—		—		Neg		100		Reaction at 6 AM
Thurs	22U 8R	4R	12R		100		120		0.5%		120		
Fri	22u 8R	4R	12R		150		—		—		150		Reaction due to delayed supper
Sat	22U 8R	4R	12R		120		180		—		100		
Sun	22U 8R	4R	12R		100		120		150		1%		Modified 7-day rule[b]

R, regular insulin; U, Ultralente insulin.

[a] Changed insulin dose underlined the first time that it is recorded.

[b] Dose of regular insulin before lunch increased to 5 U on Monday, 2/15 (see text for discussion).

increase in the amount of regular insulin taken before lunch, because the number of unsatisfactory test results before supper constituted the majority (six of nine) of those available. (Note that there were explanations for the two reactions before supper, and consequently they were not considered in the analysis.) Therefore, the amount of regular insulin was increased by 1 U before lunch on Monday of the following week. The results of the bedtime tests also indicated a need for more regular insulin before supper by the 3-day rule. Note, however, that the change was not made until Monday, February 8. The high value on Saturday was not counted because it represented the rebound of blood glucose after the severe hypoglycemic reaction. Therefore, it should be ignored in the analysis, and a modified 3-day rule applied.

Certain caveats are to be kept in mind with each of the regimens (listed in Table 7-10) used to achieve tight control. In regimens A and B, patients have the least flexibility with regard to the timing and content of meals. Hypoglycemia is most likely to occur with these two regimens if meals are delayed. In regimens A and C, the intermediate-acting insulin given before supper may have peak activity in the middle of the night rather than toward morning in some patients. In this situation, increasing the dose may lead to hypoglycemic reactions during the middle of the night before the target level of glucose before breakfast is achieved. If this should occur, switching the intermediate-acting insulin to before bedtime (regimen B) should solve the problem. In regimens C and D, if the period between lunch and supper is too prolonged (usually >5 to 7 hours), the blood glucose level before supper may be too high because the effect of the regular insulin given before lunch may have worn off. This is even more likely to occur with lispro insulin. In regimen E, because Ultralente insulin starts to work 6 to 8 hours after injection, hypoglycemia may occur between lunch and supper, especially if supper is eaten late (see Table 7-15, second Friday).

This is usually not a problem when the dose of long-acting insulin is low (approximately 10 U) but may become a problem at higher doses. In regimen F, because no intermediate- or long-acting insulin is taken by patients using insulin pumps (which use only regular or lispro insulin), interruption of these subcutaneous infusions (which is usually due to difficulties with the catheter) can lead to hyperglycemia and ketosis (in type 1 patients) relatively quickly (within 6 to 8 hours). Finally, with any regimen that does not routinely measure urinary ketone bodies, this test must be used whenever type 1 patients are sick. Many patients who rely exclusively on SMBG prefer not to test their urine at all. However, because diabetic ketoacidosis can often occur with blood glucose levels <300 mg/dl,[115] physicians must insist on urine testing for ketone bodies under these circumstances.

A delayed response to regular insulin occurs in a significant minority of patients. This situation should be suspected when premeal glucose values are low while 1- to 2-hour postprandial levels after the preceding meal are high. A delayed response can be proved by injecting regular insulin alone (with no intermediate- or long-acting insulin) at a time when glucose values are relatively high, by not eating, and by measuring glucose concentrations every hour or two until a definite response is seen. If a patient has a delayed response, short-acting insulin must be taken routinely 1 or more hours before each meal. There is not yet enough experience to determine if a delayed response can occur with lispro insulin. If it does occur with regular insulin, switching to lispro insulin should certainly be tried.

With appropriate encouragement from their physicians, many patients carry out the degree of monitoring described earlier. To minimize the time spent on the phone, every effort should be made to teach these algorithms to patients—to the degree to which they are capable of mastering them. Some may have no difficulty; others may be able to use the 3-day rule only; still others can handle adjusting only one or two components of the insulin regimen rather than all of them. Once patients are able to follow some or all of these algorithms, I have them mail or fax (e-mailing may also be a possibility for some patients and physicians) their results to me at appropriate intervals (every week or two initially and every month or two eventually) so that I can evaluate them and contact the patient at convenient times in my schedule. If patients monitor less often, I have them keep a record and send it to me every month. In that manner, I am able to adjust their insulin doses on the basis of an aggregate of data collected during a shorter period than the amount of time between office visits (every 3 to 6 months).

Two extensions of the approach just described often lead to better control. The first is to attempt to achieve 1- to 2-hour postprandial values <200 mg/dl (level 4, Table 7-11) and, if that is successful, <150 mg/dl (level 5, Table 7-11). One simply uses these postprandial values in the algorithms instead of the preprandial ones. The glucose concentration considered too low postprandially should be 100 mg/dl rather than the preprandial concentration of 70 mg/dl.

The second extension, as already mentioned, is to use prospective data to decide the amount of each injection of regular or lispro insulin. The dose of that part of the insulin regimen that is reflected in the fasting test is still determined by the retrospective method described earlier. However, the amount of regular or lispro insulin injected before each meal is composed of three components. The first one is the *basic* dose, which is what a patient takes routinely and is adjusted according to the algorithms already described. The second one is the *compensatory* dose, which is based on the prevailing blood glucose value just before the insulin injection. The amounts of the compensatory dose vary from patient to patient. Two decisions have to be made: what range of blood glucose values should be included for each

increase in the compensatory dose, and how much insulin should be assigned to each range. The final answers are always arrived at empirically. A suggested initial approach is shown in Table 7-16. For patients using visual readings, color development read as definitely <80 mg/dl should lead to decreasing the preprandial dose of regular or lispro insulin. The values 150, 200, 250, and 300 mg/dl in Table 7-16 correspond to color development on a Chemstrip read visually half-way between 120 and 180, half-way between 180 and 240, 240, and half-way between 240 and 400 mg/dl, respectively. Thus, visually read values nearer to 180 than to 150 mg/dl would lead to one extra U of regular or lispro insulin, values nearer to 240 than 180 mg/dl to 2 additional U, values nearer to 240 than to 400 mg/dl to 3 extra U, and values nearer to 400 than to 240 mg/dl to 4 additional U. After experience is gained by each patient, adjustments of both the ranges of blood glucose values and additional amounts of regular or lispro insulin for each range are frequently made. The patients monitored in our program have compensatory doses ranging from −2 to +10 U for various ranges of blood glucose.

Patients using a split/mixed regimen (regimens A or B in Table 7-10) can also use the SMBG values obtained before breakfast and supper to take compensatory doses of regular or lispro insulin before these two meals. They should not use a compensatory dose of regular or lispro insulin before lunch because both that dose and the morning NPH insulin

Table 7–16. Suggested Initial Compensatory Doses of Preprandial Regular or Lispro Insulin

Blood Glucose (mg/dl)	Insulin (U)
<70	−1
70–150	0
151–200	+1
201–250	+2
251–300	+3
>300	+4

have their peak effects at the same time and increase the chances of hypoglycemia before supper. Furthermore, the SMBG value before supper would not reflect solely the morning NPH insulin, which would invalidate using it to help adjust the dose of the morning intermediate-acting insulin.

The efficacy of instructing patients to adjust their preprandial regular insulin doses depending on the concurrent blood glucose value was clearly illustrated in an Austrian study.[116, 117] Eighty patients taking one or two injections a day, many of whom were monitored in diabetes centers and performed SMBG but were not in good control, were instructed to take morning and evening Ultralente insulin and preprandial regular insulin. The preprandial regular insulin dose was adjusted by patients in accordance with their glucose value. During the subsequent 2 years, 79 patients remained in the study and 50% attained normal Hgb A_{1c} values. The mean glucose levels of all subjects were approximately 130 mg/dl, and the mean Hgb A_{1c} values were at the upper limit of normal. Thus, to afford our patients the best chance to avoid the dire consequences of retinopathy, nephropathy, and neuropathy (see Chapter 8), we must teach and allow them to adjust their own insulin doses to the limits of their ability.

The third part of the insulin dose is the *anticipatory* one. Some patients attempt to judge the amount of food (it should be the carbohydrate content) in the upcoming meal and adjust their insulin accordingly. As one might expect, this seldom leads to a decrease in insulin because most patients attempt to compensate for extra food. The anticipatory component is not used by most of our patients, but those who do usually underestimate and end up too high before the next meal.

An example of a patient using this prospective method of adjusting insulin doses is shown in Table 7–17. She is a 45-year-old type 1 diabetic patient (112% desirable body weight) who uses a meter to perform SMBG.

She is using a four-injection regimen because her NPH insulin previously taken before supper caused her to wake up with hypoglycemic symptoms several times a week between 3 and 5 AM. Moving her NPH insulin to bedtime has solved that problem. Her target level is preprandial values of ≤120 mg/dl (level 3 in Table 7–11). On Monday, February 15, her basic regular insulin doses before breakfast, lunch, and supper were 6, 4, and 8 U, respectively. She usually eats at 8 AM, 12:30 PM, and 5:30 PM, with a bedtime snack at 10 PM just after taking her NPH insulin. Her compensatory doses have, in general, controlled her diabetes well. Note that on Tuesday and Saturday of the first week, the before supper values were high because of the delayed supper. As mentioned earlier hyperglycemia occurs under these circumstances because the action of the preprandial dose of insulin before lunch has waned and there is no effective intermediate- or long-acting insulin at this time. However, the compensatory dose before supper limits the hyperglycemia so that the patient is under reasonable control by bedtime. On Sunday of the week of February 15, the basic dose before breakfast was decreased by 1 U because of the 3-day rule. The before lunch value of 258 mg/dl on Friday was disregarded because the hypoglycemic reaction that occurred at 11 AM on that day takes precedence in using the algorithm. However, it was important to obtain that value to judge the before lunch dose of insulin. Application of the 7-day rule for the preprandial supper values might suggest a need to increase the before lunch basic dose. However, remember that a delayed supper was responsible for two of these high values, and therefore they should not be considered. During the week of February 22, no changes were made in the insulin dose based on the 3-day rule. However, using the 7-day rule, the evening NPH was increased to 12 U on Monday of the following week. Likewise, the before lunch basic dose of regular insulin dose was also increased by 1 U, using the 7-day rule on the glucose values before supper. Note that during the 2-week period described in Table 17–17, the patient took anticipatory doses of insulin before supper on three occasions, Thursday and Sunday of the first week and Tuesday of the second week. Each time, she underestimated and ended up with elevated glucose values before bed. Although this patient chose not to react to these high bedtime levels, a compensatory dose of NPH insulin (if it is taken before bed) might be suggested to sophisticated patients. Alternatively, the patient might take a compensatory dose of regular insulin. I prefer to try the former first (if possible), because in my experience, the latter approach is more likely to produce hypoglycemia overnight.

The limiting factor for monitoring patients who take insulin is the amount of information that they will furnish. Physicians should continually encourage patients to increase the frequency of their SMBG up to four times per day, to start it if they are relying only on urine testing, or to embark on urine testing if they are not monitoring themselves at all. It frequently takes me months to several years to persuade patients to monitor themselves appropriately. Continued elevated glycated hemoglobin values motivate some patients to undergo the discipline of SMBG. Once they start, a physician's approach obviously has to be tailored to the frequency of its use. The guidelines described earlier are just that—guidelines. Decisions about when and how to change insulin doses can be flexible within the general principles discussed earlier.

FASTING HYPERGLYCEMIA

In my experience, the most difficult test result to bring under control in insulin-requiring patients is the fasting glucose concentration. Assuming that no untoward event has occurred (e.g., large bedtime snack), three reasons for fasting hyperglycemia are possible: waning of insulin action, the dawn phe-

nomenon, and the Somogyi phenomenon. The first situation is due to an inadequate dose of that insulin preparation that is supposed to cover the overnight period.[118] The dawn phenomenon is caused by insensitivity to insulin between approximately 4 AM and 8 AM due to the sleep-induced surge of growth hormone secretion.[119, 120] This causes increased lipolysis (i.e., increased free fatty acid release by adipose tissue) during the next several hours, which subsequently modestly raises glucose concentrations in the period before breakfast,[121] probably via enhanced gluconeogenesis. The Somogyi phenomenon is hyperglycemia caused by the release of counterregulatory hormones after unrecognized hypoglycemia.[120] A great deal of research has led to the following conclusions. First, unrecognized nocturnal hypoglycemia in insulin-requiring diabetic patients is common, especially in type 1 diabetes.[118, 122-124] Second, this hypoglycemia rarely causes rebound fasting hyperglycemia.[122-124] Third, although the dawn phenomenon can occur in some patients, the frequency and magnitude are variable.[123] The clinical lessons from these studies are that the Somogyi phenomenon is an unusual cause of fasting hyperglycemia. Waning of insulin action is the most likely reason for fasting hyperglycemia.[118, 120] Clinically, it is not important to distinguish between insulin waning and the dawn phenomenon because both situations require provision of more insulin for the overnight period. If relatively large increases seem necessary, it is wise to have the patient perform SMBG at 2 AM to 3 AM to ascertain that hypoglycemia is not occurring at this time. If this is the case, switching the intermediate-acting insulin to bedtime (as mentioned earlier) helps reduce the fasting hyperglycemia and avoids the dangers of nocturnal hypoglycemia. If the intermediate-acting insulin is already being given at bedtime, there are three options. The bedtime snack can be increased as the insulin dose is raised. This degree of fasting hyperglycemia has to be accepted because raising the eve-

Table 7–17. Insulin Dose Adjustments Using a Prospective Method

Week beginning Monday 2/15 (Date)

Day of Week	Insulin Injections				Monitoring								
					Breakfast		Lunch		Supper				
	Break	Lunch	Supper	Bed	Before	After	Before	After	Before	After	Bedtime	Overnight	Remarks
Mon	7R (6 + 1)	4R	8R	10N	152		107		93		117		
Tues	6R	4R	13R (8 + 5)	10N	87		83		268		179		Supper 2 hours later than usual
Wed	7R (6 + 1)	3R (4 − 1)	9R (8 + 1)	10N	166		65		158		108		
Thurs	6R	3R (4 − 1)	11R (8 + 0 + 3)	10N	111		62		112		221		Went out for supper
Fri	6R	7R (4 + 3)	9R (8 + 1)	10N	108		258		161		115		Reaction at 11 AM, ? reason
Sat	7R (6 + 1)	3R (4 − 1)	9R (8 + 1)	10N	158		58		172		109		Supper 1 hour later than usual
Sun	5R[a] (6 + 1)	4R (4 − 1)	11R (8 + 0 + 3)	10N	115		103		97		222		Dose change—3-day rule; went out for supper

Week beginning Monday 2/22 (Date)

Day of Week	Insulin Injections				Monitoring								
	Break	Lunch	Supper	Bed	Breakfast		Lunch		Supper		Bedtime	Overnight	Remarks
					Before	After	Before	After	Before	After			
Mon	6R (5 + 1)	5R (4 + 1)	9R (8 + 1)	10N	165		153		158		118		
Tues	5R	4R	11R (8 + 0 + 3)	10N	118		116		110		268		Went out for supper
Wed	8R (5 + 3)	3R (4 − 1)	9R (8 + 1)	10N	210		66		179		93		
Thurs	5R	4R	11R (8 + 3)	10N	92		103		226		81		
Fri	6R (5 + 1)	4R	8R	10N	167		99		118		125		
Sat	5R	5R (4 + 1)	11R (8 + 3)	10N	116		157		212		110		
Sun	6R (5 + 1)	4R	9R (8 + 1)	10N	164		118		163		144		Dose change—7-day rule[b]

R, regular insulin
N, NPH insulin

<70 mg/dl − 1 U	201–250 mg/dl + 3 U
70–150 mg/dl − 0	251–300 mg/dl + 5 U
151–200 mg/dl + 1 U	>300 mg/dl + 7 U

[a]Changed basic insulin dose is underlined the first time that it is recorded.
[b]Dose of bedtime NPH insulin increased to 12 U and before lunch regular insulin increased to 5 U on Monday, 3/1 (see text for discussion).

ning insulin dose would subject a patient to the risk of more nocturnal hypoglycemia. The final option is to place patients on an insulin infusion pump (at least overnight) to ensure more even insulin absorption. If necessary, different infusion rates can be used for the early and late overnight periods.

MONITORING PATIENTS WHO DO NOT TAKE INSULIN

Figure 7-11 depicts the fasting blood glucose value obtained on two occasions within 1 week in 360 patients with impaired glucose tolerance and diabetes mellitus before treatment was begun. Therefore, as discussed in Chapter 5, when sulfonylurea agent or metformin therapy is being adjusted, FPG concentrations approximately 2 weeks after the dose change are sufficient to judge its effectiveness. Alternatively, if a patient is reliable and provides accurate fasting SMBG values, these can be used to adjust the doses (I prefer to have values on these 3 consecutive

days). Once the fasting target is reached (i.e., plasma or whole blood glucose concentrations of 140 mg/dl or 120 mg/dl, respectively), I use glycated hemoglobin levels measured every 2 to 3 months to evaluate diabetic control.

Although SMBG is not necessary for short-term adjustments in therapy for type 2 patients not taking insulin, it may be helpful for educational and motivational purposes. (However, as mentioned earlier, glycated hemoglobin levels were not appreciably changed.[32-34]) The immediate feedback furnished by SMBG under different dietary circumstances can teach patients better than any lectures or reading material about which foods to avoid, which ones have the least effect on the blood glucose values, and, the usual problem with these individuals, how meal size affects glucose levels. Therefore, performing SMBG 1 to 2 hours postprandially is preferable (in my view) to preprandial monitoring. Postprandial values are more instructive for meal-related effects. Furthermore, because glucose concentrations after

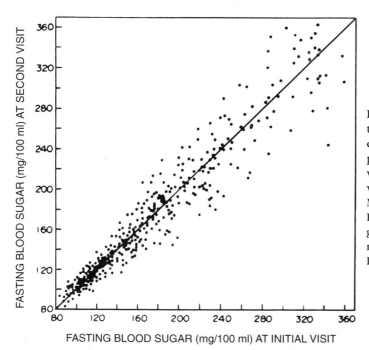

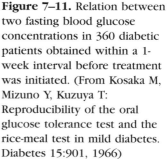

Figure 7–11. Relation between two fasting blood glucose concentrations in 360 diabetic patients obtained within a 1-week interval before treatment was initiated. (From Kosaka M, Mizuno Y, Kuzuya T: Reproducibility of the oral glucose tolerance test and the rice-meal test in mild diabetes. Diabetes 15:901, 1966)

meals (especially after breakfast because insulin is less effective in the morning than it is at other times of the day[125]) are much higher than preprandial ones, patients may be more motivated to accept the life style changes (diet and exercise) necessary for the successful treatment of type 2 diabetes. Therefore, although I do not insist on it. I do suggest SMBG to type 2 patients who seem capable of performing it. A typical schedule might involve alternating meals and measuring once or twice a day with a goal of ≤180 mg/dl if the meter is calibrated to plasma values or ≤160 mg/dl if calibrated to whole blood values. Because I do not use these results to adjust the doses of oral antidiabetic medication, patients usually choose a pattern with which they are comfortable.

If type 2 patients not on insulin are incapable of SMBG or prefer not to carry it out, I ask them to test their urine. Despite the limitations of this method of assessing diabetic control, discussed previously, it does furnish some information. Urine tests performed before meals and bedtime are more likely to yield negative results than those carried out postprandially. Therefore, patients should initially test their first-voided urines once or twice a day preprandially. The fasting test is most likely to have negative results because the glucose concentration falls overnight and is the lowest before breakfast. When the results of preprandial tests become consistently negative, urine samples passed 1 to 2 hours after meals should be tested routinely because the results are most likely to be positive postprandially. If postprandial urine results are consistently negative, testing can be limited to 1 to 2 days per week. As with SMBG, the hope is that positive urine test results will serve to motivate and educate patients.

GOALS OF THERAPY

Suggested levels of diabetic control for insulin-requiring patients who perform SMBG are listed in Table 7–11. Which level of control

to select, at least initially, is influenced by (1) the age of the patient, (2) the length of time type 1 patients have had diabetes, (3) the patient's awareness of hypoglycemic symptoms, and (4) the clinical evidence for autonomic neuropathy. Understanding the hormonal response to hypoglycemia in nondiabetic and diabetic subjects is important for arriving at this decision. In normal and type 2 diabetic individuals, four hormones are secreted in response to hypoglycemia. Glucagon and the catecholamines epinephrine and norepinephrine are released rapidly and have an immediate effect in restoring blood glucose values toward normal. The secretion of growth hormone and cortisol is delayed, and their antiinsulin effect does not occur immediately but is longlasting. Selective blockade of each of these hormones during hypoglycemia[126] revealed that (1) as long as glucagon was secreted, glucose levels were restored normally; (2) if glucagon was absent but the catecholamines were present, restoration was delayed but eventually occurred; (3) growth hormone and cortisol secretion were unnecessary for return of glucose levels to normal (at least in the short term); and (4) if both glucagon and catecholamines were absent, glucose concentrations remained at the nadir levels. This latter observation becomes extremely important in type 1 patients because within a year or two of diagnosis, the glucagon response to hypoglycemia is impaired[127] even though glucagon is hypersecreted by these patients under other circumstances. By 4 years after the diagnosis, the glucagon response is minimal.[127] Furthermore, the catecholamine response to hypoglycemia also is markedly blunted after 5 years of type 1 diabetes, even in the absence of clinical autonomic neuropathy.[128] Thus, in type 1 patients who have had their diabetes for >5 years, there is a good chance that secretion of both of the critical hormones necessary to respond to hypoglycemia is either absent or markedly impaired. Secretion of the counterregulatory hormones remains either intact or nearly so in type 2 diabetic patients.

Therefore, for those performing SMBG on a regular basis, level 1 of diabetic control in Table 7–11 is initially selected for the following: (1) type 1 patients with diabetes of >5 years' duration, (2) any patient who experiences hypoglycemia without concomitant autonomic signs and symptoms (discussed later), (3) any patient with clinical evidence of autonomic neuropathy, and (4) any patient taking insulin after age 65 years. If preprandial values ≤180 mg/dl can be achieved without inordinate difficulties with hypoglycemia, the target range is carefully advanced to level 2 in Table 7–11 for all of these groups except patients older than 80 years. Because of their more limited life expectancy and the increased dangers of hypoglycemia due to their often associated conditions of coronary artery and cerebrovascular disease, level 1 is maintained in these patients. (Younger "frail elderly" patients are also maintained at level 1.) Patients between 65 and 80 years of age have a longer life expectancy, and therefore I attempt to advance them carefully to level 2. This target level, preprandial values ≤150 mg/dl, is the initial goal for all other groups of patients. Patients with autonomic neuropathy, and especially those who experience hypoglycemia without premonitory signs and symptoms, as well as those between 65 and 80 years, are kept at level 2. All other patients who are able to achieve level 2 in Table 7–11 without too much difficulty with hypoglycemia are carefully advanced to level 3 in Table 7–11, preprandial values ≤120 mg/dl. Levels 4 and 5 in Table 7–11 require measuring blood glucose concentrations postprandially and are attempted in only a small minority of patients (unfortunately).

Important factors in achieving tight control in insulin-requiring patients are relatively constant patterns of eating (unless the patient has mastered the appropriate amount of anticipatory insulin to use) and exercise and a stable emotional state. In controlling diabetes with insulin, a balance must always be achieved between attempting to return glucose concentrations to near euglycemia and the risk of hypoglycemia. Under the present relatively crude system of replacing or supplementing endogenous insulin with exogenous insulin, some episodes of hypoglycemia are almost unavoidable if glucose concentrations are to approach normal most of the time. Because tight control has such important benefits (see Chapter 2), I ask my patients to tolerate occasional (two to three times per week) mild episodes of hypoglycemia. However, if these episodes occur more frequently, are very distressing to the patient, are not quickly aborted, and, most importantly, are not easily recognized, I reduce the insulin dose and settle for the level of control in Table 7–11 above the one at which these difficulties occurred.

These same principles apply to controlling diabetes in patients who furnish the physician with more sporadic data (e.g., glucose concentrations several times a day two to four times per week). If one can ascertain that these represent relatively consistent values, insulin doses can be adjusted appropriately. However, if these are not truly representative glucose levels (e.g., measured mostly at times of perceived hyperglycemia), hypoglycemia may become a problem and one has to decrease insulin doses and settle for looser control.

In patients who perform only urine testing, the goal of therapy is no glucosuria in all first-voided urine samples. Initially, preprandial urines are tested, and once they routinely become negative for glucose, postprandial urine should be used. In patients with an increased T_m for glucose, even negative urine test results do not ensure very good control. Conversely, in the rare (nonpregnant) patient with a lowered T_m for glucose, negative urine test results may be associated with unacceptable hypoglycemia.

The goal of therapy in regard to glycated hemoglobin levels obtained every 2 to 3 months can be simply stated: to achieve normal values. However, the closer patients are to normal, the more hypoglycemia insulin-requiring patients experience, especially severe hypoglycemia.[129, 130] Therefore, a balance must be struck between the two. Because glycated hemoglobin values do not guide day-to-day therapeutic decisions, they are used to help decide whether or not more determined efforts need to be made to optimize control. As discussed earlier, the development and progression of diabetic retinopathy and nephropathy markedly increase at glycated hemoglobin levels >2% above the upper limit of normal for the assay used. Although a target level below this value would be desirable in most patients, higher values might be more appropriate in some (e.g., those who are frail elderly or who have significant coronary artery or cerebrovascular disease, advanced microvascular complications, or hypoglycemia unawareness). Some patients are doing the best they can, and improvement is not possible. Many patients, however, are able to improve their control (or actually their compliance with the prescribed therapeutic regimen yielding better control), and glycated hemoglobin levels serve as the reminder.

"HONEYMOON PHASE" OF TYPE 1 DIABETES

Shortly after the onset of type 1 diabetes, a *temporary* remission occurs in approximately 20% of patients (even in those who were in profound DKA). This is termed the *honeymoon phase*. The clinical manifestation of this remission varies from a moderate reduction in insulin requirement to complete normalization of glucose tolerance without therapy. Secretion of endogenous insulin returns, at least in part, during the remission period.[131] The duration of the honeymoon phase usually is short, lasting from a few weeks to several months, although an occasional patient may remain in remission for many years. Although evidence suggests that

the earlier and more intensive the initial treatment, the more likely and longer the remission will be, diabetes always returns. Thus, it is important to be aware of this phenomenon in order both to anticipate the possible decrease in insulin requirements and not to offer patients false hope that the diabetes has been cured.

INSULIN TREATMENT OF GROSSLY OBESE DIABETIC PATIENTS

Treatment of obese diabetic patients who remain markedly out of control on maximal doses of oral antidiabetic medications can be a difficult problem because these patients often do not respond to conventional doses of insulin. In general, the more obese the patient, the less responsive he or she is to insulin. Hospitalization to determine an appropriate insulin dose is useless, because the imposed ingestion of a suitable hypocaloric diet in the hospital improves their control considerably. Indeed, under these dietary conditions, obese diabetic patients may not require insulin or even oral antidiabetic medication. Some physicians withhold insulin therapy from these patients, with the rationale that a weight-reducing diet is the appropriate treatment. Although this obviously is true, these patients are unable to adhere to such a diet, and their tissues remain exposed to greatly elevated levels of glucose. Therefore, I use insulin in obese diabetic patients even though it may be only partially effective. I usually use a split/mixed regimen to bring the diabetes under control.

Although one tends to become discouraged with these patients, they can be controlled if enough insulin is administered. Figure 7–12 depicts the response to insulin of 13 type 2 diabetic patients with a mean body mass index (kg/m²) of 42.6, which is an extremely obese group. They were given Ultralente insulin before breakfast and three injections of regular insulin before each meal (regimen E in Table 7–10). Doses were

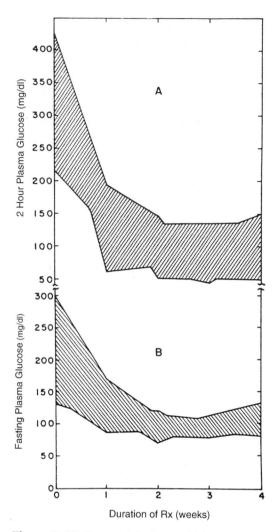

Figure 7–12. Range of fasting and 2-hour postprandial glucose concentrations in 13 obese type 2 patients during 4 weeks of insulin therapy. (From Andrews WJ, Vasquez B, Nagulesparan M: Insulin therapy in obese, non–insulin-dependent diabetes induces improvements in insulin action and secretion that are maintained for two weeks after insulin withdrawal. Diabetes 33:634, 1984)

adjusted on the basis of fasting and 2-hour postprandial glucose levels obtained throughout the day. The total amount of insulin administered varied between 99 and 322 U/day, with a mean dose of 198 U! However,

over a period of 4 weeks, fasting and postprandial glucose concentrations were markedly improved. In addition, these patients did not gain weight, probably because they were in a clinical research center in which their food intake could be controlled. In a 6-month outpatient study of obese type 2 diabetic patients uncontrolled on sulfonylurea agents (metformin was not available at that time), excellent control was achieved with insulin doses often exceeding 100 U/day.[132] In clinical practice, it can be difficult to achieve near euglycemia. However, no matter which insulin regimen is used, fasting glucose concentrations can often be decreased from the 250 to 350 mg/dl range to the 150 to 250 mg/dl range. Although this degree of control is far from good, the reduction in glucose levels is healthier for patients even if they should gain a few pounds in the process. A small amount of weight gain in an already obese patient represents little or no increased health risk, especially when compared with the benefit of lowered glycemia. It should be pointed out that almost all of the weight gain can be accounted for by the retained calories occurring as control is improved[133, 134] (i.e., they are not lost in the urine). No evidence shows that insulin per se causes weight gain. In fact, some evidence suggests that insulin may suppress appetite in the central nervous system.[135]

BRITTLE DIABETES

A pattern of extreme and frequent fluctuations in glucose concentrations occurs in a small minority of insulin-requiring patients. This situation has been variously termed *unstable, labile,* or *brittle* diabetes. Investigators disagree on the definition of this entity. Tattersall[136] suggests that a person with brittle diabetes is "any patient whose life is constantly being disrupted by episodes of hypo- or hyperglycemia whatever their cause." This is a good operational definition because this is exactly the situation a clinician encounters.

Several circumstances are associated with unstable diabetic control. First, individuals who do not secrete endogenous insulin are more likely to have labile diabetes than those with some insulin secretion.[137] Thus, brittle diabetes is rarely noted in type 2 diabetic patients or during the first year or so of type 1 diabetes. However, this cannot be the entire explanation, because most patients devoid of their own insulin secretion do not have brittle diabetes.

Second, many patients with brittle diabetes seem to have more severe emotional problems than those usually encountered in other patients.[138-140] Although it is possible that this is a result of the labile course, the present consensus does not support this view.[136, 140] It is more likely that the hormonal responses to anxiety and anger in these patients lead to rapid increases in glucose concentration that cannot be counteracted by the slow absorption of subcutaneously injected insulin. Because the emotional state of these patients varies, increasing the insulin dose to improve diabetic control at one point may cause hypoglycemia at another. Thus, identification and alleviation of emotional problems can be very helpful in treating brittle diabetes. This can be a difficult challenge, however.

In my experience, some patients with unstable diabetes are those who take relatively large amounts (>15 U per injection) of regular insulin. A rapid decline in glucose may stimulate the release of counterregulatory hormones, the effects of which last for many hours. Reduction or, in extreme cases, elimination of the dose of regular insulin is often helpful in improving control in these patients.

Schade and coworkers[139, 141] have systematically evaluated a relatively large number of patients referred for brittle diabetes. Their findings were rather surprising. Approximately half had fictitious disease—that is, they were knowingly manipulating their environment and/or their health care providers so that their diabetes would appear to be brittle. Approximately one quarter had a communication (learning) disorder such that although their vision and hearing were normal, they had difficulty processing the information received and formulating appropriate responses. Thus, their responses to unexpected variations in glucose levels were not appropriate, and this intensified the brittleness of their diabetes. These patients differed from the first group in that their aberrant responses were not intentional. Other causes of brittle diabetes in their series[139] were diabetic gastroparesis and insulin resistance syndromes (due to antibodies to the insulin molecule or to the insulin receptor). A systematic approach to ascertaining the cause of the brittle diabetes has been suggested by Schade and colleagues.[142]

The insulin management of these patients is obviously quite difficult. These type 1 patients must have continuous insulinization to prevent rapid increases in glucose levels. On the other hand, avoidance of hypoglycemia is also extremely important. Schade[141] recommends use of regular insulin four to five times a day, with the dose determined by SMBG results. I alter this approach to give the short-acting insulin before meals (using compensatory dose adjustments [discussed earlier] in small increments) and intermediate-acting insulin at bedtime for overnight control. For some patients, an insulin pump can be helpful. If preprandial regular insulin with overnight coverage provided by either bedtime NPH insulin or the basal infusion rate of an insulin pump is not satisfactory, I use NPH insulin twice a day and add regular insulin only if a relatively predictable pattern emerges indicating its need. Changes in both the intermediate- and short-acting insulin preparations are made in small increments. The insulin pump regimen paralleling this approach is to use several different basal rates covering different periods of the day and overnight, with either very small amounts of preprandial boluses or none at all. Tight control is not a realistic goal for these patients. Avoiding excessive hyperglycemia and hypoglycemia and keeping them relatively asymptomatic are success enough. Finally, isolated case reports describe brittle diabetes (1) due to high titers of insulin antibodies successfully treated with sulfated beef insulin[142a] (see Chapter 4 for rationale); (2) due to increased subcutaneous degradation[142b, 142c] successfully treated with lispro insulin[142c]; and (3) successfully treated with octreotide[142d] (the long-acting preparation of somatostatin).

HYPOGLYCEMIA

The hormonal responses to hypoglycemia were described earlier. Normal glucose counterregulation (i.e., the sequence of events and the glucose concentrations at which they occur) is depicted in Figure 7–13. As glucose concentrations decline to below approximately 80 mg/dl in normal subjects, the first response is decreased insulin secretion. At approximately 70 mg/dl, the rapid-acting counterregulatory hormones glucagon and epinephrine and the longer-

acting growth hormone are secreted and brain glucose uptake starts to diminish. At approximately 60 mg/dl, cortisol is secreted. Symptoms begin to appear at approximately 55 mg/dl, and impairment of cognition occurs when the glucose concentration falls below 50 mg/dl. As a last ditch effort to preserve glucose levels, autoregulation occurs—that is, the liver senses the low glucose concentration and produces glucose independent of external hormonal or sympathetic nervous system stimuli. Thus, as glucose concentrations fall, a well-coordinated cascade of hormonal responses ensues and early, easily recognized symptoms develop to protect the brain from glucose deprivation.

The signs and symptoms of hypoglycemia (Table 7–18) fall into two categories: autonomic (those caused by increased activity of the autonomic nervous system) and neuroglucopenic (those caused by depressed activity of the central nervous system). The brain, which has an absolute requirement for glucose, seems to accommodate to the prevailing concentration. This accounts for the fact

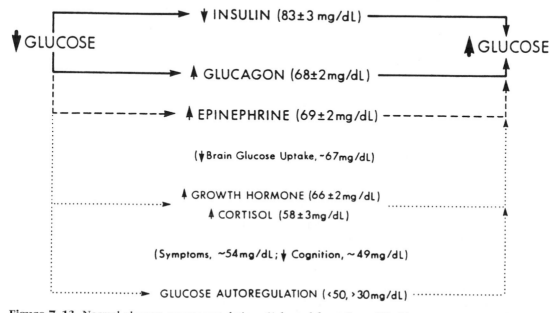

Figure 7–13. Normal glucose counterregulation. (Adapted from Cryer PE: Glucose counterregulation: The prevention and correction of hypoglycemia in humans. Am J Physiol 264:E149, 1993)

Table 7–18. Signs and Symptoms of Hypoglycemia

Autonomic[a]	Neuroglucopenic[b]
Weakness	Headache
Sweating	Hypothermia
Tachycardia	Visual disturbances
Palpitations	Mental dullness
Tremor	Confusion
Nervousness	Amnesia
Irritability	Seizures
Tingling of mouth and fingers	Coma
Hunger	
Nausea[c]	
Vomiting[c]	

[a]Caused by increased activity of the autonomic nervous system.
[b]Caused by decreased activity of the central nervous system.
[c]Unusual.

that patients in poor control brought to lower but not hypoglycemic glucose levels often experience mild autonomic symptoms.[143, 144] These invariably disappear after several weeks, and patients must be encouraged to continue their more strict diabetic control.

Hypoglycemia unawareness occurs commonly in type 1 diabetic patients, in an estimated 25% overall, and in probably more than half of those with a very long duration (>30 years) of the disease.[145] (It does not seem to be a problem in type 2 diabetic patients.) The inability to perceive the autonomic symptoms of hypoglycemia prevents type 1 patients from taking steps to avoid neuroglucopenia (commonly but incorrectly called *neuroglycopenia*), often leading to severe hypoglycemia, which is defined as a situation in which another party must intervene. At least three factors are associated with hypoglycemia unawareness: defective glucose counterregulation, intensive therapy, and recent antecedent hypoglycemia. These three tend to appear together but not necessarily in every patient. As discussed earlier, glucagon responses to hypoglycemia in type 1 diabetic patients are lost within the first 5 years of onset. The backup rapid response,

the catecholamines, may also be attenuated in patients after 5 years of the disease. This leaves patients without a rapid response to declining glucose concentrations. The fact that the brain seems to accommodate to prevailing glucose concentrations explains why lower glucose levels are necessary to activate symptoms of hypoglycemia and counterregulation in patients under intensive treatment[143, 146] (and those with insulinomas[147]).

Hypoglycemia unawareness also follows recent antecedent hypoglycemia, both in normal subjects[148-150] and in type 1 diabetic patients.[151-154] These impaired responses were not a result of prior activation of the autonomic nervous system because stimuli other than hypoglycemia (e.g., standing, exercise, meal) evoked normal responses.[154] Interestingly and of clinical importance, meticulous avoidance of hypoglycemia can reverse hypoglycemia unawareness[155, 156] and can still be compatible with strict diabetic control.[155] (As might be expected, hypoglycemia unawareness was also reversed after successful removal of insulinomas.[147])

In contrast to conventional wisdom, autonomic neuropathy does not seem to have much of a role in hypoglycemia unawareness.[151, 157, 158] For instance, type 1 diabetic patients with autonomic neuropathy documented by a battery of conventional tests did not have hypoglycemia unawareness, whereas those with hypoglycemia unawareness did not have autonomic neuropathy.[157] Regardless of the cause(s) of hypoglycemia unawareness (and the ones discussed here cannot fully account for this phenomenon[145]), we must try to reverse it if possible. Type 1 diabetic patients with hypoglycemia unawareness have an average of three episodes a year of severe hypoglycemia (defined earlier), a sixfold increase compared with those who can appreciate the autonomic symptoms of hypoglycemia.[159]

Before ending this discussion of hypoglycemia unawareness, it is necessary to comment briefly on the suggestion that patients using human insulin are more likely to suffer from hypoglycemia unawareness than those using animal insulins.[145] Suffice it to say that carefully performed studies[160] and a meta-analysis of the literature[161] do not support such a contention.

It is obvious that all patients who take insulin should carry with them a source of simple carbohydrate. What is not so obvious is that after ingestion of these items and reversal of the hypoglycemic symptoms, patients should then eat a snack containing carbohydrates and protein within the next hour to avoid recurrence of this problem. The simple carbohydrate ingested alone is absorbed rapidly and raises the plasma glucose concentration only temporarily. Glucose is deposited in the tissues or lost in the urine if the plasma concentration exceeds the T_m and may not be available in the plasma long enough to buffer the continued effect of the insulin. Therefore, it is important to provide carbohydrate in a snack that is absorbed more slowly. Amino acids from the ingested protein also help to replenish stores of hepatic glycogen via the gluconeogenic pathway.

Two studies have attempted to quantitate the response to various treatments for (laboratory-induced) hypoglycemia.[162, 163] Their conclusions were that 15 to 20 g of glucose in tablet form or in solution were appropriate for treating these patients. The responses to juices and gels were delayed in both studies. In our experience, patients often have a marked improvement in symptoms with only 10 g of glucose. Our patients are treated just to the point where they feel better rather than to the point of complete disappearance of symptoms. If the symptoms are not definitely improved in 10 to 15 minutes, another 10 g of glucose is taken, and this should be repeated every 10 to 15 minutes until the symptoms have definitely improved. This conservative approach avoids overtreatment with resultant marked hyperglycemia, an all too common occurrence. If patients perform SMBG at this time, the results can be particularly helpful. Rising values signal a suitable response. Moreover, if the

test was performed before treatment and the symptoms were not associated with a low concentration of glucose, inappropriate therapy would be avoided. If, however, the symptoms are severe, a patient cannot test, or past experience has shown that these symptoms are most always due to hypoglycemia, glucose should be taken without delay. Temporary hyperglycemia is preferable to the risk of severe hypoglycemia.

Table 7–19 lists readily available sources that contain 10 g of glucose. As just discussed, my recommendation would be that all insulin-requiring patients carry on their person (not in the car or in a special place at home) glucose tablets or packets of table sugar rather than rely on juices, gels, or food items. In this manner, a precise amount of rapidly absorbed simple carbohydrate is always available. If the next meal is more than 30 to 60 minutes away, the patient should also eat small amounts of complex carbohydrate, equivalent to 1 bread exchange, and 1 to 2 ounces of protein (see Chapter 3) to prevent the recurrence of hypoglycemia. In this manner, hypoglycemic episodes are handled appropriately and not overtreated.

Home treatment of unconscious hypoglycemic patients presents a difficult problem. Although preparations of "instant glucose" that are placed between the cheek and the teeth have been advocated in this situation, virtually no glucose is absorbed through the buccal mucosa with this technique.[164] Because these preparations must be swallowed

Table 7–19. Commonly Available Sources of 10 g of Glucose

Orange juice	1 cup[a]
Grape juice	½ cup
Table sugar	4 teaspoons[b]
Honey	3 teaspoons
Lifesavers	10
B-D glucose tablets	2
DextroEnergy glucose tablets	3
Dex 4 glucose tablets	2.5
Glutose tablets	2

[a]1 cup = 8 ounces (fluid).
[b]1 tablespoon = 3 teaspoons.

to be effective,[164] they should not be given to an unconscious patient because of the danger of aspiration. Instead, glucagon should be available, and a responsible family member or friend should be taught how to use it. Glucagon is available in two preparations (and soon may be available in a third). One glucagon preparation (Glucagon for Injection Vial) consists of 1 mg of the powdered hormone in a sterile bottle and a vial containing 1 ml of sterile diluent. After the vial is broken, the diluent should be drawn into the patient's insulin syringe and injected through the rubber stopper of the bottle. The powder dissolves quickly, and the solution should be drawn back into the syringe and injected. A second preparation (Glucagon Emergency Kit) is similar, except that a syringe containing the diluent is provided. The diluent is injected into the vial containing the powdered glucagon (with the syringe and needle remaining attached through the rubber stopper), the powder is dissolved, the resulting solution is drawn back into the syringe, and the contents are injected. Within 5 to 10 minutes, glucagon raises the blood glucose level through stimulation of hepatic glycogenolysis. Although the effect is mild (~20 to 50 mg/dl increase) and transient (lasting ~30 minutes), patients often regain consciousness. At this point, patients should immediately consume simple carbohydrates, followed by a substantial snack containing carbohydrates. Although not available in this country, intranasal glucagon is almost as effective as the parenterally administered preparation in the treatment of hypoglycemia in type 1 diabetic patients.[165-167]

Hypoglycemia secondary to the use of sulfonylurea agents usually lasts longer than insulin-induced hypoglycemia. Therefore, continued treatment for many hours may be necessary to prevent a recurrence. If moderate to marked mentation changes have occurred, hospitalization is advisable, because intravenous glucose therapy is usually necessary for several days.

Finally, it is important to reiterate that if a patient taking acarbose experiences hypoglycemia due to the concomitant administration of insulin or a sulfonylurea agent, it must be treated with glucose tablets because acarbose blocks the digestion and therefore the absorption of other sources of carbohydrate. Because acarbose does not inhibit lactase (see Chapter 5), milk might also be an appropriate treatment, although there are no published reports attesting to this.

STARVATION KETOSIS

The mechanism of starvation ketosis is similar to that of diabetic ketosis: increased breakdown of triglycerides in adipose tissue to free fatty acids, with their subsequent conversion to ketone bodies in the liver (see Chapter 2). In diabetic ketosis, the absence of insulin causes overproduction of free fatty acids; in starvation ketosis, the signal is an underutilization of carbohydrates secondary to decreased carbohydrate intake. The utilization of ~80 to 100 g of exogenous carbohydrate per day is required to prevent ketosis. If much less than that amount is available, energy requirements in tissue must be met by increased fat metabolism, which leads to ketosis as described earlier. Although decreased carbohydrate intake is usually associated with diminished ingestion of total calories, ketosis also can occur with eucaloric diets that are low in carbohydrates. Thus, the term *starvation ketosis* is not entirely accurate.

There are two ways to distinguish between diabetic and starvation ketosis. The former almost always is associated with marked glucosuria but the latter is not. However, ketonuria may interfere with the glucose reactions on Keto-Diastix, and type 1 patients thus may need an independent check of mild glucosuria occuring in the presence of moderate to large ketonuria by retesting with either Chemstrip uG, Diastix, or Clinitest tablets. Alternatively, glucose levels can be measured by SMBG, although DKA can occur with blood glucose levels <200 mg/dl.[115] The most accurate way to distinguish between diabetic and starvation ketosis is to measure plasma ketone bodies. The degree of ketosis is much greater in uncontrolled diabetic patients than in patients whose ketosis is due primarily to inadequate carbohydrate intake. Therefore, in diabetic ketosis, results of the nitroprusside test for plasma ketone bodies remain positive when the sample is diluted. In contrast, in starvation ketosis, the results almost invariably are negative after dilution. Clinically, patients with evolving DKA feel sick whereas those with starvation ketosis have relatively few symptoms.

In two situations, differentiation between diabetic and starvation ketosis is important. The first involves obese type 2 patients who maintain a hypocaloric diet whose carbohydrate content is low enough to lead to starvation ketosis. This usually is not difficult to distinguish from diabetic ketosis, because the ketosis resistance of patients will already have been established at the time of diagnosis. Furthermore, the urine test results should show little glucosuria. The other circumstance involves type 1 patients who become ill with gastrointestinal symptoms and are forced to limit their oral intake of food. This can be a difficult situation to resolve. On the one hand, gastrointestinal symptoms can be part of evolving ketoacidosis. Therefore, establishing the presence of diabetic ketosis and treating it vigorously is important in preventing hospitalization (see the later section on sick day rules). On the other hand, if the situation is really one of viral gastroenteritis associated with starvation ketosis, overtreatment with insulin may cause hypoglycemia. Although a comparison of the degrees of glucosuria and ketonuria often help in making the decision, patients may need to go to a laboratory facility for measurement of plasma ketone bodies and possibly serum bicarbonate levels.

SICK DAY RULES

In the presence of an infection of any kind, insulin action is impaired by unknown mechanisms. Therefore, in such circumstances, diabetic control usually worsens, often quickly and profoundly. Because normal food intake is diminished, patients sometimes decrease their insulin dose or omit it altogether. This is inadvisable for patients with type 1 diabetes. These patients should take the prescribed amount and often even require additional insulin. I usually have patients take their usual insulin dose and use the following regimen for supplementing it if necessary (Table 7–20). If patients are testing only their urine, these tests should be carried out before each meal or at least every 6 hours. If the urine test for glucose is 1% or 2% (and the patients know that they're infected), they should take 4 extra U of regular or lispro insulin if they are lean and 8 extra U if they are obese. For patients who also show moderate or strong ketone bodies in their urine along with this amount of glucosuria,

Table 7–20. Sick Day Rules

1. Take usual insulin dose.
2. Additional insulin based on results of urine testing.

Urine Test		Additional Regular or Lispro Insulin (U)	
Glucose (%)	Ketone Bodies	Lean	Obese
1 or 2	Negative, trace, small	4	8
½,[a] 1, or 2	Moderate, large	8	12

3. Additional insulin based on results of self-monitoring of blood glucose.

Blood Glucose	Urine Ketones	Additional Regular or Lispro Insulin (U)	
		Lean	Obese
>300 mg/dl	Negative, trace, small	4	8
>300 mg/dl	Moderate, large	8	12

[a]Because ketone bodies do not interfere with glucose results measured by Chemstrip uG or Clinitest tablets, glucosuria measured by these two methods usually is ≥1% in the presence of moderate to large ketonuria.

an additional 4 U of regular insulin should be added. However, it should be kept in mind that moderate to large ketone bodies in the urine may interfere with the glucose test measured by all test strips except Chemstrip uG. Therefore, the amount of glucosuria may only be 0.5% in the presence of large amounts of ketone bodies in the urine. On the other hand, ketonuria in the absence of glucosuria probably represents starvation ketosis, a situation due to the lack of carbohydrate intake in sick patients. This does not suggest that a patient's diabetes is in poor control.

In patients performing SMBG, I use 300 mg/dl as a level at which to add extra insulin. Patients should initially measure their glucose level before each meal. If the value is >300 mg/dl, they should take an additional 4 U of regular or lispro insulin for lean patients and 8 U for obese patients. It is extremely important to ensure that type 1 diabetic patients also measure ketones in their urine. If, in the presence of these levels of hyperglycemia, the ketone test in the urine is moderate or strong, an additional 4 U of regular or lispro insulin should be taken. Glucose measurements should be repeated in 3 to 4 hours to ascertain that a response occurred. For patients with gastrointestinal symptoms, whether due to a viral gastroenteritis or possibly secondary to evolving diabetic ketoacidosis, it is critical to ensure their ability to maintain oral fluid intake. Once the symptoms have progressed to the point where oral intake is no longer possible, patients must be admitted to a hospital for parenteral fluid therapy. This underscores the importance of frequent testing on days that patients are ill so that this eventuality can be minimized.

The approach just described for adjusting insulin doses can also be used for patients whose diabetic control deteriorates in association with other kinds of stress (e.g., emotional upsets, trauma). Effective and frequent communication between patient and physician is an important component of care dur-

ing these periods. Most hospitalizations can be avoided if adjustments in treatment are started early and continued appropriately.

Type 2 patients are less of a problem than type 1 patients. Their resistance to ketosis most often persists, and they very seldom become ketotic. The increasing hyperglycemia may need treatment, but their metabolic status does not deteriorate to the point where hospitalization is required. Because these episodes are self-limited, treatment regimens in patients on dietary therapy alone or dietary therapy supplemented with oral antidiabetes medication usually are not altered. The dose of the sulfonylurea agent can be increased temporarily if a patient becomes very symptomatic from uncontrolled diabetes. (Theoretically, one could increase the doses of metformin or acarbose temporarily, but their gastrointestinal side effects make this approach problematic.) However, the benefits of starting either oral hypoglycemic therapy (in those on diet alone) or insulin are outweighed by inconvenience and by the short period for which these new therapies should be necessary. Furthermore, because most type 2 diabetic patients are obese, the decreased food intake usually associated with illness tends to offset the worsening of control secondary to the infection in these patients.

In addition to adjusting insulin doses, three other modalities of treatment are important in infected diabetic patients: carbohydrate intake and, in patients with vomiting, diarrhea, or marked polyuria, fluid (sodium) and potassium replacement. Because most of these patients receive insulin, some carbohydrate intake is important. A method for obtaining carbohydrate from more easily digestible foods is described in detail in Chapters 3 and 10. For some patients this is not feasible because either they are not properly educated in this approach or their gastrointestinal symptoms may prevent them from eating the appropriate amounts of food. These patients should eat foods that they can tolerate from the milk, fruit, bread, and vegetable exchange lists. Liquids and soft foods are easier to digest, and patients are often able to consume six to eight smaller meals more easily than three to four larger ones. Soft drinks (not low-calorie ones) and fruit juices are good sources of carbohydrates.

Fluid losses from the kidneys or gastrointestinal tract are high in sodium. To avoid marked depletion of the intravascular volume (dehydration), replacement must be with fluids that contain relatively large amounts of sodium. As long as enough insulin and fluids can be given, hospitalization can often be avoided. When the severity of the gastrointestinal symptoms precludes oral intake of fluid, patients usually must be hospitalized. Two good sources of sodium are bouillon (1 cup contains ~40 mEq) and tomato juice (1 cup contains ~20 mEq). Other foods high in sodium are canned soups, saltine crackers, and packaged custard pudding mixes. Salt can be added to other juices. Soft drinks contain little sodium.

Sources high in potassium include orange juice, tomato juice, and prune juice (1 cup ~15 mEq). Foods with moderate potassium content (1 cup ~10 mEq) include milk, grapefruit juice, and pineapple juice. Apple juice, grape juice, and cranberry juice are low in potassium (1 cup ~5 mEq). A large banana contains ~10 mEq of potassium.

EXERCISE

Exercise is receiving more and more attention as a general health measure to prevent diabetes[168, 169] as well as a helpful adjunct in managing it.[170-172] It is helpful, however, to put the role of exercise in these patients in its proper perspective. What can realistically be achieved, and by what levels of exercise? Exercise has four main benefits: (1) It leads to a sense of well-being; (2) it aids in weight loss in obese patients; (3) it improves cardiovascular conditioning; and, in diabetic patients, (4) it improves insulin sensitivity.

The level of exercise that provides subjects with a heightened sense of well-being is obviously variable and depends on a person's usual amount of activity. For many of our obese patients, simply walking around the block a few times constitutes increased physical activity and makes patients feel better psychologically. More active people need higher levels of exercise to achieve this sense of well-being.

Exercise as the sole method of losing weight is usually unsuccessful without a concomitant reduction of food intake. This is because the amount of extra calories expended in the usual exercise program is not enough to lead to much weight loss. One pound of fat represents approximately 3,500 calories. A person running a mile uses 100 calories. (Walking a mile also expends 100 calories; it just takes longer.) Two extra cookies cancel out that 100 calories of caloric expenditure. Thus, it is apparent why the usual modest exercise programs most patients embark on do not result in much weight loss unless hypocaloric diets are also followed conscientiously.

A much greater amount of exercise is necessary to attain beneficial cardiovascular effects.[172, 173] One needs to exercise at least 30 minutes 3 times a week at a level that keeps the pulse rate at 70% to 85% of maximum. Maximum heart rate is age dependent and can be calculated by subtracting a patient's age from 220. Therefore, a 50-year-old person has a maximum heart rate of 170 and must sustain a pulse rate between 119 and 144 for 90 minutes a week during exercise. This level of exercise should result in lowered blood pressure and resting pulse rate and has a beneficial effect on the cardiovascular system. In the real world, however, diabetic patients find exercise programs very difficult to sustain,[174] and despite receiving repeated recommendations for regular exercise, they do not exercise more than people without diabetes.[175]

Exercise can be a difficult challenge in the treatment of insulin-requiring patients, especially those with type 1 diabetes. The reason for this is depicted in Figure 7–14. Normal exercise physiology regarding glucose metabolism is shown in the middle. Four factors can influence glucose levels. Blood flow increases and delivers more glucose to the exercising muscle. Muscle insulin sensitivity also increases. Secretion of the counterregulatory hormones inhibits endogenous insulin secretion and enhances hepatic glucose production. The first two lower glucose levels and are balanced by the second two, which raise them, so that in a normal individual or a diabetic patient not taking insulin, glucose concentrations remain stable. In underinsulinized diabetic patients (Fig. 7–14, top), increased insulin-mediated glucose utilization in muscle and the restraining effect of insulin on hepatic glucose production do not occur. Under these circumstances of diminished glucose utilization by muscle and overproduction of glucose by the liver, marked hyperglycemia can occur. In addition, in type 1 patients, the increased lipolysis associated with exercise can become excessive because little insulin is available to restrain it. The resultant free fatty acids produced are converted into ketone bodies in the liver (especially because exercise-induced glucagon levels are high and insulin levels are low) and can cause ketosis.

The lower part of Figure 7–14 shows the situation when excessive insulin is present. Exercise can cause this because the enhanced blood flow to the area in which the insulin has been injected increases its absorption. For this reason, an abdominal rather than an extremity site for injection is recommended before exercise, although if the intensity of the exercise is high enough, rates of absorption from these two areas may differ little. The increased circulating insulin concentrations increase muscle glucose utilization and block the enhanced hepatic glucose production, thus leading to hypoglycemia. Exercise, therefore, can place insulin-requiring patients at risk for either hyperglycemia (and possibly ketosis in type 1 patients) or hypoglycemia.

Because the conditions surrounding exercise cannot be predicted accurately, only general guidelines are offered. In terms of food, it may be beneficial to exercise shortly after eating or, if that is not feasible, to eat a small snack before starting. If the exercise is prolonged and intense, carbohydrate snacking during exercise may be necessary. Patients occasionally become hypoglycemic many hours after exercise, and extra food

INSULIN AND THE METABOLIC RESPONSE TO EXERCISE

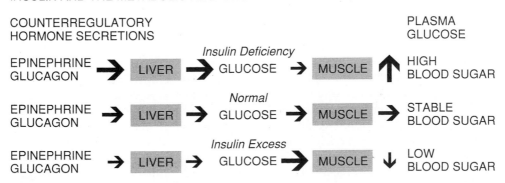

Figure 7–14. Insulin and the metabolic response to exercise. (From Doner K: Exercise and diabetes. A research perspective. JDF International Countdown. Fall, 1989, p. 16. With permission.)

needs to be eaten at these times. A general approach for balancing the amount of extra food with the anticipated level of exercise is suggested in Chapter 3. However, patients must determine for themselves whether these amounts are applicable to them or whether adjustments are necessary.

Decreasing insulin doses in anticipation of exercise has also been suggested.[174] This is more feasible if regular insulin can be decreased shortly before exercise. I usually prefer additional calories for exercise not included in the usual daily schedule instead of decreasing insulin doses. If the anticipated extra exercise is not performed, the patient will have taken too small a dose of insulin that day, and diabetic control will suffer accordingly. The more time between insulin administration and exercise, the less a repository of subcutaneous insulin is present for enhanced absorption. Thus, exercising before breakfast (and before the morning injection of insulin) is an effective way to minimize exercise-induced hypoglycemia.

Some authorities suggest avoiding exercise if glucose levels are high (e.g., >250 mg/dl) or if ketosis is present.[174] Although the principles behind this recommendation are sound (as discussed earlier), I do not *routinely* advocate this for several reasons. Patients' responses to exercise are variable and depend on, among other things, the intensity and duration of the exercise as well as the timing of the previous insulin injection. This approach has been vindicated by a study[176] in which only 5 of 74 episodes of exercise in type 1 diabetic patients begun with blood glucose concentrations exceeding 300 mg/dl resulted in increased levels at the conclusion of the exercise. Most importantly, because exercise often involves other people, canceling plans would have a detrimental effect on the patient's social interactions.

It is very helpful to perform SMBG before, after, and sometimes during exercise (e.g., between sets of tennis) in order for patients to learn their responses to various levels of exercise, insulin injection schedules, and extra food intake. Patterns that often emerge allow patients (with the help of a physician) to plan an effective and safe approach to exercise.

In conclusion, exercise can be helpful to diabetic patients, especially from a psychologic point of view. Before embarking on a strenuous exercise program, all diabetic patients older than 40 years and those adult type 1 patients with diabetes for more than 15 to 20 years should probably undergo a thorough cardiovascular evaluation. Unfortunately, intense levels of exercise are necessary to achieve the benefits of weight loss, cardiovascular conditioning, and a sustained increase in insulin sensitivity. For example, the effect of an acute bout of exercise on increasing insulin sensitivity lasted only several days in untrained individuals[177] (although it was still evident 5 days later in those who were trained, i.e., had exercised regularly for 1 hour 5 days a week[178]). Finally, although exercise must be handled judiciously by patients taking insulin, it can be included in their schedule, particularly if they are willing to undertake SMBG and to learn their response to varying degress of exercise and food intake.

FOOT CARE

Infections of the feet are a major source of morbidity among diabetic patients and often lead to death. Even though many of these infections are preventable, foot ulcers and gangrene continue to exact a tremendous toll in the diabetic population. Thus, physicians must emphasize the importance of proper foot care (see Chapter 10 for a detailed discussion of this topic). The feet of patients older than 40 years and of those who have had diabetes for >10 years should be examined at every regularly scheduled office visit for diabetes. Patients with impairment of blood flow to the feet should have their toenails cut by qualified medical personnel (i.e., podiatrist, nurse, or physician).

Calluses are an important sign of possible future trouble. They represent increased pressure on an area that a patient often cannot feel because of associated sensory neuropathy. Calluses should be shaved routinely (usually by a podiatrist, but other medical personnel can be taught how) and kept to a minimum. Unroofing an innocuous-looking callus sometimes reveals an extensive ulcer, which could have been prevented by treating the callus when it first appeared. The source of the pressure (e.g., ill-fitting shoes, collapsed metatarsal arch, hammertoe) must be identified and corrective measures taken, if possible. Softer and better-fitting shoes usually are all that is needed, although persuading patients to forgo style simply to prevent calluses is not always easy. Prophylactic surgery to correct or remove a hammertoe is indicated in some patients, because no orthopedic method can reduce the pressure on the offending digit. The evaluation and management of foot problems in diabetic patients is beyond the scope of this chapter. The important prognostic information obtained by using the 5.07 (10-g) monofilament in the examination[8] has already been mentioned. *Cost-effective* approaches to the diagnosis and treatment of diabetic foot infections and other lesions are available.[179-182]

In summary, *most foot ulcers and other infected lesions of the feet are preventable.* Although examination of the feet and instruction of patients in proper prophylactic foot care seem mundane, probably no other service that the physician performs offers as important a benefit for their diabetic patients, especially those who are older.

TRAVEL

Insulin-requiring diabetic patients who travel should be advised about their insulin. Insulin is stable at room temperature, a feature that facilitates travel for these patients. Extra insulin vials and syringes should be taken along, especially for patients going to a foreign country. It is wise for patients to carry their syringes and vials of insulin on their person in case baggage is lost. The timing and occasionally the amount of the insulin dose may need adjustment on the day of travel, especially if patients are flying into a different time zone. Patients should find out from the airline what kind of meal will be served and at what time. The insulin dose is then adjusted to the meal pattern. Traveling from north to south and vice versa is the easiest change to accommodate, because the time does not change and the eating pattern usually is not too different. Traveling from east to west and vice versa presents more of a problem because the change in time often disrupts both meal and sleeping patterns. A relatively smooth integration of the new eating and activity schedule with the insulin regimen can be accomplished by keeping both schedules geared to the patient's internal clock for the first 12 to 24 hours after arrival before shifting to the changed external time.

For example, for patients taking two insulin injections per day, an afternoon flight from Los Angeles to New York City might be handled as follows. The flight leaves at 2 PM, and a large meal is served 2 hours later. Patients would start their day ~1 hour earlier than usual. They would take the usual insulin dose and eat breakfast and lunch slightly earlier than normal. They would take their second injection of insulin on the plane just before the 4 PM meal (Los Angeles time) is served. Patients arrive in New York City at 11 PM local time (but at 8 PM according to their internal clock) and eat their bedtime snack shortly after arrival. This is necessary because they took their second injection of NPH insulin ~4 hours before. They go to sleep at 1 to 2 AM New York time (9 to 10 PM Los Angeles time). On awakening the next day at 8 AM (5 AM Los Angeles time), their fasting glucose level should still be controlled by the NPH insulin, which was taken ~12 hours earlier. They now can follow their usual schedule. Although according to their internal clock they are taking their insulin 3 hours earlier than usual, their eating and activity patterns also have shifted by 3 hours, and the relation between the two patterns has not been disrupted seriously.

Traveling from New York City back to Los Angeles requires more of an adjustment. A morning flight leaves the East Coast at 9 AM and arrives on the West Coast at noon (local time). The same patients would take their insulin and a small breakfast several hours before the flight. A large breakfast usually is served shortly after takeoff. Patients could either take a small amount of extra regular insulin to handle these calories or consume only a portion of them as a midmorning snack. Regardless of which they choose, they need to have some food available several hours before landing to serve as a small lunch. After arriving in Los Angeles at noon (3 PM by their internal clock), they should arrange to eat their major meal several hours later. Although this occurs in the middle of the afternoon on the West Coast, it is an appropriate time for their supper according to the peak action of their morning insulin injection. They should delay their second injection of NPH insulin for several more hours (5 PM Los Angeles time, 8 PM New York time). They would need to eat their bedtime snack at 8 to 9 PM (local time) to cover this injection, by which time they probably would wish to retire (approximately midnight by their internal clock). Although they might arise very early the next morning according to West Coast time, the hour would theoretically be appropriate for the East Coast, and they should delay taking their morning injection and eating until the appropriate Los Angeles time. This delay should not cause much of a problem because their last NPH injection was taken ~15 hours previously and should still be effective in controlling their fasting glucose concentration. Their insulin regimen and eating patterns are now adjusted (with respect to time, at least) back to the West Coast schedule.

Although the disruptions encountered by patients taking longer plane trips are greater, the same general approach is used to treat them during the flight and to aid their adjustment after arrival. These examples do not take into account the stress effect of changing time zones ("jet lag"), which may impair diabetic control temporarily.

An alternative method is to give patients the entire daily insulin dose as a short-acting insulin. Twenty-five percent of the total daily dose would be taken as regular insulin before each meal during travel, starting the morning of departure. The normal amount of intermediate-acting insulin should be resumed with the first breakfast at the patient's destination. The disadvantage of this approach, however, is that the timing of the meals often is not evenly spaced during a 24-hour period. Patients may need a small dose of NPH insulin after arrival if they plan to sleep for 8 hours or longer before starting a more normal eating and activity schedule. With travel, as with exercise, SMBG is extremely helpful to manage a patient's blood glucose levels.

DENTAL PROCEDURES

Dental infections, especially periodontal disease, are more common in diabetic patients than in nondiabetic individuals.[183] Therefore, diabetic patients are more likely to undergo dental procedures that impair food intake. This may be a problem for those taking insulin or sulfonylurea agents unless precautions are taken. Effective communication between the patient's physician and dentist is important so that the extent and timing of the diminished food intake and the severity of the operative stress can be judged.

If a patient taking sulfonylurea agents will miss more than one meal because of a dental procedure, the drugs should be omitted that morning and resumed when normal food intake occurs. Chlorpropamide (Diabinese) should be discontinued the previous day because of its long half-life.

Hypoglycemia is more likely to occur secondary to insulin therapy than to oral hypoglycemic agents. In these patients, dental procedures should be performed in the morning, if possible, because the effects of intermediate-acting insulins injected before breakfast peak late in the afternoon and because an insulin reaction may occur if the supper calories are decreased. If the lunch calories are diminished, regular and lispro insulin should be omitted from the morning dose. In addition, NPH insulin and breakfast might be taken a little later than usual to minimize the risk of early afternoon hypoglycemia. If the amount of food intake at supper will be decreased, the dose of morning intermediate-acting insulin should be reduced. However, type 1 patients must have some insulin to avoid ketosis and possibly ketoacidosis. Therefore, a balance must be achieved between the decreased insulin requirements caused by decreased food intake and the need for insulin caused by the stress of the dental procedure and possibly by the infection that led do it. It is important that patients monitor their control closely after the procedure and communicate with their physician. If extensive dental work that impairs food intake is necessary for ketosis-prone diabetic patients, hospitalization sometimes is advisable.

SURGICAL AND POSTOPERATIVE MANAGEMENT

The therapeutic goals during surgery in diabetic patients are to minimize fluid and electrolyte losses secondary to osmotic diuresis by limiting hyperglycemia, to prevent diabetic ketosis in type 1 patients, and to avoid hypoglycemia while patients are anesthetized. Although some anesthesiologists fear that hypoglycemia will occur during surgery if insulin is given preoperatively, this rarely happens. The stress of surgery for patients usually receiving intravenous glucose almost always leads to hyperglycemia. Indeed, in a prospective study of 58 patients receiving NPH insulin on the morning of surgery with glucose infusions begun at the time of the insulin injection and continuing throughout surgery, hypoglycemia only occurred *before* the operation when surgery was delayed until the afternoon.[184] The average glucose level at the end of surgery was 258 mg/dl, excluding three patients who were treated intraoperatively when their glucose concentrations exceeded 400 mg/dl.[184]

Although several insulin regimens have been proposed, one is clearly superior. This involves continous insulin and glucose infusions given through separate sets of tubing. Patients receive their usual insulin regimen until the morning of surgery. At this time, 5% dextrose in water is infused at 125 ml/h and insulin is piggy-backed onto the glucose line through an infusion pump. Suggested insulin infusion rates are shown in Table 7–21. Capillary blood glucose levels are measured by a bedside glucose meter every hour or two before surgery, and the insulin infusion rate adjusted accordingly. During surgery, the anesthesiologist must be able to measure glucose concentrations *hourly* and infuse insulin appropriately. This approach requires that the intravenous line infusing glucose and insulin be under the control of the anesthesiologist and a separate intravenous line be used to give saline, plasma, blood, and so on as required by the surgeon. Although the insulin infusion rates in Table 7–21 may need to be changed according to an individual patient's response, they seem to work very well in most types of operations except for kidney transplants and open heart surgery, during which higher rates are required.[185] This glucose–insulin infusion method is also ideal for the perioperative period until patients can eat. It requires, however, nurses able to use a bedside glucose meter accurately (on the ward, in the recovery room, and in the intensive care unit) and a cooperative anesthesiologist who can use a glucose meter in the operating room. If a pump to infuse insulin is not available, insulin can be added to the glucose

Table 7–21. Algorithm for Intravenous Insulin Infusion Adjustment Before, During, and After Surgery

A. Stop feeding and usual treatment with insulin or oral hypoglycemic agents 12 hours before surgery. Chlorpropamide should be discontinued 24 hours before surgery.

B. Start infusion of a solution containing 5% dextrose at a rate of 125 ml/h.

C. Start intravenous insulin infusion as follows:

Whole Blood Glucose (mg/dl)	Insulin Infusion Rate (U/h)
≤100	None
101–150	1
151–250	2
251–350	3
>350	4 (Dextrose infusion is held until blood glucose level ≤250 mg/dl.)

1. Measure blood glucose level with a glucose meter every 2 hours before and after surgery and hourly during surgery.
   a. Do not change insulin infusion rate if blood glucose level ranges between 100 and 180 mg/dl.
   b. Increase insulin infusion rate by 0.5 U/h if blood glucose level is >180 mg/dl.
   c. Hold dextrose infusion if blood glucose level >350 mg/dl. Restart once blood glucose level ≤250 mg/dl.
   d. Decrease insulin infusion rate by 0.5 U/h if blood glucose level is <100 mg/dl, and increase dextrose infusion rate by 50 ml/h.
      1) Once blood glucose level increases to >100 mg/dl, decrease dextrose infusion rate back to 125 ml/h.
2. Measure blood glucose level 1 hour after an adjustment is made to assess response, and readjust if indicated.
3. If glucose level stable postoperatively, blood glucose determinations can be carried out every 4 hours.

solution.[186] This latter modification has two drawbacks. It does not allow for separate adjustments of the infusion rates for insulin and glucose. Moreover, every time an adjustment is made, a new solution must be made up. Even so, this method is superior to the two others discussed next.

If monitoring glucose levels by bedside meters is not feasible, the following two approaches are recommended for insulin-requiring diabetic patients. In one, patients receive half of their total daily insulin dose (i.e., half of the entire amount of intermediate- and short-acting insulin taken normally) as NPH insulin on the morning of surgery. An infusion of 5% dextrose in water is administered at a rate of 125 ml/h. If surgery must be delayed for ≥4 hours after the insulin is given, the fasting glucose concentration should be measured (ordered *stat* or measured at the bedside). If this value is <150 mg/dl, the rate of glucose infusion should be increased to 200 ml/h when the value is available.

The second approach is to withhold insulin before surgery and not give patients dextrose-containing fluids until the postoperative period. This requires communication with and the cooperation of the anesthesiologist. In type 1 patients, this method works best with morning surgery. It would not be advisable in type 1 patients on one injection of insulin per day, because relatively little effective insulin would be available the following morning. In addition, if surgery were not scheduled until late morning or afternoon for type 1 patients, there might be a problem with continued insulin effectiveness even with insulin administration the evening before. Thus, this approach is most effective with type 1 patients who are undergoing relatively short (several hours) operations scheduled in the early or midmorning period.

This method also works well for type 2 patients, in whom glucose concentrations will not rise in the preoperative period because they are not eating or receiving glucose. One must ensure, however, that both type 1 and type 2 patients are not hypoglycemic on the morning of surgery in response to the previous evening's insulin dose. If this is the case, a dextrose infusion must be started and one of the alternate methods used (i.e., either giving half of the total insulin requirement as NPH insulin or starting an insulin infusion). If both insulin and glucose are withheld until after surgery, the postoperative blood glucose level is usually similar to the preoperative one.[187]

Insulin treatment after surgery depends on two factors: which insulin regimen was used and whether a patient will resume eating that day (arbitrarily defined here as *minor* surgery) or not (defined as *major* surgery). Thus, there are six possible situations, which involve three insulin regimens (intravenous insulin, half of the usual total dose given as intermediate-acting insulin, withholding insulin [and the glucose infusion] until after surgery), in patients undergoing either minor or major surgery.

Patients given an insulin infusion are the easiest to treat postoperatively irrespective of which kind of surgery they undergo. The same approach, with sampling for glucose measurements and adjustments of the insulin infusion rate every 2 to 4 hours, is used until they eat. To disrupt the usual time course of insulin for patients as little as possible, subcutaneous administration should be started at the same times as before surgery, usually before breakfast and before supper (or bedtime for the evening intermediate-acting insulin preparation). If lunch is eaten on the day of surgery, the insulin infusion can be stopped at that time and subcutaneous regular insulin given to carry patients to the evening meal. If the insulin infusion is used instead, the rate can be increased arbitrarily for the 2-hour period after the meal is started in anticipation of the postprandial rise of glucose concentrations. Consideration should be given to increasing the usual amount of the evening intermediate-acting insulin slightly because there will be no overnight effect from a morning dose. The usual amounts of regular insulin may need to be adjusted downward if caloric intake will be less than usual but upward because of postoperative discomfort. These possible changes in insulin doses need to be considered for patients undergoing minor surgery managed by the other two insulin regimens as well. (The one exception to this is the dose of the evening intermediate-acting insulin in patients who receive their usual morning insulin prescription, albeit delayed, after a short minor surgical procedure.)

Patients receiving half of their total insulin dose as NPH insulin on the morning of surgery along with a dextrose infusion should be treated postoperatively as follows. In those undergoing *minor* surgery, the glucose infusion is stopped when they eat. If the first meal is lunch, subcutaneous regular or lispro insulin is given to control the blood glucose level until supper. If patients do not eat until supper on the day of surgery, subcutaneous regular or lispro insulin is still given postoperatively (every 4 hours) to control the blood glucose level until the dextrose infusion is discontinued and patients eat. In both situations, glucose should be measured as soon as patients enter the recovery room, because not only is the glucose concentration usually elevated immediately postoperatively when this insulin regimen is used[184] but the glucose infusion is usually being continued. Therefore, the dose of regular or lispro insulin at this time must take these factors into consideration. The submaximal amount of the preoperative NPH insulin has only a minor role after surgery and should not be relied on to have a large effect on postoperative patients receiving intravenous glucose. The same principles apply in those patients who are treated with this regimen and who undergo *major* surgery—that is, their glucose concentrations are managed by subcutaneous regular insulin every 4 hours until the evening. Longer-term treatment of surgical patients unable to eat is discussed later.

Those patients who are undergoing minor surgery and in whom both a glucose infusion and insulin are withheld fall into two categories. If the procedure is short (~2 hours or less) and general anesthesia is not necessary, their usual insulin dose can be given postoperatively. This approach applies to those patients who will be able to eat soon after receiving their insulin. The usual eating and insulin administration schedule for the rest of the day should be delayed as well to minimize disruption of the relationship between the two. This method of insulin management works very well for patients undergoing minor outpatient procedures, especially those with type 2 diabetes. One needs to be certain that the delay before insulin administration will not be more than several hours for type 1 patients, who may develop hyperglycemia and possibly ketosis after a (painful) surgical procedure when the effect of the previous evening's insulin wanes. If patients will be unable to eat until supper (whether inpatient or outpatient), regular or lispro insulin should be given every 3 to 4 hours to control the blood glucose level until supper. If patients are in the hospital, a concomitant glucose infusion is preferred to lessen the chances of hypoglycemia. If patients return home after an outpatient procedure, the physician must be certain that they (or a family member) will be able to measure the blood glucose reliably and respond appropriately by giving the suggested insulin doses.

Patients undergoing major surgery, especially abdominal operations, will not be able to eat for various lengths of time postoperatively. Their parenteral nutrition should include at least 100 g of glucose (2 L of 5% dextrose in water) over each 24-hour period to avoid starvation ketosis. It is important that the physician managing the insulin regimen also write the orders concerning the glucose infusion (or for any other source of carbohydrate administration). There is a potential danger if the rate of glucose administration is changed or possibly even reduced to zero once insulin has been given on the basis of a presumed different rate of glucose infusion. I attempt to come to an agreement with the surgeons that I alone will write the orders for insulin doses *and* dextrose infusions. This may entail two intravenous lines, but this additional safeguard against a mismatch between insulin and glucose administration is well worth it.

The principle underlying the postoperative insulin management of diabetic patients is to provide continuous insulin coverage because patients are receiving a constant amount of glucose per unit of time. Three insulin regimens conveniently accomplish this. Although labor-intensive, an insulin infusion with bedside glucose monitoring and insulin rate adjustments every 2 to 3 hours leads to the least variation in glucose levels (see Table 7-21). A second approach is to administer subcutaneous regular insulin every 4 or 6 hours on the basis of the results of bedside glucose monitoring (or a very rapid turnaround time from the hospital laboratory). The least labor-intensive method of providing continuous coverage is to give NPH insulin every 12 hours with additional regular insulin at that time if necessary. This approach does not require bedside monitoring or a particularly rapid response from the laboratory. The glucose concentration obtained before each administration of NPH insulin reflects the effectiveness of the previous injection (i.e., that given 12 hours before). If that value is not available from the laboratory until several hours later, it should be used to adjust the subsequent dose of insulin. If bedside monitoring is being performed, however, and the glucose value is immediately available, the dose of NPH insulin can be adjusted on the basis of that result. As long as patients are receiving dextrose continuously (i.e., by infusion or nasogastric tube), high values should be treated with extra regular insulin as soon as they become available—for example, for glucose concentrations between 150 and 250 mg/dl, 2 to 4 U is given; between 250 and 350 mg/dl, 6 to 8 U; and for >350 mg/dl, 8 to 10 U.

For instance, if patients are receiving insulin at 0800 and 2000 in a situation in which blood samples are sent to a hospital laboratory, the morning glucose concentration should be used to judge the evening dose and the glucose value at 2000 helps to determine what adjustments (if any) should be made the following morning. Lean patients are started on 10 U of NPH every 12 hours, and obese patients (i.e., those at >120% of desirable body weight; see Appendix to this chapter for estimation) are begun on 16 U of NPH insulin at both times. (These initial amounts of insulin may be changed if patient's sensitivity to insulin, as reflected in their usual insulin regimen, suggests that different doses would be more effective.) Each dose of NPH insulin is increased by 2 to 4 U if the appropriate glucose concentration is >180 mg/dl. If the glucose level is >150 mg/dl, extra regular insulin is given when that value becomes known, as described earlier. As patients begin to eat, increasing amounts of insulin can be added to the morning injection. When intravenous glucose is no longer infused overnight (which should occur after oral caloric intake improves considerably), some of the evening dose of NPH insulin also can be shifted to the morning. In this manner, the transition from total parenteral nutrition through partial oral supplementation to normal food intake can be accomplished smoothly without large fluctuations in diabetic control. The following case should serve to illustrate this approach.

The patient is a 37-year-old woman who has had type 1 diabetes for 17 years. She is 5 feet 5 inches tall and weighs 142 pounds. Her insulin regimen consists of 28 U of NPH and 8 U of regular insulin in the morning and 12 U of NPH insulin before supper. She was admitted to the hospital for an elective cholecystectomy after intermittent episodes of colicky pain in the right upper quadrant associated with mild postprandial nausea. (Several previous abdominal operations for appendicitis and gynecologic problems precluded a laparoscopic cholecystectomy.) On the morning of surgery, she received 24 U of NPH insulin; the appropriate glucose infusion was started, and she went to the operating room at 0900. Her postoperative course is summarized in Table 7–22.

A blood sample for glucose determination was sent to the laboratory at 1300 when she arrived in the recovery room. The value of 384 mg/dl returned at 1400, for which she was given 10 U of regular insulin. Another blood sample was sent at 1800, and the result returned at 1900—227 mg/dl—for which she received 4 U of regular insulin. At 2200, another blood sample was sent and she was given 10 U of NPH insulin because she is not obese. She received 6 U of regular insulin when the results of the 2200 sample were returned 1 1/2 hours later. Unfortunately, the response to this injection of regular insulin was not evaluated and she probably remained markedly hyperglycemic throughout the night. Her morning glucose level on 7/24, the first day after surgery, revealed an inadequate response to the insulin given the previous evening, and she was given 10 U of regular insulin when the value was reported.

If the morning or evening glucose concentration exceeds 250 mg/dl, the response to the regular insulin administered should be checked 3 to 4 hours later. This ensures that marked hyperglycemia is not present throughout the 12-hour period until the sampling before the next NPH insulin injection. If glucose levels continue to exceed 250 mg/dl at these subsequent times, appropriate amounts of regular insulin can be given again. Although both the previous NPH insulin and the subsequent regular insulin doses will have their maximal effects during the same time period, hypoglycemia is very unlikely to occur given the fact that the blood glucose level exceeded 250 mg/dl when the

Table 7–22. Postoperative Course of a Type 1 Diabetic Patient After Cholecystectomy

Date	Time	Plasma Glucose (mg/dl)	Amount (U) of Insulin (Type)	Remarks
7/23	1300	384		Enters recovery room; receives 5%
	1400		10 (Reg)[a]	dextrose solution at 125 ml/h
	1800	227		
	1900		4 (Reg)[a]	
	2200	289	10 (NPH)	
	2330		6 (Reg)[a]	
7/24	0800	397	10 (NPH)	
	1000		10 (Reg)[a]	
	1400	241		
	2000	283	14 (NPH)	
	2200		8 (Reg)[a]	
7/25	0200	206		
	0800	313	14 (NPH)	
	1000		10 (Reg)[a]	
	1400	190		
	2000	275	18 (NPH)	
	2200		6 (Reg)[a]	
7/26	0200	187		
	0800	225	18 (NPH)	Bowel sounds present
	1000		4 (Reg)[a]	
	1400	168		
	2000	210	18 (NPH)	
	2130		3 (Reg)[a]	
7/27	0130	163		
	0800	178	18 (NPH)	Liquid diet started but patient vomited
	2000	164	18 (NPH)	
7/28	0800	172	18 (NPH)	Liquid diet tolerated
	2000	154	18 (NPH)	
7/29	0800	163	18 (NPH)	Soft diet started
	2000	143	18 (NPH)	
7/30	0800	174	18 (NPH)	Glucose infusion stopped; soft diet
	1600	265	12 (NPH)	continued
7/31	0800	143	22 (NPH)	
	1130	258		
	1600	225	12 (NPH)	
8/1	0800	158	26 (NPH) 2 (Reg)	Normal diet tolerated
	1130	227		
	1600	179	12 (NPH)	
	2200	284		
8/2	0800	138	26 (NPH) 4 (Reg)	Patient ambulatory
	1130	198		
	1600	183	12 (NPH) 4 (Reg)	
	2200	217		
8/3	0800	147	26 (NPH) 6 (Reg)	
	1130	156	12 (NPH) 6 (Reg)	
	1600	163		
	2200	172		
8/4	0800	153	26 (NPH) 6 (Reg)	Patient discharged after breakfast

[a]Regular insulin given according to glucose value measured several hours previously.

regular insulin was received and that glucose is being infused. On the other hand, I do not routinely measure the blood glucose level during the 12-hour period between NPH insulin administration if the last value was <250 mg/dl because marked hyperglycemia is unlikely to occur during this time. In the case under discussion (see Table 7–22), the glucose concentration 4 hours after 10 U of regular insulin was 241 mg/dl and no further regular insulin was given.

That evening, the amount of NPH insulin was increased to 14 U because the dose on the previous evening was inadequate. Because the glucose concentration that evening was 283 mg/dl, she was given 8 extra U of regular insulin at 2200, and the response to it was adequate. The morning dose of NPH insulin was increased the following day. The amounts of NPH insulin were increased gradually on 7/25 and 7/26. Decreasing amounts of regular insulin also had to be given during this period. Strict control during the immediate postoperative period, when a patient is experiencing pain and receiving infusions of glucose, can be difficult to attain.

Although the patient began a liquid diet on 7/27, the insulin doses were not changed because the glucose infusions were maintained and the initial oral intake was limited. Extra regular insulin was withheld because glucose values were mostly <200 mg/dl. On 7/30, when she could tolerate a soft diet and the intravenous dextrose was discontinued, the effect of the morning dose of NPH insulin was evaluated before supper (at 1600 instead of 2000) and the evening dose of insulin was reduced. The pattern of adjusting her subsequent insulin requirements followed the guidelines discussed in Chapter 4.

The following approach is recommended for patients who do not require insulin. Those whose diabetes is controlled by dietary therapy alone can be treated in the same way as nondiabetic patients. Monitoring of glucose concentrations is important, however, because hyperglycemia can occur secondary to the stress of surgery and postoperative discomfort. Although deterioration of diabetic control usually is temporary, glucose concentrations persistently elevated at >250 mg/dl should be treated with small doses of NPH insulin. Sulfonylurea agents should be discontinued on the day of surgery; chlorpropamide, however, should be discontinued the day before surgery because it has a long half-life (see Chapter 5). Metformin should also be discontinued 48 hours before surgery, and acarbose can simply be omitted when patients stop eating. With minor surgery, oral medication should be resumed when patients resume eating. Major surgical procedures often cause marked elevations in glucose concentration in patients who required oral antidiabetes medication before surgery. Therefore, lean individuals should receive 10 U of NPH insulin and obese individuals (>120% desirable body weight) should receive 16 U of NPH insulin on the morning of surgery. All patients should then be monitored in the manner described for insulin-requiring diabetic patients. When patients start eating again, the insulin should be withdrawn gradually and the oral antidiabetes agent resumed. Metformin and acarbose can also be resumed but may cause gastrointestinal symptoms and need to be retitrated if they have been withheld for a week or more. Patients' responses in this situation will vary.

APPENDIX

ESTIMATION OF DESIRABLE BODY WEIGHT (DBW)

For females, allow 100 pounds for the first 5 feet and 5 pounds for each additional inch.

For males, allow 106 pounds for the first 5 feet and 6 pounds for each additional inch.

Subtract 10% for a small frame size; add 10% for a large frame size.

To estimate frame size, have the patient take the predominant hand (e.g., right hand if right-handed or left hand if left-handed) and grasp the other wrist, opposing the thumb and middle (third) finger. If the two meet, the patient has a medium frame and no adjustment of the DBW calculated above is indicated. If the two overlap, the patient has a small frame and the value calculated above should be decreased by 10% to give the appropriate DBW. If there is a gap between the thumb and middle finger, the patient has a large frame and the value calculated above should be increased by 10% to give the appropriate DBW.

REFERENCES

1. American Diabetes Association: Clinical practice recommendation. Diabetes Care 20(suppl 1):S5, 1997
2. Ishihara M, Yukimura Y, Aizawa T et al: High blood pressure as risk factor in diabetic retinopathy development in NIDDM patients. Diabetes Care 10:20, 1987
3. Teuscher A, Schnell H, Wilson PWF: Incidence of diabetic retinopathy and relationship to baseline plasma glucose and blood pressure. Diabetes Care 11:246, 1988
4. Klein R, Klein BEK, Moss SE et al: Is blood pressure a predictor of the incidence or progression of diabetic retinopathy? Arch Intern Med 149:2427, 1989
5. Mogensen CE, Schmitz O: The diabetic kidney: from hyperfiltration and microalbuminuria to end-stage renal failure. Med Clin North Am 72:1465, 1988
6. Krolewski AS: The natural history of diabetic nephropathy in type I diabetes and the role of hypertension. In Noth RH (ed): Diabetic nephropathy: hemodynamic basis and implications for disease management. Ann Intern Med 110:795, 1989
7. Katz PP, Wirthlin MR, Szpunar SM et al: Epidemiology and prevention of periodontal disease in individuals with diabetes. Diabetes Care 14:375, 1991
8. McNeely MJ, Boyko EJ, Ahroni JH et al: The independent contributions of diabetic neuropathy and vasculopathy in foot ulceration. Diabetes Care 18:216, 1995
9. Rubenstein LZ, Greenfield S: The baseline ECG in the evaluation of acute cardiac complaints. JAMA 244:2536, 1980
10. Hoffman JR, Igarashi E: Influence of electrocardiographic findings on admission decisions in patients with acute chest pain. Am J Med 79:699, 1985
11. Sox HC, Garber AM, Littenberg B: The resting electrocardiogram as a screening test. A clinical analysis. Ann Intern Med 111:489, 1989
11a. Daneman D, Wolfson DH, Becker DJ et al: Factors affecting glycosylated hemoglobin values in children with insulin-dependent diabetes. J Pediatr 99:847, 1981
12. Drash AL, Kingsley LA, Doft B et al: Observations on the effects of changing therapeutic strategies on metabolic status and microvascular complications in IDDM. Pediatr Adolesc Endocrinol 17:206, 1988
13. Peter Chase H, Jackson WE, Hoops SL et al: Glucose control and the renal and retinal complications of insulin-dependent diabetes. JAMA 261:1155, 1989
14. Larsen ML, Horder M, Mogensen EF: Effect of long-term monitoring of glycosylated hemoglobin levels in insulin-dependent diabetes mellitus. N Engl J Med 323:1021, 1990
15. Daneman D: Glycated hemoglobin in the assessment of diabetes control. Endocrinologist 4:33, 1994
16. The Diabetes Control and Complications Trial Research Group: The effect of intensive treatment of diabetes on the development and progression of long-term complications in insulin-dependent diabetes mellitus. N Engl J Med 329:977, 1993
17. Ohkubo Y, Kishikawa H, Araki E et al: Intensive insulin therapy prevents the progression of diabetic microvascular complications in Japanese patients with non-insulin-dependent diabetes mellitus: a randomized prospective 6-year study. Diabetes Res Clin Pract 28:103, 1995
18. Krolewski AS, Laffel LMB, Krolewski M et al: Glycosylated hemoglobin and the risk of microalbuminuria in patients with insulin-dependent diabetes mellitus. N Engl J Med 332:1251, 1995
19. Summary of the second report of the National Cholesterol Education Program (NCEP): expert panel on detection, evaluation, and treatment of high blood cholesterol in adults treatment panel II. JAMA 269:3015, 1993
20. American Diabetes Association: Detection

and management of lipid disorders in diabetes. Diabetes Care 16:828, 1993

21. American College of Physicians, American Diabetes Association and American Academy of Ophthalmology: Screening guidelines for diabetic retinopathy. Ann Intern Med 116:683, 1992

22. The Diabetic Retinopathy Study Group: Photocoagulation treatment of proliferative diabetic retinopathy: clinical application of diabetic retinopathy study (DRS) findings, DRS report number 8. Ophthalmology 88:583, 1981

23. Early Treatment Diabetic Retinopathy Study Research Group: Photocoagulation for diabetic macular edema: early treatment diabetic retinopathy study report number 1. Arch Ophthalmol 103:1796, 1985

24. Javitt JC, Aiello LP: Cost-effectiveness of detecting and treating diabetic retinopathy. Ann Intern Med 124 (1 pt 2):164, 1996

25. Edmonds ME, Blundell MP, Morris HE et al: The diabetic foot: impact of a foot clinic. Q J Med 232:763, 1986

26. Willard JE, Lange RA, Hillis LD: The use of aspirin in ischemic heart disease. N Engl J Med 327:175, 1992

27. Steering Committee of the Physicians' Health Study Research Group: Final report on the aspirin component of the ongoing physicians' heath study. N Engl J Med 321:129, 1989

28. Fuster V, Cohen M, Halperin J: Aspirin in the prevention of coronary disease. N Engl J Med 321:183, 1989

29. Manson JE, Tosteson H, Ridker PM et al: The primary prevention of myocardial infarction. N Engl J Med 326:1406, 1992

30. EDTRS Investigators: Aspirin effects on mortality and morbidity in patients with diabetes mellitus: early treatment diabetic retinopathy study report 14. JAMA 268:1292, 1992

31. Clement S: Diabetes self-management education. Diabetes Care 18:1204, 1995

32. Wing RR, Epstein LH, Nowalk MP et al: Does self-monitoring of blood glucose levels improve dietary compliance for obese patients with type II diabetes? Am J Med 81:830, 1986

33. Klein CE, Oboler SK, Prochazka A et al: Home blood glucose monitoring. J Gen Intern Med 8:597, 1993

34. Patrick AW, Gill GV, MacFarlane IA et al: Home glucose monitoring in type 2 diabetes: is it a waste of time? Diabetic Med 11:62, 1994

35. Feldman JM, Kelley WN, Lebovitz HE: Inhibition of glucose oxidase paper tests by reducing metabolites. Diabetes 19:337, 1970

36. Johansen K, Svendsen PA, Lørup B: Variation in renal threshold for glucose in type 1 (insulin-dependent) diabetes mellitus. Diabetologia 26:180, 1984

37. Hayford JT, Weydert JA, Thompson RG: Validity of urine glucose measurements for estimating plasma glucose concentration. Diabetes Care 6:40, 1983

38. Rotblatt MD, Koda-Kimble MA: Review of drug interference with urine glucose tests. Diabetes Care 10:103, 1987

39. Feldman JM, Lebovitz FL: Tests for glucosuria. An analysis of factors that cause misleading results. Diabetes 22:115, 1973

40. Self TH, Wester VL: Noneffect of isoniazid on urine glucose tests. Diabetes Care 3:44, 1980

41. Bowers CB, Self TH: Noneffect of methyldopa on urine glucose tests. Diabetes Care 1:36, 1978

42. Caraway WT, Kammeyer CW: Chemical interference by drugs and other substances with clinical laboratory test procedures. Clin Chim Acta 41:395, 1972

43. Wolcott GJ, Hackett TN Jr: Levodopa and tests for ketonuria (letter). N Engl J Med 283:1522, 1970

44. Pocelinko R, Solomon HM, Gaut ZN: Doped dipsticks (letter). N Engl J Med 281:1075, 1969

45. Warren SE: False-positive urine ketone test with captopril (letter). N Engl J Med 303:1003, 1980

46. Guthrie DW, Hinnen D, Guthrie RA: Single-voided vs. double-voided urine testing. Diabetes Care 2:269, 1979

47. McCarthy J: Double-voided dilemma. Am J Nurs 79:1249, 1979

48. Davidson MB: The case for routinely testing the first-voided urine specimen. Diabetes Care 4:443, 1981

49. Malone JI, Rosenbloom AL, Grgic A, Weber FT: The role of urine sugar in diabetic management. Am J Dis Child 130:1324, 1976

50. Morris LR, McGee JA, Kitabchi AE: Correlation between plasma and urine glucose in diabetes. Ann Intern Med 94:469, 1981

51. Galagan RC, Strack TR, Leibel BS, Albisser AM: Urine glucose measurements: reappraisal of their clinical limitations and value. Diabetes Nutr Metab 1:89, 1988

52. Worth R, Home PD, Johnston DG et al: Intensive attention improves glycaemic control in insulin-dependent diabetes without further advantage from blood glucose monitoring: results of controlled trial. BMJ 285:1233, 1982

53. Muhlhauser I, Bruckner I, Berger M et al: Evaluation of an intensified insulin treatment and teaching programme as routine management of type-I (insulin-dependent) diabetes. Diabetologia 30:681, 1987

54. Baynes JW, Bunn HF, Goldstein D et al: National Diabetes Data Group: report of the expert committee on glucosylated hemoglobin. Diabetes Care 7:602, 1984

55. Goldstein DE, Little RR, Wiedmeyer HM et al: Glycated hemoglobin: methodologies and clinical applications. Clin Chem 32:B64, 1986

56. Jackson RL, Hess RL, England JD: Hemoglobin A_{1c} values in children with overt diabetes maintained in varying degrees of control. Diabetes Care 2:391, 1979

57. Koenig RJ, Peterson CM, Jones RL et al: Correlation of glucose regulation and hemoglobin A_{1c} in diabetes mellitus. N Engl J Med 295:417, 1976

58. Gabbay KH, Hasty K, Breslow JL et al: Glycosylated hemoglobins and long-term blood glucose control in diabetes mellitus. J Clin Endocrinol Metab 44:859, 1977

59. Schultz TA, Lewis SB, Davis JL et al: Effect of sulfonylurea therapy and plasma glucose levels on hemoglobin A_{1c} in type II diabetes mellitus. Am J Med 70:373, 1981

60. Tahara Y, Shima K: The response on GHb to stepwise plasma glucose change over time in diabetic patients. Diabetes Care 16:1313, 1993

61. Bunn HF: Evaluation of glycosylated hemoglobin in diabetic patients. Diabetes 30:613, 1981

62. Service FJ, Fairbanks VF, Rizza RA: Effect on hemoglobin A_1 of rapid normalization of glycemia with an artificial endocerine pancreas. Mayo Clin Proc 56:377, 1981

63. Boden G, Master RW, Gordon SS et al: Monitoring metabolic control in diabetic outpatients with glycosylated hemoglobin. Ann Intern Med 92:357, 1980

64. Compagnucci P, Cartechini MG, Bolli G et al: The importance of determining irreversibly glycosylated hemoglobin in diabetics. Diabetes 30:607, 1981

65. Fairbanks V: The incidence of hemoglobin variants and their effect on glycated hemoglobin assay results. In Service FJ, Sheehan J (eds): Symposium Proceedings, Isolab, Akron, OH, 1988, p. 28

66. Eberentz-Lhomme C, Ducrocq R, Intrator S et al: Haemoglobinopathies: a pitfall in the assessment of glycosylated haemoglobin by ion-exchange chromatography. Diabetologia 27:596, 1984

67. Goldstein DE, Little RR, Lorenz RA et al: Tests of glycemia in diabetes. Diabetes Care 18:896, 1995

68. Garlick RL, Mazer JS, Higgins PJ, Bunn HF: Characterization of glycosylated hemoglobins. Relevance to monitoring of diabetic control and analysis of other proteins. J Clin Invest 71:1062, 1983

69. Davie SJ, Gould BJ, Yudkin JS: Effect of vitamin C on glycosylation of proteins. Diabetes 41:167, 1992

70. Ceriello A, Giugliano D, Quatraro A et al: Vitamin E reduction of protein glycoslyation in diabetes: new prospect for prevention of diabetic complications? Diabetes Care 14:68, 1991

71. Nathan DM, Singer DE, Hurxthal K, Goodson JD: The clinical information value of the glycosylated hemoglobin assay. N Engl J Med 310:341, 1984

72. Santiago JV: Perspectives in diabetes: lessons from the Diabetes Control and Complications Trial. Diabetes 42:1549, 1993

73. McFarland KF, Catalano EW, Day JF et al: Nonenzymatic glycosylation of serum proteins in diabetes mellitus. Diabetes 28:1011, 1979

74. Jones IR, Owens DR, Williams S et al: Glycosylated serum albumin: an intermediate index of diabetic control. Diabetes Care 6:501, 1983

75. Ziel FH, Davidson MB: The role of glycosylated serum albumin in monitoring glycemic control in stable insulin-requiring diabetic outpatients. J Clin Endocrinol Metab 64:269, 1987

76. Rendell M, Kao G, Mecherikunnel P et al: Use of aminophenylboronic acid affinity chromatography to measure glycosylated albumin levels. J Lab Clin Med 105:63, 1985

77. Armbruster DA: Fructosamine: structure, analysis, and clinical usefulness. Clin Chem 33:2153, 1987

78. Smart LM, Howie AF, Young RJ et al: Comparison of fructosamine with glycosylated hemoglobin and plasma proteins as measures of glycemic control. Diabetes Care 11:433, 1988

79. Negoro H, Morley JE, Rosenthal MJ: Utility of serum fructosamine as a measure of glycemia in young and old diabetic and nondiabetic subjects. Am J Med 85:360, 1988

80. Ashby JP, Frier BM: Is serum fructosamine a clinically useful test? Diabetic Med 5:118, 1988

81. Dominiczak MH, Smith LA, McNaught J et al: Assessment of past glycemic control: measure fructosamine, hemoglobin A_1 or both? Diabetes Care 11:359, 1988

82. Watts GF, Macleod AF, Benn JJ et al: Comparison of the real-time use of glycosylated haemoglobin and plasma fructosamine in the diabetic clinic. Diabetic Med 8:573, 1991

83. Furuseth K, Bruusgaard D, Rutle O et al: Fructosamine cannot replace Hb A_{1c} in the management of type 2 diabetes (NIDDM). Scand J Prim Health Care 12:219, 1994

84. McCance DR, Coulter D, Smye M, Kennedy L: Effect of fluctuations in albumin on serum fructosamine assay. Diabetic Med 4:434, 1987

85. Schleicher ED, Mayer R, Wagner EM, Gerbitz K-D: Is serum fructosamine assay specific for determination of glycated serum protein? Clin Chem 34:320, 1988

86. Skrha J, Svacina S: Serum fructosamine and obesity. Clin Chem 37:2020, 1991

87. Windeler J, Kobberling J: The fructosamine assay in diagnosis and control of diabetes mellitus: scientific evidence for its clinical usefulness? J Clin Chem Biochem 28:129, 1990

88. Lee PDK, Sherman LD, O'Day MR et al: Comparisons of home blood glucose testing and glycated protein measurements. Diabetes Res Clin Pract 16:53, 1992

89. Aebi-Ochsner CH, Grey VL: Fructosamine measurements in the adolescent with type I diabetes. Diabetes Care 18:1619, 1995

90. Consensus statement on self-monitoring of blood glucose. Diabetes Care 10:95, 1987

91. American Diabetes Association Consensus Statement: Self-monitoring of blood glucose. Diabetes Care 19(suppl 1):S62, 1996

92. Harris MI, Cowie CC, Howie LJ: Self-monitoring of blood glucose by adults with diabetes in the United States population. Diabetes Care 16:1116, 1993

93. Hiss RG, Anderson RM, Hess GE et al: Community diabetes care: A 10-year perspective. Diabetes Care 17:1124, 1994

94. Spraul M, Sonnenberg GE, Berger M: Less expensive, reliable blood glucose self-monitoring. Diabetes Care 10:357, 1987

95. Anderson J: Effect of storage in light and dark on accuracy of blood glucose test strips. Diabetic Med 2:134, 1985

96. Cox D, Herrman J, Snyder A et al: Stability of reacted chemstrip bG. Diabetes Care 11:288, 1988

97. Mezitis NHE, Heshka S, Zappulla D et al: Stability of stored chemstrip bG. Diabetes Care 13:179, 1990

98. Gifford-Jorgensen RA, Borchert J, Hassanein R et al: Comparison of five glucose meters for self-monitoring of blood glucose by diabetic patients. Diabetes Care 9:70, 1986

99. North DS, Steiner JF, Woodhouse KM, Maddy JA: Home monitors of blood glucose: comparison of precision and accuracy. Diabetes Care 10:360, 1987

100. Clarke WL, Cox D, Gonder-Frederick LA et al: Evaluating clinical accuracy of systems for self-monitoring of blood glucose. Diabetes Care 10:622, 1987

101. Rockett M, Anderly D, Bessman A: Blue-yellow vision deficits in patients with diabetes. West J Med 146:431, 1987

102. Keeling AB, Schmidt P: Dopamine influence on whole-blood glucose reagent strips. Diabetes Care 10:532, 1987

103. Rice GK, Galt KA: In vitro drug interference with home blood-glucose-measurement systems. Am J Hosp Pharm 42:2202, 1985

104. Atkin SH, Dasmahapatra A, Jaker MA et al: Fingerstick glucose determination in shock. Ann Intern Med 114:1020, 1991

105. Mazze RS, Shamoon H, Pasmantier R et al: Reliability of blood glucose monitoring by patients with diabetes mellitus. Am J Med 77:211, 1984

106. William CD, Scobie IN, Till S et al: Use of memory meters to measure reliability of self blood glucose monitoring. Diabetic Med 5:459, 1988

107. Ziegler O, Kolopp M, Got I et al: Reliability of self-monitoring of blood glucose by CSII-treated patients with type I diabetes. Diabetes Care 12:184, 1989

108. Graber AL, Wooldridge K, Brown A: Effects of intensified practitioner-patient communication on control of diabetes mellitus. South Med J 79:1205, 1986

109. Pirart J: Diabetes mellitus and its degenerative complications: a prospective study of 4,400 patients observed between 1947 and 1973. Diabetes Care 1:168, 1978

110. Olsson P-O, Hans A, Henning VS: Miscibility of human semisynthetic regular and lente insulin and human biosynthetic regular and NPH insulin. Diabetes Care 10:473, 1987

111. Robert JJ, Chevenne D, Debray M: The contribution of intermediate-acting insulin preparations to daytime insulin treatment. Diabetic Med 6:531, 1989

112. Mühlhauser I, Broermann C, Tsotsalas M, Berger M: Miscibility of human and bovine ultralente insulin with soluble insulin. BMJ 289:1656, 1984

113. Torlone E, Pampanelli S, Lalli C et al: Effects of the short-acting insulin analog [Lys(B8), Pro(B29)] on postprandial blood glucose control in IDDM. Diabetes Care 19:945, 1996

114. Package Insert. Humalog: insulin lispro injection (rDNA origin). Eli Lilly & Co, Indianapolis, IN, 1996

115. Munro JF, Campbell IW, McCuish AC, Duncan LJP: Euglycaemic diabetic ketoacidosis. BMJ 2:578, 1973

116. Waldhäusl W, Howorka K, Derfler K et al: Failure and efficacy of insulin therapy in insulin dependent (type I) diabetic patients. Acta Diabetol Lat 22:279, 1985

117. Waldhäusl WK: The physiological basis of insulin treatment—clinical aspects. Diabetologia 29:837, 1986

118. Gale EA, Kurtz AB, Tattersall RB: In search of the Somogyi effect. Lancet 2:279, 1980

119. Gerich JE: Dawn phenomenon: pathophysiology, diagnosis, and treatment. Clin Diabetes 6:1, 1988

120. De Feo P, Perriello G, Bolli GB: Somogyi and dawn phenomena: mechanisms. Diabetes Metab Rev 4:31, 1988

121. Davidson MB, Harris MD, Ziel FH et al: Suppression of sleep-induced growth hormone secretion by anticholinergic agent abolishes dawn phenomenon. Diabetes 37:166, 1988

122. Lerman IG, Wolfsdorf JI: Relationship of nocturnal hypoglycemia to daytime glycemia in IDDM. Diabetes Care 111:636, 1988

123. Stephenson JM, Schernthaner G: Dawn phenomenon and Somogyi effect in IDDM. Diabetes Care 12:245, 1989

124. Hirsch IB, Smith LJ, Havlin CE et al: Failure of nocturnal hypoglycemia to cause daytime hyperglycemia in patients with IDDM. Diabetes Care 13:133, 1990

125. Clarke WL, Haymond MW, Santiago JV: Overnight basal insulin requirements in fasting insulin-dependent diabetics. Diabetes 29:78, 1980

126. Cryer PE: Glucose counterregulation in man. Diabetes 30:261, 1981

127. Bolli G, De Feo P, Compagnucci P et al: Abnormal glucose counterregulation in insulin-dependent diabetes mellitus: interaction of anti-insulin antibodies and impaired glucagon and epinephrine secretion. Diabetes 32:134, 1983

128. Kleinbaum J, Shamoon: Impaired counterregulation of hypoglycemia in insulin-dependent diabetes mellitus. Diabetes 32:493, 1983

129. Goldstein DE, Parker KM, England JD et al: Clinical application of glycosylated hemoglobin measurements. Diabetes 31(suppl 3):70, 1982

130. Lorenz RA, Santiago JV, Siebert C et al: Epidemiology of severe hypoglycemia in the Diabetes Control and Complications Trial. Am J Med 90:450, 1991

131. Park BN, Soeldner JS, Gleason RE: Diabetes in remission. Insulin secretory dynamics. Diabetes 23:616, 1974

132. Henry RR, Gumbiner B, Ditzler T et al: Intensive conventional insulin therapy for type II diabetes. Diabetes Care 16:21, 1993

133. Carlson MG, Campbell PJ: Intensive insulin therapy and weight gain in IDDM. Diabetes 42:1700, 1993

134. Shank ML, Del Prato S, DeFronzo RA: Bedtime insulin/daytime glipizide: effective therapy for sulfonylurea failures in NIDDM. Diabetes 44:165, 1995

135. Woods SC, Porte D, Bobbioni E et al: Insulin: its relationship to the central nervous system and to the control of food intake and body weight. Am J Clin Nutr 42:1063, 1985

136. Tattersall R: Brittle diabetes. Clin Endocrinol Metab 6:403, 1977

137. Yue DK, Baxter RC, Turtle JR: C-peptide secretion and insulin antibodies as determinants of stability in diabetes mellitus. Metabolism 27:35, 1978

138. Pickup J, Williams G, Johns P, Keen H: Clinical features of brittle diabetic patients unresponsive to optimized subcutaneous insulin therapy (continuous subcutaneous insulin infusion). Diabetes Care 6:279, 1983

139. Schade DS, Drumm DA, Duckworth WC, Eaton RP: The etiology of incapacitating, brittle diabetes. Diabetes Care 8:12, 1985

140. Gill GV, Walford S, Alberti KGMM: Brittle diabetes—present concepts. Diabetologia 29:579, 1985

141. Schade DS: Brittle diabetes: strategies, diagnosis, and treatment. Diabetes Metab Rev 4:371, 1988

142. Schade DA, Eaton RP, Drumm DA, Duckworth WC: A clinical algorithm to determine the etiology of brittle diabetes. Diabetes Care 8:5, 1985

142a. Davidson MB, Kumar D, Smith W: Successful treatment of unusual case of brittle diabetes with sulfated beef insulin. Diabetes Care 14:1109, 1991

142b. Amiel SA, Sherwin RS, Simonson DC, Tamborlane WV: Effect of intensive insulin therapy on glycemic thresholds for counterregulatory hormone release. Diabetes 37:901, 1988

142c. Henrichs HR, Unger H, Fittkau T et al: Treatment of a case of severe subcutaneous insulin resistance using the insulin analogue Lys(B28),Pro(B29) for facilitated subcutaneous absorption. Diabetologia 37(suppl 1):A168, 1994

142d. Falko BF, O'Dorisio JM, Osei K: The use of continuous octreotide infusion in brittle type I diabetic patients. Diabetic Med 8:385, 1991

143. Boyle PJ, Schwartz NS, Shah SD et al: Plasma glucose concentrations at the onset of hypoglycemic symptoms in patients with poorly controlled diabetes and in nondiabetics. N Engl J Med 318:1487, 1988

144. Jones TW, Boulware SD, Kraemer DT et al: Independent effects of youth and poor diabetes control on responses to hypoglycemia in children. Diabetes 40:358, 1991

145. Cryer PE, Fisher JN, Shamoon H: Hypoglycemia. Diabetes Care 17:734, 1994

146. Amiel SA, Pottinger RC, Archibald HR et al: Effect of antecedent glucose control on cerebral function during hypoglycemia. Diabetes Care 14:109, 1991

147. Mitrakou A, Fanelli C, Veneman T et al: Reversibility of unawareness of hypoglycemia in patients with insulinomas. N Engl J Med 329:834, 1993

148. Heller SR, Cryer PE: Reduced neuroendocrine and symptomatic responses to subsequent hypoglycemia after one episode of hypoglycemia in nondiabetic humans. Diabetes 40:223, 1991

149. Widom B, Simonson DC: Intermittent hypoglycemia impairs glucose counterregulation. Diabetes 41:1597, 1992

150. Hvidberg A, Fanelli CG, Hershey T et al: Impact of recent antecedent hypoglycemia on hypoglycemic cognitive dysfunction in nondiabetic humans. Diabetes 45:1030, 1996

151. Dagogo-Jack SE, Craft S, Cryer PE: Hypoglycemia-associated autonomic failure in insulin-dependent diabetes mellitus. J Clin Invest 91:819, 1993

152. Lingenfelser T, Renn W, Sommerwerck U et al: Compromised hormonal counterregulation, symptom awareness, and neurophysiological function after recurrent short-term episodes of insulin-induced hypoglycemia in IDDM patients. Diabetes 42:610, 1993

153. Lingenfelser T, Buettner U, Martin J et al: Improvement of impaired counterregulatory hormone response and symptom perception by short-term avoidance of hypoglycemia in IDDM. Diabetes Care 18:321, 1995

154. Rattarasarn C, Dagogo-Jack S, Zachwieja JJ et al: Hypoglycemia-induced autonomic failure in IDDM is specific for stimulus of hypoglycemia and is not attributable to prior autonomic activation. Diabetes 43:809, 1994

155. Fanelli C, Pampanelli S, Epifano L et al: Long-term recovery from unawareness, deficient counterregulation and lack of cognitive dysfunction during hypoglycaemia, following institution of rational, intensive insulin therapy in IDDM. Diabetologia 37:1265, 1994

156. Dagogo-Jack S, Rattarasarn C, Cryer PE: Reversal of hypoglycemia unawareness, but not defective glucose counterregulation, in IDDM. Diabetes 43:1426, 1994

157. Ryder REJ, Owens DR, Hayes TM et al: Unawareness of hypoglycaemia and inadequate hypoglycaemic counterregulation: no casual relation with diabetic autonomic neuropathy. BMJ 301:783, 1990

158. Hepburn DA, MacLeod KM, Frier BM: Physiological, symptomatic and hormonal responses to acute hypoglycaemia in type I diabetic patients with autonomic neuropathy. Diabetic Med 10:940, 1993

159. Gold AE, MacLeod KM, Frier BM: Frequency of severe hypoglycemia in patients with type I diabetes with impaired awareness of hypoglycemia. Diabetes Care 17:697, 1994

160. Colagiuri S, Miller JJ, Petocz P: Double blind crossover comparison of human and porcine insulins in patients reporting lack of hypoglycaemia awareness. Lancet 339:1432, 1992

161. Nellmann Jorgensen L, Dejgaard A, Pramming SK: Human insulin and hypoglycaemia: a literature survey. Diabetic Med 11:925, 1994

162. Brodows RG, Williams C, Amatruda JM: Treatment of insulin reactions in diabetics. JAMA 252:3378, 1984

163. Slama G, Traynard P-Y, Desplanque N et al: The search for an optimized treatment of hypoglycemia: carbohydrates in tablets, solution, or gel for the correction of insulin reactions. Arch Intern Med 150:589, 1990

164. Gunning RR, Garber AJ: Bioactivity of instant glucose, failure of absorption through oral mucosa. JAMA 240:1611, 1978

165. Pontiroli AE, Calderara A, Pajetta E et al: Intranasal glucagon as remedy for hypoglycemia: studies in healthy subjects and type I diabetic patients. Diabetes Care 12:604, 1989

166. Slama G, Alamowitch C, Desplanque N et al: A new non-invasive method for treating insulin-reaction: intranasal lyophylized glucagon. Diabetologia 33:671, 1990

167. Stenninger E, Aman J: Intranasal glucagon treatment relieves hypoglycaemia in children with type I (insulin-dependent) diabetes mellitus. Diabetologia 36:931, 1993

168. Helmrich SP, Ragland DR, Leung RW et al: Physical activity and reduced occurrence of non-insulin-dependent diabetes mellitus. N Engl J Med 325:147, 1991

169. Manson JE, Nathan DM, Krolewski AS et al: Exercise and incidence of diabetes among U.S. male physicians. JAMA 268:63, 1992

170. Schneider SH, Ruderman NB: Exercise and NIDDM. Diabetes Care 13:785, 1990

171. Wasserman DH, Zinman B: Exercise in individuals with IDDM. Diabetes Care 17:924, 1994

172. Schneider SH, Morgado A: Effects of fitness and physical training on carbohydrate metabolism and associated cardiovascular risk factors in patients with diabetes. Diabetes Rev 3:378, 1995

173. Oberman A: Healthy exercise. West J Med 141:864, 1984

174. Schneider SH, Khachadurian AK, Amorosa LF et al: Ten-year experience with an exercise-based outpatient life-style modification program in the treatment of diabetes mellitus. Diabetes Care 15(suppl 4):1800, 1992

175. Selam JL, Casassus P, Bruzzo F et al: Exercise is not associated with better diabetes control in type I and type II diabetic subjects. Acta Diabetol 29:11, 1992

176. Hanisch R, Snyder A: Exercise in insulin dependent diabetes (IDDM) may be safe with starting glucose >16.7 mM. Diabetes 45(suppl 2):107A, 1996

177. Mikines KJ, Sonne B, Farrell PA et al: Effect of physical exercise on sensitivity and responsiveness to insulin in humans. Am J Physiol 254:E248, 1988

178. Mikines KJ, Sonne B, Tronier B et al: Effects of training and detraining on dose-response relationship between glucose and insulin secretion. Am J Physiol 256:E588, 1989

179. Young MJ, Veves A, Boulton AJM: The diabetic foot: aetiopathogenesis and management. Diabetes Metab Rev 9:109, 1993

180. Caputo GM, Cavanagh PR, Ulbrecht JS et al: Assessment and management of foot disease in patients with diabetes. N Engl J Med 331:854, 1994

181. Grayson ML, Gibbons GW, Balogh K et al: Probing to bone in infected pedal ulcers: a clinical sign of underlying osteomyelitis in diabetic patients. JAMA 273:721, 1995

182. Eckman MH, Greenfield S, Mackey WC et al: Foot infections in diabetic patients: deci-

sion and cost-effectiveness analyses. JAMA 273:712, 1995

183. Williams RC: Periodontal disease. N Engl J Med 322:373, 1990

184. Walts LF, Miller J, Davidson MB, Brown J: Perioperative management of diabetes mellitus. Anesthesiology 55:104, 1981

185. Rosenstock J, Raskin P: Surgery! Practical guidelines for diabetes management. Clin Diabetes 5:62, 1987

186. Alberti KGMM, Gil GV, Elliott MJ: Insulin delivery during surgery in the diabetic patient. Diabetes Care 5(suppl 1):65, 1982

187. Fletcher J, Langman MJS, Kellock TD: Effect of surgery on blood-sugar levels in diabetes mellitus. Lancet 2:52, 1965

COMPLICATIONS OF DIABETES MELLITUS: PRIMARY CARE IMPLICATIONS

Diabetes mellitus affects approximately 6% of the population of the United States (>15 million people), and it is estimated that half of these cases remain undiagnosed. The prevalence of diabetes rises with age, with a major increase starting after 40 years of age, reaching approximately 10% in the seventh decade, 15% in the eighth decade, and 20% or greater in the ninth decade.

Although by definition diabetes is characterized by elevated glucose concentrations, the impact of diabetes, on both the health of individuals and on the health care systems of industrialized countries, resides almost entirely in the "complications" of diabetes. The effect of acute hyperglycemia and its associated ketoacidosis in type 1 patients has a very small role in the total mortality, morbidity, and costs ascribed to diabetes mellitus. It has been estimated that diabetes and its associated vascular complications are the fourth leading cause of death in this country. Diabetes is the leading cause of blindness in individuals between 20 and 74 years of age in industrialized countries. Almost half of new patients undergoing dialysis have diabetic nephropathy. More than half of all lower extremity amputations take place in diabetic patients. On a relative basis, people with diabetes are 25 times more likely to develop blindness, 17 times more likely to develop kidney disease, 20 times more likely to develop gangrene, 30 to 40 times more likely to undergo a major amputation, two (males) or four (females) times more likely to develop coronary artery disease, and twice as likely to suffer a stroke than are individuals without diabetes. The total cost of diabetes is approximately 100 billion dollars per year,[1, 2] which accounts for one of every seven health care dollars spent in this country!

Because >90% of diabetic patients are cared for by primary care physicians, it is obvious that major inroads into improving this dismal situation for diabetic patients will have to be initiated by nonspecialists. In the past, it was not clear if anything could be done to ameliorate these complications. As discussed in Chapter 2, it has now been irrefutably demonstrated that strict diabetic control has an important beneficial effect on delaying (and possibly preventing) the appearance of the early changes in diabetic retinopathy, nephropathy, and neuropathy, as well as in reversing them. In addition, primary care physicians should take a number of other approaches to help prevent, recognize, and/or treat diabetic complications.

The complications of diabetes are best considered in three separate categories: (1) macrovascular (large vessel or atherosclerotic) disease, the clinical manifestations of which are angina and myocardial infarctions, cerebrovascular accidents, and peripheral vascular disease; (2) microvascular (small vessel) disease, the clinical manifestations of which are diabetic retinopathy and diabetic nephropathy; and (3) neuropathy (involvement of both the peripheral and autonomic nervous systems), the clinical manifestations of which can lead to various problems.

MACROVASCULAR COMPLICATIONS

Six independent risk factors for macrovascular disease are identified in the general population (smoking, hypertension, hyperlipidemia, obesity, genetic factors, and diabetes mellitus). Whatever the degree of risk an individual has, smoking approximately doubles it. Smoking is obviously a reversible risk factor. Hypertension eventually occurs in approximately 50% of diabetic patients. Although appropriate treatment of hypertension eliminates it as a risk factor, it is estimated that at least 25% of all hypertensive patients do not take their medications. Like diabetes, hypertension is a silent killer without symptoms. Many patients do not bother with treatment. However, if a patient complies with proper treatment, hypertension is also a reversible risk factor. (Controlling hypertension is extremely important in slowing the progression of renal insufficiency. Treatment of hypertension is discussed in the description of diabetic nephropathy.)

The evidence regarding elevated cholesterol levels as a risk factor is very strong. To be more specific, increased levels of low-density lipoproteins (LDL) show the strongest association with macrovascular disease. Low levels of high-density lipoproteins (HDL) are also associated with macrovascular disease. LDL and HDL are usually quantitated by measuring their cholesterol content. HDL cholesterol levels may be measured directly. Although a method of measuring LDL cholesterol concentrations directly has become available in most laboratories, the LDL cholesterol level is calculated from the results of a lipoprotein analysis in which total and HDL cholesterol as well as triglyceride (TG) concentrations are measured. LDL cholesterol concentrations are estimated from the following relationship:

$$\text{LDL cholesterol} = \text{total cholesterol} - \text{HDL cholesterol} - \text{triglycerides}/5$$

TG levels must be measured after an overnight fast (12 hours or more is preferable). If TG concentrations are $\geq$400 mg/dl, the relationship depicted earlier becomes less and less accurate, and the formula should not be used.

The second report of the National Cholesterol Education Program (NCEP), called the *Adult Treatment Panel* II (ATP II),[3] recommended certain changes in their initial report. The revised, rather complicated guidelines for the *general population* are depicted in Figure 8-1. Table 8-1 lists the threshold levels of LDL cholesterol for both initiating dietary treatment and considering drug therapy in subjects with and without coronary artery disease. It also includes goal levels to be achieved.

The greater propensity for coronary artery disease in patients with diabetes is shown in Figure 8-2. Diabetes imposes an increased risk for cardiovascular disease mortality over and beyond what would be expected in the presence of one to three of the more important classic risk factors. Although it is not known for certain what causes this enhanced tendency for macrovascular disease in diabetic patients, a clue may be found in the association of coronary artery disease with a number of other factors. Because insulin resistance seems to be the underlying feature, this clustering of risk factors (in addition to the classic ones mentioned earlier) has been termed the *insulin resistance syndrome*.[4] (Another name is *syndrome X*.) The components of the insulin resistance syndrome are listed in Table 8-2. The association between coronary artery disease and circulating insulin concentrations is noted in some studies involving white middle-aged men. It does not seem to hold in women, older white men, or non-Caucasian populations. Cardiovascular risk is associated with central obesity—that is, android or "apple" obesity—not with gynoid or "pear" obesity. A clinical approach to determine which kind of obesity a patient has is to measure the waist-to-hip ratio (i.e., the circumference at the umbilicus divided by the circumference at the iliac crests). Values >0.85 are considered to represent central obesity in Caucasian populations.

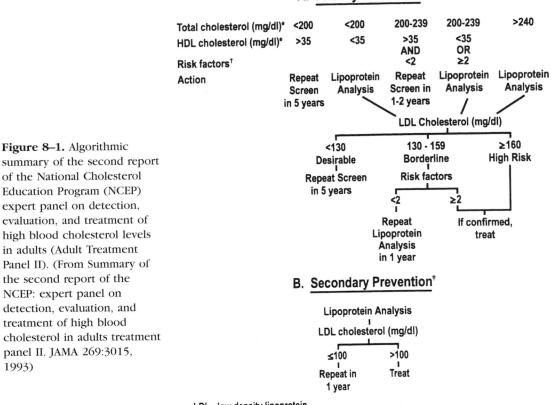

A. Primary Prevention

Total cholesterol (mg/dl)*	<200	<200	200-239	200-239	>240
HDL cholesterol (mg/dl)*	>35	<35	>35 AND <2	<35 OR ≥2	
Risk factors†					
Action	Repeat Screen in 5 years	Lipoprotein Analysis	Repeat Screen in 1-2 years	Lipoprotein Analysis	Lipoprotein Analysis

LDL Cholesterol (mg/dl)

<130 Desirable	130 - 159 Borderline	≥160 High Risk
Repeat Screen in 5 years	Risk factors	

<2	≥2
Repeat Lipoprotein Analysis in 1 year	If confirmed, treat

Figure 8–1. Algorithmic summary of the second report of the National Cholesterol Education Program (NCEP) expert panel on detection, evaluation, and treatment of high blood cholesterol levels in adults (Adult Treatment Panel II). (From Summary of the second report of the NCEP: expert panel on detection, evaluation, and treatment of high blood cholesterol in adults treatment panel II. JAMA 269:3015, 1993)

B. Secondary Prevention†

Lipoprotein Analysis

LDL cholesterol (mg/dl)

≤100	>100
Repeat in 1 year	Treat

LDL - low density lipoprotein
HDL - high density lipoprotein
*Screen consists of total and HDL cholesterol
†Risk factors - age (≥45 years old in men and ≥55 years old in women); family history of premature coronary artery disease, cigarette smoking; hypertension; low HDL cholesterol levels (<35 mg/dl); diabetes mellitus; high HDL cholesterol level (≥60 mg/dl) is a negative risk factor and one other risk factor is subtracted.
†Coronary artery disease or other atherosclerotic disease present.

The dyslipidemia characterizing the insulin resistance syndrome (and found in many patients with type 2 diabetes) does not include elevated LDL cholesterol levels. The prevalence of high LDL concentrations is not increased in patients with type 1 diabetes compared with an appropriately matched nondiabetic control group. Elevated levels of LDL cholesterol were found more often in patients with type 2 diabetes compared with nondiabetic persons in some but not all studies.[5, 6] The dyslipidemia associated with type 2 diabetes is characterized by high TG

and low HDL cholesterol concentrations. In addition to these more familiar alterations in lipid levels, two other changes are more commonly noted in type 2 diabetic patients. These are smaller, dense LDL particles and postprandial large TG-rich lipoprotein particles. Both of these lipid particles increase the risk of coronary artery disease.

The size and density of LDL particles are heterogeneous. Larger particles (pattern A) predominate in the majority of individuals, whereas a minority of subjects have a predominance of smaller particles (pattern B).

Table 8–1. Treatment Decisions Based on LDL Cholesterol Levels

Type of Treatment	Initiation Level	LDL Goal
Dietary therapy		
Without CAD and with fewer than two risk factors	≥160 mg/dl	<160 mg/dl
Without CAD and with two or more risk factors	≥130 mg/dl	<130 mg/dl
With CAD	>100 mg/dl	≤100 mg/dl
	Consideration Level	**LDL Goal**
Drug treatment		
Without CAD and with fewer than two risk factors	≥190 mg/dl[a]	<160 mg/dl
Without CAD and with two or more risk factors	≥160 mg/dl	<130 mg/dl
With CAD	≥130 mg/dl[b]	≤100 mg/dl

LDL, low-density lipoproteins; CAD, coronary artery disease.

[a]In men <35 years old and premenopausal women with LDL cholesterol levels of 190 to 219 mg/dl, drug therapy should be delayed except in high-risk patients such as those with diabetes.

[b]In patients with CAD and LDL cholesterol levels of 100 to 129 mg/dl, the physician should exercise clinical judgment in deciding whether to initiate drug treatment.

From Summary of the Second Report of the National Cholesterol Education Program (NCEP): Expert panel on detection, evaluation, and treatment of high blood cholesterol in adults, treatment panel II. JAMA 269:3015, 1993.

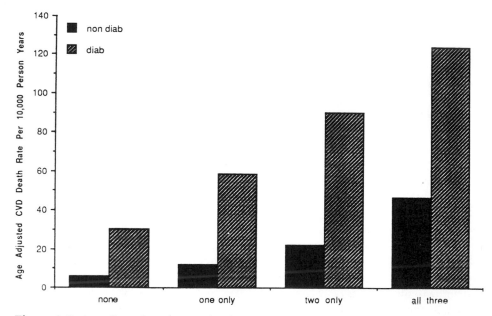

Figure 8–2. Age-adjusted cardiovascular disease (CVD) by presence of number of risk factors (smoking, systolic blood pressure, total cholesterol levels) for men screened for the Multiple Risk Factor Intervention Trial (MRFIT) with and without diabetes at baseline. (From Stamler J, Vaccaro O, Neaton JD et al: Diabetes, other risk factors, and 12-yr cardiovascular mortality for men screened in the Multiple Risk Factor Intervention trial. Diabetes Care 16:434, 1993)

Table 8–2. Insulin Resistance Syndrome—1995[a]

Insulin resistance
Compensatory hyperinsulinemia
   Normal glucose tolerance
   Impaired glucose tolerance
   Mild type 2 diabetes mellitus[b]
Central obesity
Hypertension
Dyslipidemias
   Increased fasting triglyceride concentration
   Decreased high-density lipoprotein cholesterol concentration
   Small, dense, low-density lipoprotein cholesterol particles[a]
   Large postprandial triglyceride-rich lipoprotein particles[a]
Coronary artery disease
Hyperuricemia[a]
Increased plasminogen activator inhibitor, type 1[a]
Decreased plasminogen activator activity[a]
Microvascular angina (in absence of large vessel coronary artery disease)[a]

[a]These factors are recent additions and require further studies for confirmation.

[b]Insulin concentrations are no longer elevated in more severe type 2 diabetes mellitus (e.g., fasting plasma glucose levels approximately >180 mg/dl).

People with pattern B often have higher fasting TG concentrations and lower HDL cholesterol levels. Furthermore, those with elevated fasting TG concentrations also have increased amounts of intestinally derived, TG-rich lipoprotein particles postprandially. Thus, the dyslipidemia associated with type 2 diabetes is characterized by increased fasting TG concentrations, low HDL cholesterol levels, a predominance of small dense LDL particles (pattern B), and accumulation of large, TG-rich lipoprotein particles after a meal.

The possible pathogenetic relationships among the various components of the insulin resistance syndrome (see Table 8-2) and *coronary artery disease* is depicted in Figure 8-3. *Insulin resistance* itself is mainly genetically determined, but obesity (central) and, to a lesser extent, a sedentary life style increase it further. Insulin resistance is responsible for a *compensatory hyperinsuli-* *nemia, glucose intolerance,* and probably (through mechanisms that have not been entirely worked out) *hypertension.* The *dyslipidemia,* elevated blood pressure, and changes in the *plasminogen activator* system have been shown to have a direct effect on coronary artery disease. Hyperinsulinemia may contribute to the dyslipidemia, although several studies have shown significant relationships between TG levels and insulin resistance independent of insulin concentrations.[5] In addition, hyperinsulinemia is unlikely to be a causal factor in the development of coronary artery disease for the following reasons (and discussed in more detail elsewhere).[4] First, as mentioned earlier, the statistical association between insulin levels and coronary artery disease seems to hold in middle-aged white men but not in elderly white men, women, or non-Caucasian populations. Second, with one exception, the in vitro studies demonstrating an insulin effect on lipid synthesis in vessel walls used extremely high insulin concentrations. Third, the cholesterol in atheromatous plaques is not synthesized there but delivered by circulating lipoproteins, and thus the physiologic significance of the in vitro studies on lipid synthesis is questionable. Fourth, although smooth muscle cell proliferation in arterial walls is an important pathologic event in plaque formation, the in vitro insulin effect (also using large concentrations) on this process is thought to represent a generalized trophic change rather than an in vivo physiologic action. Glucose intolerance is definitely associated with coronary artery disease, but it is far from clear how this mild metabolic abnormality could directly affect the vasculature. One assumes that insulin resistance somehow causes the alterations in the plasminogen system and *uric acid* metabolism as well as the development of *microvascular angina* (assuming that the latter two are confirmed), but the mechanisms by which this may occur are obscure.

Because of the increase in coronary artery

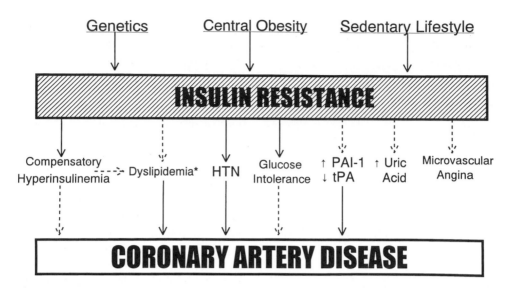

Figure 8–3. Components of insulin resistance syndrome (syndrome X). → Indicates probable or established causal relationship. ⋯⋗ Indicates association present but causal relationship not determined. *Dyslipidemia includes increased triglyceride levels, decreased HDL cholesterol levels, small dense LDL particles, and large postprandial triglyceride-rich lipoprotein particles. HTN, hypertension; PAI-1, plasminogen activator inhibitor, type 1; tPA, tissue plasminogen activator. (From Davidson MB: Clinical implications of insulin resistance. Am J Med 99:420, 1995)

disease imposed by diabetes (approximately three quarters of deaths in patients with type 2 diabetes are due to macrovascular disease), it behooves all of us (physicians, other health care providers, and, most importantly, patients) to reduce the reversible risk factors as much as possible. In regard to lipids, I (along with many other diabetologists) alter the recommendations of the ATP II (see Fig. 8-1) for testing, levels at which treatment is initiated, target levels to be achieved, and therapy for persons with diabetes. A lipoprotein analysis is performed initially and, if results are normal (i.e., no action needs to be taken), is repeated yearly. Table 8-3 lists the lipid levels at which treatment should be initiated and the target levels to be achieved. Note that the action and target levels are the same. This avoids the perplexing situation in which in one patient treatment is initiated and doses of drug are increased at a lipid value that would not be treated in another patient. For instance, under the ATP II rec-

ommendations (see Table 8-1), drug therapy would be started at an LDL concentration of 175 mg/dl and the dose would be increased when a subsequent value returns at 150 mg/dl in order to achieve a target level of <130 mg/dl. Another patient (with the same number of risk factors) whose initial LDL cholesterol concentration was 150 mg/dl would not receive drug treatment. Yet the risk attributable to the LDL concentration of 150 mg/dl is the same in the two patients.

Note also that some of the action/target levels in Table 8-3 are less than those recommended for the general population (see Table 8-1), reflecting the increased risk for coronary artery disease in diabetic patients. Action is recommended for diabetic patients with coronary artery disease and LDL cholesterol concentrations exceeding 100 mg/dl because several studies have shown regression of coronary artery plaques when these values are reduced to this level.[7, 8] Table 8-3 shows only one action level for treatment,

Table 8–3. Action/Target Levels for the Treatment of Dyslipidemias in Diabetic Patients

LDL Cholesterol Concentrations (mg/dl)			
CAD	Risk Factors[a]	Action Level	Target Level
Yes	None or any	100	100
No	One or more	130	130
No	None	160	160

Triglyceride Concentrations (mg/dl)		
CAD	Action Level	Target Level
Yes	200	200
No	400	400

CAD, coronary artery disease; LDL, low-density lipoprotein.

[a]Risk factors are the same as listed at the bottom of Figure 8-1. Note, however, that because these recommendations are for people with diabetes, every patient for whom these guidelines are used already has this risk factor, which is not considered in the table.

not one for initiating dietary therapy and another one for drug therapy. Furthermore, because all of these patients have at least one risk factor (i.e., diabetes), the number of risk factors to be considered is one less than for the general population.

The influence of TG levels on coronary artery disease is more complex. Although some studies have demonstrated a significant relationship between the two, in few of them were HDL cholesterol concentrations measured.[6] Therefore, it is not clear whether elevated TG levels are an independent risk factor. When low HDL cholesterol levels, an important risk factor for coronary artery disease, were present, high TG concentrations did not add any additional risk in type 2 diabetic patients.[6] However, given the overwhelming morbidity and mortality of coronary artery disease in type 2 diabetes and the difficulty in raising low HDL cholesterol levels, expert panels[3, 9] have recommended treating elevated TG concentrations.

NONPHARMACOLOGIC TREATMENT

The initial treatment of dyslipidemia should be nonpharmacologic (except for the chy-

lomicronemia syndrome, discussed later) and consists of diet, exercise, and glycemic control. Exercise and glycemic control have more effect on lowering elevated TG than LDL cholesterol levels. Consumption of alcohol should be avoided by patients with elevated TG levels. Diet (especially if weight loss occurs in obese patients) and exercise also help to lower glucose concentrations. Although some have cautioned against the use of insulin in type 2 diabetic patients because of the potential for accelerating macrovascular disease, in my view this is ill advised. Not only is the case for a direct effect of insulin on atherogenesis weak, as discussed earlier, but at least six studies have shown that better diabetic control lessens both cardiovascular events and mortality in type 2 diabetic patients (many of whom were treated with insulin).[10] Therefore, if insulin is necessary for glycemic control, it should not be withheld, even if macrovascular disease is present. If nonpharmacologic treatment for dyslipidemia has not lowered the elevated TG and/or LDL cholesterol levels into an acceptable range (see Table 8–3) in 2 months, drug therapy should be strongly considered. An exception is patients without coronary artery or other atherosclerotic disease, a normal HDL cholesterol level, and a total cholesterol concentration <300 mg/dl. Nonpharmacologic treatment can be tried for 6 months in these patients.

A detailed discussion of dietary therapy can be found in Chapter 3. A few guiding principles[5] are mentioned here. Most dietary studies of type 2 diabetic patients have found that replacing fat with foods containing complex carbohydrates and high fiber decreases both total and LDL cholesterol concentrations. Significant increases in fasting or postprandial TG levels have not been noted (for the most part) in type 2 diabetic patients ingesting high-carbohydrate diets containing adequate amounts of soluble fiber. An added advantage for obese individuals is that for comparable portion sizes, foods high in complex carbohydrates are less caloric than if they contained fat. Some have suggested replacing dietary saturated fat with monounsaturated fat because this substitution also results in comparable reductions of LDL cholesterol in patients with type 2 diabetes.[11] Substituting with monounsaturated fat rather than with complex carbohydrate may lead to less hyperglycemia. Unfortunately, only three foods—nuts, olives, and avocados—contain large amounts of monounsaturated fats. Although certain oils can be used as other sources of monounsaturated fat, they still represent a high-calorie food, which may be problematic for obese patients who need to lose weight. For patients with high TG levels, increased intake of ω-3 polyunsaturated fatty acids has been recommended. These fatty acids, which are constituents of fish oils, lower TG levels. In some but not all studies, however, LDL cholesterol levels have increased and/or glycemia has worsened. Finally, abstinence from alcohol often lowers TG levels.

PHARMACOLOGIC TREATMENT— DESCRIPTION OF DRUGS

Five classes of drugs are used in the treatment of hyperlipidemia (Table 8–4). These are (1) bile acid resins, (2) nicotinic acid, (3) hydroxymethylglutaryl–coenzyme A (HMG-CoA) reductase inhibitors; (4) fibric acid derivatives, and (5) probucol. Not all are recommended for patients with diabetes. Estrogen might be considered a drug to be used in postmenopausal patients. It reduces LDL cholesterol levels by approximately 15% in nondiabetic women and can increase HDL cholesterol levels as much as 15% as well. Estrogens can also increase TG concentrations, however, and some consider the hormone contraindicated if TG levels exceed 500 mg/dl.[11]

Bile acid resins are not absorbed. They act in the gastrointestinal tract by binding bile acids. This interferes with the enterohepatic circulation of cholesterol and forces the liver to utilize stored cholesterol. The result is an up-regulation of LDL receptors that increases LDL clearance. Side effects include constipation, bloating, flatulence, nausea, abdominal pain, hemorrhoids, and drug interactions. Therefore, these drugs should not be used by patients with autonomic neuropathy and constipation. Because the bile

Table 8–4. Recommended Lipid-Lowering Drugs for Diabetic Patients

Generic Name	Brand Name	Tablet Size (mg)	Initial Dose (mg)	Maximum Dose (mg)
Statins[a]				
Lovastatin	Mevacor	10, 20, 40	10	80[b]
Pravastatin	Pravachol	10, 20, 40	10	40
Simvastatin	Zocor	5, 10, 20, 40	5	40
Fluvastatin[c]	Lescol	20, 40	20	40
Atorvastatin[d]	Lipitor	10, 20, 40	10	80
Fibric Acid Derivative				
Gemfibrozil	Lopid	300, 600	1200[e]	1200
Bile Acid Resin				
Cholestyramine	Questran	4 g per packet	8 g	24 g
Colestipol	Colestid	5 g per packet	10 g	30 g

[a]HMG-CoA reductase inhibitors.

[b]Up to 40 mg is given at bedtime, and the rest taken in the morning; the other statins are usually taken only at bedtime.

[c]Fluvastatin is slighlty less effective than the other statins; it is the only one to bind to the bile acid resins and therefore should be taken 4 hours after the evening dose of the resin when that combination is used.

[d]More effective than other statins; also lowers triglyceride levels.

[e]The usual dose is 600 mg bid except when combined with a statin. When a combination of statin and gemfibrozil is used, statin should be started at the lowest dose and gemfibrozil given at 300 mg bid to minimize the risk of rhabdomyolysis. The dosage for both drugs should be increased cautiously if LDL cholesterol or triglyceride levels remain elevated.

acid resins interfere with the absorption of other drugs (e.g., digoxin, warfarin, diuretics, β-blockers, iron, thyroid hormone, tetracycline, vancomycin, barbiturates), it is recommended that other drugs be taken at least 1 hour before or 4 hours after these cholesterol-lowering agents. Bile acid resins raise TG concentrations and are (relatively) contraindicated in patients with TG levels exceeding 400 mg/dl.

Nicotinic acid lowers both LDL cholesterol and TG concentrations and raises HDL cholesterol levels. Its mechanism of action is not clear. The drug has significant side effects including flushing, pruritus, gastritis, peptic ulcer, hepatitis, cholestatic jaundice, hyperuricemia, and, in doses ≥3.0 g, worsening of glycemia. For the last reason, it is not recommended for use by diabetic patients.

The *HMG-CoA reductase inhibitors (statins)* inhibit the rate-limiting enzyme of cholesterol synthesis. This decrease of cellular cholesterol, especially in the liver, up-regulates LDL receptors and thus increases the clearance of LDL cholesterol. As a single-drug therapy, the statins are the most effective LDL cholesterol–lowering agents. TG levels may decrease slightly and HDL concentrations increase somewhat, but these effects are not consistent. Because hepatic cholesterol synthesis is more active overnight, these drugs are more effective if taken at bedtime. Side effects are uncommon and include abnormal results of liver function tests, headaches, sleep disturbances, and rarely creatine phosphokinase (CPK) elevations and myositis (especially with gemfibrozil, nicotinic acid, cyclosporine, erythromycin, or renal failure). There is no effect on glycemia.

The only *fibric acid derivative* recommended and available in this country is gemfibrozil. The drug lowers TG concentrations by increasing their clearance, although the mechanism is not clear. HDL cholesterol levels rise slightly. In general, LDL cholesterol concentrations increase in hypertriglyceri-

demic patients but decrease in normotriglyceridemic patients. The increase in LDL cholesterol levels, however, is associated with a potentially favorable change in the composition of the LDL particle, which increases in size and decreases in density (i.e., a shift from pattern B to pattern A—see the earlier discussion of dyslipidemia in insulin resistance syndrome for significance). Side effects include rash, nausea, abdominal pain, and cholelithiasis. Myositis occurs rarely in patients in renal failure or also taking a statin.

Probucol is an antioxidant. It lowers LDL cholesterol concentrations but unfortunately also decreases HDL cholesterol levels as much as 25%. It is carried in LDL particles and protects them against oxidation. (Oxidized LDL particles are more likely to be taken up by macrophages, whose interaction with the vessel wall leads to atherosclerosis.) Because of its profound effect on HDL levels, it is not usually recommended except for patients with markedly elevated LDL cholesterol levels resistant to statins and bile acid resins used in combination.

PHARMACOLOGIC TREATMENT—GENERAL APPROACH

If nonpharmacologic methods have failed to lower TG and/or LDL concentrations to below target levels in 2 months (or in 6 months in patients with normal HDL cholesterol levels, no vascular disease, and total cholesterol concentrations <300 mg/dl), drug therapy should be considered. The approach to the drug treatment of the dyslipidemia in diabetes is complex and is depicted in Figure 8–4. The TG concentration determines the initial decision. If the value is >400 mg/dl (invalidating calculation of an LDL cholesterol concentration), gemfibrozil 600 mg bid is started if hepatic transaminase values are less than twice normal. The effect of the drug is evident in 1 month, at which time a repeat lipoprotein analysis is performed and hepatic transaminases remeasured. If the TG level remains ≥400 mg/dl, every effort should be

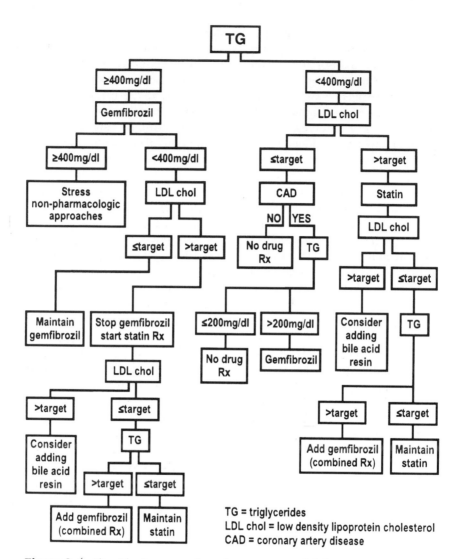

Figure 8–4. Algorithmic approach to the treatment of diabetic patients with hyperlipidemia.

made to optimize glycemia and emphasize exercise and diet (including abstention from alcohol). If the patient's diabetes is well controlled—or controlled as well as possible, given the circumstances for that patient— and no further improvement with diet and exercise is deemed likely, an extremely low-fat diet (10% to 20%) should be considered. This is particularly important for patients with a history of TG-induced pancreatitis.

If after 1 month of gemfibrozil therapy TG levels decrease to <400 mg/dl, the LDL cholesterol concentration can be calculated, and that value drives the next decision. If it is less than the target level (see Table 8-3), gemfibrozil is maintained and lipoprotein analyses and hepatic transaminases are measured every 4 months for the first year and every 6 months thereafter. Gemfibrozil is discontinued if the liver enzyme levels rise to greater than twice normal. If, on the other hand, the LDL concentration exceeds the target level, gemfibrozil is discontinued and a statin (see Table 8-4) is started. Again, a lipoprotein analysis is performed and hepatic transaminases are measured in 1 month, when the maximal effect of that dose of the drug would be evident. If the LDL concentration exceeds the target level at that time, the dose of the statin is increased gradually, with monthly evaluations until either the target level is met or a maximal dose is reached. If the target level has not been met with a maximal dose of a statin, consideration should be given to adding a bile acid resin.

If the LDL cholesterol target level has been met, the TG concentration drives the next decision. The statin dose is maintained if the TG target level has been met. If it has not, combination therapy with a statin and gemfibrozil is begun. Because rhabdomyolysis, although unusual, is more common with this combination than with either drug alone, a baseline CPK level should be measured. CPK levels can fluctuate, and minor elevations may result from minor soft tissue injury. Elevated levels should be remeasured before withholding combination therapy. Although no guidelines are found in the literature, I use 5 times the upper limit of normal to withhold treatment and 10 times to discontinue it. To minimize the possibility of rhabdomyolysis, gemfibrozil is either started at one half of the usual dose (300 mg bid) or halved to that dose if the patient had been taking it, and the lowest dose of the statin is used. A CPK level is added to the monthly measurement of hepatic transaminases and lipoprotein analysis. Because the LDL cholesterol concentration is probably a greater risk factor than the TG level, the statin dose is increased gradually to achieve the appropriate target level. If that has been achieved or the maximal dose is reached, the gemfibrozil dose may be doubled if the TG target level is not met. The CPK level should be measured after every dose increase, along with the lipids and hepatic transaminases. When stable doses are achieved, these measurements are carried out every 4 months

during the first year and every 6 months thereafter. Patients should be warned to report any unexplained muscle soreness and, especially, any darkening of their urine. Additionally, both the physician and the patient should be aware of the other drugs (e.g., macrolide antibiotics, cyclosporine) and conditions (i.e., renal failure) mentioned earlier that increase the possibility of rhabdomyolysis.

If the initial TG concentration is <400 mg/dl, the LDL cholesterol level can be calculated, and that value drives the decision. If the LDL cholesterol concentration meets the target level, the next decision involves whether to treat the TG concentration. For patients with coronary artery disease and a TG level between 200 and 400 mg/dl, gemfibrozil is started. All other patients in this arm of the algorithm would have been successfully treated by nonpharmacologic methods. If the initial TG level is <400 mg/dl but the LDL cholesterol concentration does not meet the target level, a statin is started. Treatment of a patient at this point is the same as described earlier when gemfibrozil was discontinued and a statin introduced.

TG levels exceeding 1,000 mg/dl are occasionally found in patients with uncontrolled diabetes. These patients are at increased risk for pancreatitis. Therefore, drug therapy with gemfibrozil should be started immediately without waiting for a lower-fat diet and treatment of the hyperglycemia to have an effect on the TG levels.

In addition to abdominal pain (with or without documented pancreatitis), they may also have eruptive xanthomata, lipemia retinalis, mental confusion, myalgias, and arthralgias (often in the hands). This is termed the *chylomicronemia syndrome* and is potentially very serious. In this situation, fat intake may need to be decreased to <20% of total calories until the TG levels fall to three-digit numbers. Treatment of the uncontrolled diabetes (usually with insulin) is also important. TG levels of this magnitude are invariably superimposed on either a familial or another cause of hypertriglyceridemia.

Thus, hyperlipidemia is a potentially reversible risk factor. Intensive dietary treatment alone or in combination with one or several drugs can usually improve the lipid status of the patient and lower or eliminate this risk.

Although obesity is associated with elevated TG levels, hypertension, and diabetes mellitus, multivariate analysis of the results in large epidemiologic studies has identified obesity as an independent risk factor for macroangiopathy. It is a reversible one if patients can sustain weight loss.

A strong family history of coronary artery disease is an irreversible risk factor. Unfortunately, diabetes mellitus may be one as well. As mentioned in Chapter 2, no convincing evidence shows that strict diabetic control has a direct effect on macroangiopathy. On the other hand, as mentioned earlier, prospective studies have demonstrated fewer cardiovascular events and less mortality in type 2 diabetic patients in good control compared with those less well controlled.[10] However, the fact that accelerated atherogenesis also characterizes individuals with impaired glucose tolerance in whom hyperglycemia is obviously much less marked than in patients with diabetes suggests that factors other than glucose concentration are responsible for the macroangiopathy in both groups.

DIABETIC EYE DISEASE

Diabetes can affect the outer (lens), middle (vitreous), and inner (retina) parts of the eye. The lens can change shape with marked changes in blood glucose concentration, leading to temporary blurring of vision. Glucose concentrations equilibrate between the lens and the aqueous humor surrounding it, leading to shifts in water that alter the shape of the lens. Hyperglycemia in the aqueous humor draws fluid out of the lens, resulting in an artificial myopia or nearsightedness.

Return of glucose levels to a more normal concentration in the aqueous humor causes water to move into the lens. This results in a transient hyperopia, or farsightedness. Both can occur, the former when a patient's hyperglycemia is evolving and the latter as treatment lowers glucose levels. It can take up to 1 month before baseline vision is restored, although most patients note a significant improvement within a few weeks.

The lens is also more prone to cataract formation in diabetic patients. A rare occurrence is a snowflake or Christmas tree type of cataract (sometimes called the *diabetic cataract*) in which a pattern resembling these kinds of structures can be seen in the middle of the lens. Because this type of cataract was usually associated with episodes of severe diabetic ketoacidosis, it is rarely seen today. Although more typical "senile" cataracts may not be more common in the diabetic population, they are approximately five times more likely to develop at a younger age than in the normal population. Diabetic control (as reflected in glucose levels) does not seem to have a role in the development of these cataracts.

The first observable diabetic changes on the retina are a subtle dilatation of the major retinal veins. The retinal veins normally are 1.5 times the size of the retinal arteries (a 2:3 artery-to-vein ratio). In these early changes, the arteries remain normal but the veins become distended and may become two to three times the size of the arteries. This phase, termed *preretinopathy,* is generally present for <2 years before the retinal changes progress to the classic background stage.

The next phase is called *background, simple,* or *nonproliferative* diabetic retinopathy. These changes occurring within the retina are characterized by microaneurysms, hemorrhages, and hard exudates (Fig. 8–5). Microaneurysms, usually the first sign of background retinopathy, appear as tiny round red dots, which, as the name implies, are small aneurysmal outpouchings or sacculations of

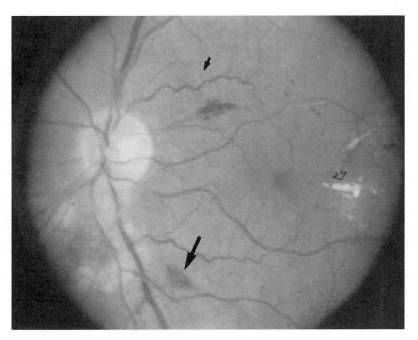

Figure 8–5. Background diabetic retinopathy. Note the microaneurysm (short dark arrow), hard exudate (open arrow), and hemorrhage (long dark arrow). (Courtesy of Albert Sheffer, MD)

the retinal capillaries. If hemorrhage from these weakened areas of the capillary occurs in the superficial retinal layers, they appear flame shaped. Those occurring in the deeper retinal layers have the appearance of dots and blots. Although the smaller ones may be difficult to distinguish from microaneurysms, most are large enough to be differentiated. In addition, the capillaries become permeable to plasma, which leaks out and precipitates in the retinal layers. This leads to the formation of hard exudates, which are seen as sharply defined, glistening, yellowish deposits. Such leakage involves only plasma, not red blood cells. These changes (microaneurysms, hemorrhages, and exudates) wax and wane. They do not impair vision unless the plasma leakage occurs near or in the macular area. There, the pattern is often of a ring of hard exudates surrounding the macula (Fig. 8-6). Because this is the central vision area, exudates here with the associated swelling (termed *macular edema*) can

diminish vision. Macular edema is much more common in older patients. Background retinopathy is not usually seen until approximately 10 years after the diagnosis of diabetes. (However, because the diagnosis is often delayed in persons with type 2 diabetes, background retinopathy is found in approximately 20% of patients when first diagnosed.) With our current results of controlling glucose levels, it eventually appears in up to 80% of diabetic patients.

The next stage is called *preproliferative diabetic retinopathy.* The veins now have an irregular caliber, often looking like a string of sausages. A particularly important sign is the appearance of cotton wool spots or soft exudates (Fig. 8-7). They represent evidence of capillary closure with resultant hypoxia (lack of oxygen) to parts of the retina. Soft exudates are pale yellow patches with poorly defined margins that do not contrast well with the normal retina (i.e., they may be difficult to see with an ophthalmoscope).

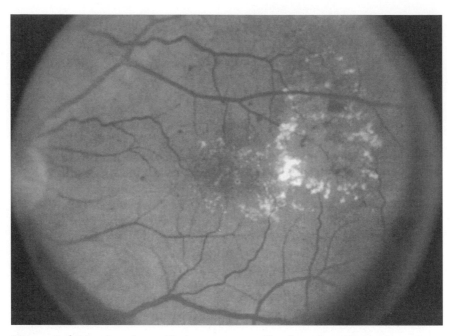

Figure 8–6. Macular edema. Circinate pattern of hard exudates in macular area. Note the other characteristics of background retinopathy (microaneurysms, hemorrhage). (Courtesy of Albert Sheffer, MD)

The other finding of particular significance is intraretinal microvascular abnormalities (IRMAs). IRMAs are tufts of new capillaries that are still located beneath the inner limiting membrane of the retina—that is, they have not yet broken through to lie on the surface of the retina.

Although it may be difficult (except by special tests) to distinguish between IRMAs and neovascularization (i.e., new vessels that either lie on the surface of the retina or are growing out into the vitreous), the differentiation is not clinically important because either one should trigger an immediate referral to a qualified ophthalmologist.

These preproliferative changes are the immediate forerunner to proliferative diabetic retinopathy (in which changes take place outside of the retina), which occurs in 5% to 10% of patients with diabetic retinopathy. New vessel growth occurring on the surface of the retina or growing from there into the vitreous is its distinguishing feature. These

new vessels (Fig. 8-8) are structurally weak and likely to hemorrhage, thereby obscuring vision. This often leads to formation of fibrous tissue as the blood is resorbed. This scar tissue obscures the retina and places traction on it, and a retinal detachment can result. If the process is allowed to continue untreated, the neovascularization can eventually involve the front part of the eye—namely, the iris and the anterior chamber angle. This angle is functionally very important because it contains a channel that drains to the outside the aqueous humor that is constantly secreted in the eye. If neovascularization occurs in the angle, this drainage channel becomes occluded, resulting in a drastic rise in the intraocular pressure (i.e., neovascular glaucoma), which usually leads to a blind and painful eye.

Fortunately, the natural history of diabetic retinopathy does not have to occur in appropriately screened and treated patients. Photocoagulation has been shown to slow and

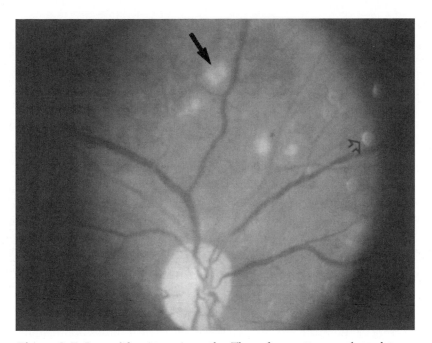

Figure 8–7. Preproliferative retinopathy. The soft or cotton wool exudate (dark arrow) has indistinct margins in contrast to the hard exudates in Figures 8-5 and 8-6, which have sharp margins and are brighter. The round structures with distinct margins (open arrow) are artifacts. (Courtesy of Albert Sheffer, MD)

Figure 8–8. Proliferative retinopathy with a large area of neovascularization. Note the presence of background retinopathy (microaneurysms, hard exudates, hemorrhage) as well.

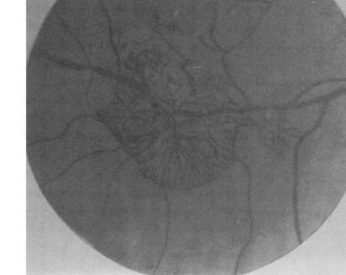

often arrest the two processes that lead to severe visual loss. These are the proliferation of new vessels with subsequent bleeding (leading to vitreous opacities, the formation of scar tissue obscuring the retina and possibly causing a retinal detachment) and macular edema. In regard to the former mechanism, 1,727 patients with proliferative retinopathy were randomized to receive either immediate photocoagulation or careful observation in the Diabetic Retinopathy Study.[12] Severe visual loss was defined as vision <5/200 at two or more consecutively completed visits at 4-month intervals. The incidence of severe visual loss was decreased by 50% throughout a 6-year follow-up starting almost immediately. After 6 years, approximately 30% of the untreated eyes had suffered severe visual loss, compared with approximately 15% of the treated eyes.

The results of therapy for macular edema in the Early Diabetic Retinopathy Study[13] were similar. Focal photocoagulation of the macular area was carried out in 754 eyes with macular edema, and 1,490 untreated eyes served as controls. The endpoint was a 50% deterioration of vision (e.g., 20/40 to 20/80) when evaluated by a visual acuity chart. At the end of 3 years, 12% of the treated eyes compared with 24% of the untreated eyes had deteriorated. Further analysis revealed that only eyes with "clinically significant macular edema" needed to be treated because the rate of visual loss was very low in eyes with milder macular changes, and there was no evidence of benefit from treatment of this earlier process. Retinal thickening that occurs at or near the center of the macula is the hallmark of clinically significant macular edema. This can only be assessed by stereo contact lens biomicroscopy and stereo photography, procedures not available to nonophthalmologists. To complicate matters further, initial visual acuity does not help select patients for further investigation. Even patients with normal visual acuity and clinically significant macular edema were helped by focal macular photocoagulation. Thus, appropriate treatment might be denied patients who were not referred to an ophthalmologist either until some visual loss occurred or until lesions could be appreciated by direct ophthalmoscopy.

What then is the role of primary care physicians in regard to diabetic eye disease? Strict diabetic control forestalls the development of diabetic retinopathy (see Chapter 2 and Fig. 2–6) and it is the physician's responsibility to discuss this fact with patients and to give direct diabetic care to achieve the best control possible, given the limitations of patients' compliance and intelligence. In regard to the diagnosis of diabetic retinopathy, most primary care physicians do not dilate the pupils before examination with an ophthalmoscope if they examine the retina at all. Even if direct ophthalmoscopy is performed through dilated pupils, diabetic retinopathy is diagnosed poorly by nonophthalmologists, including diabetologists. For instance, senior medical residents and board-certified internists missed proliferative retinopathy approximately 50% of the time, and diabetologists missed it 33% of the time.[14] These and similar observations lead to the conclusion that diabetic retinopathy should be diagnosed (at an early stage for appropriate follow-up and treatment) by an ophthalmologist, preferably one who is a retinal specialist.

The American Diabetes Association[15] has promulgated the following guidelines: (1) Care of the eyes in a diabetic patient reflects a partnership between the primary care physician and the ophthalmologist; (2) the former has a fundamental role in the medical management, appropriate referrals, and coordination of care, and the latter determines the diagnosis and treatment of diabetic retinopathy; and (3) it is the responsibility of the primary care physician to inform the patient of the potential for visual loss in diabetes and that early detection and treatment greatly reduce this risk and to refer the patient appropriately to a qualified ophthalmologist. In regard to the latter, type 1 patients should be referred after 5 years of diabetes and type 2 patients should see an ophthalmologist at the time of diagnosis. The latter procedure is recommended because many of these patients will have had their disease for approximately 10 years before the diagnosis is made.[16]

Primary care physicians may interact with the patient in one more circumstance regarding diabetic retinopathy. They are often called when a patient develops a vitreous hemorrhage. This typically involves a rather sudden, painless loss of vision, the amount depending on the size of the hemorrhage. If total vision is not obscured, the patient describes a dark area moving around in the field of vision. The hemorrhage tends to spread out inferiorly, especially if the patient remains upright. Activity should be restricted, and the head should be elevated during sleep. Patients who note the sudden onset of floaters (possible small vitreous hemorrhage) or the sudden onset of blurring of vision (possible large vitreous hemorrhage) should be referred immediately to an ophthalmologist, preferably a retinal specialist. Although many may have hemorrhages that are too large (thus obscuring the vitreous) for immediate treatment, some may have small hemorrhages that are easier to treat early while the clot is organized and has not yet had the opportunity to spread out diffusely throughout the vitreous space. Gradual onset of blurring of vision may be due to changes in the lens secondary to changing glucose concentrations or to macular edema.

DIABETIC NEPHROPATHY[17]

The clinical course of diabetic nephropathy for type 1 patients is depicted in Figure 8–9. Although less information is available on type 2 patients, it is assumed that the sequence of events is the same because the prevalence of overt diabetic nephropathy is similar in the two types of diabetes for a given duration of disease.

CLASSIFICATION

Diabetic nephropathy can be divided into five stages.[18, 19] Stage I occurs at the onset of the disease (and is not shown in Fig. 8–9). It is characterized by a 30% to 40% increase in the glomerular filtration rate (GFR) above normal. The elevated GFR does not reverse acutely with institution of insulin therapy

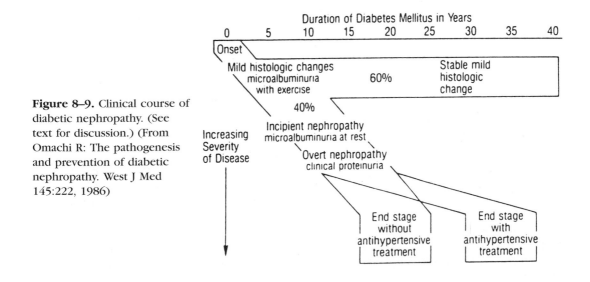

Figure 8–9. Clinical course of diabetic nephropathy. (See text for discussion.) (From Omachi R: The pathogenesis and prevention of diabetic nephropathy. West J Med 145:222, 1986)

but may return to normal within several weeks to a few months. This hyperfiltration is associated with enlarged kidneys and increased intraglomerular pressure, which may cause a transient increase in albumin excretion. One current theory about the development of renal insufficiency involves intraglomerular hypertension causing subsequent nephron loss. This has several important prognostic and therapeutic implications (discussed later).

Stage II is characterized by normal excretion of albumin (<20 μg/min or 30 mg/24 h) regardless of the duration of the disease. Some patients maintain their hyperfiltration, which may be a poor prognostic indicator for subsequent development of diabetic nephropathy.[20] In general, these individuals are usually in poor diabetic control whereas those whose GFRs return to normal have generally lower glycated hemoglobin levels.[19]

Stage III or incipient diabetic nephropathy is characterized by microalbuminuria at rest. This is defined as elevated excretion rates of albumin between 20 and 200 μg/min (30 and 300 mg/24 h). In general, patients with lower amounts of microalbuminuria (20 to 70 μg/min) have either elevated or normal GFRs that are higher than those with more microalbuminuria (70 to 200 μg/min). In a 2-year prospective study,[21] patients with either normal albumin excretion rates (<30 mg/24 h) or mild microalbuminuria (30 to 100 mg/24 h) had no change in their GFR whereas those with more marked microalbuminuria (101 to 300 mg/24 h) showed a significant reduction. This suggests that the GFR begins to decline during the incipient stage of diabetic nephropathy. At this stage, blood pressures are often higher (although in the normal range) than in nondiabetic subjects and may increase to abnormally high levels during exercise. In general, blood pressures increase 3 to 4 mm Hg per year. In the past, approximately 80% of patients with microalbuminuria progressed within 7 to 14 years to clinical proteinuria or overt diabetic nephropathy (discussed later); only 5% without

microalbuminuria did so.[19] Control of glucose levels and blood pressure reduces or eliminates microalbuminuria.[17] More recently, with strict diabetic control, $<20\%$ of type 1 patients with microalbuminuria progressed to overt nephropathy in a 10-year period.[22] The majority reverted to normoalbuminuria. This is very encouraging because patients with normal albumin excretion rates maintain normal GFR and blood pressure even after 20 years of follow-up.[17]

Stage IV or overt diabetic nephropathy is characterized by clinical proteinuria—that is, a level of urinary protein that is detectable (dipstick positive) by simple tests. These semiquantitative methods are much less sensitive than the specially developed ones used to measure microalbuminuria. Thus, overt diabetic nephropathy is defined by urinary protein excretion exceeding 0.5 g/24 h. Because albumin is not the only protein excreted at this stage, clinical proteinuria corresponds to albumin excretion rates exceeding 200 μg/min or 300 mg (0.3 g)/24 h. Overt diabetic nephropathy develops in approximately 30% to 40% of type 1 diabetic patients,[17, 23] although more recently, when patients were kept in strict diabetic control, $<10\%$ did so.[24] Genetics also has a role at least in type 1 diabetes. Two independent predictors for type 1 diabetic patients to develop overt nephropathy are positive family histories of renal disease[25] or hypertension.[26] Smoking is also an independent risk factor in both type 1[27] and type 2[28] diabetes.

Early in the clinical course of overt diabetic nephropathy, the GFR may be in the normal range but usually declines slowly but steadily. Although the rate of fall in GFR may vary markedly among patients, the decrease in GFR is fairly constant within each patient. This is shown in Figure 8–10, where the GFR is approximated by the inverse of the serum creatinine concentration. There is a linear relationship between the two once the serum creatinine level reaches 2.3 mg/dl (200 μmol/L). The average GFR decline is approximately 1 ml/min/month. During this stage

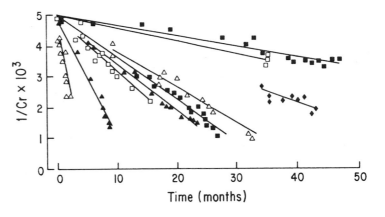

Figure 8–10. Progression of renal failure in nine diabetic patients. Inverse of serum creatinine (μmol/L) plotted against time. (From Jones RH, McKay JD, Hayakawa H et al: Progression of diabetic nephropathy. Lancet 1:1105, 1979)

of diabetic nephropathy, blood pressure increases approximately 7 mm Hg per year, and thus hypertension eventually occurs in almost all patients. Aggressive treatment of elevated blood pressure slows the rate of decline of the GFR[17] (Fig. 8–11). At this point, aggressive treatment of elevated glucose concentrations has little impact. Once the process of nephron destruction is under way, it seems independent of the inciting cause (in many types of renal disease, not just diabetic nephropathy), although lowering the blood pressure is definitely helpful.

Stage V or end-stage renal disease (ESRD) is similar to kidney failure due to any other cause. However, a disproportionate share have diabetic nephropathy. Although only 3% of the population is known to have diabetes, nearly 50% of patients starting dialysis have renal failure due to diabetes. Signs and symptoms include progressive weakness, lethargy, fluid retention (possibly leading to congestive heart failure), anorexia, nausea, vomiting, diarrhea, hiccups, pruritus, difficulty in controlling hypertension, anemia, and electrolyte disturbances. The clinical impression, however, is that patients with ESRD due to diabetes are more symptomatic at higher levels of GFR than patients with non-diabetic causes of kidney failure—that is, the GFR does not have to be as low for diabetic patients to start experiencing difficulties. Therefore, dialysis is usually started earlier in patients with diabetes. I usually refer dia-

betic patients with renal insufficiency to a nephrologist when the serum creatinine level reaches 3 mg/dl or when a patient starts to experience the symptoms of kidney failure, whichever occurs first. Diabetic patients undergoing dialysis have a worse prognosis than nondiabetic patients. For this reason, kidney transplantation is considered the preferred method of treatment, especially if a close relative will donate a kidney. Despite successful treatment for ESRD, many of these patients succumb to their associated macrovascular disease.

With this background for the development of diabetic nephropathy, what part can the primary care physician play? Medical management of diabetic patients is a critical factor not only in their propensity to develop but also in the subsequent course of their diabetic nephropathy. As discussed in Chapter 2 and shown in Figure 2–10, tight diabetic control has a marked impact on delaying and possibly preventing clinical proteinuria. Once persistent proteinuria occurs, elevation of serum creatinine levels is much more likely in hypertensive patients than in normotensive ones.[29] The 10-year mortality in diabetic patients with overt diabetic nephropathy is three to four times lower if effective hypertensive treatment is given.[30] Thus, the primary care physician has an overriding responsibility (in my view, even a duty) to ensure that the blood glucose and blood pressure are meticulously con-

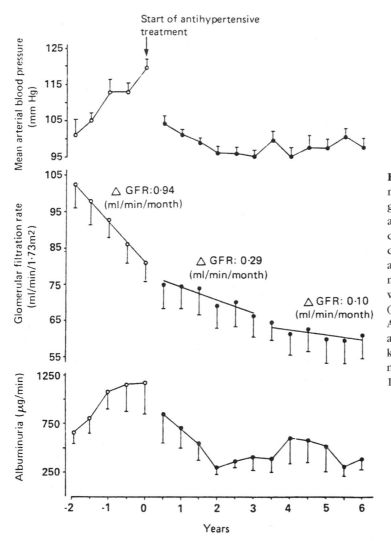

Figure 8–11. Changes in mean arterial pressure, glomerular filtration rate, and albuminuria before (open circles) and during (closed circles) long-term effective antihypertensive treatment of nine type 1 diabetic patients with diabetic nephropathy. (From Parving HH, Andersen AR, Smidt UM et al: Effect of antihypertensive treatment on kidney function in diabetic nephropathy. BMJ 294:1443, 1987)

trolled to the level that patients' compliance and disease allow. The limiting factor should be the patient, not the physician.

TREATMENT OF HYPERTENSION[31]

Ideally, antihypertensive agents should not increase insulin resistance, promote hypoglycemia, mask the symptoms of hypoglycemia, potentiate impotence, enhance orthostatic hypotension, aggravate macrovascular disease, or increase dyslipidemia, and they should offer specific preservation of renal function. The ideal drug is not yet available, and the choice of antihypertensive agents represents a compromise based on these considerations. The Fifth Report of the Joint National Commission on Detection, Evaluation, and Treatment of High Blood Pressure (JNC-V) recommended using thiazide diuretics and β-blockers.[32] This recommendation is based on the extensive experience garnered since the late 1950s (diuretics) and late 1960s (β-blockers) from large randomized trials demonstrating that treatment with these drugs erases the excess risk for stroke and reduces by half the risk of heart disease associated with hypertension. Large long-term studies evaluating these clinical end-points are not yet available for the other classes of antihypertensive agents. The recommendations of the JNC-V did include a caveat that other drugs should be considered for patients with contraindications to the use of diuretics or β-blockers or with a specific indication for another agent. This is indeed the situation in diabetic patients, as seen in the following discussion of each class of antihypertensive agents (in alphabetic order).

When given as monotherapy, the *angiotensin-converting enzyme (ACE) inhibitors* are equally as effective as diuretics, β-blockers, and calcium antagonists in lowering blood pressure. They enhance insulin sensitivity (i.e., decrease insulin resistance) and have no adverse effects on lipids. Although lowering insulin or sulfonylurea agent doses in an occasional patient is necessary to avoid hypoglycemia, for the most part this is unnecessary. Indeed, in large studies of use of ACE inhibitors in diabetic patients, few have shown improvements in long-term glycemic control. ACE inhibitors, more than any other class of antihypertensive agents, reduced urinary protein excretion.[33] This included both clinical proteinuria and microalbuminuria. Furthermore, ACE inhibitors retarded the deterioration of renal function (Fig. 8–12).[34]

ACE inhibitors are usually well tolerated. They are contraindicated in pregnancy because they may cause anomalies of the genitourinary tract in the fetus. Acute renal failure may occur in patients who have renal artery stenosis and are given these drugs. It is reversible if they are discontinued in time. Acute renal failure may also occur in a rare patient without renal stenosis, but renal insufficiency is usually present before initiation of ACE inhibitor therapy. Hyperkalemia may also occur, especially in patients with hyporeninemic hypoaldosteronism, a condition more common in diabetic patients with mild renal insufficiency (discussed later). For

these reasons, serum creatinine and potassium concentrations should be measured several weeks after starting an ACE inhibitor. Other side effects include a dry cough, rash, orthostatic hypotension, and rarely angioedema.

Although few direct comparisons have been made between α₁-*adrenoceptor blockers* and other antihypertensive agents in diabetic patients, almost all studies with these drugs have shown good efficacy in persons with diabetes. This class of agents has the added advantage of slightly improving insulin sensitivity, glycemic levels, the lipid profile, and urinary flow in older men, and it has the lowest prevalence of sexual dysfunction. The main drawback is postural hypotension, especially after the initial dose. Therefore, it is recommended that the first dose of one of these drugs be given just before going to bed. Extra caution should be exercised in patients with nocturia. These agents may not be able to be tolerated by patients with autonomic neuropathy and a tendency toward orthostatic hypotension.

β-*Adrenoceptor blockers* have been used to lower blood pressure since the late 1960s. Although they are considered preferred therapy for hypertension by the JNC-V, the Working Group Report on Hypertension in Diabetes (WGRHD) does not agree on their use for diabetic patients.[35] This is because (1) they have adverse effects on glucose and lipid levels, (2) they reduce the recognition of and prolong the recovery from hypoglycemia, and (3) they decrease peripheral blood flow. In discussing β-blockers, it should be remembered that there are important differences among them. Some block both the β₁- and β₂-adrenoceptors (nonselective); others preferentially inhibit the β₁-adrenoceptor (selective), although in high doses they also affect the β₂-adrenoceptors; a few have intrinsic sympathomimetic activity; and one (labetalol) also has α₁-adrenoceptor blocking activity. It should also be recognized that there are indications for β-blockers other than hypertension. These include angina,

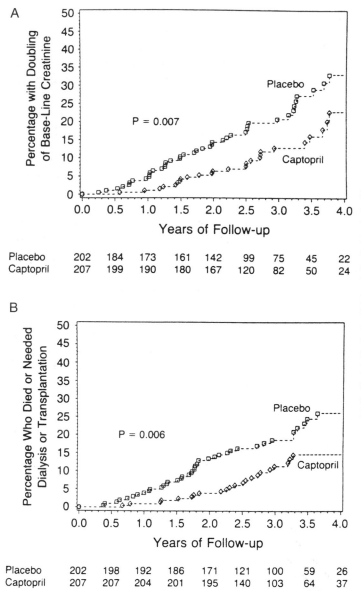

Placebo	202	184	173	161	142	99	75	45	22
Captopril	207	199	190	180	167	120	82	50	24

Placebo	202	198	192	186	171	121	100	59	26
Captopril	207	207	204	201	195	140	103	64	37

Figure 8–12. Cumulative incidence of events in patients with diabetic nephropathy receiving either captopril (an angiotensin-converting enzyme inhibitor) or placebo. Differences between the captopril and placebo groups were significant for both doubling of the serum creatinine (P < 0.007) and death, dialysis, or transplantation (P < 0.006) (From Lewis EJ, Hunsicker LG, Bain RP et al: The effect of angiotensin-converting-enzyme inhibition on nephropathy. N Engl J Med 329:1456, 1993)

some cardiac dysrhythmias, migraine headache prophylaxis, tremors, and prevention of recurrent myocardial infarctions. If the indications are strong enough and other drugs would not be as effective, β-blockers should be used for these nonhypertensive reasons in diabetic patients despite their potential adverse effects mentioned earlier. This is especially true for the prevention of a recurrent myocardial infarction.

The efficacy of β-blockers as antihypertensive agents in diabetic patients is good, especially in young Caucasian individuals. However, glycemia can worsen in type 2 diabetic patients taking β-blockers, especially the nonselective ones. This is, in part, because insulin secretion is mediated by the β_1-adrenoceptor. Additionally, although no studies of the effects on diabetic patients have been reported, β-blockers decrease insulin sensitivity in nondiabetic subjects. β-Blockers also increase TG concentrations and reduce HDL cholesterol levels. This is especially likely with the nonselective ones. Their effect on LDL cholesterol levels is less consistent. The agents with intrinsic sympathomimetic activity have little effect on lipid levels.

Not surprisingly, β-blockers can impair the recognition of the adrenergic symptoms of hypoglycemia and prolong the restoration of normal glucose concentrations. These adverse effects are more troublesome in diabetic patients seeking near euglycemia; in these patients, hypoglycemia is more common. Again, nonselective agents are more likely to have this effect because both hepatic glycogenolysis and gluconeogenesis are mediated by the β_2-adrenoceptor. High doses of the selective ones, however, can also affect the recognition of and recovery from hypoglycemia.

Other adverse effects of β-blockers must also be considered; some may be more of a problem in patients with diabetes. These include decreased exercise tolerance (again, the nonselective agents are more likely to have this effect than the selective ones), less weight loss, bronchospasm, worsening of congestive heart failure, fatigue, lethargy, depression, altered sleep patterns, and hyperkalemia. (The latter is related to the fact that β-blockers decrease renin production by the juxtaglomerular apparatus in the kidneys and that β_2-adrenoceptors help mediate the shift of potassium from the extracellular to the intracellular space.) Therefore, potassium levels should be monitored in patients receiving β-blockers, especially those also taking nonsteroidal antiinflammatory agents, those with renal impairment, and elderly individuals.

The two general types of *calcium channel blockers* are dihydropyridine derivatives and nondihydropyridine compounds. The nondihydropyridine drugs in this class are verapamil and diltiazem. The other calcium channel blockers are dihydropyridine compounds. All calcium channel blockers

cause peripheral vasodilation, which decreases peripheral vascular resistance, thereby lowering blood pressure. Both dihydropyridine and nondihydropyridine calcium channel blockers have a mild natriuretic effect, which is helpful because many diabetic patients have increased total body sodium content (although generally not increased plasma volumes). These drugs are effective antihypertensive agents in diabetic patients. All racial/ethnic subgroups respond equally. They have little effect on glycemic and lipid levels. Diltiazem has the extra benefit of decreasing proteinuria (both microalbuminuria and clinical proteinuria). Verapamil and some of the dihydropyridine derivatives have also shown this effect in some but not all studies.

Calcium channel blockers are generally well tolerated, especially at low doses. The dihydropyridine derivatives may cause pedal edema, facial flushing, and tachycardia. Diltiazem and verapamil have negative inotropic and chronotropic effects on the heart. Both may precipitate or exacerbate congestive heart failure, especially in patients with decreased ejection fractions. In low doses, diltiazem is considered the best tolerated of the calcium channel blockers. The most common side effect at high doses is an atrioventricular conduction defect. Constipation is the most common side effect of verapamil at high doses. Both dihydropyridine and nondihydropyridine calcium channel blockers occasionally cause sexual dysfunction, orthostatic hypotension, and gingival hyperplasia. Finally, concern has been raised[36] (and disputed[37]) that short-acting calcium channel blockers, especially in high doses, may increase major cardiovascular events. No long-term studies with the sustained-release preparations are available.

The other class of drugs preferred by the JNC-V was *diuretics* because they have been shown to significantly reduce myocardial infarctions, strokes, and other cardiovascular events. Furthermore, they are inexpensive, are very effective, have few symptomatic side effects (especially when used in low doses), and have an additive effect when used with other antihypertensive agents. They are a good choice for diabetic patients because the hypertension associated with diabetes is linked to increased total body sodium, and therefore, not surprisingly, diuretics are as effective in diabetic patients as any other drug. Although somewhat less response is observed in young Caucasian males, diuretics work well in older individuals, African Americans, and obese patients, as well as those with diabetes. In patients with renal impairment (GFR <50 ml/min), however, thiazide diuretics are ineffective and loop diuretics must be used to control volume and blood pressure.

A number of side effects have been associated with use of diuretics. These include glucose intolerance in nondiabetic individuals, worsening glycemia in diabetic patients, transient increases in cholesterol and TG concentrations, sexual dysfunction, cardiac dysrhythmias, and even increased mortality in diabetic patients. It is now generally accepted, however, that these side effects are associated with high doses of thiazide diuretics and are minimal at doses equivalent to ≤25 mg hydrochlorothiazide.

Other available antihypertensive agents are not usually used in diabetic patients. These include centrally acting α_2-adrenergic agonists, other adrenergic antagonists, and vasodilators. The α_2-*adrenergic agonists* (e.g., clonidine, α-methyldopa) lower blood pressure by decreasing peripheral sympathetic nervous system activity. They are effective in diabetic patients but are limited by their side effects, especially sedation, dry mouth, and male sexual dysfunction. They have little effect on glucose and lipid metabolism. Some reports have described a beneficial effect of clonidine on orthostatic hypotension, painful peripheral neuropathy, and diabetic enteropathy,[32] suggesting a role for this drug in a small subset of diabetic patients (albeit not necessarily to lower blood pressure). Other *adrenergic antagonists*

(e.g., reserpine, guanethidine) reduce blood pressure, but their side effects (sedation, postural hypotension, sexual dysfunction) make these a poor choice. They are not recommended as first-line agents by either the JNC-V or the WGRHD. *Vasodilators* (e.g., hydralazine, minoxidil) are third-line agents that if used are typically given with diuretics to combat fluid retention and/or β-blockers to control reflex tachycardia. Minoxidil is particularly helpful in resistant hypertensive patients but has not been formally evaluated in patients with diabetes.

Finally, a new class of drugs, *angiotensin II antagonists,* has been introduced. These drugs block the angiotensin II receptor and thus would be expected to have properties similar to the ACE inhibitors. Although no studies have been directed at diabetic patients, the first drug to be approved (losartan) was as equally effective as enalapril and β-blockers in mild to moderate essential hypertension.[38] Like ACE inhibitors, they seem to be less effective in African Americans. Early reports suggest that they reduce proteinuria, do not affect glucose or lipid metabolism, and do not induce cough. Not surprisingly, based on their mechanism of action, these drugs can raise potassium levels.

A complete list of available antihypertensive agents can be found in the *Medical Letter.*[39]

The recommendations of the WGRHD for treating hypertension in diabetic patients (published before the calcium channel blocker controversy[36, 37]) are shown in Figure 8–13. The goal is to achieve a blood pressure of <130/85 mm Hg in persons with diabetes. My preference is to use lower doses of two or more antihypertensive agents to reach this target level rather than higher doses of a single agent in order to reduce potential side effects. This may be particularly helpful with calcium channel blockers and diuretics, for which evidence exists that their adverse effects are dose related. If there are no contraindications, my initial therapy is an ACE inhibitor because of its renal pro-

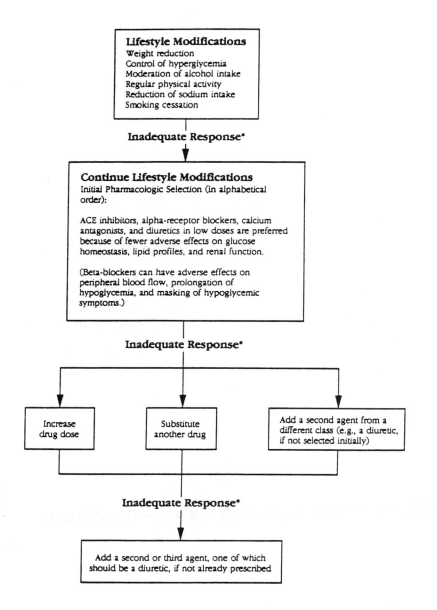

Lifestyle Modifications
Weight reduction
Control of hyperglycemia
Moderation of alcohol intake
Regular physical activity
Reduction of sodium intake
Smoking cessation

Inadequate Response*

Continue Lifestyle Modifications
Initial Pharmacologic Selection (in alphabetical order):

ACE inhibitors, alpha-receptor blockers, calcium antagonists, and diuretics in low doses are preferred because of fewer adverse effects on glucose homeostasis, lipid profiles, and renal function.

(Beta-blockers can have adverse effects on peripheral blood flow, prolongation of hypoglycemia, and masking of hypoglycemic symptoms.)

Inadequate Response*

| Increase drug dose | Substitute another drug | Add a second agent from a different class (e.g., a diuretic, if not selected initially) |

Inadequate Response*

Add a second or third agent, one of which should be a diuretic, if not already prescribed

*Response means achieved goal blood pressure or considerable progress toward this goal.

Figure 8–13. Algorithmic approach to the treatment of hypertension in diabetic patients suggested by the Working Group Report on Hypertension in Diabetes. ACE, angiotensin-converting enzyme inhibitor. (From the National High Blood Pressure Education Program Working Group on Hypertension in Diabetes. Hypertension 23:145, 1994)

tective effect. I would then add a diuretic, and if this combination were not effective, the third drug would be either a calcium channel blocker or an α_1-adrenoceptor blocker. The calcium channel blockers are usually better tolerated than the α_1-blockers. If an ACE inhibitor were contraindicated (keep in mind that losartan could be substituted if cough were the reason an ACE inhibitor could not be used), my initial choice would be a calcium channel blocker. If cardiovascular considerations (e.g., congestive heart failure, arrhythmias) were not present, I would favor one of the nondihydropyridine drugs because of their positive renal effects. It must be kept in mind that achievement of the blood pressure goal is more important than the means by which it is reached.

The issue of isolated systolic hypertension needs to be addressed. In the Systolic Hypertension in the Elderly Program,[40] 10% of the participants had diabetes. The relative risk reductions of stroke, myocardial infarctions, and mortality associated with diuretic therapy were similar in diabetic patients and subjects without diabetes. Thus, reducing

systolic blood pressure in diabetic patients to <160 mm Hg should be pursued. If an older patient (≥65 years old) has microalbuminuria or clinical proteinuria, I attempt to lower the blood pressure to <130/85 mm Hg. If the patient has no evidence of renal disease, I am satisfied to achieve a blood pressure of <160/90 mm Hg.

MICROALBUMINURIA

The development of ESRD proceeds along a continuum from normoalbuminuria to microalbuminuria to clinical proteinuria to a progressive decline in renal function (Fig. 8–14). Virtually all of the longitudinal studies have been carried out on type 1 diabetic patients because the onset of diabetes can usually be accurately determined. The few studies enrolling type 2 diabetic patients strongly suggest that in general, the same progression occurs in these patients as well, although the high prevalence of hypertension has an additional important role.[41] Microalbuminuria is rare during the first 5 years of diabetes. It generally occurs 8 to 10 years

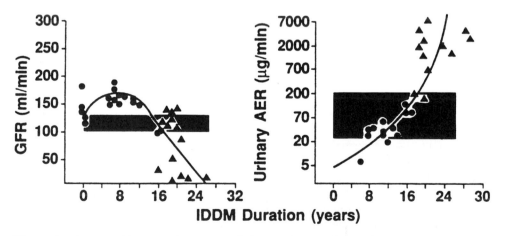

Figure 8–14. Natural history of 20 type 1 diabetic patients who progressed to overt diabetic nephropathy (see text for definition of overt nephropathy) in a 12-year period. IDDM, insulin-dependent diabetes mellitus (type 1 diabetes); GFR, glomerular filtration rate; AER, albumin excretion rate; initial values (●); follow-up values (▲); shaded areas show normal range. (From DeFronzo RA: Diabetic nephropathy etiologic and therapeutic considerations. Diabetes Rev 3:510, 1995)

after the onset of diabetes and precedes clinical proteinuria by 5 to 8 years. Thus, as discussed earlier, the microalbuminuria, if left untreated, predicted the subsequent development of clinical proteinuria in approximately 30% of patients after 5 years and in as many as 80% 10 to 14 years later. Fewer than 5% of diabetic patients without microalbuminuria developed clinical proteinuria 7 to 14 years later.[19]

Because of these considerations and the fact that microalbuminuria is treatable (discussed later), it is very important for the primary care physician to accurately assess whether microalbuminuria is present or not. Other nondiabetic causes of microalbuminuria must be kept in mind, and before microalbuminuria is assumed to reflect incipient diabetic nephropathy, they must be ruled out. These causes are (1) poor diabetic control, (2) systemic or urinary tract infection, (3) fever (per se), (4) congestive heart failure, (5) elevated blood pressure, and (6) exercise.

Five methods are available for assessing for the presence of microalbuminuria: (1) measuring albumin in urine collected during a 24-hour period, (2) measuring albumin in a specifically timed shorter urine collection period (e.g., over 4 hours), (3) measuring albumin in urine collected overnight (i.e., between going to sleep and waking up in the morning), (4) measuring the albumin-to-creatinine ratio in a random urine sample, and (5) measuring the albumin concentration. The latter can be performed either quantitatively or semiquantitatively with a strip (Micral, Boehringer Mannheim, Indianapolis, IN) specifically adapted to very low concentrations of albumin. A concentration ≥ 20 mg/L has been accepted as being positive for microalbuminuria. However, an albumin concentration exceeding this value must be confirmed by one of the other methods before a diagnosis of microalbuminuria can be made. Because urinary volume is so critical to the concentration of albumin measured, simply measuring the albumin concentration is not generally recommended as

a screening test if one of the other approaches is available.[42]

A single abnormal value is not sufficient to make the diagnosis of microalbuminuria. Because of as much as a 40% to 50% day-to-day variation in albumin excretion, an abnormal result mandates a repeat test to confirm the abnormal value. This is especially important in patients whose results are in the lower microalbuminuric range. Timed urine collections and 24-hour urine collections are the least convenient for patients. An overnight urine collection is less inconvenient, but because of recumbency and little activity, the albumin excretion rate overnight is approximately 25% less than during the day (upright posture and exercise increase albumin excretion). This may not be a drawback because an abnormal value in an overnight collection is more certain to be a valid diagnosis (values in the lower microalbuminuric range are much more likely to be normal on retesting). The albumin-to-creatinine ratio is the simplest of the four valid tests to assess microalbuminuria. Albumin-to-creatinine ratios ≥ 30 μg/mg (3.5 μg/μmol) have a high degree (95% to 100%) of both sensitivity and specificity in predicting microalbuminuria when measured by 24-hour or timed urine collections.[43, 44] A ratio measured in a sample collected on rising in the morning correlates much more closely with microalbuminuria measured by other means than does a sample collected randomly during the day.[45] The Council on Diabetes Mellitus of the National Kidney Foundation[46] has recommended the simpler albumin-to-creatinine ratio over other methods. A diagnosis of microalbuminuria requires two values between 30 and 300 μg/mg within a 3-month period. Values ≥ 300 μg/mg diagnose clinical proteinuria. However, a more cost-effective approach is to initially test a random urine sample with a standard dipstick for protein. If that result is positive (and confirmed), the patient has clinical proteinuria and further work-up for microalbuminuria is unnecessary. The distinction between the upper end of the microalbuminuric range and the lower end of the clinical proteinuria range is not important because the clinical approach is the same. All diabetic patients, with the exception of those with type 1 diabetes within the first 5 years of diagnosis, should be tested for the presence of albumin in the urine. If the test result for microalbuminuria is negative, evaluation should be repeated on a yearly basis.

Four modalities of treatment improve or reverse microalbuminuria. One is aggressive antihypertensive therapy. The second is achieving near euglycemia. One of many studies supporting this statement was a retrospective analysis of glycated hemoglobin (Hgb A_{1c}) levels and the presence of microalbuminuria in >1,600 type 1 diabetic patients. It revealed that the latter increased

sharply with values of the former that were equivalent to a Hgb A_{1c} level >8.0% (Fig. 8–15).[47] The third modality is use of ACE inhibitors. As mentioned earlier, strong evidence shows that intraglomerular pressure is increased in the kidneys of diabetic patients. Increased urinary albumin excretion results from this increased intraglomerular pressure. A major reason for the intraglomerular hypertension is vasoconstriction of the efferent arteriole. ACE inhibitors relieve this vasoconstriction. These drugs prevent the progression from microalbuminuria to clinical proteinuria in normotensive patients with both type 1[48-51] and type 2[52] diabetes. When the ACE inhibitor was discontinued (by the patient's choice), clinical proteinuria developed.[53] Therefore, an ACE inhibitor should be prescribed for all diabetic patients with

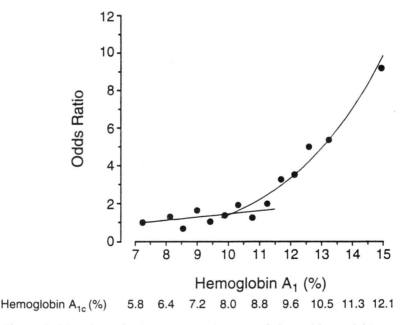

Figure 8–15. Relation between geometric mean of glycated hemoglobin values and the risk of developing microalbuminuria in 1,419 patients with type 1 diabetes. Glycated hemoglobin levels were measured repeatedly in the 4-year period before testing for microalbuminuria. An odds ratio of one indicates no increased risk for microalbuminuria. (From Krolewski AS, Laffel LMB, Krolewski M et al: Glycosylated hemoglobin and the risk of microalbuminuria in patients with insulin-dependent diabetes mellitus. N Engl J Med 332:1251, 1995)

microalbuminuria unless there is a contraindication. As stated earlier, an ACE inhibitor
should be used in the antihypertensive regimen and in patients with clinical proteinuria
(almost all of whom have hypertension). I
am unaware of any data showing that increasing the amount of the ACE inhibitor
beyond a dose equivalent to 100 mg of captopril or 10 mg of enalapril has any effect
other than blood pressure reduction. Therefore, if a patient is already taking an ACE
inhibitor, I do not routinely measure the
amount of urinary albumin because I would
use no additional therapy beyond aggressive
glycemic and blood pressure control.

The fourth modality is a low-protein diet.
Because high-protein intake increases intraglomerular pressure,[17] reduced dietary protein might be expected to have a beneficial
effect on renal function in diabetic patients.
Indeed, low-protein diets in type 1 diabetic
patients with incipient nephropathy reduce
microalbuminuria.[54, 55] In patients with clinical proteinuria and renal insufficiency, low-
protein diets also decrease urinary protein
excretion and, more importantly, slow the
deterioration of renal function.[56–58] Because
of the difficulty in sustaining a low-protein
diet and the availability of other effective
therapies for microalbuminuria (aggressive
glycemic and blood pressure control), I usually reserve a low-protein diet for patients
with clinical proteinuria, at which point renal function has already started to decline
even if the serum creatinine concentration is
still within the normal range. In the past, the
amount of protein prescribed in the low-
protein diet was usually 0.6 g/kg. Dietary
histories revealed that most of these patients
ingested approximately 0.85 g/kg (and still
derived beneficial results). Given that some
have questioned whether 0.6 g/kg is enough
protein to continually sustain lean body
mass, that the usual American diet contains
1.2 to 1.5 g/kg of protein, and that the recommended daily allowance for protein is 0.8
g/kg, it seems reasonable to prescribe the
latter amount of protein for a low-protein

diet. The type of protein in the diet may also
have an important role in influencing renal
function. Albuminuria decreased further
when vegetable protein was substituted for
animal protein without a change in total
protein intake in type 1 diabetic patients.[59]
Certainly, the older practice of increasing
protein intake in patients with clinical
proteinuria or the nephrotic syndrome
should be discarded.

In summary, the salient features of diabetic
nephropathy are as follows: (1) The progression from normal albumin excretion to microalbuminuria (incipient nephropathy) to
clinical proteinuria (overt nephropathy) to
deterioration of kidney function (renal insufficiency or failure) to ESRD requiring dialysis
or renal transplantation occurs along a continuum. (2) Near euglycemia is extremely
beneficial in preventing or reversing microalbuminuria but is ineffective once renal insufficiency and/or clinical proteinuria has su-
pervened. (3) Aggressive blood pressure
control is helpful in preventing or reversing
microalbuminuria and slowing the progression of clinical proteinuria and renal deterioration. (4) Because of their effect on reducing intraglomerular pressure (in addition to
their systemic effect on blood pressure), ACE
inhibitors (unless contraindicated) should be
part of the antihypertensive regimen and
should also be prescribed for normotensive
diabetic patients (both type 1 and type 2)
with either microalbuminuria or clinical proteinuria (almost all of the latter require antihypertensive medications). (5) Low-protein
diets reverse (and, although not studied,
probably prevent) microalbuminuria and
slow the progression of clinical proteinuria
and renal deterioration. I do not prescribe
an ACE inhibitor for a normotensive patient
with normal albumin excretion to prevent
diabetic nephropathy because, to date, no
evidence supports this approach.

Another aspect of microalbuminuria is
intriguing.[17, 60] It predicts not only the development of clinical proteinuria but also cardiovascular mortality in type 2 diabetic pa-

tients. For instance, Figure 8–16 shows a progressive increase in mortality after 9.5 years as the level of microalbuminuria increased in type 2 diabetic patients compared with age-matched controls. Although these patients have other risk factors for cardiovascular disease, the excess mortality is only partially explained by them. It has long been well documented that clinical proteinuria in type 1 diabetes is a powerful predictor of mortality due to coronary artery disease.

Microalbuminuria and clinical proteinuria also predict increased cardiovascular mortality in nondiabetic populations. One hypothesis to explain this association is that albuminuria simply reflects vascular damage that has occurred throughout the body.[21] The increased permeability of vessels would allow atherosclerotic lipoproteins to penetrate the walls of large vessels and would account for the leakiness of retinal blood vessels in diabetic patients. This theory is supported by the markedly increased transcapillary escape of albumin[61] and fibrinogen in diabetic patients with microalbuminuria.

HYPORENINEMIC HYPOALDOSTERONISM

Another situation with which primary care physicians may have to deal is the syndrome of hyporeninemic hypoaldosteronism.[62] Patients with this condition present with hyperkalemia that is asymptomatic approximately 75% of the time. Symptoms in the other 25% are muscle weakness and/or cardiac arrhythmias. Approximately half of patients have a hyperchloremic acidosis. This syndrome usually occurs in older patients. This fact may not be surprising because aging is associated with decreased secretion of both renin and aldosterone. Most patients have mild to moderate renal insufficiency and/or diabetes mellitus.

The pathogenesis of this enigmatic syndrome is not clear, and this is not the place to discuss the various hypotheses. The problem for primary care physicians is one of management. One must keep in mind that most of these patients are older and have associated medical conditions such as diabetes, renal failure, macroangiopathy, and/or hypertension. Therefore, the side effects of

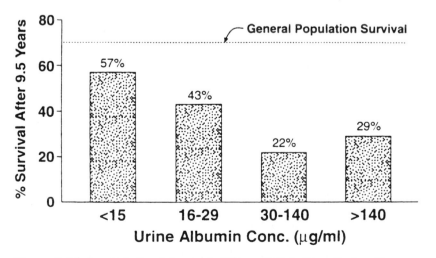

Figure 8–16. Survival after 9.5 years in 76 type 2 diabetic patients with various degrees of microalbuminuria (based on urinary albumin concentration) compared with an age-matched population. (From DeFronzo RA: Diabetic nephropathy: Etiology and therapeutic considerations. Diabetes Rev 3:510, 1995)

any therapeutic interventions must be weighed against the possible benefits of lowering the serum potassium level. Obviously, drugs that may raise potassium levels (e.g., potassium-sparing diuretics, ACE inhibitors) should be avoided. Because β-blockers and calcium channel blockers suppress renin secretion and vasodilatory prostaglandins stimulate renin secretion, it has been suggested that these two classes of antihypertensive agents and nonsteroidal antiinflammatory drugs be avoided.[63] I usually do not treat an asymptomatic patient with a potassium level <6 mEq/L as long as no changes of hyperkalemia are noted on the electrocardiogram. If therapy is deemed necessary, either mineralocorticoid (fludrocortisone acetate or Florinef) administration or sodium-potassium exchange resins can be tried. Sodium retention leading possibly to congestive heart failure may occur with both therapies (high doses of Florinef [0.2 to 0.5 mg] are often required). Potassium-wasting diuretics may be helpful. The mild acidosis may be treated with oral sodium bicarbonate, which may also improve potassium excretion, but once again an increased sodium load may be a problem.

The final circumstance to be discussed involving diabetic nephropathy concerns radiocontrast-induced acute renal failure. Because of their coronary artery and peripheral vascular diseases, diabetic patients are likely to undergo dye studies. Unfortunately, patients with diabetes, congestive heart failure, and/or renal insufficiency are at an increased risk for radiocontrast-induced renal dysfunction. Diabetic patients with renal insufficiency are particularly susceptible.[64] The higher the prestudy serum creatinine concentration, the more likely it is that acute renal failure will occur and that dialysis may be necessary for temporary treatment.[65, 66] For example, in a cohort of patients with a mean serum creatinine level of 2.4 mg/dl, 40% manifested radiocontrast-induced renal failure despite previous hydration.[65] In two other studies,[64, 67] the prevalence of acute renal failure was 2% to 5% in low-risk patients and 9% to 16% in high-risk patients, with high risk defined as the presence of diabetes mellitus, preexisting renal insufficiency, or congestive heart failure. None of these patients required dialysis. Unfortunately, using the newer, nonionic, low-osmolality radiocontrast materials did not protect the patients from acute renal failure.[64, 67, 68]

What then is the role of primary care physicians under these circumstances? First, be certain that the dye study is really necessary and that equivalent information could not be obtained by other imaging techniques. Second, because plasma volume contraction and decreased renal plasma flow are extremely important risks, withhold diuretics, nonsteroidal antiinflammatory agents, and metformin (which decrease renal blood flow) the day before the procedure. Third, ensure adequate hydration by infusing saline to induce a gentle diuresis (≥75 ml/h).[65, 69] Some physicians begin this several hours before the study; others begin the hydration after the study is completed. In either case, it should be continued for approximately 4 hours after the procedure. Although centers also use concomitant administration of furosemide or mannitol, a prospective controlled study demonstrated that these agents may actually increase nephrotoxicity.[69]

DIABETIC NEUROPATHY

Diabetic neuropathy (Table 8–5) has an important role in the increased morbidity and mortality suffered by individuals with diabetes. Although the exact mechanism is not known, it is generally believed that long-term hyperglycemia is the cause (except as noted).

PERIPHERAL NEUROPATHY

Peripheral neuropathy is the earliest, most widely recognized, and probably the most common form of diabetic neuropathy. It is a

Table 8–5. Classification of Diabetic Neuropathy

Peripheral neuropathy
Autonomic neuropathy
  Cardiovascular
  Gastrointestinal
  Genitourinary
  Sudomotor
  Hypoglycemia unawareness
Acute-onset neuropathies
  Mononeuropathy
  Mononeuropathy multiplex
  Radiculopathy
  Plexopathy
Neuropathic diabetic cachexia

common complication intimately related to the duration of diabetes (Fig. 8–17). Note that 20% of type 2 diabetic patients have peripheral neuropathy at the time of diagnosis, reflecting the preceding many years of asymptomatic hyperglycemia. The overall prevalence in the diabetic population is 25% to 35%.[70, 71]

Peripheral neuropathy is a generalized, sensorimotor polyneuropathy of gradual onset that is usually progressive. The legs are almost always affected earlier than the hands. Patients initially experience sensory manifestations (e.g., paresthesias, burning sensations, and hyperesthesia), which can be quite uncomfortable. On examination, early loss of tendon reflexes, decreased vibration sense, and sense of touch are noted. As the peripheral neuropathy progresses, the feet become numb and the patient is unable to appreciate trauma. Additionally, involvement of motor fibers can cause muscle weakness and atrophy. This can cause deformities of the feet, leading to areas that receive increased pressure and are manifested initially by callus formation. A further serious cause of foot deformities and areas receiving increased pressure is Charcot's arthropathy (joint destruction secondary to unappreciated trauma). This repeated unrecognized trauma to the foot may destroy the joint structures, with subsequent flattening of the

foot arch (Fig. 8–18). Because patients have decreased sensation in the foot, these areas can ulcerate. Once the integrity of the skin has been breached, the chances for a serious infection are increased, especially if a patient is very hyperglycemic. Any impairment of circulation to the foot because of peripheral vascular disease compounds the problem. The combination of loss of sensation leading to ulceration of the skin (whether foot deformities are involved or not) and diminished circulation is the root cause of the large number of lower extremity amputations in diabetic patients (50% to 75% of total nontraumatic amputations in the United States).

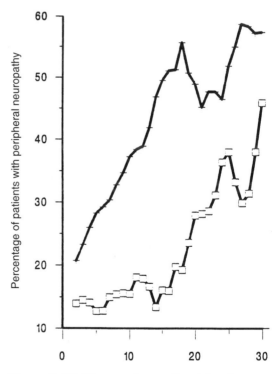

Figure 8–17. The prevalence of peripheral neuropathy in type 1 (□) and type 2 (+) diabetic patients by duration of disease. (From Young MJ, Boulton AJM, Macleod AF et al: A multicentre study of the prevalence of diabetic peripheral neuropathy in the United Kingdom hospital clinic population. Diabetologia 36:150, 1993)

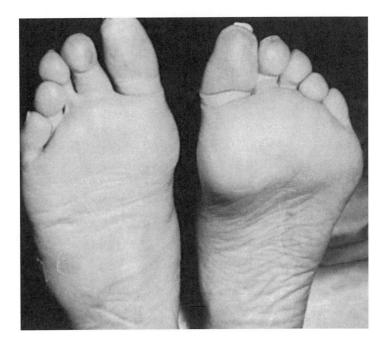

Figure 8–18. Charcot's joint resulting in flattening of the arch.

AUTONOMIC NEUROPATHY

Although various tests may reveal abnormalities in the functioning of the autonomic nervous system (both sympathetic and parasympathetic) early in the course of diabetes, clinical signs and symptoms appear much later and almost always after peripheral neuropathy is established. Normally, parasympathetic activity decreases the heart rate while sympathetic activity increases the heart rate and the force of cardiac contraction (leading to a rise in cardiac output) and redirects blood flow from the viscera to skeletal muscle by increasing splanchnic resistance more than peripheral resistance. The parasympathetic arm of the autonomic nervous system is often affected earlier and more profoundly than the sympathetic one. Therefore, a *resting tachycardia* is usually the initial clinical cardiovascular effect of autonomic neuropathy. *Exercise intolerance* may occur when the sympathetic nervous system is affected, because the necessary increase in cardiac output and skeletal blood flow is blunted. When one arises from a lying to sitting to standing position, the sympathetic nervous system is responsible for the maintenance of the blood pressure via stimuli from the baroreceptors. Therefore, autonomic neuropathy may cause *postural (orthostatic) hypotension,* which has been defined in two ways: either a 30 mm Hg decrease in systolic blood pressure or a 10 mm Hg fall in diastolic blood pressure 2 minutes after standing. Clinically, patients complain of sudden dizziness (lightheadedness), weakness, nausea, and occasionally vomiting or syncope after standing up quickly.

Autonomic neuropathy can involve all parts of the gastrointestinal tract: esophagus, stomach, gallbladder, small intestine, and large intestine. Esophageal and gallbladder dysfunction do not usually cause any symptoms.

In patients with gastric involvement *(gastroparesis diabeticorum),* the stomach is large, dilated, and hypotonic. (Smooth muscle contractions of the gastrointestinal tract are mediated by the parasympathetic nervous system.) Symptoms include anorexia, postprandial bloating, early satiety, nausea, vomiting, and gastric reflux. Because the ingested food remains in the stomach and is delayed in entering the small intestine, the vomitus may include undigested food eaten many hours earlier. This problem is a particularly difficult one for insulin-requiring patients, who need a predictable response to meals to cover the action of the injected insulin. Autonomic neuropathy of the intestine leads to constipation (most common) or diarrhea or alternating constipation and diarrhea. Diabetic diarrhea is often nocturnal and can be associated with fecal incontinence (due to neurogenic impairment of rectal sensation).

Bladder dysfunction and, in males, retrograde ejaculation and impotence are the result of autonomic neuropathy involving the genitourinary tract. As in the intestinal tract, the parasympathetic nervous system mediates the sensation of bladder fullness and contraction of bladder smooth muscle. The necessary involuntary relaxation of the bladder sphincters during urination is under control of the sympathetic nervous system. The initial symptom is decreased frequency of urination as the bladder capacity increases before contraction occurs. This progresses to overflow incontinence associated with urgency and dribbling, incomplete emptying of the bladder, and finally inability to void. The retained urine is a prime source for infection, which, if it travels in a retrograde direction up the ureter, can lead to serious kidney infections.

Unfortunately, impotence (*erectile dysfunction*) is a common problem in male diabetic patients and can eventually occur in >50%. The usual situation is a slowly progressive inability initially to maintain and eventually to achieve a satisfactory erection. This usually occurs (at least initially) in association with normal libido and ejaculation. However, as satisfactory intercourse becomes more difficult, the accompanying anxiety and depression may secondarily impair libido. Other causes of impotence must be ruled out, especially a primary psychogenic

cause and, importantly in diabetic patients, vascular insufficiency. As mentioned earlier, certain antihypertensive medications may be a contributing factor.

Normal functioning of the parasympathetic nervous system is necessary for an erection by dilating the penile blood vessels. The sympathetic nervous system is responsible for muscle contractions resulting in ejaculation. If the internal bladder sphincter (which is innervated by the sympathetic nervous system) does not close appropriately during orgasm, the ejaculate enters the bladder *(retrograde ejaculation)*. The sensory component of orgasm (as opposed to the ejaculatory aspect) is mediated by nervous pathways that are not part of the autonomic nervous system. Thus, the pleasurable sensation of orgasm remains intact. Involvement of the parasympathetic nervous system occurs more readily than impairment of the sympathetic component. Therefore, the inability to achieve a satisfactory erection to complete the act of sexual intercourse successfully is much more common than retrograde ejaculation. The latter is uncommon by itself. When it does occur, it is almost always in conjunction with erectile dysfunction.

Patients with autonomic dysfunction may also have *sudomotor dysfunction*. Areas of anhidrosis and hyperhidrosis are usually distributed over the body, with the former more common in the lower extremities and the latter usually occurring over the trunk and face. The probable explanation is that lack of perspiration over one area leads to a compensatory increase over other areas to accomplish overall heat regulation. Regrowth of damaged autonomic nerve fibers has also been suggested. Excessive sweating often occurs at mealtime, at night, or under stress. Although sudomotor dysfunction is usually not bothersome, an uncommon but troublesome symptom is profuse facial perspiration when the patient starts to eat (*gustatory sweating*).

The final manifestation of autonomic dysfunction may be *hypoglycemic unaware-ness*. As discussed in Chapter 7, autonomic neuropathy is but one cause of hypoglycemic unawareness. Hypoglycemic unawareness secondary to autonomic neuropathy is mainly restricted to type 1 diabetic patients for the following reason. The normal hormonal counterregulatory responses to hypoglycemia are secretion of glucagon from the α-cells in the pancreatic islets of Langerhans, epinephrine from the adrenal medulla, cortisol from the adrenal cortex, and growth hormone from the pituitary gland. The first two are secreted rapidly and have immediate but short-lived effects to restore glucose levels toward normal. Not only is there an approximately 30-minute delay before the latter two are secreted, but their effects are also delayed and prolonged. As long as the glucagon response is intact, glucose concentrations will be restored. If glucagon is not secreted, epinephrine will raise glucose levels. If both of these normal responses are absent, hypoglycemic levels will be maintained (or continue to drop) because the effects of growth hormone and cortisol are too delayed to reverse the situation.

For unknown reasons, the glucagon response to hypoglycemia starts to wane shortly after the onset of type 1 (but not type 2) diabetes and is mostly gone 5 years later. Epinephrine secretion remains as the patient's only effective rapid counterregulatory response to combat hypoglycemia. Secretion of epinephrine also causes the autonomic signs and symptoms of hypoglycemia (weakness, sweating, tachycardia, palpitations, hunger, tremor, nervousness, tingling of mouth and fingers). Because epinephrine secretion by the adrenal medulla is mediated by autonomic innervations, autonomic neuropathy blunts and eventually abolishes this counterregulatory response. Not only does this leave patients without any warning of hypoglycemia so that they may eat to counteract it, but epinephrine is not present to reverse the hypoglycemia. Therefore, the neuroglucopenic signs and symptoms (visual disturbances, bizarre behavior, mental dullness, confusion, amnesia, seizures, coma) often occur without warning in these patients. Even though autonomic neuropathy would also impair the catecholamine response to hypoglycemia in type 2 diabetic patients, preservation of the glucagon response usually prevents severe hypoglycemia (i.e., assistance by another person required) by increasing hepatic glucose production before glucose concentrations fall to extremely low levels. Severe hypoglycemia does occasionally occur in sulfonylurea agent–induced hypoglycemia because the effect of the drug persists and overwhelms the ability of the liver to produce enough glucose.

ACUTE-ONSET NEUROPATHIES

Certain neuropathies seem to develop rapidly. In addition to their rather acute onset, they are usually associated with pain and a self-limited course of 1 to 3 months' duration for cranial nerve palsies but up to 1 year or more for the others, with eventual spontaneous resolution of both cranial and peripheral nerve dysfunction. They may occur in patients without peripheral or autonomic neuropathy. Indeed, the most common one, a third cranial nerve palsy (Fig. 8–19) (fourth, sixth, and rarely seventh nerve palsies may also occur), may herald the onset of diabetes. Also classified under acute-onset neuropathies are lesions of several nerves (mononeuropathy multiplex) and focal lesions of the lumbosacral (or rarely brachial) plexus (plexopathy) or of the nerve roots (radiculopathy). In addition to the pain in the distribution of the affected nerve structures, motor weakness in the muscles innervated by involved nerve(s) also commonly occurs. The descriptive term *amyotrophy* is sometimes used to describe a syndrome of asymmetric pain and weakness usually involving the pelvic girdle and thigh muscles. It is commonly encountered in older individuals and could be the result of lesions classified as a mononeuropathy, mononeuropathy multiplex, or

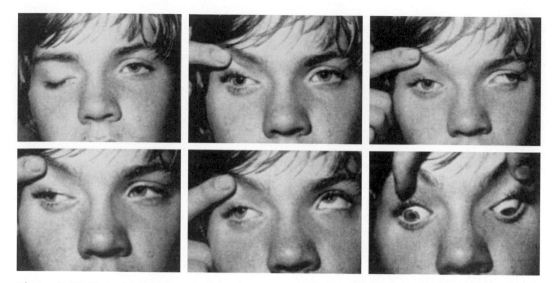

Figure 8–19. Right third nerve palsy in a diabetic patient. Note ptosis of the lid and sparing of the pupil (which is a distinguishing characteristic of diabetic origin compared with more serious causes, which usually affect the pupil). The patient is unable to turn the eye inward. Although the eye can turn outward, it cannot be raised or lowered normally in the lateral position. (From Miller NR: Walsh and Hoyt's Clinical Neuro-Ophthalmology, 3rd ed. Williams & Wilkins, Baltimore, 1969, p. 668)

plexopathy. The acute-onset neuropathies are likely caused by acute thrombosis or ischemia of the vessels nourishing the particular nervous system structures involved rather than by chronic hyperglycemia.

NEUROPATHIC DIABETIC CACHEXIA

A very unusual syndrome, occurring mostly in older men with relatively mild type 2 diabetes, consists of anorexia, painful neuropathy, depression, and profound weight loss (neuropathic diabetic cachexia). The weight loss is so dramatic that an occult malignancy is usually suspected. Spontaneous recovery occurs gradually within 12 to 18 months.

PREVENTION

Given this litany of the deleterious effects of diabetic neuropathy, what can primary care physicians do to help their patients with this complication of diabetes? The primary role is one of prevention, for once manifestations of diabetic neuropathy occur, our interventions are palliative at best. As discussed in Chapter 2 and shown in Figure 2–11, tight diabetic control not only forestalls (and possibly prevents) the development of diabetic neuropathy but also reverses the early painful symptoms. Once the peripheral neuropathy progresses to numbness of the feet, patients are at an increased risk of developing diabetic foot ulcers over areas receiving increased pressure (Fig. 8–20). These are entirely preventable by appropriate education and by examination of the feet. Unfortunately, physicians examine the feet of their diabetic patients only approximately 15% of the time![72, 73] Even when a nurse or aide removes the patient's shoes and socks, examinations were performed only two thirds of the time.[72] Callus formation should alert physician to increased pressure. Appropriate advice about properly fitting shoes and general foot care[74] should be given, and possible referral to a qualified podiatrist should be considered.

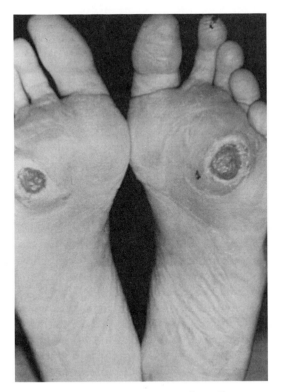

8–20. Diabetic foot ulcers. Note the callus formation surrounding the ulcerations.

TREATMENT

The *pain of peripheral neuropathy* is particularly vexing to the patients and not easy to treat. The first thing to emphasize to patients is that near euglycemia often alleviates the pain of peripheral diabetic neuropathy,[75] especially in its early stages. This discomfort often motivates patients to work with you to achieve strict diabetic control. Although many patients do not respond to ordinary analgesics, these should be tried first (as a patient is attempting to improve diabetic control) because some will respond.[76] Nonsteroidal antiinflammatory drugs, however, should not be used on a long-term basis because of their potential to reduce renal function. Narcotics should be avoided because these drugs often do not satisfactorily control the pain and addiction is a potential problem. However, if other approaches fail,

small doses, best given intermittently, can take the edge off the pain.

Most patients with marked pain have difficulty sleeping through the night and are often depressed as well. Sleeping medication is usually not helpful. However, small amounts of the tricyclic antidepressants imipramine (Tofranil) or amitriptyline (Elavil) may improve the pain, disturbed sleeping patterns, and associated depression.[77-79] The beneficial effect of the tricyclic antidepressants on the pain of diabetic peripheral neuropathy is independent of their antidepressant effects.[79] Because nighttime pain is usually more severe, the drugs are given before bed, starting with small doses and gradually increasing up to 150 mg if necessary. Patients should be warned about the side effects (sedation and anticholinergic symptoms). Patients usually respond within 1 week (which is faster than the antidepressant effect of higher doses). Therefore, I usually increase the dose weekly. If the pain is significant during the day, a small amount can be given on arising, but many patients prefer the discomfort of the neuropathy to the side effects of the drug during the day. If the side effects limit the use of amitriptyline or imipramine, desipramine may be substituted. This metabolite of imipramine has less anticholinergic and sedative action than its parent compound but has a comparable effect on the pain of diabetic neuropathy.[80] For this reason, it may be the drug of choice for elderly patients who may be particularly sensitive to these side effects. The tricyclic antidepressants are contraindicated in patients with heart block, recent myocardial infarctions, congestive heart failure, urinary tract obstruction, orthostatic hypotension, or narrow-angle glaucoma. They should be tapered slowly to avoid withdrawal symptoms (e.g., rebound insomnia, headache, excessive salivation, diarrhea, malaise, anorexia, and fatigue), although these are less likely with the lower doses used to treat diabetic neuropathy.

A locally applied cream, 0.075% capsaicin,

may be helpful for the superficial (as opposed to the deep, gnawing, "toothache") type of pain of diabetic peripheral neuropathy.[81] Capsaicin (naturally found in red peppers and used as a folk remedy for centuries to treat pain) is thought to work by depleting substance P, a neurotransmitter of pain, from peripheral nerve endings. It should be applied to the painful areas three to four times a day. Patients should be cautioned not to use excessive amounts because of its tendency to aerosolize and induce coughing and sneezing. Great care must be taken to avoid exposing mucous membranes (e.g., eyes and mouth) to the drug by either wearing gloves when applying it or thoroughly washing one's hands afterward to prevent a burning sensation in those areas. Because the mechanism of action of capsaicin is to deplete the nerve endings of substance P, thereby alleviating pain, it is not surprising that many patients experience a local exacerbation of pain after the initial applications until the neurotransmitter has been depleted. This usually abates after the first week if the patient uses the cream consistently. Although statistically significant differences have been found between capsaicin and its vehicle in published studies, the high placebo response (approximately 50%) makes interpretation difficult. Its role in the treatment of painful diabetic neuropathy remains uncertain because it can take up to 4 weeks to be effective and many patients stop using it during the initial stages when the pain increases at the sites of application. Furthermore, anecdotal experience has suggested that it is not helpful for many patients.

If a tricyclic antidepressant and capsaicin (for superficial pain) have not alleviated the problem to the extent that a patient can tolerate it, a second-line drug should be considered. Although phenytoin (Dilantin) was advocated many years ago[82] (and carried along in textbooks and reviews ever since), a small double-blind placebo-controlled study refuted the value of the drug.[83] Anecdotal experience (mine included) supports this lack of an effect, and I do not routinely use it.

The second-line drug most often used is carbamazepine (Tegretol). Several double-blind studies have demonstrated its efficacy in painful diabetic neuropathy.[84, 85] The usual effective dose of carbamazepine ranges between 400 and 800 mg/day in divided doses, although for some patients up to 1200 mg/day may be required. The initial dose is 100 mg bid; this should be gradually increased every day or two to yield therapeutic plasma levels of 4 to 10 μg/ml. Baseline blood and platelet counts, urinalysis, and hepatic and renal function tests are advisable before starting treatment. Because of the number of potential side effects (some of which can be quite serious), I refer these patients to a neurologist who has had much more experience with this drug.

Another second-line drug is mexiletine (the oral congener of lidocaine), which has been shown to be effective in some patients with painful diabetic peripheral neuropathy.[86, 87] Obtaining an electrocardiogram with a long rhythm strip before initiating treatment is essential because this drug may worsen cardiac arrhythmias. To minimize the common side effects of nausea and dizziness, mexiletine should be given after meals and in gradually increasing doses every 2 or 3 days. The initial dose is 75 to 200 mg tid, with dose increments of 50 to 100 mg. The effective dose is stated to be 10 mg/kg/day[86] or 450 mg/day.[87] The drug should be discontinued if a patient develops ectopic beats.

Finally, two other second-line drugs, clonidine[88] (an α_2-adrenergic agonist) and baclofen[89] (a γ-aminobutyric acid analogue), may be tried, although the usefulness of neither is supported by controlled studies, only anecdotal reports. Both should be started at low doses and increased gradually to minimize side effects—clonidine at 75 to 100 μg before retiring to avoid the effects of hypotension and drowsiness and baclofen at 5 to 15 mg/day to minimize drowsiness, dizziness, and ataxia. Even if drug therapy is not very helpful, patients are often comforted to know their pain is self-limited, although it may take up to a year or two until it abates completely.

Diabetic patients often complain of *leg cramps.* These can occur at rest (and therefore are not related to intermittent claudication) and seem to be more frequent overnight. It is commonly stated that these may be a manifestation of diabetic neuropathy, although little direct evidence supports this. In any event, quinine sulfate, 200 to 300 mg given at bedtime, has proved to be helpful.[90, 91]

The treatment of *Charcot's arthropathy* previously was total immobilization (usually by casting) and surgery to correct the deformities due to bone destruction. Although in the early stages immobilization can arrest the condition, it most often recurs on weight bearing. An anecdotal report[92] described a beneficial effect (decreased temperature and improvement in symptoms) in six patients given pamidronate, a second-generation bisphosphonate.

Although many of the problems caused by *autonomic neuropathy* may be handled by the appropriate specialist (neurologist, urologist, gastroenterologist, cardiologist), primary care physicians should be aware of certain treatment options in which they may be involved. Most of the cardiovascular manifestations of the autonomic nervous system do not require treatment except for the *orthostatic hypotension.* A number of non-pharmacologic measures can be very helpful in this difficult situation.[93] If drugs are necessary, the use of Florinef (0.05 to 0.1 mg daily) to increase the intravascular volume is usually tried first. If a small dose is ineffective, larger amounts may be tried, but excessive sodium retention with edema and possibly congestive heart failure often limit this approach. Other drugs that may be helpful are midodrine[94, 94a] (an orphan drug), diltiazem,[95] erythropoietin,[96] and octreotide (somatostatin).[97, 98] If drug therapy is ineffective or only partially effective, use of Jobst stockings should be considered and usually helps to some extent.[99]

Treatment of symptomatic *gastroparesis diabeticorum*[100] can be difficult and frustrating. The modalities of treatment are diet, glycemic control, drugs, and in severe cases nutritional support. Although hyperglycemia delays gastric emptying, near euglycemia improves it. Dietary treatment consists of frequent small meals (six to eight feedings per day) with a low-fat and low-fiber content. Liquids and foods of soft consistency are best. Because absorption of carbohydrate is delayed, it may be helpful not only to inject regular insulin just before eating or even after the meal (instead of the recommended 30 minutes prior) but also to move the site of injection from the abdomen to the arms, thighs, or buttocks, where absorption of insulin is slower. Drug treatments include metoclopramide (Reglan), cisapride (Propulsid), and erythromycin.

Metoclopramide is cholinergic and antidopaminergic. The former action increases gastric emptying and the latter accounts for its antiemetic properties by inhibiting the central vomiting center. Metoclopramide has little effect on gastric emptying of a liquid meal, and many patients develop tachyphylaxis to the effect of the drug on accelerating gastric emptying of more solid meals. Despite this, metoclopramide often produces sustained relief of symptoms, probably related to its central antiemetic properties. The usual dose is 5 to 20 mg given 15 to 60 minutes before each meal and at bedtime. It can also be administered as a suppository. If the symptoms are mild and intermittent, the drug should be given only during symptomatic intervals to avoid the long-term side effects. These occur in as many as 20% of patients, in whom reversible neurologic symptoms (sedation, restlessness, anxiety, fatigue) develop. Extrapyramidal signs (tremor and even tardive dyskinesia) can be a problem, as can the neuroendocrine side effects of hyperprolactinemia and occasionally galactorrhea.

Cisapride increases gastric emptying of both liquid and solid meals by a cholinergic effect. The drug has no antidopaminergic activity and few side effects. The dose is 10 mg 30 to 60 minutes before meals and at bedtime. In contrast to metoclopramide, gastric emptying remains improved during long-term administration of cisapride.

Erythromycin stimulates gastrointestinal motor activity via its binding to the motilin receptor. Through that mechanism, it accelerates gastric emptying of both liquid and solid meals and improves the symptoms related to gastroparesis diabeticorum.[101, 102] The dose varies from 125 to 500 mg three to four times a day. The side effects (nausea, bloating, abdominal cramps, diarrhea) seem to be dose related, allowing the possibility that a dose reduction might alleviate the side effects without eliminating the beneficial therapeutic effect.[100]

Diabetic diarrhea is a diagnosis of exclusion to be made only when other causes of diarrhea have been ruled out. Because the pathogenesis is unknown, treatment is necessarily empirical. The antidiarrheal agents loperamide and diphenoxylate can decrease the number of stools per day. Some cases have been associated with bacterial overgrowth, and use of broad-spectrum antibiotics (tetracycline, cephalosporins, quinolones, metronidazole) can be helpful. Rather than attempt to document bacterial overgrowth, it is easier to treat these patients empirically with antibiotics on a rotating basis for 10 to 14 days per month (to avoid bacterial resistance).[103] Clonidine (started in a low dose, 0.1 mg bid and gradually increased up to 0.5 or 0.6 mg bid as necessary) has been effective.[104] Others have successfully used topical clonidine[105, 106] to avoid the side effects of the oral formulation that would be particularly troublesome in these patients (orthostatic hypotension and delay of gastric emptying). Finally, 50 to 75 µg of octreotide, the long-acting somatostatin analogue, injected twice a day has been very

beneficial in some patients[97, 98, 107] and may be given in the same syringe with insulin.[107]

Constipation is more common than diarrhea and can be very difficult for patients. Management should include bulk or osmotic laxatives, but cathartics should be avoided. Stimulants of colonic motility, such as cisapride and cholinergic agonists (e.g., bethanechol) may be helpful in some patients. If all else fails and the constipation is severe, an enema program may be necessary.

Most genitourinary complications are managed by a urologist. However, the problem of *impotence* is almost always shared first with the primary care physician. Although the work-up of impotence[108] is beyond the scope of this chapter, the primary cause usually falls within the following categories: endocrine, psychogenic, autonomic neuropathy, vascular, or drug related. In diabetic patients, two or all three of the latter three may be involved. The first step is to evaluate whether drugs[109] (usually antihypertensive agents) may be contributing. Assuming that this is not the case and that an appropriate evaluation rules out endocrine and primarily psychogenic causes, one needs to discuss treatment options. Although sophisticated evaluation by urologists for impotence is sometimes able to pinpoint a vascular cause for which surgical intervention may be helpful, a National Institutes of Health consensus conference on impotence recommended that this approach be limited to very select patients (e.g., those with congenital or traumatic vascular abnormalities) and restricted to clinical investigation settings in medical centers with experienced personnel.[110] Therefore, the treatment for erectile dysfunction is necessarily nonspecific. Because the sensation of orgasm is retained, it is possible for both the patient and his wife or sexual partner to achieve sexual gratification in ways not requiring vaginal penetration by the erect penis. I point this out and, in a sense, give them "permission" to consider this alternative as one option.

I also discuss two other options, vacuum

tumescence devices and intracavernosal injection of vasodilators.[108, 110] Vacuum tumescence devices produce erections by creating a vacuum around the penis, causing blood to flow into it. The erection is maintained by placing a constricting band around the base of the penis. The constriction should not be maintained for more than 30 minutes. These devices are effective in approximately 70% of couples who use them. Drawbacks include the need for some dexterity to put them on correctly, the lack of spontaneity, and in some men discomfort due to impairment of ejaculation.

Injection of vasodilatory substances, papaverine, phentolamine, and alprostadil[111] (a synthetic prostaglandin E_1) alone or in various combinations is successful in 65%[112] to 85%[111] of patients with various causes of erectile dysfunction. However, in a small study of diabetic men, age was an important predictor of success, which was less than in the general population of impotent men.[113] Only 1 of 14 patients older than 60 years had a satisfactory response to phentolamine-papaverine intracavernosal injections, whereas 11 of 19 younger than 60 years did. Solutions containing prostaglandin E_1 are replacing those with papaverine because of a lower incidence of priapism and penile scarring. Priapism and penile fibrosis occur in <5% of patients, but dose-related pain occurs at the injection site 10% of the time after injection of the prostaglandin E_1 analogue. The first injection of these agents should take place under a physician's supervision in a private examination room while instructing the patient to administer the injections at home. This initial demonstration often helps to alleviate some of the patient's anxiety about self-administering intracavernosal injections and helps to determine the appropriate dose to achieve an erection. Recently, transurethral instillation of prostaglandin E_1 has been used successfully in approximately 70% of men with erectile dysfunction.[114]

Implantation of a penile prosthesis is considered second-line therapy for erectile dysfunction.[110] Use of testosterone is indicated only in patients in whom a hypogonadal state has been documented; it is ineffective otherwise. Similarly, oral yohimbine, an α_2-blocker, although widely used, was shown to be ineffective in the single double-blind study carried out.[108]

Finally, for the *acute-onset neuropathies* and *neuropathic diabetic cachexia,* the primary care physician can only provide reassurance about the eventual outcome and palliative measures (as discussed earlier) for the associated pain and depression.

REFERENCES

1. Rubin RJ, Altman WM, Mendelson DN: Health care expenditures for people with diabetes mellitus, 1992. J Clin Endocrinol Metab 78:809A, 1994
2. American Diabetes Association: Direct and indirect costs of diabetes in the United States in 1992. American Diabetes Association, Alexandria, VA, 1993
3. Summary of the second report of the National Cholesterol Education Program (NCEP): Expert panel on detection, evaluation, and treatment of high blood cholesterol in adults treatment panel II. JAMA 269:3015, 1993
4. Davidson MB: Clinical implications of insulin resistance syndromes. Am J Med 99:420, 1995
5. Howard BV, Howard WJ: Dyslipidemia in non-insulin-dependent diabetes mellitus. Endocr Rev 15:263, 1994
6. Laakso M: Epidemiology of diabetic dyslipidemia. Diabetes Rev 3:408, 1995
7. Brown G, Albers JJ, Fisher LD et al: Regression of coronary artery disease as a result of intensive lipid-lowering therapy in men with high levels of apolipoprotein B. N Engl J Med 323:1289, 1990
8. Blankenhorn DH, Azen SP, Kramsch DM et al: Coronary angiographic changes with lovastatin therapy. Ann Intern Med 119:969, 1993
9. American Diabetes Association: Detection

and management of lipid disorders in diabetes. Diabetes Care 16:828, 1993

10. Davidson MB: The case for control in type II diabetes. Endocr Pract 3:145, 1997

11. Garg A, Grundy SM: Treatment of dyslipidemia in patients with NIDDM. Diabetes Rev 3:433, 1995

12. The Diabetic Retinopathy Study Group: photocoagulation treatment of proliferative diabetic retinopathy: clinical application of diabetic retinopathy study (DRS) findings. DRS report number 8. Ophthalmology 88:583, 1981

13. Early Treatment Diabetic Retinopathy Study Research Group: photocoagulation for diabetic macular edema: early treatment diabetic retinopathy study report number 1. Arch Ophthalmol 103:1796, 1985

14. Sussman EJ, William GT, Soper KA: Diagnosis of diabetic eye disease. JAMA 247:3231, 1982

15. American Diabetes Association: Screening for diabetic retinopathy. Diabetes Care 20 (suppl 1):S28, 1997

16. Harris MI, Klein R, Welborn TA et al: Onset of NIDDM occurs at least 4-7 yr before clinical diagnosis. Diabetes Care 15:815, 1992

17. DeFronzo RA: Diabetic nephropathy: etiologic and therapeutic considerations. Diabetes Rev 3:510, 1995

18. Selby JV, FitzSimmons SC, Newman JM et al: The natural history and epidemiology of diabetic nephropathy. JAMA 263:1954, 1990

19. Mogensen CE, Schmitz O: The diabetic kidney: from hyperfiltration and microalbuminuria to end-stage renal failure. Med Clin North Am 72:1465, 1988

20. Rudberg S, Persson B, Dahlquist G: Increased glomerular filtration rate as a predictor of diabetic nephropathy: results from an 8-year prospective study. Kidney Int 41:822, 1992

21. Deckert T, Feldt-Rasmussen B, Borch-Johnsen K et al: Albuminuria reflects widespread vascular damage: the Steno hypothesis. Diabetologia 32:219, 1989

22. Bojestig M, Arnqvist HJ, Karlber BE et al: Glycemic control and prognosis in type 1 diabetes patients with microalbuminuria. Diabetes Care 19:313, 1996

23. Rossing P, Rossing K, Jacobsen P et al: Un-changed incidence of diabetic nephropathy in IDDM patients. Diabetes 44:739, 1995

24. Bojestig M, Arnqvist HJ, Hermansson G et al: Declining incidence of nephropathy in insulin-dependent diabetes mellitus. N Engl J Med 330:15, 1994

25. Seaquist ER, Goetz FC, Rich S et al: Familial clustering of diabetic kidney disease: evidence for genetic susceptibility to diabetic nephropathy. N Engl J Med 320:1161, 1989

26. Krolewski AS, Canessa M, Warram JH et al: Predisposition to hypertension and susceptibility to renal disease in insulin-dependent diabetes mellitus. N Engl J Med 318:140, 1988

27. Sawicki PT, Didjurgeit U, Muhlhauser I et al: Smoking is associated with progression of diabetic nephropathy. Diabetes Care 17:126, 1994

28. Klein R, Klein BEK, Moss SE: Incidence of gross proteinuria in older-onset diabetes. Diabetes 42:381, 1993

29. Hassalacher Ch, Stech W, Wahl P et al: Blood pressure and metabolic control as risk factors for nephropathy in type I (insulin-dependent) diabetes. Diabetologia 28:6, 1985

30. Parving HH, Hommel E: Prognosis in diabetic nephropathy. BMJ 299:230, 1989

31. Elliott WJ, Stein PP, Black HR: Drug treatment of hypertension in patients with diabetes. Diabetes Rev 3:477, 1995

32. The fifth report of the Joint National Committee on detection, evaluation and treatment of high blood pressure (JNC V). Arch Intern Med 153:154, 1993

33. Kasiske BL, Kalil RSN, Ma JZ et al: Effect of antihypertensive therapy on the kidney in patients with diabetes: a meta-regression analysis. Ann Intern Med 118:129, 1993

34. Lewis EJ, Hunsicker LG, Bain RP et al: The effect of angiotensin-converting-enzyme inhibition on diabetic nephropathy. N Engl J Med 329:1456, 1993

35. National high blood pressure education program working group on hypertension in diabetes. Hypertension 23:145, 1994

36. Furberg CD: Should dihydropyridines be used as first-line drugs in the treatment of hypertension? The con side. Arch Intern Med 155:2157, 1995

37. Epstein M: Calcium antagonists should continue to be used for first-line treatment of

hypertension. Arch Intern Med 155:2150, 1995

38. Losartan for hypertension. Med Lett Drugs Ther 37:57, 1995

39. Drugs for hypertension. Med Lett Drugs Ther 37:45, 1995

40. Systolic Hypertension in the Elderly Program Cooperative Research Group: Implications of systolic hypertension in the elderly program. Hypertension 21:335, 1993

41. Ravid M, Savin H, Lang R et al: Proteinuria, renal impairment, metabolic control, and blood pressure in type 2 diabetes mellitus. Arch Intern Med 152:1225, 1992

42. Kouri TT, Viikari JSA, Mattila KS et al: Microalbuminuria; invalidity of simple concentration-based screening tests for early nephropathy due to urinary volumes of diabetic patients. Diabetes Care 14:591, 1991

43. Gatling W, Knight C, Hill RD: Screening for early diabetic nephropathy: which sample to detect microalbuminuria? Diabet Med 2:451, 1985

44. Nathan DM, Rosenbaum C, Protasowicki VD: Single-void urine samples can be used to estimate quantitative microalbuminuria Diabetes Care 10:414, 1987

45. Gatling W, Knight C, Mullee MA et al: Microalbuminuria in diabetes: a population study of the prevalence and an assessment of three screening tests. Diabet Med 5:343, 1987

46. Bennett PH, Haffner S, Kasiske BL et al: Screening and management of microalbuminuria in patients with diabetes mellitus: recommendations to the scientific advisory board of the National Kidney Foundation from an ad hoc committee of council on diabetes mellitus of the National Kidney Foundation. Am J Kidney Dis 25:107, 1995

47. Krolewski AS, Laffel LMB, Krolewski M et al: Glycosylated hemoglobin and the risk of microalbuminuria in patients with insulin-dependent diabetes mellitus. N Engl J Med 332:1251, 1995

48. Marre M, Chatellier G, Leblan H et al: Prevention of diabetic nephropathy with enalapril in normotensive diabetics with microalbuminuria. BMJ 297:1092, 1988

49. Mathiesen ER, Hommel E, Giese J et al: Efficacy of captopril in postponing nephropa-thy in normotensive insulin dependent diabetic patients with microalbuminuria. BMJ 303:81, 1991

50. Viberti GC, Mogensen CE, Groop LC et al: Effect of captopril on progression to clinical proteinuria in patients with insulin-dependent diabetes mellitus and microalbuminuria. JAMA 271:275, 1994

51. Laffel LMB, McGill JB, Gans DJ et al: The beneficial effect of angiotensin-converting enzyme inhibition with captopril on diabetic nephropathy in normotensive IDDM patients with microalbuminuria. Am J Med 99:497, 1995

52. Ravid M, Savin H, Jutrin I et al: Long-term stabilizing effect of angiotensin-converting enzyme inhibition on plasma creatinine and on proteinuria in normotensive type II diabetic patients. Ann Intern Med 118:577, 1993

53. Ravid M, Lang R, Rachmani R et al: Long-term renoprotective effect of angiotensin-converting enzyme inhibition in non-insulin-dependent diabetes mellitus. Arch Intern Med 156:286, 1996

54. Cohen D, Dodds R, Viberti G: Effect of protein restriction in insulin dependent diabetics at risk of nephropathy. BMJ 294:795, 1987

55. Dullaart RP, Beusekamp BJ, Meijer S et al: Long-term effects of protein-restricted diet on albuminuria and renal function in IDDM patients without clinical nephropathy and hypertension. Diabetes Care 16:483, 1993

56. Barsotti G, Ciardella F, Morelli E et al: Nutritional treatment of renal failure in type 1 diabetic nephropathy. Clin Nephrol 29:280, 1988

57. Evanoff G, Thompson C, Brown J et al: Prolonged dietary protein restriction in diabetic nephropathy. Arch Intern Med 149:1129, 1989

58. Pedrini MT, Levey AS, Lau J et al: The effect of dietary protein restriction on the progression of diabetic and nondiabetic renal disease: a meta-analysis. Ann Intern Med 124:627, 1996

59. Viberti GC, Walker JD: Diabetic nephropathy: etiology and prevention. Diabetes Metab Rev 4:147, 1988

60. Alzaid AA: Microalbuminuria in patients with NIDDM: an overview. Diabetes Care 19:79, 1996

61. Nannipieri M, Rizzo L, Rapuano A et al: Increased transcapillary escape rate of albumin in microalbuminuric type II diabetic patients. Diabetes Care 18:1, 1995

62. DeFronzo RA: Hyperkalemia and hyporeninemic hypoaldosteronism. Kidney Int 17:118, 1980

63. Williams G: Hyporeninemic hypoaldosteronism. N Engl J Med 314:1041, 1986

64. Parfrey PS, Griffiths SM, Barrett BJ et al: Contrast material-induced renal failure in patients with diabetes mellitus, renal insufficiency, or both: a prospective controlled study. N Engl J Med 320:143, 1989

65. Brezis M, Epstein FH: A closer look at radiocontrast-induced nephropathy. N Engl J Med 320:179, 1989

66. Manske CL, Sprafka M, Suon JT et al: Contrast nephropathy in azotemic diabetic patients undergoing coronary angiography. Am J Med 89:615, 1990

67. Schwab SJ, Hlatky MA, Pieper KS et al: Contrast nephrotoxicity: a randomized controlled trial of a nonionic and an ionic radiographic contrast agent. N Engl J Med 320:149, 1989

68. Moore RD, Steinberg EP, Powe NR et al: Nephrotoxicity of high-osmolality versus low-osmolality contrast media: randomized clinical trial. Radiology 182:649, 1992

69. Solomon R, Werner C, Mann D et al: Effects of saline, mannitol, and furosemide on acute decreases in renal function induced by radiocontrast agents. N Engl J Med 331:1416, 1994

70. Young MJ, Boulton AJM, Macleod AF et al: A multicentre study of the prevalence of diabetic peripheral neuropathy in the United Kingdom hospital clinic population. Diabetologia 36:150, 1993

71. Harris M, Eastman R, Cowie C: Symptoms of sensory neuropathy in adults with NIDDM in the U.S. population. Diabetes Care 16:1446, 1993

72. Cohen SJ: Potential barriers to diabetes care. Diabetes Care 6:499, 1983

73. Bailey TS, Yu HM, Rayfield EJ: Patterns of foot examination in a diabetes clinic. Am J Med 78:371, 1985

74. Mooney V, Gottschalk F, Powell H: The diabetic foot ulcer: treating one, preventing the next. Clin Diabetes 3:36, 1985

75. Boulton AJM, Drury J, Clarke B et al: Continuous subcutaneous insulin infusion in the management of painful diabetic neuropathy. Diabetes Care 5:386, 1982

76. Cohen KL, Harris S: Efficacy and safety of nonsteroidal anti-inflammatory drugs in the therapy of diabetic neuropathy. Arch Intern Med 147:1442, 1987

77. Kvinesdal B, Molin J, Froland A et al: Imipramine treatment of painful diabetic neuropathy. JAMA 251:1727, 1984

78. Young RH, Clarke BF: Pain relief in diabetic neuropathy: the effectiveness of imipramine and related drugs. Diabetic Med 2:363, 1985

79. Max MB, Culnane M, Schafer SC et al: Amitriptyline relieves diabetic neuropathy pain in patients with normal or depressed mood. Neurology 37:589–596, 1987

80. Max MB, Lynch SA, Muir J et al: Effects of desipramine, amitriptyline, and fluoxetine on pain in diabetic neuropathy. N Engl J Med 326:1250, 1992

81. The Capsaicin Study Group: Treatment of painful diabetic neuropathy with topical capsaicin: a multicenter, double-blind, vehicle-controlled study. Arch Intern Med 151:2225, 1991

82. Ellenberg M: Treatment of diabetic neuropathy with diphenylhydantoin. N Y State J Med 68:2653, 1968

83. Saudek CD, Werns S, Reidenberg MM: Phenytoin in the treatment of diabetic symmetrical polyneuropathy. Clin Parmacol Ther 22:196, 1977

84. Rull RA, Quibrera R, Gonzalez-Millan H et al: Symptomatic treatment of peripheral diabetic neuropathy with carbamazepine (Tegretol): double blind crossover trial. Diabetologia 5:215, 1969

85. Wilton TD: Tegretol in the treatment of diabetic neuropathy. S Afr Med J 48:869, 1974

86. Dejgard A, Petersen P, Kastrup J: Mexiletine for treatment of chronic painful diabetic neuropathy. Lancet 1:9, 1988

87. Stracke H, Meyer UE, Schumacher HE et al: Mexiletine in the treatment of diabetic neuropathy. Diabetes Care 15:1550, 1992

88. Tan Y-M, Croese J: Clonidine and diabetic patients with leg pains. Ann Intern Med 105:633, 1986

89. Anghinah R, Oliveira AS, Gabbai AA: Effect of baclofen on pain in diabetic neuropathy. Muscle Nerve 17:958, 1994

90. Fung MC, Holbrook JH: Placebo-controlled trial of quinine therapy for nocturnal leg cramps. West J Med 151:42, 1989

91. Man-Son-Hing M, Wells G: Meta-analysis of efficacy of quinine for treatment of nocturnal leg cramps in elderly people. BMJ 310:7, 1995

92. Selby PL, Young MJ, Boulton AJM: Bisphosphonates: a new treatment for diabetic Charcot neuroarthropathy? Diabet Med 11:28, 1994

93. Onrot J, Goldberg MR, Hollister AS et al: Management of chronic orthostatic hypertension. Am J Med 80:454, 1986

94. Jankovic J, Gilden JL, Hiner BC et al: Neurogenic orthostatic hypotension: a double-blind placebo-controlled study with Midodrine. Am J Med 95:38, 1993

94a. Low PA, Gilden JL, Freeman R et al, for the Midodrine Study Group: Efficacy of midodrine vs placebo in neurogenic orthostatic hypotension: a randomized, double-blind multicenter study. JAMA 277:1046, 1997

95. Meyerhoff C, Sternberg F, Bischof F et al: Diltiazem for tachycardiac orthostatic hypotension in NIDDM. Diabetes Care 16:1628, 1993

96. Hoeldtke RD, Streeten DHP: Treatment of orthostatic hypotension with erythropoietin. N Engl J Med 329:611, 1993

97. Dudl RJ, Anderson DS, Forsyth AB et al: Treatment of diabetic diarrhea and orthostatic hypotension with somatostatin analogue SMS 201-995. Am J Med 83:584, 1987

98. Nakabayashi H, Fujji S, Miwa U et al: Marked improvement of diabetic diarrhea with the somatostatin analogue octreotide. Arch Intern Med 154:1863, 1994

99. Sheps SG: Use of an elastic garment in the treatment of orthostatic hypotension. Cardiology 61(suppl 1):271, 1976

100. Nilsson P-H: Diabetic gastroparesis: a review. J Diabetes Complications 10:113, 1996

101. Richards RD, Davenport K, McCallum RW: The treatment of idiopathic and diabetic gastroparesis with acute intravenous and chronic oral erythromycin. Am J Gastroenterol 88:203, 1993

102. Erbas T, Varoglu E, Erbas B et al: Comparison of metoclopramide and erythromycin in the treatment of diabetic gastroparesis. Diabetes Care 16:1511, 1993

103. Valdovinos MA, Camilleri M, Zimmerman BR: Chronic diarrhea in diabetes mellitus: mechanisms and an approach to diagnosis and treatment. Mayo Clin Proc 68:691, 1993

104. Fedorak RN, Field M, Chang EB: Treatment of diabetic diarrhea with clonidine. Ann Intern Med 102:197, 1985

105. Sacerdote A: Topical clonidine for diabetic diarrhea. Ann Intern Med 105:139, 1986

106. Roof LW: Treatment of diabetic diarrhea with clonidine. Am J Med 83:603, 1987

107. Tsai S-T, Vinik Al, Brunner JF: Diabetic diarrhea and somatostatin. Ann Intern Med 104:894, 1986

108. Korenman SG: Advances in the understanding and management of erectile dysfunction. J Clin Endocrinol Metab 80:1985, 1995

109. Drugs that cause sexual dysfunction: an update. Med Lett Drugs Ther 34:73, 1992

110. NIH Consensus Conference: Impotence. JAMA 270:83, 1993

111. Linet OI, Ogring FG, for the Alprostadil Study Group: Efficacy and safety of intracavernosal alprostadil in men with erectile dysfunction. N Engl J Med 334:873, 1996

112. Virag R, Shoukry K, Floresco J et al: Intracavernous self-injection of vasoactive drugs in the treatment of impotence: 8-year experience with 615 cases. J Urol 145:287, 1991

113. Bell DSH, Cutter GR, Hayne VB et al: Factors predicting efficacy of phentolamine-papaverine intracorporeal injection for treatment of erectile dysfunction in diabetic males. Urology 40:36, 1992

114. Padma-Nathan H, Hellstrom WJG, Kaiser FE et al: Treatment of men with erectile dysfunction with transurethral alprostadil. N Engl J Med 336:1, 1997

DIABETES AND PREGNANCY

JOHN L. KITZMILLER

MAYER B. DAVIDSON

PREPREGNANCY COUNSELING

Any discussion of diabetes and pregnancy must begin with prepregnancy counseling. Ideally, any woman who is of childbearing age and who has diabetes should be informed of the risks of pregnancy, to both her and her fetus. Effective contraception should be practiced until a woman and her partner are ready for pregnancy. At this point, more detailed prepregnancy counseling and care should take place. If a referral to an obstetrician for this purpose is not possible, this information must be provided by the woman's primary care physician (or endocrinologist/diabetologist if one is involved in her care).[1]

IMPACT OF MATERNAL DIABETES ON THE FETUS

Diabetes in a pregnant woman can be detrimental to her fetus for four reasons. First, diabetic women have an increased spontaneous abortion rate compared with the rate in nondiabetic pregnant women. This increase, however, can be eliminated if near euglycemia is achieved at the time of conception[2, 3] and during the first trimester.[4, 5] Second, 6% to 8% prevalence of major congenital anomalies has been found in the newborns of type 1 diabetic women compared with the nondiabetic rate of approximately 2%.[6, 7] The usual major malformations involve neural tube defects and cardiac anomalies; affected tissues are formed during the early part of the first trimester period of organogenesis. Therefore, it is perhaps not too surprising that the rate of major congenital anomalies can be returned to the nondiabetic rate if near euglycemia can be achieved at the time of conception.[6, 8-10] The goal is to lower the glycated hemoglobin level to a value <1% above the upper limit of normal (or within 4 standard deviations of the mean) for the assay used at the time of conception. If this degree of strict control is difficult to reach, a realistic goal might be <2% above the upper limit of normal.

The other two negative consequences that diabetes may have on a fetus are macrosomia and certain neonatal morbidities, such as respiratory distress syndrome (RDS), hypoglycemia, hyperbilirubinemia, and hypocalcemia. Macrosomia can make delivery more difficult and thus can lead to increased rates of cesarean sections or shoulder dystocias during vaginal deliveries. Although both macrosomia[11-13] and neonatal morbidity[11] are associated with maternal hyperglycemia, near euglycemia needs to be achieved during the second and third trimesters to reduce these outcomes rather than at the time of conception and during the first trimester. Nevertheless, these relationships should be discussed with a diabetic woman contemplating pregnancy to prepare her for the challenges ahead.

IMPACT OF DIABETES ON THE PREGNANT WOMAN

In addition to emphazing the importance of achieving near euglycemia before conception and throughout pregnancy, prepregnancy counseling should include a frank discussion of how pregnancy will affect the complications of diabetes in both the near term and long term. Background retinopathy often worsens, probably because of the rapid imposition of near euglycemia,[14, 15] a situation commonly observed in nonpregnant diabetic patients. Although background retinopathy may progress during pregnancy, it usually regresses to the prepregnant baseline status after delivery.[7] If the vision-threatening changes of proliferative retinopathy or macular edema are treated with laser before or during pregnancy, the eyes remain quiescent without further deterioration.[7] For these reasons, it is extremely important that a patient be evaluated by an ophthalmologist as soon as pregnancy is established and her eyes monitored periodically until delivery.

The situation regarding diabetic nephropathy is similar to that of retinopathy. For the most part, pregnancy does not affect the typical progression of renal disease. Fortunately, <5% of diabetic women who become pregnant have overt nephropathy (i.e., dipstick positive or clinical proteinuria).[7] Because total protein excretion increases by 50% to 100% during normal pregnancy up to 200 mg/day,[16] evaluation of incipient nephropathy during pregnancy in women with diabetes mellitus is difficult. (See Chapter 8 for the distinction between incipient and overt diabetic nephropathy.) Total protein excretion >190 mg/day but below the level of overt nephropathy (500 mg/day) is associated with the same increased prevalence of preeclampsia as in women with clinical proteinuria.[17] It is likely that some of the women with this level of protein excretion have incipient nephropathy. However, we are unaware of any data about how pregnancy affects the natural history of pregestational incipient diabetic nephropathy.

Clinical proteinuria usually increases during pregnancy but returns to prepregnancy levels after delivery.[7, 18] Hypertension often becomes more of a problem, and stringent efforts must be made to control it because it may lead to preeclampsia and hydramnios. In contrast to clinical proteinuria with normal renal function, if a woman has azotemia (almost always accompanied by hypertension) before pregnancy, she may have further loss of renal function during pregnancy, and this may not regress after delivery.[7] Although angiotensin-converting enzyme (ACE) inhibitors are particularly suited to treat hypertension in diabetic patients (see Chapter 8), they *must* be avoided in pregnancy because of their association with fetal renal damage, oligohydramnios, and congenital anomalies.[7] Fortunately, no increased fetal problems were found in pregnant women inadvertently treated with ACE inhibitors in the first trimester.[7]

Peripheral neuropathy has no bearing on the outcome of pregnancy. However, symptomatic autonomic neuropathy involving the stomach (gastroparesis diabeticorum—see Chapter 8) can cause intractable vomiting, with its attendant risks to metabolic control and nutrition.

Macrovascular disease per se presents no risk to a fetus but has led to the death of pregnant diabetic women who have it.[19] Therefore, a careful cardiac evaluation is recommended for such women contemplating pregnancy. Although rare, coronary artery bypass surgery may be required to ensure a successful outcome.[19]

CONTRACEPTION[20]

Because only 25% of pregnancies in diabetic women are planned,[21] information on contraception is a vital part of prepregnancy counseling. Sexual activity with no protection leads to an 85% chance of pregnancy within 1 year. Table 9-1 lists available methods of contraception. There is no evidence that the failure rate or adverse effects of any method are different between women with and without diabetes. The choice depends on a couple's preference because the presence of diabetes does not dictate one method over another. Because contraception is necessary only until near euglycemia is achieved, a readily reversible, highly effective method should be chosen. The choice usually is between an oral contraceptive or a barrier method.

Although high-dose estrogen preparations have been associated with increased vascular sequelae, including hypertension, large prospective studies using low-dose estrogen preparations have not shown such an association. Therefore, except for older women who smoke, oral contraceptives with doses of estrogen $\leq 35 \mu g$ of ethinyl estradiol or its methylated derivative, mestranol, and low doses of a progestin offer a safe, very effective, and usually readily reversible contraceptive. An attractive alternative is a low dose of a progestin only.

Barrier methods have a higher failure rate than oral contraceptive agents (see Table 9-1). They are most effective when combined with a spermicide or foam. If conception occurs, it is almost always due to user failure rather than inadequacy of the method itself. A condom is the only method that protects against sexually transmitted diseases.

After pregnancy, longer-term contraception may be a consideration. The only intrauterine device (IUD) that was associated with increased rates of infection was the Dalkon shield, which is no longer marketed. No evidence shows that the two IUDs listed in Table 9-1 are associated with increased rates of infection in women with diabetes. The costs of the Norplant system and 5 years of oral contraceptives are similar, but be-

Table 9–1. Contraceptive Methods

Type	Effectiveness (%)	Disadvantages/Comments
Oral contraceptives		
Combined (estrogen and progestin or sequential)	98	Associated with increased risk of thromboembolism, stroke, and myocardial infarction in past; no increased risk demonstrated with current low-dose estrogens ($\leq 35 \mu g$)
Progestin alone	94	May increase serum lipid values
Norplant system	99	Menstrual irregularities
Barrier methods		
Diaphragm plus spermicide	82	High failure rate
Condom plus foam	88	High failure rate; prevents some sexually transmitted diseases
Contraceptive sponge	72	High failure rate
Cervical cap	82	Increased rate of abnormal findings on Papanicolaou smear?
Intrauterine devices		
Progesterone containing	97	Pain, irregular bleeding, perforation of uterus, infection(?), and possibly increased failure rate
Copper device	97	Does not require annual removal and reinsertion
Rhythm	80	Diabetic women may not be regular and thus have an increased failure rate
Sterilization	99 +	Essentially irreversible

Adapted from American Diabetes Association: Contraception. In Jovanovic-Peterson L (ed): Medical Management of Pregnancy Complicated by Diabetes. American Diabetes Association, Alexandria, VA, 1993, pp 14–18.

cause the cost of the former is borne all at once at the time of insertion of the Silastic capsules, it appears to be more expensive. Some method of contraception should be instituted post partum because breast-feeding (if carried out) is a relatively ineffective method of protection against pregnancy.

HORMONAL AND METABOLIC ALTERATIONS DURING PREGNANCY[22]

HORMONAL CHANGES

Concentrations of circulating hormones during pregnancy (which are produced by the placenta) are depicted in Figure 9–1. Placenta production of human chorionic gonadotropin (hCG) peaks early in pregnancy and plateaus at low levels after the first trimester.

Its action is similar to that of the gonadotropins of pituitary origin, which have little direct effect on carbohydrate metabolism. The rise in the other three hormones—estrogen, progesterone, and human chorionic somatomammotropin (hCS) (also known as human placental lactogen—hPL)—occurs gradually, paralleling the growth of the placenta. All of these antagonize the action of insulin, especially hCS, which has many of the properties of pituitary growth hormone. Thus, increasing insulin resistance characterizes the second and third trimesters of pregnancy. Therefore, the pattern of insulin secretion (Fig. 9–2) is expected to parallel the changes of hormone secretion during pregnancy. Increased concentrations of insulin are necessary to overcome the hormonally induced state of insulin resistance. Failure of the pancreatic β-cells to meet this increased demand is responsible for the development

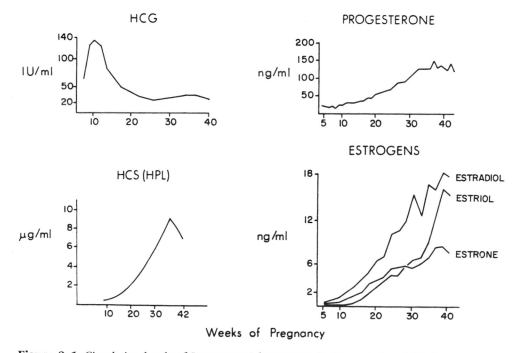

Figure 9–1. Circulating levels of "pregnancy" hormones during gestation. hCG, human chorionic gonadotropin; hCS, human chorionic somatomammotropin; hPL, human placental lactogen. (From Freinkel N: Of pregnancy and progeny, Diabetes 29:1023, 1980)

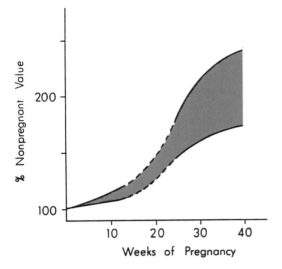

Figure 9–2. The effects of pregnancy on glucose-stimulated insulin secretion. The increments above fasting values of insulin concentrations after a glucose challenge have been summated to derive an index of the secretory response. The figure compares the range of published values during pregnancy and in nongravid women. (From Freinkel N: Of pregnancy and progeny. Diabetes 29:1023, 1980)

of gestational diabetes mellitus (GDM) (discussed later).

METABOLIC CHANGES

To compare the metabolic changes in pregnancy with the nongravid state, it is helpful to consider separately the normal fed and fasted states. After an overnight fast, plasma glucose concentrations are maintained fairly constant by an equilibrium between glucose utilization and hepatic glucose production, occurring mainly via the pathways of gluconeogenesis (synthesis of glucose from noncarbohydrate precursors, i.e., amino acids, lactate, and glycerol). The majority of glucose utilization in the fasting state occurs in tissues that are not insulin sensitive, and therefore insulin levels are low. After food consumption, glucose and amino acid concentrations rise, triggering increased insulin

secretion. This results in storage of ingested glucose and amino acids in muscle and liver and cessation of hepatic glucose production.

Both maternal glucose and amino acids enter the fetus through the placenta. Glucose is transported via facilitated diffusion, the same process that occurs in the insulin-sensitive tissues of muscle and fat. Although this process is not influenced by insulin (insulin is destroyed by the placenta), the ability of the placenta to transport glucose by facilitated diffusion results in greater entrance of glucose into the fetus than would be the case if glucose uptake simply occurred down its concentration gradient as it does in most other tissues (e.g., brain, liver). Amino acids are transported across the placenta *against* their concentration gradient. In this manner, the fetus serves as a trap for maternal glucose and amino acids. A normal fasting glucose concentration cannot be maintained for two reasons. More glucose is siphoned off to serve the fetus (increased glucose utilization), and an important gluconeogenic precursor, the amino acid alanine, is not as available (decreased hepatic glucose production). This results in a lowering of the fasting glucose concentration in normal pregnancy.

Other changes occur in the fasting state as well. These are termed *accelerated starvation*. In addition to the lower concentrations of glucose and alanine mentioned earlier, higher levels of free fatty acids and ketone bodies are found in pregnant women than in nongravid controls after extending an overnight fast by several hours. These changes are caused, in part, by the lipolytic action (i.e., the hydrolysis of adipose tissue triglycerides) of hCS. The increased tendency to develop ketosis in pregnancy has some implications for the subsequent intellectual development of the child (discussed later).

Changes also occur in the fed state owing to the increasing insulin resistance during the second and third trimesters. Although insulin secretion increases markedly (Fig. 9–3), glucose concentrations are often in-

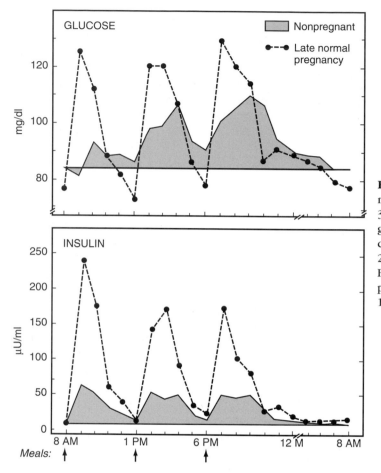

Figure 9–3. The effect of normal late pregnancy (weeks 33 to 39 of gestation) on glucose and insulin concentrations throughout a 24-hour period. (From Freinkel N: Of pregnancy and progeny. Diabetes 29:1023, 1980)

creased (albeit still in the normal range) compared with the nongravid state. If insulin secretion cannot meet this increased demand, the resulting hyperglycemia of GDM can have important detrimental effects on the fetus (discussed later).

PREGESTATIONAL DIABETES

CLASSIFICATION

Diabetic pregnant women were classified on the basis of duration and severity of diabetes (Table 9–2) by Priscilla White,[23] a pioneer in the management of diabetes in pregnancy who worked for 50 years at the Joslin Clinic

in Boston. Her classification system was originally used to estimate prognosis for perinatal outcome and to determine some aspects of obstetric management, such as timing of delivery. The system is no longer used for that purpose because perinatal outcome has improved for many reasons in women of all White classes. It is now recognized that the major determinants of outcome are the degrees of glycemic control, hypertension, and impaired renal function that exist before and during pregnancy. The White classification system is now used to describe and compare populations of diabetic pregnant women. For example, class B patients probably have residual islet β-cell function, and control of hyperglycemia may be easier than in class C

Table 9–2. Classification of Diabetes During Pregnancy

Class	Characteristics	Implications
A	Impaired glucose tolerance diagnosed before pregnancy (as compared with GDM diagnosed during pregnancy). Any age at onset	Treated with diet to produce euglycemia and optimal weight gain. If insulin is needed, manage as in classes B, C, and D.
B	Onset age ≥20 years; duration <10 years	Can be type 1 or 2 diabetes mellitus; maternal insulin secretion may persist, but exogenous insulin prescription is usually necessary for euglycemia to reduce fetal and neonatal risks.
C	Onset age 10 to 19 years or duration 10 to 19 years	Usually type 1 insulin-deficient diabetes, but MODY is possible. Glycemic control is major focus.
D	Onset before age 10, or duration >20 years, or chronic hypertension, or background retinopathy	Fetal growth depends on balance of diabetic microvascular disease and glycemic control. Retinal microaneurysms, dot hemorrhages, and exudates may progress during pregnancy, then regress after delivery.
F	Diabetic nephropathy with clinical proteinuria	With control of glycemia, hypertension, and anemia, renal function is usually stable, but proteinuria increases and then declines after delivery. Fetal growth restriction, superimposed preeclampsia common. Perinatal survival can exceed 90%.
H	Coronary artery disease	Serious maternal risk.
R	Proliferative retinopathy	Neovascularization, with risk of vitreous hemorrhage or retinal detachment; laser photocoagulation needed.

MODY, maturity-onset diabetes of the young (see Chapter 1 for description); GDM, gestational diabetes mellitus.
From Hare JW, White P: Gestational diabetes and the White classification. Diabetes Care 3:394, 1980.

or D patients. On the other hand, obesity in some women in class B may have independent effects on perinatal outcome. Finally, the most complicated and difficult pregnancies occur in women with cardiovascular, renal, or retinal disease.

Another pioneer in the management of diabetes in pregnancy was Jorgen Pedersen, an internist who worked at the Rigshospital Obstetrics Department in Copenhagen. He developed a classification system known as Prognostically Bad Signs in Pregnancy, which served to alert health care providers to patients requiring special attention.[24] His classification concerned complications that became evident during pregnancy. The bad signs were (1) clinical pyelonephritis, (2) ketoacidosis, (3) preeclampsia, and (4) neglector (failure to follow the recommended regimen). As with the White classification, use of Pedersen's system has been co-opted by the present emphasis on control of glycemia and hypertension to optimize perinatal outcome.

NONMETABOLIC MATERNAL COMPLICATIONS IN DIABETIC WOMEN

The hormonal changes of early pregnancy stimulate nausea and vomiting in many pregnancies, and *hyperemesis* can be devastating in diabetic women with autonomic neuropathy and gastroparesis diabeticorum (see Chapter 8).[25] Weight loss and ketonemia are common indications for hospitalization and intravenous hydration. Medications that can help include promethazine, hydroxyzine, and metoclopramide (oral, intravenous, or by subcutaneous pump). It may be useful to administer cisapride or odansetron intravenously or orally before meals, although information related to potential teratogenesis is lacking. Despite pharmacologic treatment, occasional diabetic women continue to be unable to retain oral feedings, and total parenteral nutrition via a central line is necessary to provide adequate substrates for normal fetal growth and development.

Clinically detected *polyhydramnios* was formerly quite common (15% to 30%) in women with poorly controlled diabetes.[26] In these series, the diagnosis was based on dramatically increased maternal abdominal girth due to excess amniotic fluid. This was sometimes associated with maternal dyspnea, or preterm labor due to overdistention of the uterus. Using ultrasonography, the diagnosis of polyhydramnios has been defined as a four-quadrant amniotic fluid index of >20 cm, but most cases defined this way are not clinically significant.

Studies of the cause of polyhydramnios in diabetic women, in the absence of fetal anomalies such as open neural tube defects or tracheoesophageal fistulas, are inconclusive. The concentration of solutes is not greater in the amniotic fluid in cases of polyhydramnios. The hypothesis that the polyhydramnios is due to fetal glucosuria and excess urine output is not supported by ultrasonographic studies of fetal bladder emptying in diabetic women with and without excessive amniotic fluid volume.[27] However, polyhydramnios is clearly associated with maternal hyperglycemia and fetal macrosomia, but the primary causal mechanisms remain unclear.

Treatment of severe polyhydramnios by transabdominal drainage is usually not successful for more than a short time owing to reaccumulation of amniotic fluid. The role of maternal indomethacin therapy, which reduces fetal urine output and amnionic fluid volume, has not been evaluated in diabetic women. Because treatment is difficult, it is fortunate that prevention is possible by intensified maternal glycemic control, which is shown to reduce the frequency of polyhydramnios to ~12%.

Some evidence shows that *preterm labor* (PTL) may be more common in diabetic than nondiabetic women, even without polyhydramnios, but the causes are obscure.[26] Various frequencies of PTL or of tocolytic treatment (5% to 30%) in different studies of diabetes and pregnancy may be due to the use of different criteria for diagnosis.[28] PTL should be diagnosed on the basis of changes in the cervix: effacement or shortening, with or without dilatation, in response to uterine contractions, which may be subtle. Many factors predict an increased risk of PTL, including more than 5 uterine contractions per hour, cervical length <3 cm or funneling seen on ultrasound studies, and fetal fibronectin measured in cervical secretions as a response to inflammatory changes in the amniotic membranes.

Because the degree of preterm birth (by gestational age) is a major determinant of mortality, morbidity, and cost of care of infants of diabetic mothers, effective identification and treatment of PTL is essential. The first-choice uterine tocolytic agent should be magnesium sulfate given intravenously to avoid the hyperglycemic effects of β-adrenergic agents such as ritodrine and terbutaline. Total intravenous fluid volume should be carefully controlled to 100 to 125 ml/h to avoid iatrogenic pulmonary edema. The dosage of tocolytic drug is titrated to keep the frequency of uterine contractions under the threshold that causes cervical change. This amount seems specific for each patient. If additional tocolytic effect is needed in the acute management of an episode of PTL at <30 weeks' gestation, oral indomethacin is effective and does not impair glycemic control. Its effectiveness must be balanced against a possible association with intracranial bleeding or bowel perforation in very low-birth-weight infants born to indomethacin-treated mothers. Beyond 30 weeks' gestation, maternal use of indomethacin can result in significant narrowing of the fetal ductus arteriosus.

Limited evidence suggests that continued long-term tocolytic treatment, in addition to bed rest, can reduce the likelihood of recurrent episodes of PTL. Oral nifedipine (10 to 20 mg q 4 h) may be successful in controlling contractions and may allow a patient to be monitored at home. Long-term oral terbutaline (2 to 5 mg q 4 to 6 h) may induce desensitization of uterine adrenergic responses with failed tocolytic effect. However, low-dose subcutaneous terbutaline pump therapy (0.5 to 1.0 mg/h, with boluses of 0.25 mg/h q 4 to 6 h) probably avoids down-regulation of the uterine β-adrenergic receptors. The moderate hyperglycemic side effects can be counteracted with increased insulin doses.

For cases of possible preterm birth before 34 weeks' gestation in diabetic women, it is presumed that the corticosteroid betamethasone given intramuscularly to gravidas stimulates fetal surfactant production and decreases neonatal mortality and morbidity due to RDS. However, betamethasone also stimulates marked maternal hyperglycemia, which can lead to ketoacidosis. To prevent this, insulin dose should be doubled by 4 hours after the initial injection of betamethasone for a duration of 48 to 72 hours. This also prevents the possible harmful result of fetal hyperglycemia and fetal hyperinsulinemia, which may block the hoped-for effect of the corticosteroid on the surfactant system in the fetal alveolar type II cells.[29, 30] Another potentially harmful result of fetal hyperglycemia and hyperinsulinemia is fetal hypoxia and acidosis.[31] Therefore, be vigilant in preventing maternal hyperglycemia while managing PTL or preterm ruptured membranes in diabetic women.

The *preeclamptic toxemic* syndrome (PET) of acute hypertension, proteinuria, variable edema, but reduced plasma volume and potential end-organ damage due to vasospasm and intravascular coagulation in liver, brain, and kidneys is a frequent and serious complication of pregnancy in diabetic women. The prevalence of PET ranges from 8% to 14% in women with gestational or established diabetes without microalbumin-uria, to 30% to 40% in women with diabetic microalbuminuria, and up to 50% to 60% in diabetic women with overt nephropathy (i.e., those with clinical proteinuria) or renal transplants.[17] The causes of preeclampsia are still obscure but probably relate to uteroplacental vascular insufficiency, although the placenta-related "toxins" that damage the peripheral maternal vasculature remain to be identified.[32] Some evidence suggests that the risk of developing PET is greater with poor glycemic control.[33] Diagnosis of PET in diabetic women with prior hypertension and proteinuria is difficult, but the rapid acceleration of hypertension and proteinuria in the third trimester with or without laboratory evidence of end-organ damage should be managed as superimposed preeclampsia to protect the gravida and fetus.

The dangerous effects of preeclampsia are related to reversible ischemia of regional vascular beds. Decreased glomerular filtration and tubular dysfunction are marked by rising serum creatinine and uric acid levels and falling creatinine clearance and urine output. Hematuria is possible, and renal cortical necrosis is an avoidable end-stage result. Ischemia of hepatocytes is marked by rising serum transaminase values. Periportal microhemorrhages can lead to epigastric and right upper quadrant pain due to distention of the liver capsule. Here spontaneous rupture of the liver is the avoidable end-stage result. Foci of ischemia and perivascular hemorrhage in the brain are associated with generalized convulsions (eclampsia) or coma. Pulmonary endothelial changes, fluid retention, and left heart failure due to increased afterload can lead to acute pulmonary edema. Finally, decreased uteroplacental blood flow in diabetic gravidas with PET is associated with placental infarction, fetal growth restriction, and fetal asphyxia, with the possible end result of stillbirth.

The objective of management of PET in diabetic women is to recognize and prevent progression of the maternal or placental vascular damage. The only known cure for severe preeclampsia is to deliver the placenta, which is the reason PET is a leading cause of premature birth in diabetic women. Short of that, sequential monitoring of blood pressure, proteinuria, creatinine clearance, platelet counts, and transaminase levels and estimation of fetal growth and hypoxia are used to determine how long a preterm pregnancy can safely be continued. Intravenous infusions of magnesium sulfate have been shown to be the most effective therapy to prevent convulsions and improve maternal and fetal outcomes,[34] and magnesium sulfate may have beneficial hemodynamic effects as well.[35] In diabetic women, the blood pressure should be kept below 140/90 to minimize retinal and renal damage, and long-term antihypertensive therapy with methyldopa, diltiazem, prazosin, and clonidine is usually effective and safe for a woman and her fetus. ACE inhibitors should not be used in pregnancy because they cause fetal renal damage. For severe acute hypertension (>160/110) in the peripartum situation, epidural anesthesia, intravenous labetalol, or nitroglycerin infusions can be quite effective.

METABOLIC MATERNAL COMPLICATIONS IN DIABETIC WOMEN

The metabolic complications of diabetes in pregnant women are the same as in the nongravid state—that is, hyperglycemia, diabetic ketoacidosis (DKA), and hypoglycemia. As opposed to the acute symptoms of marked hyperglycemia (i.e., polyuria, polydipsia, blurred vision, and fungal infections), the consequences of hyperglycemia (i.e., retinopathy, nephropathy, and neuropathy) are not evident for years. In pregnancy, the long-term consequences of maternal hyperglycemia involve the fetus (e.g., congenital anomalies, stillbirths, macrosomia, RDS, and neonatal hypoglycemia) and obviously occur in months, not years. Thus, pregnant diabetic women do not have the luxury of gradually achieving near euglycemia; they must do it quickly and sustain it.

The diagnosis and treatment of DKA are discussed in detail in Chapter 6 and are the same whether a patient is pregnant or not. An urgent concern, however, is either prompt recognition of impending DKA or, if it develops, rapid treatment of the pregnant woman because fetal demise commonly follows the episode. Prevention, of course, is preferred and is maximized by frequent communication between the patient and the health care provider, especially when the woman is feeling ill. Particularly challenging is the situation (usually in the first trimester) of nausea and sometimes vomiting in association with ketonuria. This could either be morning sickness with "starvation" ketosis secondary to decreased carbohydrate intake or mild DKA. Unfortunately, the blood glucose (BG) concentration may not be entirely helpful to distinguish between the two because near normal or even normal levels are sometimes found in patients in DKA.[36] This seems to be more common in those who are vomiting. Because the consequences of delaying the treatment of DKA can be so dire to a fetus, it is better to err on the side of caution and measure a serum bicarbonate level whenever the distinction between these two diagnoses is in doubt. Even if the diagnosis is hyperemesis, a type 1 diabetic patient with protracted vomiting often requires hospitalization to receive appropriate fluids and to balance the administration of glucose and insulin.

Maternal hypoglycemia does not harm a fetus. Therefore, considerations regarding hypoglycemia are similar in the gravid and nongravid states, with one potential difference. One of the causes of hypoglycemia unawareness is lowered thresholds for both the symptoms and the release of counterregulatory hormones. The brain accommodates to the prevailing level of BG to which it is exposed. Thus, patients who are chronically hyperglycemic (e.g., average BG concentrations of 250 mg/dl) experience symptoms of hypoglycemia at BG levels that are not low (e.g., 125 mg/dl). Conversely, in patients whose average BG levels are lower than usual (e.g., in pregnancy and/or those achieving very strict control), hypoglycemic symptoms and counterregulatory hormones do not appear at the usual BG concentrations (50 to 60 mg/dl) but do so at lower values (30 to 40 mg/dl). Thus, the possibility that a patient may experience the consequences of severe hypoglycemia (e.g. confusion, seizures, or coma) is enhanced because the milder signs and symptoms did not warn the patient to initiate actions to avoid this outcome. (See Chapter 7 for a detailed discussion of hypoglycemia and hypoglycemia unawareness.) This is another reason why frequent self-monitoring of BG (SMBG) is necessary in pregnancy, so that asymptomatic hypoglycemia can be recognized and appropriate adjustments made.

TREATMENT—DIET[37]

The goal of appropriate dietary management for a pregnant diabetic woman is to provide adequate nutrition for both the woman and fetus and to achieve near euglycemia. Pregnancy imposes certain nutritional demands that necessitate alterations in the diet.

Calories

To determine the appropriate caloric intake during pregnancy, one must estimate the desirable body weight (DBW) of the woman. The relationship between height and DBW for both men and women is generally the following:

	Women	*Men*
First 5 feet	100 pounds	106 pounds
Each inch over 5 feet	5 pounds	6 pounds

Ten percent is added for large-framed individuals, and 10% is subtracted for small-framed subjects. Frame size can be grossly estimated by having the patient's predominant hand grasp the other wrist and oppose the thumb and middle finger. If these two fingers meet, the patient has a medium frame. If they overlap appreciably, the patient is small framed. If they fail to meet, the patient is large framed. Appropriate adjustments are made to the DBW in the latter two circumstances.

Women within 90% to 120% of DBW before becoming pregnant should gain between 25 and 30 pounds to minimize obstetric complications and premature births. Women who are <90% of DBW prepregnancy should gain between 28 and 40 pounds to ensure delivery of an infant of appropriate size. Overweight women do not need to gain as much weight to ensure delivery of a healthy baby. Recommended weight gain for those between 120% and 150% of DBW before pregnancy should be between 15 and 25 pounds. Appropriate weight gain for women >150% of DBW is approximately 15 pounds. Any indicated weight loss should be deferred until the postpartum period. However, as long as a pregnant diabetic woman is eating a nutrtionally adequate diet, BG levels are being maintained in an acceptable range, and parameters of maternal and fetal health are normal, the amount of weight gain does not need to be an overriding issue.

The normal pattern of weight gain is a gradual one. A 2- to 5-pound increase in the first trimester represents the growth of the uterus and expansion of the maternal blood volume. Appropriate weight gain during the second and third trimesters is 0.5 to 1 pound per week. In the second trimester, the weight gain represents mostly maternal changes to support the pregnancy. During the third trimester, the weight gain is mainly due to the growth of the placenta and fetus. On average, a nonpregnant woman of normal weight ingests approximately 2,200 kilocalories (kcal)/day. To support the necessary weight gain of pregnancy, an additional 300 kcal/day is required (Table 9–3). However, these additional calories are necessary during only the latter two trimesters. Caloric

Table 9–3. Dietary Allowances for Women 25 to 50 Years of Age

Constituent	Nonpregnant	Pregnant	Increase
Protein (g)	50	60	10
Average kcal[a]	2,200	2,500	300
Vitamin C (mg)	60	70	10
Vitamin B$_6$ (mg)	1.6	2.2	0.6
Folate (μg)	180	400	220
Calcium (mg)	800	1,200	400
Magnesium (mg)	280	320	40
Iron (mg)	15	30	15
Zinc (mg)	12	15	3

[a]Additional calories are needed during the second and third trimesters only.

Adapted from American Diabetes Association: Nutritional management during pregnancy in preexisting diabetes. In Jovanovic-Peterson L (ed): Medical Management of Pregnancy Complicated by Diabetes. American Diabetes Association, Alexandria, VA, 1993, pp 47-56.

recommendations are summarized in Table 9-4.

Protein

Additional protein is required for growth of the fetus and the increased size of the maternal blood volume, uterus, and breasts. Proteins in the placenta and fetus are synthesized from amino acids supplied by the mother. An additional 10 g of protein per day is required for this purpose (see Table 9-3).

Table 9–4. Recommended Daily Caloric Intake During the Second and Third Trimesters of Pregnancy

Prepregnancy Weight	Kilocalories/ kg/Day	Kilocalories/ Pound/Day
90% to 120% DBW	30	14
>120% DBW	24	11
<90% DBW	36 to 40	16 to 18

DBW, desirable body weight.

Adapted from American Diabetes Association: Nutritional management during pregnancy in preexisting diabetes. In Jovanovic-Peterson L (ed): Medical Management of Pregnancy Complicated by Diabetes. American Diabetes Association, Alexandria, VA, 1993, pp 47-56.

Carbohydrate

Postprandial glucose concentrations are mainly dependent on the carbohydrate content of the preceding meal. Because achieving maternal euglycemia is so important in avoiding fetal complications and macrosomia, the carbohydrate content of the diet in a pregnant diabetic women is often less than in the prepregnant state—for instance, 40% to 50% instead of 50% to 60%. This is the recommendation of the California Diabetes and Pregnancy Sweet Success Program.[38] However, carbohydrate intake must be enough to avoid "starvation" ketosis (i.e., ketosis due to insufficient carbohydrate intake) because maternal ketosis, especially during the third trimester, is associated with a small but statistically significant decrease in the subsequent intelligence quotient of the child measured between 2 and 5 years after birth.[39] Although the principle of adjusting the timing and number of meals to accommodate the life style and physical activity of the patient applies, three daily meals and three snacks during pregnancy seem to be optimal. Distributing the carbohydrate intake throughout the day not only blunts the higher postprandial rise that occurs if the carbohydrate is ingested in only three meals and a bedtime snack but also prevents hypoglycemia. Because the postprandial rise of glucose is often greater in the morning than during other times of the day, carbohydrate intake is usually restricted at breakfast. One example of the distribution of calories during the day is as follows:

- 10% of calories at breakfast
- 20% to 30% of calories at lunch
- 30% to 40% of calories at supper
- 30% of calories as snacks

Fat

Decreasing the carbohydrate content of the diet to achieve normoglycemia results in increased fat intake, sometimes to as much as 40%. Whatever the final amount of dietary fat, less than one third should be saturated fat, no more than one third should be polyunsaturated fat, and the remainder should be monounsaturated fat.

Fiber

Soluble fibers form gels that delay the absorption of carbohydrate from the gastrointestinal tract. This tends to blunt the postprandial rise of glucose. Therefore, consumption of foods high in soluble fibers, such as fruit, beans, and oat bran, should be encouraged. Insoluble fibers, such as wheat bran, are not digested and thereby increase fecal bulk, which contributes to regularity, also a favorable outcome.

Vitamins and Minerals

The extra requirements of certain vitamins and minerals imposed by pregnancy are summarized in Table 9–3. Additional calcium is necessary for calcification of fetal bones and teeth, especially during the third trimester, when most of the calcium is deposited. If this extra amount is not supplied by the diet, maternal demineralization occurs. Additional iron is needed for the development of erythrocytes, to supply iron to the fetus, and to replace blood loss during delivery. Most of the additional requirements are necessary during the second and third trimesters because the conservation of iron stores due to the cessation of menstruation balances the smaller increased need during the first trimester. The extra 15 mg of iron per day cannot be supplied by the typical American diet, and one daily 30-mg tablet of ferrous sulfate is recommended. The folate requirement during pregnancy more than doubles. Folate supplementation (prenatal vitamins by prescription contain 100 to 400 μg of folate) markedly decreases neural tube defects and the rate of small-for-date neonates. Women eating a well-balanced, nutritious diet need only iron and folate supplementation. A multivitamin-mineral preparation containing vitamins B_6, C, D, and folate and the minerals iron, zinc, copper, and calcium is often given, however, especially to women with inadequate dietary intakes or with special problems.

TREATMENT—INSULIN

If the prepregnancy insulin regimen incorporates two or more insulin injections a day, it may be suitable to achieve the near euglycemia necessary for a successful outcome of the pregnancy. Indeed, if appropriate prepregnancy counseling has occurred and near euglycemia had been achieved before conception, the physician and patient will have arrived at an insulin regimen that has the potential of meeting the target levels during pregnancy (Table 9–5). (Note that these blood glucose goals are lower than ones in the nongravid state because they reflect the changes in carbohydrate metabolism that occur during pregnancy, as discussed earlier.) Several caveats should be recognized in choosing an insulin regimen, however. A split/mixed regimen (NPH and regular or lispro insulin given in the morning and evening) in which NPH insulin is given before supper has the likelihood of producing overnight hypoglycemia as the dose is increased to control the next morning's fasting value (even though the patient eats a bedtime snack). This happens because the peak action of the intermediate-acting insulin occurs during the middle of the night. Moving the injection of the evening NPH insulin to bedtime shifts the time of peak action toward breakfast and minimizes the possibility of

Table 9–5. Blood Glucose Target Levels During Pregnancy in Women with Prepregnancy Diabetes

Fasting, 60 to 90 mg/dl	1-hour postprandial, 100 to 130 mg/dl
Preprandial, 60 to 105 mg/dl	2-hour postprandial, 90 to 120 mg/dl
0200 to 0600, 60 to 120 mg/dl	

overnight hypoglycemia. Injecting NPH insulin in the morning, however, limits a patient's flexibility in regard to eating and exercise patterns. Unanticipated changes are more difficult to deal with because once the intermediate-acting insulin is given, it exerts its preordained effect for many hours. Using three injections of regular or lispro (see Chapter 4) insulin before each meal gives a patient more flexibility in regard to eating and exercise. For instance, if lunch is delayed, the short- or rapid-acting insulin taken before breakfast will have mostly been expended and preprandial hypoglycemia is unlikely. On the other hand, if a patient had taken NPH insulin before breakfast, it would be starting to work before lunch and the delayed meal might precipitate a hypoglycemic reaction. Preprandial regular or lispro insulin can be particularly helpful during the first trimester, when nausea and anorexia (morning sickness) are common.

Controlling the fasting BG concentration requires either evening NPH insulin or ultralente insulin, a longer-acting preparation. Because several days are required before reaching the full effect of changing the dose of ultralente, NPH insulin is preferred. During the second and third trimesters, rapid changes in insulin doses are sometimes necessary (because of the increasing insulin resistance discussed earlier), making it difficult to use the long-acting insulin. No evidence shows that insulin pump therapy produces better diabetic control during pregnancy than intensive insulin management with two to four subcutaneous injections per day.[40]

SMBG (see Chapter 7 for a thorough discussion) eight times a day is considered ideal during pregnancy.[41] This should occur before and between 1 and 2 hours after each meal and before the bedtime snack. It should also be performed in the middle of the night whenever nocturnal hypoglycemia is suspected or during the second and third trimesters when insulin doses are being increased frequently. How to adjust insulin doses based on the results of *both* prepran-

dial and postprandial SMBG values is not always obvious. This is because the same component of the insulin regimen affects both the postprandial BG level of a meal and the preprandial value of the subsequent one (see Table 4-2 in Chapter 4). These two results can sometimes dictate contradictory actions. Table 9-6 lists the combination of possible values and suggested actions in each case. In addition to adjusting doses of insulin, changing the timing of injections of regular insulin before meals can be helpful for the following reason. Regular insulin is usually given 1/2 hour before a meal because it does not start to work until approximately 30 minutes after injection. The timing of injection is often used in intensive insulin management protocols to help achieve near euglycemia. For instance, if the BG concentration is high before eating, delaying the start of the meal beyond 1/2 hour allows the short-acting insulin to achieve a lower, more appropriate BG level before starting to eat so that the postprandial rise is attenuated. In this case, the action of the preprandial regular insulin may wane before the next meal. This may be helpful if those values were below target. Alternatively, if the preprandial BG concentration is low, eating immediately after the injection prevents a further lowering and a possible hypoglycemic reaction. Changing the timing in this direction allows more of an effect before the next meal, and this may be helpful if those values were high.

Adjusting insulin doses probably is easier than changing the timing between injection and eating. However, if dose adjustments to ameliorate one problem (e.g., too high a postprandial value) cause unacceptable BG levels at another time (e.g., too low a preprandial value before the next meal), changing the timing between injection and eating may be helpful. In instances in which contradictory changes in the dose of insulin would seem indicated (e.g., postprandial values above target levels with preprandial values before the next meal too low or vice versa), changes in the timing of injection relative to

Table 9–6. Suggested Responses to Various Patterns of Blood Glucose Concentrations

Postprandial BG Pattern	Preprandial BG Pattern Before Next Meal	Action[a]
Above target	Above target	Increase insulin dose
Above target	Within target	Increase insulin dose *or* delay meal after injection
Above target	Below target	Delay meal after injection
Within target	Above target	Increase insulin dose *or* eat immediately after injection
Within target	Within target	No change
Within target	Below target	Decrease insulin dose *or* delay meal
Below target	Above target	Eat immediately after injection
Below target	Within target	Decrease insulin dose *or* eat immediately after injection
Below target	Below target	Decrease insulin dose

BG, blood glucose.

[a]Changing the timing between insulin injections and eating applies to only regular insulin; thus, this approach cannot be used to affect the patterns of postprandial lunch and preprandial supper values in patients taking morning NPH insulin to control afternoon BG concentrations.

eating should be tried (see Table 9-6). On the other hand, if the new rapid-acting insulin, lispro, is used in place of regular insulin, delaying the meal after injecting it is not an option because it starts to act within 10 to 15 minutes.

Several centers specializing in the care of pregnant diabetic women recommend monitoring only four times a day,[42, 43] before each meal and the bedtime snack. Performing SMBG in the middle of the night is still recommended if overnight hypoglycemia is suspected. This approach is simpler, is more likely to be acceptable to a patient, and avoids the possible situation in which preprandial and postprandial SMBG values lead to contradictory adjustments of the insulin dose. To the best of our knowledge, no data show that monitoring eight times a day leads to better outcomes as long as acceptable levels of control are achieved by whatever schedule of monitoring is used. Adjusting insulin doses is simpler with monitoring only four times a day because each component of the insulin regimen affects only one SMBG value (see Table 4-2 in Chapter 4). However, we recommend monitoring before breakfast and 1 to 2 hours postprandial because birth weight is related more closely to postpran-

dial glycemia than to preprandial glucose concentrations.[12, 13, 44]

During the first trimester, fluctuations of glucose concentrations often increase. Hypoglycemia may be more common, especially overnight. Insulin requirements commonly decrease at the end of the first trimester. The insulin resistance that characterizes pregnancy becomes apparent by 18 to 24 weeks, and insulin requirements start to increase gradually. As long as the physician realizes that insulin requirements need to be progressively increased, controlling glycemia is usually easier during the final two trimesters. Final doses may be up to twice the prepregnancy requirement. At approximately 36 weeks, placental growth ceases and contrainsulin hormone production plateaus. Thus, insulin requirements increase very little and may even decline. At this point in the pregnancy, a decrease in the insulin dose does not necessarily mean that the fetoplacental unit is failing.

Because of rapidly changing insulin requirements, frequent SMBG is necessary during pregnancy. The insulin dose is adjusted if a consistent pattern is observed at the same time (e.g., before lunch) during a 3-day period. If no consistent pattern develops over 3 days, 7 days of results are evaluated. If the majority of values (i.e., at least four of seven at the same time of day fail to meet the target level, the appropriate adjustment is made. Motivated patients can be taught to self-adjust their own doses, especially using the 3-day rule. The principles of intensively managing diabetes in pregnant women are no different from the ones used in nonpregnant patients. The 3- and 7-day rules for intensive management are discussed in Chapter 7.

TREATMENT—ORAL DIABETIC DRUGS

Patients with type 2 diabetes at the time of (unplanned) conception are often taking a sulfonylurea agent and/or metformin. Although some believe that sulfonylurea agents, at least, are associated with increased congenital malformations,[45] others have not found this to be the case.[46-50] Coetzee and Jackson[50] have not noted increased congenital anomalies in pregnant type 2 diabetic women treated with metformin. Nevertheless, these drugs are not recommended during pregnancy in this country. They should be discontinued as soon as pregnancy is confirmed and the woman placed on insulin. If a pregnancy is planned by a woman with type 2 diabetes, the oral antidiabetic medication can be discontinued and the patient begun on insulin before conception.

GESTATIONAL DIABETES

SCREENING AND DIAGNOSIS

The initial impetus to test for glucose intolerance during pregnancy was the recognition that women who developed diabetes many years after childbearing had excessive fetal loss and large babies in their prior pregnancies. The "prediabetes" was then studied prospectively during pregnancy, and O'Sullivan and colleagues[51] and others[52] found that women in the top 2.5% of BG

levels after being given 100 g of oral glucose had increased perinatal mortality and morbidity (often related to fetal islet hyperplasia and macrosomia) compared with women with normal glucose tolerance. The pregnant women with glucose intolerance also had an increased likelihood of developing clinical diabetes during 5 to 15 years of follow-up after pregnancy,[53, 54] and thus the potential prediabetic state during pregnancy was termed *gestational diabetes mellitus.*

Pregnant women at highest risk for glucose intolerance include those with glucosuria (especially in the fasting state), obesity, a family history of diabetes in first-degree relatives, or any prior fetal macrosomia, stillbirth, or diagnosis of GDM. However, it is not sufficient to screen only high-risk women because these factors are not present in 40% to 50% of pregnant women who have glucose intolerance and who do have risks of perinatal morbidity if undiagnosed and untreated.[55] Pregnant women with high-risk factors for GDM should be screened at 12 to 14 weeks' gestation, and if the screening test result is negative, the test should be repeated at 24 to 26 weeks' gestation because insulin resistance induced by placental hormones increases the diagnostic yield in the third trimester. All other pregnant women should be screened routinely at 24 to 26 weeks except those who meet *all* of the following criteria: <25 years of age, normal body weight, no first degree relative with diabetes, *and* not of Hispanic, Native American, Asian-American, or African-American origin.[55a]

To avoid giving a 3-hour oral glucose tolerance test (OGTT) to most pregnant women, O'Sullivan and associates[55] and others[56] suggested a screening test of plasma glucose measured 1 hour after a 50-g glucose load. Even simpler fasting or random glucose measurements lack sensitivity and precision, and assays for glycated hemoglobin are not sensitive enough to detect modest hyperglycemia. If the screening test is performed in the morning after an overnight fast, a 1-hour plasma glucose value >140 mg/dl (7.8 mM) is a sensitive threshold, predicting >90% of women with GDM. If the screening test is performed in the fed state, the screening threshold should be reduced to >130 mg/dl (7.2 mM) to retain adequate sensitivity.[57] If the appropriate screening values exceed these thresholds, then the diagnostic test that should be performed is the 3-hour 100-g OGTT. However, if the 1-hour screening value is >200 mg/dl (11.1 mM), the diagnosis of GDM (or type 2 diabetes) is so probable that it is not necessary to perform the full OGTT. In this situation, it is wise to obtain a glycated hemoglobin level to determine if hyperglycemia has been prolonged and to start treatment promptly.

In North America (in contrast to other areas of the world), the standard diagnostic test for GDM is the 3-hour 100-g OGTT, studied extensively by O'Sullivan and Mahan[58] and others.[59] The diagnosis of GDM is made if two or more values exceed the set limits (Table 9-7). O'Sullivan's and colleagues criteria (2 SD above the mean for a large population of pregnant subjects) identified women at risk of stillbirth, fetal macrosomia, and subsequent diabetes.[60, 61] Their original criteria were based on measurements of reducing substances in whole blood by the Somogyi-Nelson technique. The National Diabetes Data Group (NDDG) adjusted the values upward by 14% to account for the higher glucose concentration in plasma samples in which glucose-poor red blood cells are excluded.[62] However, they did not consider the effect of the more specific glucokinase or hexokinase assays for glucose measurements in current use. Carpenter and Coustan[56] calculated a conversion of O'Sullivan's criteria based on hexokinase measurements of glucose in plasma or serum (see Table 9-7). The validity of these modified criteria was confirmed experimentally by Sacks and co-workers,[63] who compared both types of measurements in paired whole blood and plasma samples from 995 pregnant women. Thus, the modified criteria most accurately reflect the values originally determined by O'Sul-

Table 9–7. Diagnosis of Gestational Diabetes Mellitus Using 3-Hour 100-g Oral Glucose Tolerance Test

Indication: Positive results of screening test (see text for discussion).

Procedure: After 3 days with carbohydrate intake of at least 150 g/day, in the fasting state, measure fasting plasma glucose and give 100 g of glucose by mouth. If two or more values equal or exceed the following criteria, diagnose GDM and start treatment. If one value is met or exceeded, the OGTT should be repeated in 4 weeks.

Criteria:	Time	NDDG[a] (mg/dl)[mM]	Modified[b] (mg/dl)[mM]
	Fasting	105 (5.8)	95 (5.3)
	1 hour	190 (10.5)	180 (10.0)
	2 hour	165 (9.2)	155 (8.6)
	3 hour	145 (8.0)	140 (7.7)

GDM, gestational diabetes mellitus; OGTT, oral glucose tolerance test; NDDG, National Diabetes Data Group.

[a]O'Sullivan's original criteria[58] are adapted based on 14% increase due to measurement in plasma rather than whole blood.

[b]O'Sullivan's original criteria[58] are adapted for current methods of measurement by Carpenter and Coustan.[56]

livan and Mahan.[58] Support for this view comes from the study by Magee and colleagues,[64] who compared the effect of using the two different OGTT criteria on predicting fetal hyperinsulinemia, macrosomia, and perinatal morbidities in a large group of pregnant women. In this study, pregnancies with OGTT values above the diagnostic levels of the modified criteria but below the NDDG levels (see Table 9-7) had perinatal morbidity equivalent to that predicted by using the traditional criteria. Kaufmann and colleagues[65] also found that OGTT values similar to the criteria of Carpenter and Coustan[56] but lower than the NDDG[62] were more efficient at identifying pregnant women who would develop diabetes observed for 7 years after pregnancy. Therefore, we believe that the modified 3-hour OGTT criteria (see Table 9-7) should be used for the diagnosis of GDM.

MATERNAL COMPLICATIONS OF GESTATIONAL DIABETES MELLITUS

The nonmetabolic complications are similar to those occurring in women with pregestational diabetes and were discussed earlier. The metabolic complications are also similar, except that DKA is not a problem and hypoglycemia occurs only in those women treated with insulin.

TREATMENT—DIET

Although the nutritional principles discussed earlier for pregestational diabetes apply in general for GDM, more controversy surrounds the dietary approach to the latter. This is probably because these women are often obese, sometimes markedly so, and only if diet alone fails is insulin required. Because insulin therapy represents such a marked change in life style, a more varied approach to diet has been tried to avoid insulin. The areas of controversy include the relative amounts of carbohydrate and fat in the diet, the distribution of calories throughout the day, and the use of calorie-restricted diets for obese patients.

The disagreement about the carbohydrate and fat content in the diet mirrors a similar controversy in the nutritional approach in type 2 diabetes. The higher the carbohydrate content, the greater is the postprandial rise of BG concentrations. This has specifically been demonstrated in GDM.[66] To maintain a 1-hour postprandial BG level <140 mg/dl, the percent of carbohydrate in meals needs to be approximately 50% or less. To achieve a 1-hour postprandial BG level <120 mg/dl, the carbohydrate content should be approximately 40% or less. This is especially important at breakfast because of the increased insulin resistance at that time.[66] On the other hand, because fat is more than twice as calorically dense as carbohydrate, to achieve a similar calorie level with a high-fat diet, less food would be required. This might lead to less satiety and increased hunger as well as the possibility of starvation ketosis because of the lowered carbohydrate intake. Controlling weight gain in these (often already obese) women with a diet high in fat might also pose a problem. In practice, recommen-

dations concerning the carbohydrate content of the diet in women with GDM have been <40%,[67] 40% to 50%,[68] to 55%.[69] Conversely, recommendations for the fat content range from 20% to 40%.

The second controversy concerns the distribution of calories throughout the day.[68] Many advocate three meals and three snacks a day to spread out the carbohydrate intake and lessen postprandial hyperglycemia. Others believe that obese patients with GDM are better served regarding glycemic control and weight gain by ingesting only three meals and a bedtime snack (to limit ketone body production overnight).

The third controversy concerns the safety of calorie restriction in obese patients with GDM. Limiting calories would be helpful in terms of maternal obesity but might be detrimental to fetal development because of impaired nutrient flow across the placenta and/or starvation ketosis. Although a 50% reduction in caloric intake in obese women with GDM resulted in ketonemia and ketonuria, a 33% reduction did not.[70] A clinical study in which calorie intake in women with GDM was 30% less than their prepregnancy diet resulted in a frequency of macrosomia in their infants similar to that of normal women.[71] Furthermore, none of the infants of the mothers with GDM were below the 10th percentile for weight even though the mean maternal weight gain after the 28th week of gestation was less than 4 pounds.

Because no clear-cut evidence favors one particular regimen over another, we have selected the following approach to nutritional therapy for women with GDM. Those whose pregestational weight was 80% to 120% of DBW are prescribed 30 kcal/kg of their present (pregnant) weight. If their pregestational weight had been 120% to 150% of DBW, 24 kcal/kg of present weight is recommended. If their pregestational weight exceeded 150% of DBW, only 12 kcal/kg of present weight is given. Diet composition consists of 40% to 50% carbohydrate, 30% to 40% fat, and the remainder protein. The majority of the fat intake should be monounsaturated and polyunsaturated fat. Calories are distributed in three meals and three snacks. The results of postprandial SMBG are used to adjust the foods containing carbohydrate so that insulin therapy can be avoided if possible. Approximately 75% of women with GDM achieve acceptable levels of glycemia with this dietary regimen.[68, 72] More liberal intake of carbohydrate results in approximately 50% of patients' requiring insulin.[73]

TREATMENT—EXERCISE

Several small studies have evaluated exercise in the treatment of women with GDM. Potential drawbacks to exercise in pregnancy include increased uterine contractions, fetal distress, small-for-gestational-age (SGA) infants, and maternal hypertension.[68] Exercise that uses lower body muscles and puts stress on the trunk region does increase uterine contractions, whereas exercises that use either upper extremity muscles or lower extremity muscles while recumbent do not.[74, 75] A 6-week exercise program using upper extremity muscles in women with GDM treated with diet lowered the fasting plasma glucose concentration modestly and the plasma glucose concentration markedly 1 hour after a 50-g glucose challenge.[74] In a second study,[75] patients with GDM who had failed diet therapy were randomized either to receive insulin or to enroll in an exercise program that used a recumbent bicycle. The glycemic and clinical outcomes were similar in the two groups, suggesting that appropriate exercise for patients who fail diet therapy may prevent insulin therapy.

TREATMENT—INSULIN

The treatment of GDM with insulin requires several decisions. What criteria should be used to add insulin to the dietary regimen? Related to this, what pattern of monitoring should be recommended? If a woman is started on insulin, what should the glycemic

goals be? In a normal (nondiabetic) pregnancy, the fasting plasma glucose (FPG) concentration ranges between 55 and 70 mg/dl, the 1-hour postprandial glucose level is <120 mg/dl, and glycated hemoglobin values are less than normal (e.g., a glycated hemoglobin level of 3.8% to 4.5% in an assay in which the normal nonpregnant range is 4.3% to 6.1%.)[76] (The glycated hemoglobin level is less than the normal nonpregnant range because not only are glucose concentrations lowered in pregnancy but red blood cell turnover is increased—see Chapter 7 for reasons why this leads to decreased glycated hemoglobin levels.)

Various criteria have been proposed for the initiation of insulin therapy (Table 9–8). To interpret these values, one must take into account the relationship between plasma and whole BG concentrations, the site of sampling, and whether the value is a fasting one or a postprandial one. For our purposes here, it is enough to realize that a plasma value is approximately 12% (depending on the hematocrit) higher than a whole blood value. A finger stick yields arterialized blood, which does not influence the fasting glucose concentration because in the fasting state there is little glucose uptake by muscle tissue. After eating, however, muscle glucose utilization becomes a factor. Measurement of glucose concentrations in blood samples obtained by a finger stick yields higher values than if a venous sample had been ob-

Table 9–8. Criteria Recommended for the Initiation of Insulin Therapy in Women with Gestational Diabetes

Fasting[a]	Postprandial[a]	Reference
>80	1 hour >140	Jovanovic-Peterson and Peterson[67]
>105[b]	none	Metzger[77]
>95	2 hour >120	Langer et al[73]
>100	1 hour >130	Ramus and Kitzmiller[72]
>90	1 hour >120	Jovanovic-Peterson[76]

[a]Glucose concentrations (mg/dl) measured in finger-stick whole blood samples unless designated otherwise.
[b]Venous plasma sample.

tained. This is because the arterialized blood in the sample has not yet traversed muscle and glucose removal by this tissue has not occurred. The increase due to the site of sampling is balanced by the decrease due to the fact that the sample is whole blood and not plasma. Therefore, in the postprandial state, the glucose concentration measured in a sample obtained by finger stick is comparable to a plasma venous value.

The simplest way to monitor women with GDM is to measure their FPG concentration every week in the office or laboratory and not initiate insulin treatment unless their value exceeds 105 mg/dl.[77] Indeed, Huddleston and colleagues[78] questioned the need for measuring postprandial glucose levels. They demonstrated that only 17% of women with FPG concentrations <105 mg/dl had 2-hour postprandial values >120 mg/dl and in only 5% were they >140 mg/dl. In their hands, mean birth weight, macrosomia, delivery by cesarean section, and shoulder dystocia were similar in the infants of these women whether their 2-hour glucose concentrations exceeded 120 mg/dl or not. On the other hand, Goldberg and colleagues[79] showed almost a threefold reduction in macrosomia in women who performed SMBG compared with those who were monitored by weekly glucose measurements only. Measuring postprandial rather than preprandial glucose concentrations by SMBG in women who did require insulin resulted in significant decreases in glycated hemoglobin levels, cesarean sections for cephalopelvic disproportion, macrosomia, large-for-gestational-age (LGA) babies, and neonatal hypoglycemia.[44]

In our view, performing SMBG before breakfast and postprandially maximizes the chance for a successful outcome. If the FPG concentration on the OGTT is ≥120 mg/dl, the patient is started on insulin immediately. Others are seen by a dietitian within 3 days and are also taught SMBG to be performed before breakfast and between 1 and 2 hours after each meal. Insulin is started within 1 to 2 weeks if the majority (i.e., at least four of

seven per week) of fasting BG values exceed 90 mg/dl. Similarly, if the majority of postprandial values after a particular meal exceed 120 mg/dl, insulin is started. Either a split/mixed regimen or preprandial regular insulin with evening NPH insulin is appropriate (see Chapter 4), with the decision being left up to the patient after a thorough discussion. Depending on which regimen is selected and which glucose concentration needs to be lowered (see Table 4-2 in Chapter 4 for the relationship between the various components of insulin regimens and which glucose values they affect), one or more of the following insulin doses are started: 10 U of NPH insulin before breakfast; 6 U of NPH insulin in the evening; 4 U of regular or lispro insulin before breakfast and supper. If the preprandial short- or rapid-acting insulin regimen is selected, 4 U of regular or lispro insulin is started before lunch instead of the morning dose of NPH insulin. The patient should contact the physician or program frequently (daily or every other day if possible) during the first week and then once or twice a week subsequently for insulin dose adjustments. The goals of therapy are to keep the glucose concentrations below the levels used to initiate insulin therapy. In contrast to pregnant women with type 1 diabetes, in whom insulin requirements often decrease during the last month of pregnancy, the need for insulin in insulin-requiring women with GDM continually increases.

FETAL MONITORING AND TIMING OF DELIVERY

Many decades ago, clinicians recognized a threat of fetal demise late in pregnancies complicated by diabetes.[81] The risk was 50% in the presence of ketoacidosis, 7% to 14% in women with type 1 or type 2 diabetes, and 3% to 6% in women with GDM (vs. 1% to 2% in nondiabetic women in that era). Because the risk increased as gestation approached full term, pioneer investigators such as White[23] and Pedersen[24] recommended that diabetic women be delivered at 35 to 37 weeks to prevent stillbirth. Unfortunately, this policy contributed to neonatal morbidity and mortality due to hyaline membrane disease (also termed RDS), which was also much more common in near-term infants of diabetic mothers than in control infants. Thus, the risk of stillbirth and neonatal death was frightening to diabetic patients and daunting to their clinicians.

In order to prevent unnecessary preterm births in infants of diabetic mothers, investigators developed techniques to estimate fetal well-being and to predict risk of stillbirth, so that only those babies at high risk would be delivered early. The first tests were the measurement of maternal urinary or plasma estriol levels, which usually reflected fetoplacental function, based on fetal adrenal production of an androgen that was sulfated in the fetal liver and converted to estrogen in the placenta. Sensitivity was good but specificity was not, so the biochemical assays were supplanted by biophysical methods to predict acute changes in fetal well-being.[82] Because uterine contractions transiently decrease placental oxygen transfer to the fetus and fetal heart rate (FHR) *decelerations* following the peak of the contractions reflect the degree of fetal hypoxia, a *stress test* was developed in which contractions were produced by infusion of oxytocin or by maternal nipple stimulation. Fetuses at risk of demise in utero (to be considered for delivery) were those with late decelerations, and the remainder of pregnancies could be allowed to continue. Greater diagnostic specificity was attained by assessment of FHR *accelerations* and variability between (or in the absence of) contractions, which reflect a normoxic brain and a nonacidotic fetus. This led to the application of *nonstress tests* to diabetic pregnant women. Finally, *real-time ultrasonography* was used to measure fetal body and limb movements and chest wall motion ("fetal breathing"), as well as amniotic fluid volume, all of which indicate normal fetal oxygenation. Combined with antepartum FHR monitoring (nonstress tests), this schema of testing became known as the fetal *biophysical profile,* which was shown to be valuable in the management of diabetic and other high-risk pregnancies.[82] Indeed, many medical centers demonstrated that frequent systematic use of these measures of fetal well-being in various combinations, independent of maternal glycemic control, reduced the risk of stillbirth to <2% in pregnancies complicated by diabetes.[81]

During the period that fetal monitoring was developed, clinical studies of pregnant diabetic women demonstrated that the risk of fetal distress and stillbirth was clearly associated with the degree of maternal hyperglycemia and that the risk was very low when euglycemia was attained.[81] Experimental studies demonstrated that infusions of glucose into pregnant animals or their fetuses decreased the fetal blood oxygen content and pH, which could explain the association of fetal distress and hyperglycemia. These studies provide the basis for the modern management of diabetes and pregnancy (Table 9-9), in which intensive fetal monitoring and consideration of early delivery are applied to cases with persistent hyperglycemia or other possible maternal causes of fetal hypoxia, such as hypertension, severe stress, uterine vascular lesions, or illicit drug use. On the other hand, uncomplicated cases with verified euglycemia can be managed as normal pregnancies and allowed to continue to full term.

In cases with persistent maternal hyperglycemia (>20% of postprandial values >130 mg/dl), another possible reason for early delivery is fetal macrosomia. The hypothesis that excessive fetal growth and fat deposition are due to the causal chain of maternal hyperglycemia → fetal hyperglycemia → fetal hyperinsulinemia is amply supported by experimental and clinical studies. Because a macrosomic infant of a diabetic mother is at extra risk for birth trauma due to increased shoulder dimensions, ultrasonography is

Table 9–9. Evaluation During Pregnancy for Women with Type 1 and Type 2 Diabetes

Time of Gestation	Low Risk	High Risk[a]
Baseline	Glycated hemoglobin, CBC, TSH, urine culture, 24-hour urine test for microalbumin and creatinine clearance, retinal examination	Same plus ECG
Every 4–12 weeks	Glycated hemoglobin	Glycated hemoglobin 24-hour urine
16 weeks	Expanded serum α-fetoprotein	Same
20–22 weeks	Targeted fetal US survey for anomalies, including echocardiogram	Same
25–26 weeks		Fetal growth and umbilical Doppler flow by US q 3–4 wk; NST/CST or BPP weekly
28–32 weeks	Fetal growth by US Retinal examination	Retinal examination
34–36 weeks	NST/CST or BPP weekly	
Before delivery at term	Fetal size by US study	Amniocentesis Fetal size by US

CBC, complete blood count; TSH, thyroid-stimulating hormone; US, ultrasound; NST, nonstress test of fetal heart rate pattern; CST, contraction stress test; BPP, biophysical profile (fetal motion and amniotic fluid volume by US); ECG, electrocardiogram.
[a]Definitions of high-risk categories:
  Baseline—women at risk for coronary artery disease
  Every 4–12 weeks—women with microalbuminuria or clinical proteinuria
  25–26 weeks—women with hypertension or nephropathy
  Before delivery at <39 weeks—women wtih hyperglycemia need amniocentesis; all diabetic women may need amniocentesis before delivery <36 weeks

widely used to estimate fetal weight, with only fair accuracy demonstrated.[81] If the estimated fetal weight is 3,800 to 4,100 g at 37 to 38 weeks' gestation, it may be best to induce labor, using intravaginal prostaglandins to ripen the cervix as needed. If the estimated fetal weight is >4,200 g and the maternal pelvis is untested for a large baby, it is best to perform a primary cesarean section at 39 weeks' gestation owing to the high risk of shoulder dystocia in these cases.[83]

If maternal hyperglycemia has been present in the third trimester, another possible result of fetal hyperinsulinemia is delay in the production of components of the fetal alveolar surfactant system. This helps to explain the previous high risk of RDS in infants of diabetic mothers delivered before 39 weeks' gestation. The measurement of surfactant in amniotic fluid obtained by amniocentesis is a major advance in the perinatal management of pregnancies complicated by diabetes.[84] A low risk of RDS is predicted by an amniotic fluid lecithin-to-sphingomyelin ratio of >3.4 (supranormal ratio required in diabetes, probably because of low surfactant apoprotein with ratios of 2.2 to 3.4),[85] or positive phosphatidylglycerol content, or a mature fluorescence polarization test result. In cases of verified maternal euglycemia, amniocentesis is not necessary for delivery at 37 to 38 weeks' gestation because the risk of RDS is quite low.

The management of labor in diabetic women is based on standard obstetric principles, with an emphasis on prevention of maternal-fetal hyperglycemia or hypoglycemia by intravenous infusions of insulin and dextrose and careful FHR monitoring to detect signs of fetal hypoxia.[86] To decrease the chance of shoulder dystocia and birth trauma in term pregnancies, it is wise not to attempt operative vaginal deliveries in cases of failure of descent in the second stage of labor.

Special postpartum concerns for diabetic women include prevention of plasma glucose excursions >200 mg/dl to decrease the risk of problems with infections or wound healing and recognition that insulin requirements are usually substantially lower after deliver (discussed later). As with women without diabetes, diabetic women are encouraged to breast-feed their babies. The breast milk is normal in well-controlled diabetes.

INSULIN TREATMENT DURING DELIVERY

Metabolic studies of nondiabetic pregnant women during labor revealed that glucose turnover increased fourfold with little change in insulin levels.[87] This strongly suggests that muscle contractions (probably both uterine and skeletal) independent of insulin are the predominant determinant of glucose utilization during labor. These data are consistent with the results obtained in type 1 diabetic pregnant women in labor attached to an artificial endocrine pancreas (Biostator), which delivers appropriate amounts of insulin and glucose to maintain the glucose concentration at a preset level. During active labor, the insulin requirement was zero while glucose requirements were relatively constant at 2.6 mg/kg/min or approximately 10 g/h in a 60-kg woman.[88]

Based on these considerations, the following approach (modified from that of Jovanovic and Peterson[88]) is suggested for treating an insulin-requiring woman with *pregestational* diabetes as she progresses through labor and delivery. If labor is to be induced, induction should start in the morning. The usual dose of evening NPH insulin is taken, but no morning insulin is given. The goal is to maintain the glucose concentration between 70 and 100 mg/dl. Most labor and delivery units have the ability to measure finger-stick glucose concentrations, and this should be done every hour. If labor is to be induced, intravenous saline is infused until active labor begins unless the

initial glucose concentration is <70 mg/dl. If this should be the case, 5% dextrose is infused at 100 ml/h until the glucose level is in the appropriate range. If the initial blood glucose concentration is between 100 and 150 mg/dl, insulin at a rate of 1 U/h is infused. If the initial glucose concentration is >150 mg/dl, insulin is infused at a rate of 2 U/h. In case the glucose concentration remains >100 mg/dl 2 hours after starting an insulin infusion, the rate should be increased by 0.5 U/h. This should be repeated every 2 hours as long as the glucose concentration remains >100 mg/dl. Insulin is discontinued when the glucose concentration decreases to <100 mg/dl. When active labor begins, 5% dextrose is infused at a rate of 200 ml/h (or 10% dextrose at 100 ml/h). If the glucose level falls to <60 mg/dl during active labor, the glucose infusion is doubled during the subsequent hour. No insulin is usually required during active labor, but the same insulin infusion rate described earlier is used, depending on the glucose concentration at this time as well.

If labor is spontaneous, the same approach as described earlier can be used—that is, 5% dextrose infusion rate of 100 ml/h if the glucose concentration is <70 mg/dl or 200 ml/h when active labor occurs. If the glucose concentration remains >100 mg/dl 2 hours after starting an insulin infusion, the rate should be increased by 0.5 U/h. This should be repeated every 2 hours if the glucose concentration remains >100 mg/dl. Once the glucose falls into the 70 to 100 mg/dl range, insulin can be stopped and the hourly monitoring continued.

In contrast, a woman with *GDM* does not require insulin once labor begins. If labor is to be induced, the usual evening NPH insulin should be taken the night before, but no subcutaneous insulin is given the following morning when induction begins. The same approach described earlier regarding dextrose and insulin infusions can be used if the glucose concentrations are not between 70 and 100 mg/dl until active labor ensues.

Table 9–10. Neonatal Complications

Macrosomia	Polycythemia/hyperviscosity
Hypoglycemia	Hyperbilirubinemia
Respiratory distress syndrome	Cardiomyopathy
	Small for gestational age
Hypocalcemia	Congenital anomalies

Women scheduled for an elective cesarean section can be treated as any other insulin-requiring patient undergoing major surgery (see Chapter 7).

NEONATAL MORBIDITIES[89]

Table 9–10 lists the neonatal morbidities that are possible in both pregestational and gestational diabetes. The pathogenesis of many (but not all) of them are shown in Figure 9–4. Maternal insulin is degraded by the placenta and never reaches the fetus, and under euglycemic conditions, fetal insulin concentrations are low. The β-cells typically start to respond to glucose several days after birth. The Pedersen hypothesis[24] holds that maternal hyperglycemia leads to fetal hyperglycemia, which in turn causes fetal β-cell hyperplasia and increased insulin secretion. Freinkel[22] later extended this hypothesis to include other maternal substrates reaching the fetus (especially amino acids, which also stimulate fetal insulin secretion) because of inadequate maternal insulin levels. This surfeit of mixed nutrients in the presence of elevated fetal insulin concentrations is responsible for *macrosomia*. The carryover of fetal hyperinsulinemia after birth and the hyperresponsiveness of the β-cells in newborns cause *hypoglycemia*. Hyperinsulinemia decreases hepatic glucose production, increases glucose utilization by the insulin-sensitive (mostly muscle) tissues, and blunts the rise of the rapid-acting counterregulatory hormones, glucagon and catecholamines. Neonatal hypoglycemia, defined as a plasma glucose concentration of <40 mg/dl, occurs within the first 4 to 6 hours of life in at

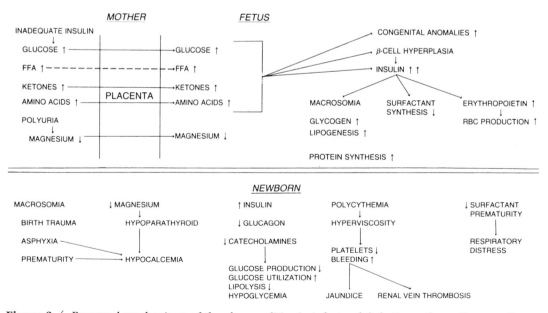

Figure 9–4. Proposed mechanisms of the abnormalities in infants of diabetic mothers. (See text for discussion.) (From Sperling MA: Diabetes mellitus. In Kaplan SA [ed]: Clinical Pediatric Endocrinology. WB Saunders, Philadelphia, 1990, p. 127)

least 20% to 25% of infants of poorly treated diabetic mothers.

Fetal hyperinsulinemia is also responsible for *RDS* by inhibiting the synthesis of various phospholipids that are components of surfactant. This feared neonatal complication is much less common today because of the emphasis on maintaining near euglycemia during pregnancy and the enhanced ability to monitor a fetus accurately to forestall early delivery. Fetal hyperinsulinemia probably also causes neonatal *polycythemia* by stimulating erythropoietin production. This can lead to *hyperviscosity* (red blood cell sludging), which can damage any organ. Finally, fetal hyperinsulinemia may underlie neonatal *cardiomyopathy.* Thickened heart muscle is found in many infants of diabetic mothers. Although most of them are asymptomatic, a few may develop congestive heart failure as a result of left ventricular outflow obstruction. Because insulin stimulates the growth of cardiac muscle, it is believed that increased insulin levels late in pregnancy may be responsible for this lesion.

The remaining neonatal complications are not secondary to fetal hyperinsulinemia. *Hypocalcemia* is probably related to the blunted secretion of parathyroid hormone during the first 4 days of life in infants of diabetic mothers compared with infants of nondiabetic mothers. Impaired secretion of parathyroid hormone may be due to neonatal hypomagnesemia that is secondary to maternal hypomagnesemia. This is thought to occur because of urinary magnesium loss associated with maternal hyperglycemia and resultant polyuria. (The renal threshold for glucose is lowered in pregnancy, and therefore even mild hyperglycemia causes a diuresis.) *Hyperbilirubinemia* may be a result of increased catabolism of red blood cell membranes. Why this should occur is not clear. Bruising of a macrosomic infant at delivery as well as possible bleeding in the hyperviscosity syndrome could also contribute. As discussed earlier, *congenital anomalies* are two to four times more common in infants

of diabetic mothers, especially if hyperglycemia is present during the first 2 months after conception. In vitro studies show that the anomalies are related to the increased availability of fetal fuels (glucose and probably other substrates), the presence of which in vivo is nicely explained by the Pedersen-Freinkel hypothesis. *SGA* infants of diabetic mothers are much less common today than in the past. If growth retardation occurs early within the first trimester, it is termed *early growth delay,* and some of these fetuses have congenital anomalies.[90] Subsequent growth seems normal. Growth retardation in the third trimester is theorized to be due to uteroplacental vascular insufficiency, although it also occurs in women whose postprandial glucose concentrations are controlled too tightly.[13, 91]

Table 9–11 shows the neonatal morbidities of offspring of pregestational diabetic and gestational diabetic women registered in the California Statewide Diabetes and Pregnancy Program in 1986 to 1988. In general, and as might be expected, neonatal morbidities were fewer in babies born to women with GDM than to those with pregestational diabetes and fewer in offspring with mothers in classes A, B, and C of the White classification compared with classes D, F, and R (see Table 9–2).

POSTPARTUM

WOMEN WITH PREGESTATIONAL DIABETES

An immediate and profound decrease in insulin requirements follows delivery. One obvious reason is that the insulin-antagonistic hormones produced by the placenta are suddenly removed, reversing the insulin resistance that characterizes pregnancy. This is probably not the entire explanation because the lowered insulin requirement during the immediate postpartum period is far less than the pregestational insulin dose. Some women may not even need insulin for several

Table 9–11. Prevalence of Neonatal Morbidities in Infants Born to Diabetic Women in the California Statewide Diabetes and Pregnancy Program in 1986–1988

	White's Classification		
Morbidity	*GDM* *(n = 1,456)*	*A, B, and C* *(n = 290)*	*D, F, R, etc.* *(n = 80)*
Hyperbilirubinemia:			
Mild/moderate/severe	27.1%	46.6%	55.0%
Moderate/severe	9.8%	21.4%	35.0%
Severe	1.2%	2.1%	3.8%
Hypertrophic cardiomyopathy	0.4%	1.7%	1.3%
Hypocalcemia	0.6%	1.0%	3.8%
Hypoglycemia	8.0%	24.5%	26.3%
Polycythemia/hyperviscosity	1.5%	3.4%	3.8%
Respiratory distress	2.1%	4.5%	11.3%
Transient tachypnea	2.3%	4.1%	5.0%

The criteria for hyperbilirubinemia, hypoglycemia, and hypocalcemia were adjusted according to gestational age. Severe hyperbilirubinemia was defined as 20 mg/dl or more at 34 or more weeks' gestation, 20 mg/dl or more at 30-33 weeks' gestation, and 12 mg/dl or more at <30 weeks' gestation. Mild hyperbilirubinemia was defined as 6-15 mg/dl at 38 weeks or more, 6-10 mg/dl at 34-37 weeks, 6-8 mg/dl at 30-33 weeks, and 5-6 mg/dl at <30 weeks. Moderate hyperbilirubinemia criteria were intermediate between those for severe and mild hyperbilirubinemia. Hypoglycemia was defined as two plasma glucose values <30 mg/dl (1.7 mmol/L) during the first 48 h of life in term infants or two plasma glucose levels <20 mg/dl (1.1 mmol/L) during the first 48 h or <30 mg/dl (1.7 mmol/L) after the first 48 h in preterm infants. Hypocalcemia was defined as a serum calcium <2.0 mmol/L in term and <1.75 mmol/L in preterm infants. Polycythemia was defined as a hematocrit of 65% or more.

From Cousins L: The California Diabetes and Pregnancy Program: a statewide collaborative program for the preconception and prenatal care of diabetic women. Bailliere's Clinical Obstet Gynecol 5:443, 1991.

days. Two explanations have been offered to account for this consistently noted phenomenon. Some of the large amounts of insulin administered during the third trimester became bound to circulating insulin antibodies and are now leaking off to supply free insulin. With the introduction of purified insulins (which include all human insulin preparations), titers of insulin antibodies are extremely low, making this explanation untenable. During pregnancy, the placental production of hCS (which has growth hormone–like actions) suppresses pituitary secretion of growth hormone. After delivery, a lag period intervenes before growth hormone release by the pituitary returns to normal. Growth hormone is a potent insulin antagonist, and patients lacking it (e.g., type 1 diabetic patients after hypophysectomy, an older treatment for proliferative diabetic retinopathy) are extremely sensitive to insulin. This seems more likely than the first explanation, but whether it can account for near euglycemia for several days without any insulin in some women with type 1 diabetes is not certain.

It is better not to attempt to achieve near euglycemia in the immediate postpartum period because too many factors are changing (e.g., insulin sensitivity, food intake, sleep patterns if the new mother is nursing, and so on). If the delivery was a vaginal one and the woman can soon eat, the simplest approach is to measure her BG concentration before each meal and give 4 U of regular or lispro insulin if the value is >150 mg/dl. If the fasting glucose level exceeds this value, 6 U of NPH insulin is given that evening. If the before bedtime BG concentration is >150 mg/dl on the day of delivery (assuming that no dextrose is being infused), it is probably safe to give 6 U of NPH insulin that first evening. If it is desired to place the patient immediately back on a split/mixed regimen, half of the pregestational dose of intermediate-acting insulin (NPH or lente) can be given the next morning. However, the patient must be monitored carefully to ensure that this amount of insulin is not excessive during this early postpartum period of enhanced insulin sensitivity. Whichever regimen is used, once BG concentrations start to rise on these low doses of insulin, doses need to be gradually increased as dictated by the BG values until the insulin dose stabilizes. This usually occurs within 2 weeks.

If delivery is by cesarean section and the patient is unable to eat for several days, the management is similar to that described in Chapter 7 for patients undergoing major surgery. Bear in mind, however, the increased insulin sensitivity in the immediate postpartum period and select and adjust the insulin doses accordingly.

If a new mother breast-feeds, which should be encouraged because diabetes itself is not a contraindication, she should ingest an additional 500 kcal/day.[37] The effect of breast-feeding on insulin requirements is variable, and some patients experience a more erratic pattern of SMBG values and more hypoglycemia. These episodes seem to occur overnight (necessitating periodic measurements of BG concentrations during that period) and an hour or so after breast-feeding. Decreasing the evening dose of intermediate-acting insulin is appropriate for the former, and a snack before breast-feeding prevents the latter.

WOMEN WITH GESTATIONAL DIABETES MELLITUS

Insulin-requiring women with GDM do not need insulin after delivery. The issue for these patients is the increased possibility that they will develop type 2 diabetes in the future. Within 5 to 15 years, approximately half of them do so.[53, 92, 93] Pregnancy acts as stress on the pancreatic β-cells, and those women who cannot respond because of impaired insulin secretion develop GDM.[94] Therefore, it is to be expected that these individuals would be susceptible to the subsequent development of type 2 diabetes. Not surprisingly, predictive factors for this outcome include pregestational weight, maternal hyperglycemia, insulin secretion both during and shortly after pregnancy, and the gestational age at which GDM was diagnosed.[92, 93, 95] A few Caucasian[96] but not African American[97] women with GDM have a defect in the pancreatic β-cell glucokinase gene that codes for an important enzyme involved in insulin secretion (see Chapter 1 for discussion of maturity-onset diabetes of the young). Therefore, more than 95% of the diabetes that subsequently develops in women with GDM is the usual type 2 diabetes.

To ascertain their carbohydrate status after pregnancy, women with GDM should have a 75-g OGTT 6 weeks after delivery. They should be fasting, and only two samples need to be drawn, before and 2 hours after the glucose load. The 2-hour glucose concentration identifies a woman as being either normal (<140 mg/dl), having impaired glucose tolerance (140 to 199 mg/dl), or having diabetes (≥ 200 mg/dl). As stated earlier, the higher this glucose concentration, the more likely type 2 diabetes is to develop in the future. For instance, 80% of Latino women with impaired glucose tolerance 6 weeks after delivery develop type 2 diabetes within 5 years.[93]

Women with a history of GDM should be monitored yearly and counseled strongly to achieve DBW. Lean women with a history of GDM developed type 2 diabetes at only half the rate of their obese counterparts.[53]

REFERENCES

1. American Diabetes Association Position Statement. Preconception care of women with diabetes, Diabetes Care 20 (suppl 1):S40, 1997
2. Dicker D, Feldberg D, Samuel N et al: Spontaneous abortion in patients with insulin-dependent diabetes mellitus: the effect of preconceptional diabetic control. Am J Obstet Gynecol 158:1161, 1988.
3. Mills JL, Simpson JL, Driscoll SG et al: Inci-

dence of spontaneous abortion among normal women and insulin-dependent diabetic women whose pregnancies were identified within 21 days of conception. N Engl J Med 319:1617, 1988

4. Key TC, Giuffrida R, Moore TR: Predictive value of early pregnancy glycohemoglobin in the insulin-treated diabetic patient. Am J Obstet Gynecol 16:1096, 1987

5. Hanson U, Persson B, Thunell S: Relationship between haemoglobin A_{1c} in early type I (insulin-dependent) diabetic pregnancy and the occurrence of spontaneous abortion and fetal malformation in Sweden. Diabetologia 33:100, 1990

6. Kitzmiller JL, Buchanan TA, Kjos S et al: Preconception care of diabetes, congenital malformations, and spontaneous abortions. Diabetes Care 19:514, 1996

7. Lowy C: Management of diabetes in pregnancy. Diabetes Metab Rev 9:147, 1993

8. Goldman JA, Dicker D, Feldber D et al: Pregnancy outcome in patients with insulin-dependent diabetes mellitus with preconceptional diabetic control: a comparative study. Am J Obstet Gynecol 155:293, 1986

9. Steel JM, Johnstone FD, Hepburn DA et al: Can pregnancy care of diabetic women reduce the risk of abnormal babies? BMJ 301:1070, 1990

10. Kitzmiller JL, Gavin LA, Gin GD et al: Preconception care of diabetes: glycemic control prevents congenital anomalies. JAMA 265:731, 1991

11. Landon MB, Gabbe SG, Piana R et al: Neonatal morbidity in pregnancy complicated by diabetes mellitus: predictive value of maternal glycemic profiles. Am J Obstet Gynecol 156:1089, 1987

12. Jovanovic-Peterson L, Peterson C, Reed GF et al: Maternal postprandial glucose levels and infant birth weight: the diabetes in early pregnancy study. Am J Obstet Gynecol 164:103, 1991

13. Combs CA, Gunderson E, Kitzmiller JL et al: Relationship of fetal macrosomia to maternal postprandial glucose control during pregnancy. Diabetes Care 15:1251, 1992

14. Phelps RL, Sakol P, Metzger BE et al: Changes in diabetic retinopathy during pregnancy: correlations with regulation of hyperglycemia. Arch Opthalmol 104:1806, 1986

15. Klein BEK, Moss SE, Klein R: Effect of pregnancy on progression of diabetic retinopathy. Diabetes Care 13:34, 1990

16. Davison JM: The effect of pregnancy on kidney function in renal allograft recipients. Kidney Int 27:74, 1985

17. Combs CA, Rosenn B, Kitzmiller JL et al: Early-pregnancy proteinuria in diabetes related to preeclampsia. Obstet Gynecol 82:802, 1993

18. Reece EA, Coustan DR, Hayslett JP et al: Diabetic nephropathy: pregnancy performance and fetomaternal outcome. Am J Obstet Gynecol 159:56, 1988

19. Reece EA, Egan JFX, Coustan DR et al: Coronary artery disease in diabetic pregnancies. Am J Obstet Gynecol 154:150, 1986.

20. American Diabetes Association: Contraception. In Jovanovic-Peterson L (ed): Medical Management of Pregnancy Complicated by Diabetes. American Diabetes Association, Alexandria, VA, 1993, pp. 14–18

21. St James PJ, Younger MD, Hamilton BD et al: Unplanned pregnancies in young women with diabetes. Diabetes Care 16:1572, 1993

22. Freinkel N: Of pregnancy and progeny. Diabetes 29:1023, 1980

23. Hare JW, White P: Gestational diabetes and the White classification. Diabetes Care 3:394, 1980

24. Pedersen J, Molsted-Pedersen L: Prognosis of the outcome of pregnancies in diabetes. A new classification. Acta Endocrinol Kbh 50:70, 1965

25. Maceold AF, Smith SA, Sonksen PH et al: The problem of autonomic neuropathy in diabetic pregnancy. Diabetic Med 7:80, 1990

26. Cousins LM: Pregnancy complications among diabetic women: review 1965–1985. Obstet Gynecol Surv 42:140, 1987

27. VanOtterlo I, Wladimiroff J, Wallenberg H: Relationship between fetal urine production and amniotic fluid volume in normal pregnancy and pregnancy complicated by diabetes. Br J Obstet Gynaecol 84:205, 1977

28. Mimouni F, Miodovnik M, Siddiqi TA et al: High spontaneous premature labor rate in insulin-dependent diabetic pregnant women: an association with poor glycemic control and urogenital infection. Obstet Gynecol 175:1988, 1972

29. Smith BT, Giroud CJP, Robert M et al: Insulin

antagonism of cortisol action on lecithin synthesis by cultured fetal lung cells. J Pediatr 87:983, 1975

30. Snyder JM, Mendelson CR: Insulin inhibits the accumulation of the major lung surfactant apoprotein in human fetal lung explants maintained in vitro. Endocrinology 120:1250, 1987

31. Carson BS, Phillips AF, Simmons MA et al: Effects of a sustained insulin infusion upon glucose uptake and oxygenation in the ovine fetus. Pediatr Res 14:147, 1980

32. Rosenn B, Miodovnik M, Combs CA et al: Poor glycemic control and antepartum obstetric complication in women with insulin-dependent diabetes. Int J Gynaecol Obstet 43:21, 1993

33. Combs CA, Katz MA, Kitzmiller JL et al: Experimental preeclampsia produced by chronic constriction of the lower aorta: validation with longitudinal blood pressure measurements in conscious rhesus monkeys. Am J Obstet Gynecol 169:215, 1993

34. Lucas MJ, Leveno KJ, Cunningham FG: A comparison of magnesium sulfate with phenytoin for the prevention of eclampsia. N Engl J Med 333:201, 1995

35. Scardo JA, Hogg BB, Newman RB: Favorable hemodynamic effects of magnesium sulfate in preeclampsia. Am J Obstet Gynecol 173:1249, 1995

36. Munro JF, Campbell IW, McCuish AC et al: Euglycaemic diabetic ketoacidosis. BMJ 2:578, 1973

37. American Diabetes Association: Nutritional management during pregnancy in preexisting diabetes. In Jovanovic-Peterson L (ed): Medical Management of Pregnancy Complicated by Diabetes. American Diabetes Association, Alexandria, VA, 1993, pp. 47–56

38. State of California, Department of Health Services, Maternal and Child Health Branch: Sweet Success, California Diabetes and Pregnancy Program Guidelines for Care. State Printing Office, Sacramento, CA, 1992

39. Rizzo T, Metzger BE, Burns WJ et al: Correlation between antepartum maternal metabolism and intelligence of offspring. N Engl J Med 325:911, 1991

40. Coustan DR, Reece A, Sherwin RS et al: A randomized clinical trial of the insulin pump vs intensive conventional therapy in diabetic pregnancies. JAMA 255:631, 1986

41. American Diabetes Association: Monitoring. In Jovanovic-Peterson L (ed): Medical Management of Pregnancy Complicated by Diabetes. American Diabetes Association, Alexandria, VA, 1993, pp. 31–38

42. Matheson D, Efantis J: Diabetes and pregnancy: need and use of intensive therapy. Diabetes Educator 15:242, 1989

43. Metzger B, Freinkel N: Diabetes and pregnancy: metabolic changes and management. Clin Diabetes 8:4, 1990

44. De Veciana M, Major CA, Morgan MA et al: Postprandial versus preprandial blood glucose monitoring in women with gestational diabetes mellitus requiring insulin therapy. N Engl J Med 33:1237, 1995

45. Piacquadio K, Hollingsworth DR, Murphy H: Effects of in-utero exposure to oral hypoglycaemic drugs. Lancet 338:866, 1991

46. Jackson WPU, Campbell GD, Notelovitz M et al: Tolbutamide and chlorpropamide during pregnancy in human diabetes. Diabetes 2(suppl):98, 1962

47. Dolger H, Bookman JJ, Nechemias C: The diagnostic and therapeutic value of tolbutamide in pregnant diabetes. Diabetes 2(suppl):97, 1962

48. Douglas CP, Richards R: Use of chlorpropamide in the treatment of diabetes in pregnancy. Diabetes 16:60, 1967

49. Sutherland HW, Bewsher PD, Cormack JD et al: Effect of moderate dosage of chlorpropamide in pregnancy on fetal outcome. Arch Dis Child 49:283, 1974

50. Coetzee EJ, Jackson WPU: The management of non-insulin-dependent diabetes during pregnancy. Diabetes Res Clin Pract 1:281, 1986

51. O'Sullivan JB, Charles D, Mahan CM et al: Gestational diabetes and perinatal mortality rate. Am J Obstet Gynecol 116:901, 1973

52. Carrington ER, Reardon HS, Shuman CR: Recognition and management of problems associated with prediabetes during pregnancy. JAMA 166:245, 1958

53. O'Sullivan JB: Body weight and subsequent diabetes mellitus. JAMA 248:949, 1982

54. Gregory KD, Kjos SL, Peters RK: Cost of non-insulin-dependent diabetes in women with a history of gestational diabetes: implications for prevention. Obstet Gynecol 81:782, 1993

55. O'Sullivan JB, Mahan CM, Charles D et al:

Screening criteria for high-risk gestational diabetic patients. Am J Obstet Gynecol 116:895, 1973

55a. Report of the expert committee on the diagnosis and classification of diabetes mellitus. Diabetes Care 20:1183, 1997

56. Carpenter MW, Coustan DR: Criteria for screening tests for gestational diabetes. Am J Obstet Gynecol 144:768, 1982

57. Coustan DR, Widness JA, Carpenter MW et al: Should the fifty-gram, one-hour plasma glucose screening test for gestational diabetes be administered in the fasting or fed state? Am J Obstet Gynecol 154:1031, 1986

58. O'Sullivan JB, Mahan CM: Criteria for the oral glucose tolerance test in pregnancy. Diabetes 13:278, 1964

59. Mestman JH: Outcome of diabetes screening in pregnancy and perinatal morbidity in infants of mothers with mild impairment in glucose tolerance. Diabetes Care 3:447, 1980

60. O'Sullivan JB, Gellis SS, Dandrow RV et al: The potential diabetic and her treatment in pregnancy. Obstet Gynecol 27:683, 1966

61. O'Sullivan JB, Mahan CM, Charles D: Medical treatment of the gestational diabetic. Obstet Gynecol 43:817, 1974

62. National Diabetes Data Group: Classification and diagnosis of diabetes mellitus and other categories of glucose intolerance. Diabetes 28:1039, 1979

63. Sacks DA, Abu-Fadil S, Greenspoon JS et al: Do the current standards for glucose tolerance testing in pregnancy represent a valid conversion of O'Sullivan's original criteria? Am J Obstet Gynecol 161:638, 1989

64. Magee MS, Walden CE, Benedetti TJ et al: Influence of diagnostic criteria on the incidence of gestational diabetes and perinatal morbidity. JAMA 269:609, 1993

65. Kaufmann RC, Schleyhahn FT, Huffman DG et al: Gestational diabetes diagnostic criteria: long-term maternal follow-up. Am J Obstet Gynecol 172:621, 1995

66. Peterson CM, Jovanovic-Peterson L: Percentage of carbohydrate and glycemic response to breakfast, lunch, and dinner in women with gestational diabetes. Diabetes 40(suppl 2):172, 1991

67. Jovanovic-Peterson L, Peterson CM: Dietary manipulation as a primary treatment strategy for pregnancies complicated by diabetes. J Am Coll Nutr 9:320, 1990

68. Gestational diabetes. In Jovanovic-Peterson L (ed): Medical Management of Pregnancy Complicated by Diabetes. American Diabetes Association, Alexandria, VA, 1993, pp. 79–90

69. Langer O; Gestational diabetes: a contemporary management approach. Endocrinologist 5:180, 1995

70. Knopp RH, Magee MS, Raisys V et al: Metabolic effects of hypocaloric diets in management of gestational diabetes. Diabetes 40(suppl 2):165, 1991

71. Dornhorst A, Nicholls JSD, Probst F et al: Calorie restriction for treatment of gestational diabetes. Diabetes 40(suppl 2):161, 1991

72. Ramus RM, Kitzmiller JL: Diagnosis and management of gestational diabetes. Diabetes Rev 2:43, 1994

73. Langer O, Berkus M, Brustman L et al: Rationale for insulin management in gestational diabetes mellitus. Diabetes 40(suppl 2):186, 1991

74. Jovanovic-Peterson L, Peterson CM: Is exercise safe or useful for gestational diabetic women? Diabetes 40(suppl 2):179, 1991

75. Bung P, Artal R, Khodiguian N et al: Exercise in gestational diabetes: an optional therapeutic approach? Diabetes 40(suppl 2):182, 1991

76. Jovanovic-Peterson L: The diagnosis and management of gestational diabetes mellitus. Clin Diabetes 13:32, 1995

77. Metzger BE: Summary and recommendation of the Third Internal Workshop-Conference on gestational diabetes mellitus. Diabetes 40(suppl 2):197, 1991

78. Huddleston JF, Cramer MK, Vroon DH: A rationale for omitting two-hour postprandial glucose determinations in gestational diabetes. Am J Obstet Gynecol 169:257, 1993

79. Goldberg JD, Franklin B, Lasser D: Gestational diabetes: impact of home glucose monitoring on neonatal birthweight. Am J Obstet Gynecol 154:546, 1986

80. McManus RM, Ryan EA: Insulin requirements in insulin-dependent and insulin-requiring GDM women during final month of pregnancy. Diabetes Care 15:1323, 1992

81. Kitzmiller JL: Sweet success with diabetes. The development of insulin therapy and glycemic control for pregnancy. Diabetes Care 16(suppl 3):107, 1993

82. Landon MB, Gabbe SG: Fetal surveillance and timing of delivery in pregnancy complicated

by diabetes mellitus. Obstet Gynecol Clin North Am 23:109, 1996

83. Langer O, Berkus MD, Huff R et al: Shoulder dystocia: should the fetus weighing ≥4000 grams be delivered by cesarean section? Am J Obstet Gynecol 165:831, 1991

84. Mueller-Heuach E, Caritis SN, Edelestone DI et al: Lecithin/sphingomyelin ratio in amniotic fluid and its value for the prediction of neonatal respiratory distress syndrome in pregnant diabetic women. Am J Obstet Gynecol 30:28, 1978

85. Kaytal SL, Amenta JS, Singh G et al: Deficient lung surfactant apoproteins in amniotic fluid with mature phospholipid profile from diabetic pregnancies. Am J Obstet Gynecol 148:48, 1984

86. Mimouni F, Miodovnik M, Siddiqi TA et al: Glycemic control and prevention of perinatal asphyxia. J Pediatr 113:345, 1988

87. Maheux PC, Bonin B, Dizazo A et al: Glucose homeostasis during spontaneous labor in normal human pregnancy. J Clin Endocrinol Metab 81:209, 1996

88. Jovanovic L, Peterson CM: Optimal insulin delivery for the pregnant diabetic patient. Diabetes Care 5(suppl 1):24, 1982

89. Ogata ES: Perinatal morbidity in offspring of diabetic mothers. Diabetes Rev 3:652, 1995

90. Pedersen JF, Molsted-Pedersen L: Early fetal growth delay detected by ultrasound marks increased risk of congenital malformation in diabetic pregnancy. BMJ 283:269, 1981

91. Langer O, Brustman L, Anyaegbunam A et al: Glycemic control in gestational diabetes—how tight is tight enough: small for gestational age versus large for gestational age? Am J Obstet Gynecol 161:646, 1989

92. Metzger BE, Cho NH, Roston SM et al: Prepregnancy weight and antepartum insulin secretion predict glucose tolerance five years after gestational diabetes mellitus. Diabetes Care 16:1598, 1993

93. Kjos SL, Peters RK, Xiang A et al: Predicting future diabetes in Latino women with gestational diabetes: utility of early postpartum glucose tolerance testing. Diabetes 44:586, 1995

94. Catalano PM, Tyzbir ED, Wolfe RR et al: Carbohydrate metabolism during pregnancy in control subjects and women with gestational diabetes. Am J Physiol 264:E60, 1993

95. Damm P, Kuhl C, Hornnes P et al: A longitudinal study of plasma insulin and glucagon in women with previous gestational diabetes. Diabetes Care 18:654, 1995

96. Stoffel M, Bell KL, Blackburn CL et al: Identification of glucokinase mutations in subjects with gestational diabetes mellitus. Diabetes 42:937, 1993

97. Chiu KC, Go RCP, Aoki M et al: Glucokinase gene in gestational diabetes mellitus: population association study and molecular scanning. Diabetologia 37:104, 1994

CHAPTER 10

PATIENT EDUCATION

CAROL ROSENBERG

ANNE PETERS

The purpose of this chapter is to provide an overview of material that a diabetes educator can use in teaching and treating patients with diabetes. In many of the sections the information is divided into two levels—the more advanced identified as information "for the diabetes educator" and the more basic information labeled "patient education." The advanced sections may be useful for patients interested in and capable of learning more detailed information. In addition, diabetes educators desiring more in-depth information are encouraged to locate topics of interest in other chapters of this book.

GOALS OF DIABETES EDUCATION

The main goals of diabetes education include helping patients and their families to

- Understand the physiology of diabetes and its complications
- Comprehend, master, and, it is hoped, participate in choosing the treatment options
- Identify the consequences, both negative and positive, of any health care choices made
- Deal with the far-ranging psychosocial impact that diabetes can have on their lives

TEACHING/LEARNING PROCESS

ASSESSMENT

The approach taken by a diabetes educator working with patients and families is influenced by many factors related to the learner, the educator, and the environment in which the education is taking place. Preteaching assessment is an important first step in the teaching/learning process. A diabetes educator needs to be flexible enough to adapt the teaching approach to factors that may influence patients' ability and willingness to learn about diabetes. In addition, it is important for educators to recognize their own particular beliefs about and approaches to learning and to health issues in general.

The preteaching assessment entails collecting information about patients' medical history, social history, diet/medication schedule, current level of diabetes knowledge, cultural issues, emotional/coping issues, and general learning abilities (e.g., visual, motor, reading, and intellectual abilities). Assessment can be performed through chart review or use of formal written questionnaires. A brief conversation at the beginning of the teaching session can reveal helpful information. In addition, frequent questioning of patients during the course of a session helps the educator to identify previously undiscovered barriers to learning.

MEDICAL HISTORY

Medical issues most relevant to the diabetes educator include the type of diabetes, duration of diabetes, current treatment regimen, medications, symptoms of hyperglycemia, frequency of hypoglycemia (for patients already taking sulfonylurea agents and/or insulin), concurrent illness, infections, impending or recent surgeries/procedures; and history of any chronic diabetic complications.

This information may be obtained through chart review, discussion with the referring health care provider, and/or questioning of the patient. A form such as the one shown in Figure 10–1 may help educators to organize the information.

SOCIAL HISTORY

Information about the social situation of patients helps to identify household members, neighbors, or coworkers who may be able to assist with diabetes management or who need to learn such skills as recognition and treatment of hypoglycemia. It is also important to find out the general typical daily schedule of patients, including the times of meals and snacks, work schedule, activity level at work (i.e., sedentary versus physically demanding work), activity level at home (e.g., housework, exercise, shopping), and variations in the daily schedule on days off. Information about unusual schedules (e.g., night shift work) or erratic schedules needs to be communicated to the physician and dietitian so that the diabetes treatment plan can be adapted accordingly.

Financial and insurance issues should also be discussed. This information is used in helping patients and families purchasing equipment needed for diabetes care, obtaining tools for ongoing education (e.g., books, journal subscriptions), and registering for health education classes and exercise programs.

DIET/MEDICATION SCHEDULE

During the course of reviewing patients' daily work and mealtime schedules, an educator can also ask about meal content and (for previously diagnosed diabetic patients) timing of diabetes medication. As discussed in sections ahead, this information can help an educator prioritize the teaching content if certain safety concerns are revealed. For example, if a patient is injecting insulin at home and then driving to work before eating breakfast, a discussion of rearranging the diet and medication schedule takes priority for hypoglycemia prevention. If a brief diet history reveals that a patient typically drinks several glasses of juice or eats excessive amounts of another carbohydrate food each day (perhaps not realizing that nondessert carbohydrates may cause dramatic elevations in blood glucose), priority may be given to discussion of immediate diet changes that may dramatically change the glucose results.

CURRENT LEVEL OF KNOWLEDGE

A patient's current level of knowledge can be assessed through use of a pretest, a questionnaire, a brief interview, and/or observation of techniques of any procedures that patients or their families already perform at home. (Relying on *observation* rather than simple verbal description of technique, especially for glucose monitoring and insulin injection, is critical in evaluating patients' technique.)

A form such as the one shown in Figure 10-2 may be used to organize and document assessment information as well as material covered in teaching sessions.

EMOTIONAL/COPING ISSUES

Asking patients and family members a few broad, open-ended questions can help open dialogue or allow them to admit uncomfortable feelings. Examples of this type of questioning include, "What concerns you most

Social History

Name _____ Age _____ Height/weight _____

Occupation _____ Lives with _____

Daily schedule (usual meal/work/exercise times) _____
_____
_____

Past diabetes education _____

Medical History

Type of diabetes: Type 1 _____ Type 2 _____ Duration _____

Other illnesses/infections _____

Hyperglycemia symptoms _____

Hypoglycemia symptoms/frequency _____

Medications taken at home _____

Insulin (type/doses/usual times) _____

Insulin sites used _____ Syringe size _____

Frequency of missed or altered dosages _____

Lab glucose/glycated Hgb/SMBG results _____
_____

Complications of Diabetes

1. Cardiovascular: MI _____ Angina _____ HTN _____ CHF_____
             Hyperlipidemia _____ CABG _____
2. Cerebrovascular: CVA _____ TIA _____ Bruits _____
3. Peripheral vascular: Leg pain (on exercising/at rest) _____
             Ulcer _____ Amputations _____
             Bypass surgery _____
4. Retinopathy: Yes/no _____ Vision affected _____ Laser tx _____
5. Other eye problems: Cataracts _____ Glaucoma _____
6. Nephropathy: Protein in urine _____ Dialysis _____ Other _____
7. Neuropathy:
   a. Peripheral: Numbness _____ Tingling _____ Burning sensations _____
   b. Autonomic: Bladder problems _____
             Feeling full after eating small amounts _____
             Nausea after eating _____
             Intermittent diarrhea _____
             Impotence _____
             Orthostatic hypotension (dizzy on rising) _____

Figure 10–1. Patient assessment form. Hgb, hemoglobin; SMBG, self-monitoring blood glucose; MI, myocardial infarction; HTN, hypertension; CHF, congestive heart failure; CABG, coronary artery bypass graft; CVA, cerebrovascular accident (stroke); TIA, transient ischemic attack (prestroke); tx, treatment.

Note: Enter code and initial for each entry		Assessment		Education—*Comments on Back*									
I = **INSTRUCTED** **RA** = **REQUIRES ASSISTANCE** **C** = **COMPETENT**		Initial											
		Date											
	Patient can verbalize/demonstrate:	Yes	No										
General Info	1. Definition of DM and normal blood sugar values												
	2. Effect of food on blood sugar												
	3. Effect of insulin/oral agents on blood sugar												
	4. Effect of physical activity on blood sugar												
	5. Effect of illness on blood sugar												
Insulin	1. Action of insulin												
	2. Differentiation of types of insulin												
	3. Medication schedule—amounts and times taken												
	4. Correct technique for insulin prep—one type: a. Rotates bottle to mix (cloudy insulin) b. Withdraws proper amount of insulin												
	5. Correct technique for insulin prep—two types: a. Rotates bottle to mix (cloudy) insulin b. Withdraws proper amount of first insulin c. Adds proper amount of second insulin												
	6. Correct technique for insulin administration: a. Cleans site with alcohol b. Pinches skin and inserts needle all the way c. Injects insulin, holding needle steady d. Rotates injection site: abdomen, arm, leg (list site demonstrated)[a]												
Orals	1. Action of oral medication												
	2. Name of medication and schedule												
Hypoglycemia	1. Definition and causes of hypoglycemia												
	2. Symptoms of hypoglycemia												
	3. Treatment of hypoglycemia/Medic Alert I.D.												

[a]Focus instruction on rotation of injections within <u>one</u> area, preferably the abdomen.

Figure 10–2 Diabetes assessment and education record.

Note: Enter code and initial for each entry	Assessment		Education—*Comments on Back*									
I = **INSTRUCTED** **RA** = **REQUIRES ASSISTANCE** **C** = **COMPETENT**	Initial											
	Date											
Patient can verbalize/demonstrate:	Yes	No										
Hyperglycemia 1. Definition and causes of hyperglycemia												
2. Symptoms of hyperglycemia												
3. Illness and "sick day" rules a. Need for taking insulin when ill b. When and how to test urine ketones c. When to call doctor d. Sick day diet												
Monitoring 1. Capillary blood glucose monitoring: a. Loads and operates lancing device b. Obtains large hanging drop of blood c. Places blood on strip properly d. Appropriately removes blood (if applicable) e. Reads visually and records results f. Uses meter correctly to obtain result g. Changes meter code h. Cleans meter i. Compares meter result to lab												
Complications 1. Reasons for foot care												
2. Daily cleansing of feet												
3. Inspection of feet												
4. Do's and don'ts for protection of feet												
5. Reasons for yearly eye examination												
6. Need for yearly urine testing												
7. Role of blood sugar and blood pressure control a. Knows normal glycated hemoglobin b. Knows own glycated hemoglobin c. Knows normal blood pressure d. Knows own blood pressure												
8. Role of control of other cardiac risk factors a. Weight control b. Lipid control c. Exercise												
9. Skin and dental care												
Follow-up 1. Community resources for information and support												

Figure 10–2 *Continued*

about the diabetes? How do your family, friends, and coworkers react to the diabetes? Do you feel supported by them?" For patients uncomfortable about expressing these types of feelings, an educator may help by giving examples such as, "Diabetes can be really overwhelming (or scary, or depressing, or can make you feel angry). Are you having any of these feelings?"

Engaging in this line of questioning and discussion may be difficult for some educators. They may fear opening up a whole line of dialogue that they are not prepared to handle. Nevertheless, such discussions are an important part of assessing patients' and families' responses to diabetes education and to identifying potential barriers to successful learning and coping. Some educators may be able to refer patients and families as needed for professional mental health intervention. In other situations, the only opportunity a patient may have to discuss emotions/coping issues may be with a diabetes educator.

CULTURAL ISSUES

In the broadest sense, the cultural background of a patient (and of a diabetes educator) provides the context in which the patient develops certain values, beliefs, behaviors, and relationships with family and health care providers. If an educator works with a large population of patients who belong to a unique group (e.g., based on country of origin, language, or religion), these patients may have some common beliefs or behaviors that influence the health-related behaviors. However, caution is advised in assuming that certain beliefs or behaviors apply to all members of a particular group, because this could lead to inappropriate stereotyping of patients. In addition, an educator needs to appreciate that a simple translation of information (e.g., diet information and food choices) into a patient's native language does not necessarily represent a culturally sensitive approach to diabetes education.

The best method for determining how patients' cultural background is affecting health-related behaviors is simply to ask general questions that allow patients to voice their unique beliefs and behaviors. The general line of questioning mentioned in the previous preteaching assessment sections would contribute to a cultural assessment of patients. An educator should make note of any comments relative to a patient's or family's beliefs about the causes of diabetes and its complications; the effect that diabetes treatments may have on the patient's life; the use of certain foods or herbs for perceived health benefits; the role of certain family members regarding health care decisions and responsibilities; and the importance of certain customs or observances that may influence the diabetes treatment plan.

It is important to remain nonjudgmental when exploring the beliefs of patients and families. Educators' attempts to correct what they believe to be erroneous beliefs can hinder establishment of rapport. Instead, an educator and the diabetes team can use this information when negotiating a treatment plan or when trying to discover why a certain plan of care has not been effective.

GENERAL LEARNING ABILITIES (VISUAL, READING, MOTOR, COMPREHENSION ABILITIES)

An informal assessment of a patient's visual and reading abilities can be performed at the beginning of the teaching session by having the patient read from readily available printed material (e.g., lines from a diabetes information pamphlet, numbers on a syringe, or instructions on a vial of visual strips for glucose testing). Further information on working with a visually impaired patient is presented later.

Fine motor skills and depth perception may be quickly assessed by watching patients insert the insulin needle through the tip of the insulin bottle or apply a control solution or a drop of blood to a strip for blood glucose testing.

Range of motion and other motor abilities required for foot inspection may be assessed by having patients attempt to visualize the bottoms of their feet (with a mirror) and touch all aspects of their feet as if washing or applying lotion.

Comprehension of information (and ability to apply the information) should be assessed at frequent intervals throughout the teaching session. The diabetes team may be quite surprised to discover, for example, that some patients lack understanding of basic mathematic concepts (e.g., addition required for mixing insulins or comparing a blood glucose result with a desired goal range). Other patients may be able to repeat information given but may not be able to apply it to practical situations. Examples of questions and explanations tailored to assessment of patients' comprehension (and adjustment of teaching as needed) are given in several sections of this chapter.

EDUCATOR SELF-ASSESSMENT

Each educator has his or her own unique beliefs, values, and experiences that influence the teaching approach. A lack of clarity about differences between the patient and the educator can sometimes impair communication and learning. Following are some examples of areas in which differences in style or approach may hinder the teaching/learning process.

PERSONAL LEARNING STYLE

Many of us tend to *teach* in the way that we *learn* the best. For example, if we find detailed written instructions personally helpful, we tend to use them in teaching. If we find analogies useful for our own learning, we tend to use them when we teach. If we find learning easiest through a particular medium (e.g., visual or auditory or hands-on instruction), we tend to favor that approach in teaching.

We need to be open to adapting our teaching methods to a particular patient's learning ability. As mentioned previously, questioning a patient at frequent intervals throughout the teaching session helps the educator assess comprehension. If problems arise, changes in the teaching approach may improve patients' comprehension.

PERSONAL LIFE STYLE

We each have our own personal approach toward issues such as time management, eating habits, timing of meals, work habits, exercise habits, role of family, and so on. We need to avoid assuming that patients have a similar approach or should have a similar view of life style issues. A classic example in diabetes care is the patient who is started on insulin injections with the assumption that mealtimes and snack times will be at approximately 7 to 8 AM, 12 to 1 PM, 5 to 6 PM, and 9 to 10 PM. Patients may feel unduly forced into completely changing their normal schedule because of feelings of guilt or embarrassment about certain habits such as eating or sleeping late. Another example is a patient who feels strongly that taking care of basic family needs (childcare, food preparation, and so on) takes precedence over certain health-related behaviors that the educator views as priorities (e.g., keeping all appointments or buying health care supplies).

A nonjudgmental approach by the educator is crucial in negotiating a treatment plan that is acceptable to all involved. Having an awareness and acceptance of differences in life style approach helps keep communication open.

PERSONAL HEALTH PHILOSOPHY

Many health care professionals receive training from the perspective of a methodic, scientific approach to solving health problems. We may have personal experience demonstrating the success of combining knowledge with self-discipline in adapting certain health behaviors in our own lives. We may firmly believe that self-care and independence represent the appropriate approach to managing health issues. We may feel strongly that patients must learn to function independently in terms of health care behaviors such as insulin injections, glucose monitoring, or food planning, but a patient's background may focus on the role of other family members in taking over these tasks. Educators need to learn to avoid promoting their own personal approach to health care without knowing what will work best for a patient.

FORMULATING A TEACHING PLAN

TEACHING PHILOSOPHY

The underlying approach to teaching that is the basis for this chapter is that diabetes educators need to be *flexible, practical,* and *realistic.* Dogmatic and rigid approaches to teaching are not appropriate, especially when attempting to train patients and their families to deal with many details and responsibilities within the context of continually changing life challenges. Having a detailed, organized approach to diabetes teaching sessions is very helpful but can be limiting if an educator is not comfortable with spur-of-the-moment changes. It is very efficient to have prepackaged educational materials to be used in a specific order. However, a mismatch between the educator's approach and the patient's or family's interest and abilities can seriously hamper the quality of learning.

A flexible, practical, and realistic approach to diabetes education demands balancing a number of different variables and being willing to make compromises between competing demands. A physician may request patient education on certain topics, but the preteaching assessment of a patient or other factors such as available teaching time may dictate a different plan for patient education. Certain situations may afford more latitude

in allowing a patient to select the order of topics covered, but other situations may present pressing medical concerns that require immediate attention to certain aspects of diabetes education regardless of a patient's desire.

A diabetes educator's assessment of a patient provides important input into formulating the actual plan of care. For example, a patient's medical situation may indicate the need for starting two injections of mixed insulin per day. However, an educator's assessment of the patient may indicate that the regimen prescribed is simply not practical or realistic and that a less intensive insulin regimen be used initially. Challenging the status quo, questioning routine practices, and advocating on behalf of diabetic patients are important roles for diabetes educators.

EVALUATION AND REASSESSMENT

Conventional educational theory suggests that learners may retain only a small percentage of what is taught to them. Retention can be increased by using several teaching modalities, providing ample opportunity for practical application, and allowing learners to guide the teaching session as much as possible. Repetition, reassessment, and evaluation of a patient's knowledge of diabetes information and skills are crucial. This is often not practical, but it must be built into the practice of every diabetes educator as much as possible. Other members of the medical team dealing with diabetic patients need to be made aware that simply attending a diabetes teaching class or individual session does not usually translate into immediate changes in behavior or a knowledge base of a patient. At each medical visit, constant reinforcement of information that patients need to know helps with retention of information.

In addition, flexibility in the approach to diabetes care helps patients with self-learning. An educator should encourage learners to experiment and explore (e.g., by trying different foods, different medication schedules, different sleeping schedules, variable glucose-monitoring schedules), provided the behavior has no immediate detrimental consequences. This type of discovery learning is often the most powerful and motivating for patients. Even if a temporary worsening of blood glucose control results from experimentation, the benefits (i.e., lessons learned by the patient, feelings of more control, freedom to try new approaches, feelings of comfort with the diabetes team) usually outweigh the temporary risks.

TEACHING TOOLS

Various teaching tools are available to help patients master new information and skills. Drug companies and diabetes organizations provide a wide selection of teaching materials. Videotapes, samples, and models of equipment are useful supplements to individual or group teaching sessions. Written instructions that reinforce information covered in teaching sessions are helpful for many patients. Some patients prefer comprehensive booklets that cover a wide variety of topics. Other patients may become overwhelmed with excessive written materials and should be given simple handouts that cover the basic information on topics addressed.

Individualizing the written information as much as possible helps with comprehension and application of skills in the home setting. An educator may want to consider having some patients write down in their own words the steps to be followed.

The Appendix at the end of the chapter provides some resources that educators can use in collecting a wide array of teaching materials. Mixing different materials from different sources may provide the best personalized diabetes education packet for patients. In addition, educators should encourage patients to pursue ongoing diabetes education through referral to a specialized diabetes education center, encourage them to join the American Diabetes Association (ADA) and other local diabetes organizations, refer them to diabetes support groups or camps, and encourage them to subscribe to diabetes magazines published for laypeople.

DIABETES TEACHING CONTENT

In 1993, a national task force published revised standards for diabetes self-management education programs. The standards were endorsed by several organizations, including the ADA and the American Association of Diabetes Educators. A proposed curriculum is outlined as follows:[1]

Standard 12. Based on the needs of the target population, the program shall be capable of offering instruction in the following content areas:

1. Diabetes overview
2. Stress and psychosocial adjustment
3. Family involvement and social support
4. Nutrition
5. Exercise and activity
6. Medications
7. Monitoring and use of results
8. Relationships among nutrition, exercise, medication, and blood glucose levels
9. Prevention, detection, and treatment of acute complications
10. Prevention, detection, and treatment of chronic complications
11. Foot, skin, and dental care
12. Behavior change strategies, goal setting, risk factor reduction, and problem solving
13. Benefits, risks, and management options for improving glucose control
14. Preconception care, pregnancy, and gestational diabetes
15. Use of health care systems and community resources

The following sections of this chapter focus on diabetes pathophysiology, basic treatment modalities (diet, exercise, monitoring, medication), acute and chronic complications, and special situations (e.g., travel, visual impairment) and populations. For more detailed information on specific aspects such as intensive insulin therapy, insulin pump therapy, chronic diabetic complications, pregnancy, and pediatrics, educators are encouraged to look elsewhere in this book and to obtain relevant information (both for educators and for patients) from resources listed in the Appendix.

DIABETES PATHOPHYSIOLOGY

FOR THE DIABETES EDUCATOR

DEFINITION

Diabetes mellitus is a metabolic syndrome characterized by hyperglycemia (elevated blood glucose levels). The two general types of diabetes, type 1 and type 2, differ greatly in their pathophysiology, but both produce hyperglycemia and the complications associated with it. These complications include microvascular, neuropathic, and macrovascular ones. Microvascular complications are abnormalities of small blood vessels that are manifested in diabetic retinopathy (diabetic eye disease) and nephropathy (diabetic kidney disease). The neuropathic complications cause loss of function of both peripheral and autonomic nerves, and the macrovascular (large blood vessel) complications include myocardial infarction (heart attack), peripheral vascular disease, and stroke. Hypertension is commonly associated with diabetes, especially type 2.

The microvascular and neuropathic complications of diabetes occur because of prolonged exposure to hyperglycemia for many years. The Diabetes Control and Complications Trial (DCCT), in addition to numerous other studies, proved that maintaining near euglycemia (near normal blood glucose levels) for many years considerably reduces the risk of developing these complications of diabetes. The macrovascular complications are not as clearly linked to the levels of blood glucose control, but controlling blood glucose levels in addition to treating lipid abnormalities and hypertension and assisting patients in smoking cessation lower the risk of these complications as well.

DIAGNOSIS*

Diabetes is diagnosed either in a patient who has symptoms of diabetes (such as polyuria, polydipsia, nocturia, blurring of vision, involuntary weight loss, and vaginal infections in women or more severe manifestations such as diabetic ketoacidosis [DKA]) or in an asymptomatic person. In asymptomatic individuals, diabetes is usually diagnosed by measuring a fasting plasma glucose (FPG) concentration (Table 10–1). If a patient has an FPG concentration ≥126 mg/dl or a random blood glucose concentration ≥200 mg/dl

*For a complete discussion of the 1997 classification and diagnosis criteria, see Chapter 1.

Table 10–1. Official Criteria for the Diagnosis of Diabetes Mellitus

1. Symptoms of diabetes plus casual plasma glucose concentrations ≥200 mg/dl (11.1 mmol/L). (Casual = any time of day without regard to time since last meal. The classic symptoms of diabetes include polyuria, polydipsia, and unexplained weight loss.)

    or

2. Fasting plasma glucose (FPG) ≥126 mg/dl (7.0 mmol/L). Fasting is defined as no caloric intake for at least 8 hours.

    or

3. Two-hour plasma glucose (2hPG) >200 mg/dl during an oral glucose tolerance test (OGTT). The test should be performed as described in reference 3 or 5 using a load of 75 g anhydrous glucose.

In the absence of unequivocal hyperglycemia with acute metabolic decompensation, these criteria should be confirmed by repeat testing on a different day.

The third measure (OGTT) is not recommended for routine clinical use.

Adapted from Report of the Expert Committee on the Diagnosis and Classification of Diabetes Mellitus. Diabetes Care, 20:1, 1997.

with symptoms of hyperglycemia, the diagnosis of diabetes is established.

Although not officially recommended, in some patients, Hgb A_{1c} level is measured to diagnose diabetes. An Hgb A_{1c} level is a measure of a patient's overall glucose concentration throughout the past 2 to 3 months. It is the best measure of a patient's diabetic control over time. Although Hgb A_{1c} levels correlate poorly with results from oral glucose tolerance tests (OGTTs), if the Hgb A_{1c} is $\geq 7.0\%$ it is likely that the patient has diabetes and particularly indicates that the patient has treatment-requiring diabetes (diet and exercise with or without medication, depending on the clinical circumstances).

CLASSIFICATION

Diabetes mellitus can be divided into several different types. One kind is called *type 1 diabetes*. This type is defined by the presence of serum (blood) ketones in the absence of exogenous insulin. This almost complete lack of effective insulin means that without insulin therapy, these patients usually develop DKA and die. Although most of these patients are children and young adults (i.e., <30 years of age), the older terminology, *juvenile-onset diabetes*, was not entirely accurate because some lean adult and elderly patients can also have ketosis-prone diabetes. Of the 6% of the total population, or approximately 6 million Americans who have diabetes, only 10% or approximately 1 million have type 1 diabetes.

The second kind of diabetes is called *type 2 diabetes*. The important metabolic characteristic of this type of diabetes is the absence of ketosis. Older terms were *adult-onset, maturity-onset,* or *ketosis-resistant diabetes.* The fact that these patients do not develop DKA signifies that they have at least some effective insulin. Eighty percent to 90% of type 2 diabetic patients are obese. Non–insulin-dependent diabetes is a confusing designation because approximately 25% of these patients receive insulin. The difference

is that they do not need insulin to sustain life as type 1 diabetic patients do. Obesity and older age are two independent risk factors for this kind of diabetes. It is estimated that the chance of developing type 2 diabetes doubles for every 20% increase over desirable body weight (see Chapter 9 for calculation of desirable body weight) and for each decade after the fourth, regardless of weight. The prevalence of diabetes mellitus in persons age 65 to 74 years is nearly 20%. It is likely that a higher percentage of people in the 9th and 10th decades of life have diabetes mellitus.

A third kind of diabetes is termed *other specific types*. It was formerly called *secondary diabetes* and included (1) diseases of the pancreas that destroyed the β-cells (e.g., hemochromatosis, pancreatitis, cystic fibrosis); (2) hormonal syndromes (e.g., acromegaly, Cushing's syndrome, pheochromocytoma) that interfere with insulin secretion and/or inhibit insulin action; (3) disease caused by drugs that may interfere with insulin secretion (e.g., phenytoin [Dilantin]) or that may inhibit insulin action (e.g., glucocorticoids, estrogens); (4) rare conditions involving abnormalities of the insulin receptor; (5) various rare genetic syndromes in which diabetes mellitus inexplicably occurs more frequently than in normal persons; and (6) diabetes in very rare families that inherit an inability to make normal insulin but make an abnormal insulin molecule that is ineffective.

The results of OGTTs that are higher than normal but fail to meet the criteria for diabetes mellitus (see Table 1–2) are classified as *impaired glucose tolerance* (IGT). Ten percent to 30% of the population >65 years of age have IGT (in addition to the 15% to 20% with diabetes mellitus). Former terminology included chemical, latent, subclinical, borderline, and asymptomatic diabetes. When the subjects are retested with an OGTT, even after many years, approximately 30% have reverted to normal, 50% continue to show IGT, and the remaining 20% are diabetic. Progression to overt diabetes in this latter population occurs at 5% to 7% per year. Conversely, patients with type 2 diabetes can revert to IGT (especially obese patients who lose weight). Patients with IGT are unlikely to develop the neuropathic and microvascular complications of diabetes. However, these patients are especially prone to the macrovascular complications: coronary artery disease, peripheral vascular disease, and cerebrovascular disease.

Gestational diabetes is really IGT that occurs in pregnancy (see Chapter 9). Thus, diabetic patients who subsequently become pregnant are not included in this class. In normal pregnancy, hormones that are produced by the placenta interfere with the action of insulin. In 2% to 5% of pregnant women, the increased demands on the pancreatic β-cells to produce more insulin cannot be met and abnormal carbohydrate metabolism develops. Gestational diabetes is associated with increased perinatal risks to the offspring and an increased risk to the mother for progression to type 2 diabetes mellitus within the next 10 to 15 years.

PATHOGENESIS (CAUSE)

The onset of type 1 diabetes is associated with a combination of genetic, immunologic, and in some cases viral factors. The genes involved produce certain human leukocyte antigens (HLA), whereas the immunologic abnormality involves autoimmunity (i.e., the production of antibodies against one's own tissue). It is believed that patients with a particular genetic predisposition (i.e., type 1) have some sort of environmental stress (e.g., virus, toxin, or other) that causes their immune system to make antibodies against their own insulin-producing cells in the pancreas (the β-cells). Once the β-cells are destroyed, patients can no longer make insulin and type 1 diabetes develops.

Less is known about the causes of type 2 diabetes, although heredity is a strong influence and both obesity and aging increase the risk of developing it. The factors that are involved in causing hyperglycemia in patients with type 2 diabetes include peripheral insulin resistance (i.e., the inability of insulin to exert its normal effect on the tissues that should respond to it), a relative decrease in the secretion of insulin from the pancreas, and increased glucose production by the liver. A more detailed discussion of the pathogenesis of types 1 and 2 diabetes can be found in Chapter 2.

FOR THE DIABETIC PATIENT

BASIC PATIENT EDUCATION

For patients who have limited learning capacity, who are very anxious, or who do not believe that they actually have diabetes, try the following approach:

Having diabetes means that your blood sugar is too high. The normal blood sugar is about 100 (mg/dl). Your blood sugar is _____. Having high blood sugar can make you feel tired and thirsty and can give you other problems such as blurry vision, excess urination, and infections, but it's also possible for you to feel fine when your blood sugar is too high. Our biggest concern is that if your blood sugar stays high for a while, it can cause permanent damage to your eyes, kidneys, feet, and sexual function.

INTERMEDIATE PATIENT EDUCATION

For patients capable of hearing more.

Normal Physiology

It is normal for your blood sugar to go up and down all day long. It usually goes up about 50 points after you eat—even when you eat healthy food. Insulin is a substance that your body is supposed to make to help process the food you eat. Food makes the blood sugar go up. Insulin makes the blood sugar go (back) down.

Diabetes Physiology

When someone has diabetes, it means that something is wrong with their insulin. So when a person with diabetes eats, the blood sugar goes up (that's normal) but it doesn't come back down properly.

In type 1 diabetes, the insulin is missing completely. The body just stops making insulin. This is most common in children and thin young adults. The main treatment for this type of diabetes is to give insulin shots.

In type 2 diabetes, there is still insulin in the body but the body doesn't make enough insulin (or strong enough insulin). This is most common in older adults and in people who are overweight. The treatments for type 2 diabetes are supposed to help the body make more insulin and use it better. The most important treatments for type 2 diabetes are weight loss and exercise. Pills that help the body to make and use its own insulin are started if diet and exercise fail, and insulin shots are added if the pills don't work.

Symptoms of Diabetes

When the blood sugar goes up and stays up, the extra sugar goes into the urine and you urinate more. When your body makes extra urine, you can become very thirsty. Your vision can also become temporarily blurry. The loss of sugar can make you lose weight and feel very hungry, and it can make you very tired (Fig. 10–3).

When you are first found to have diabetes, you may feel all of these symptoms, just one or two of the symptoms, or no symptoms at all. It depends how high your blood sugar has been and how long it's been high. If you had very few or no symptoms of diabetes when it was first diagnosed, it does not mean that you just have mild or borderline diabetes. No matter how or when your diabetes was discovered, it is important to learn to control your blood sugar as much as possible even if you feel fine. If the blood sugar level runs too high, it can damage the blood vessels and nerves, causing problems with the eyes, kidneys, legs, and sexual functions (in men).

QUESTIONS TO TEST KNOWLEDGE/ STIMULATE THOUGHTS

The purpose of this line of questioning is to ascertain a patient's very basic understanding of diabetes and to make sure a patient (especially an asymptomatic patient) is aware that diabetes treatment measures might not seem related to any immediate symptoms or problems but are for prevention of future problems. In addition, it is hoped that questions will encourage patients to express some concerns about which they may feel some embarrassment or anxiety, such as questions about diabetic complications that they may have seen in relatives or acquaintances. Some patients may harbor guilt or may be accused by family members of bringing on the diabetes by eating too much sugar, and the hope is that this discussion will clarify any misconceptions regarding the causes and treatment of diabetes.

- Does having diabetes mean that your blood sugar level is too high or too low?
- What would happen if you ignored the diabetes and decided not to treat it?
- Is diabetes caused by eating too much sugar?
- What is your biggest fear/concern about having diabetes?
- Why does high blood sugar sometimes cause problems like thirst and frequent urination?
- If you just stop eating sweets, would that be enough to take care of the diabetes?

Table 10–2 presents some common misconceptions that patients may have about diabetes and offers some suggested responses. Later in the chapter, common mis-

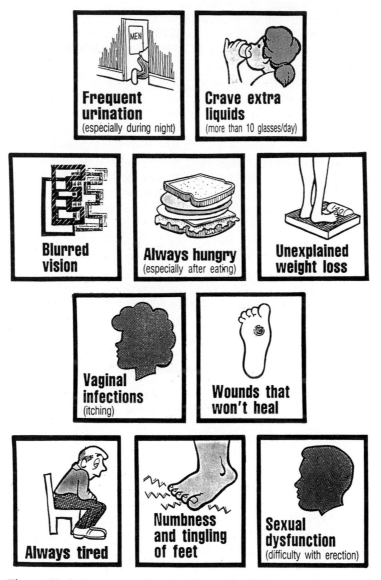

Figure 10–3. Symptoms of marked hyperglycemia.

Table 10–2. Misconceptions Related to Diabetes or Its Treatment

Misconception	Educator's Response
Diabetes is caused by eating too much sugar.	Diabetes happens because you have a problem with the insulin in your body, not because you ate too much sugar. *For patients with type 1 diabetes or lean patients with type 2 diabetes:* The pancreas is the organ in your body that is supposed to make insulin, but the part of your pancreas that's supposed to make the insulin stopped working properly. We're not exactly sure why the pancreas stopped making insulin—it may be a combination of a problem inherited from your family and something that harmed the pancreas, like a virus (for type 1 diabetes). Eating sugar did not harm your pancreas. However, once diabetes develops, eating too much sugar can make your blood sugar level go too high. *For overweight patients with type 2 diabetes:* Diabetes was not caused by eating too much sugar per se but because you ate too many calories and gained too much weight. Eating foods that contain a lot of fat causes more of a problem with weight gain than eating sugar. In addition to the genes for developing diabetes, being overweight helped cause you to develop diabetes. If you learn to follow a lower-calorie diet, start to exercise, and begin to lose weight, your diabetes will improve.
The only diet change needed in the treatment of diabetes is just to stop eating sugar.	First it's important to know that sugar and desserts are not the only foods that can cause your blood sugar to go up. Many nutritious foods like starch (bread, pasta, corn), fruit, and milk also make your blood sugar rise. You don't need to completely *stop* eating any one type of food—try to have smaller servings of the foods that make blood sugar go up. It also helps your blood sugar stay more balanced if you eat a variety of foods including vegetables and low-fat or no-fat protein foods. If you take medication to treat your diabetes, it is important to try to eat meals or snacks on a regular basis without skipping meals. If you need to lose weight, the most important diet change is to eat less fat. It is acceptable for people with diabetes to eat foods that contain sugar as long as you have been taught how to balance sugar foods with the rest of your diet and your medication.
If I only have to watch my diet or take pills then I just have "mild" or "borderline" diabetes.	The diagnosis of diabetes is based on results of a blood sugar test. No matter what you have to do to treat the diabetes and to control your blood sugar, you still have actual diabetes. People who just have to watch their diet or take pills can have the same problems from diabetes as people who take insulin shots. No matter how you feel or what you have to do to treat your diabetes, it's important to see your medical team regularly so that you can be tested for any problems with your heart, circulation, feet, kidneys, and eyes. (Sometimes people who do *not* take insulin shots can have more problems with their diabetes because they may think it's not a serious problem and may ignore it for many years).
Blood sugar levels remain the same throughout the day.	Blood sugar levels normally swing up and down during the day. They are usually the lowest before meals and the highest 1 to 2 hours after eating. The goal of the diabetes treatment plan is to prevent the sugar from going too high or low, not to stop the normal up-and-down swings in sugar. You and/or your doctor should be testing your blood sugar at different times and should do a special blood test in the laboratory (glycated hemoglobin) to make sure the average amount of sugar in your blood is not too high.

conceptions and concerns about insulin treatment are addressed (see Table 10–6).

TREATMENT OF DIABETES

Although specific goals may vary from patient to patient, the main goal is to lower blood glucose levels safely to as near normal as possible and to keep blood glucose levels in a desirable range throughout a patient's lifetime. This takes persistent follow-up and reinforcement of the principles of diabetes management. The five components of the management of diabetes are

- Education
- Diet
- Exercise
- Glucose monitoring
- Antidiabetic medication

Additionally, patients with diabetes need to have meticulous control of hypertension and elevated lipid levels because these are conditions commonly found in patients with type 2 diabetes. Other health concerns, such as smoking cessation, compliance with vaccinations, and stress management, should also be emphasized.

Treatment needs may change throughout the course of the disease, with changes in a patient's life style and physical status. In addition, advances in therapy resulting from research necessitate periodic updating of the treatment regimen. The diabetes management plan therefore involves frequent assessment and modification by health professionals as well as daily adjustments in therapy by patients themselves. For these reasons, education (including repeated assessment of patients' knowledge and provision of ongoing, in-depth diabetes teaching) is listed as an essential component of treatment for all diabetic patients.

DIET

FOR THE DIABETES EDUCATOR

Regulating food intake is essential to successful management of diabetes. This does not mean that patients must eat the same food every day or must never vary their mealtimes. Rather, patients should be encouraged to learn as much as possible about the nutritional content of the foods they eat and the effect that foods have on their blood glucose levels. Generally, the more that patients know about diet, the more flexible their meal plan can be (see Chapter 3 for more details).

To increase the chances of dietary adherence, individualizing the meal plan and incorporating as many current eating habits as is safe and practical are important. If at all possible, patients should be referred to a nutritionist (preferably one who has special knowledge of and interest in diabetes).

Assessment

As part of the overall preeducation assessment, it is useful to obtain at least a general diet history and a report of the range of times of meals, medication, and exercise. Even if patients are to see a nutritionist at a future time, a diabetes educator can give patients some immediate feedback about their current dietary habits that may place them at risk for pronounced hyperglycemia or hypoglycemia. For example, frequent hyperglycemia may occur in patients who avoid sweets but who consume large quantities of juice or fruit or milk with the assumption that these healthy foods do not have a negative impact on blood glucose control. Conversely, patients may be in the habit of skipping certain meals or having a prolonged delay between medication and meals or exercising before (rather than after) a meal, and this practice may put them at risk for hypoglycemia.

When asking a patient about current eating habits, an accepting, nonjudgmental attitude promotes rapport and honesty. An educator can ask patients what they like to eat for breakfast, lunch, dinner, and snacks. If patients seem to be vague or seem to be describing a meal plan that may be what they think the educator wants to hear, it may be useful to obtain a 24-hour recall of food intake.

Reassurance by the educator is helpful—letting patients know that it is human nature to be imperfect and to go off the diet sometimes. This may be a good time to introduce the concept that the current approach to the diabetes diet is not to give patients a standard diet. Rather, the educator wants to help patients make a few adjustments in their current diet. Favorite foods need not be eliminated, but changes in portion size or food combinations or timing of certain food intake may be suggested. Reassure patients that dietary indiscretion that results in elevated blood glucose levels, although not advisable on a regular basis, does not cause immediate onset of long-term complications or hyperglycemic coma.

Basic Patient Education

For patients who are beginning oral agents or insulin and who seem overwhelmed with the diabetes treatment plan.

Provide a few general principles:

1. Limit concentrated sweets, juices, milk, and fruit.
2. Eat something, either a meal or snack, every 4 to 5 hours while awake.
3. If a meal must be delayed, eat a small snack at the usual mealtime.
4. Try to eat meals and snacks consisting of a mixture of different types of food (give patients examples: sandwich with fruit; low-fat cheese and crackers; cottage cheese with crackers or fruit; chicken or fish with vegetables and starches; convenience foods—list specific meals readily available in your community).
5. Limited amounts of sugar, honey, and candy are acceptable (as are products with sugar listed as an ingredient). The patient does not need to eliminate every source of sugar from the diet.
6. For patients starting insulin, emphasize the importance of not skipping meals. Teach

patients that it is better to eat a meal or snack that is less than ideal than to skip a meal altogether.
7. For all patients, encourage an increase in intake of water and vegetables.
8. For patients who need to lose weight, discuss decreasing portion sizes and overall fat intake.

Questions to Stimulate Discussion and Assess Patients' Comprehension

When reviewing the foregoing general guidelines with patients, test patients' comprehension by asking very practical questions. For example,

- Based on our discussion today, name three changes that you think you can make in your diet.
- What would you like to eat for dinner tonight?
- If you get hungry tomorrow between meals, what do you think would be a good snack?
- When you go to the store, what types of fluids will you buy?
- What do you think would happen if you ate a piece of cake?
- Are you worried about the diet?
- How do you feel about having to make some changes in the food you eat?
- What is the food you fear you will miss the most? (And then try to help patients incorporate their favorite food back into their meal plan.)

Intermediate Patient Education

For patients who are able to absorb more than just the very basic information.

1. Introduce patients to the six different food groups (lists, exchanges)—starch, fruit, milk and protein, vegetable, and fat (Table 10-3). One effective way to organize this information is to explain that the first three groups listed can be called sugar foods (i.e., contain the most carbohydrate) and the last

Table 10–3. Food Groups

Carbohydrate Food Groups (Will Affect Sugar)	Non-Carbohydrate Food Groups (Minimum Effect on Sugar)
Starch	Protein (meat)
Fruit	Vegetables
Milk	Fat
(Nutritive sweeteners, e.g., fructose, corn syrup, fruit juice)	(Nonnutritive sweeteners, e.g. aspartame, saccharin, acesulfame-K)

three groups listed are nonsugar foods (i.e., contain less carbohydrate). At this point, the focus is on helping patients identify the groups to which their usual foods belong.

2. Explain to patients that even healthy foods such as fruit, bread, and nonfat milk cause the blood sugar to go up. This can be very confusing or surprising to many patients. Reassure them that they do not need to eliminate these foods, but they may need to eat starch, fruit, and milk in smaller portions at one time. Have patients identify the foods they ate in the past 24 hours that would be considered sugar foods.

3. Teach patients that even though the nonsugar food such as proteins and fats have minimal impact on blood sugar, they need to be limited to avoid problems with cholesterol and heart disease.

4. Introduce patients to the concept that the amount of starch, fruit, and milk that they will be able to consume depends on the degree of blood sugar rise after meals. An increase of up to 50 to 60 mg/dl 2 hours after a meal would be considered acceptable. (The exact amount of increase considered acceptable may vary from setting to setting, but the general concept that food normally causes a rise in blood sugar can be universally taught.) Show patients sample blood sugar records with premeal and 2-hour postmeal pairs (Fig. 10–4) and help them to identify the meals in which blood sugar increased

more than 50 to 60 mg/dl. Have patients identify the foods in that meal responsible for the increase.

5. Reassure patients that experimenting with food is essential to help establish a sound meal plan. Patients are sometimes more willing to limit or eliminate certain foods once they have discovered on their own just how much their blood sugar increases after consuming these foods.

Patient Education for Previously Diagnosed Diabetic Patients

1. To establish knowledge level: After taking a 24-hour (or typical daily) food history, ask patients to identify the foods eaten that would cause a rise in the blood sugar. Ask patients to identify the foods eaten that would increase the body weight or serum lipids. If patients are not able to answer these questions appropriately, instruct them as described earlier.

2. To identify behavioral issues: Ask patients to identify their trouble spots in terms of diet. Ask them which part of the diet is most challenging or where they think they have room for improvement. Find out if family, friends, or coworkers help or hinder them when it comes to diet. Negotiate a plan involving a few behaviors that address patients' trouble spots. For example, if patients consume a high-fat and/or high-sugar snack daily, would they consider a lower-fat, sugar-free alternative and/or reducing the portion size of their usual snack and/or reducing the frequency of the snack to every other day. Working with patients to consider several options may promote behavior change more effectively than telling patients that they must completely eliminate the snack in question.

EXERCISE

Exercise is an integral part of diabetes management. In the preinsulin era, exercise was recommended along with carbohydrate re-

Date	Breakfast Before	Breakfast 2 Hours After	Lunch Before	Lunch 2 Hours After	Dinner Before	Dinner 2 Hours After	Comments
			Blood Glucose Tests				
Monday	135	182					
Monday	2 eggs, 2 sausages, 1 biscuit, coffee						
Tuesday			166	244			
Tuesday			2 bread, pork, corn, milk				
Wednesday					198	195	
Wednesday					chicken, stuffing, vegetables		Exercised after dinner
Thursday	149	186					
Thursday	½ grapefruit, 1 toast, cheese, coffee						
Friday			139	192			
Friday			tuna sandwich, salad, diet soda				
Saturday					146	271	
Saturday					salad, spaghetti, bread, apple		
Sunday	158	280					
Sunday	milk, cereal, banana, 1 toast, OJ						

Figure 10–4. Sample blood glucose record.

striction to control blood glucose levels. The general increase in the popularity of exercise and conditioning has created an awareness of the importance of exercise in the treatment of diabetes. Regular exercise is beneficial to almost everyone. The benefits are primarily the same for patients with diabetes, with a few added benefits and some risks. The mechanisms by which exercise influences glucose levels are discussed in Chapter 7.

Benefits of Exercise

1. Increased efficiency of the heart and lungs.
2. Decreased "bad" cholesterol (low-density lipoprotein [LDL]) and triglyceride levels, which increase the risk for coronary artery disease, and increased "good" cholesterol (high-density lipoprotein [HDL]), which decreases the risk for coronary artery disease.

3. Changes in body composition that cause an increase in muscle mass and a decrease in body fat. Increased energy expenditure causes a decrease in weight if there is no compensatory increase in caloric intake.

4. Decreased blood glucose levels during and after exercise. (However, the effect on overall glucose control may be only slight if not combined with weight loss.)

5. Increased sensitivity of muscle and fat tissue to insulin.

6. Improved self-image and stress management.

General Guidelines

1. *Consult a physician* to determine whether or not a patient has any medical problems that would be a contraindication to certain forms of exercise. These include heart disease, poor diabetic control, proliferative diabetic retinopathy, untreated hypertension, or hypoglycemia unawareness. A heart stress test (treadmill test) may be required for evaluating cardiac function.

2. *Select an appropriate exercise program.* An appropriate exercise program is one that patients will adhere to and that conforms to their life style. Some patients may be best suited to an individual exercise program; others may prefer group activities. For many, walking is the most convenient, safest, and most economical form of exercise. It is also a good starting point for the initiation of a more rigorous exercise program. If patients have no special exercise limitations, they should contact community facilities such as the YMCA/YWCA and senior citizen centers. Some hospitals offer low-impact aerobic classes, and some cardiac rehabilitation programs have excellent exercise facilities. Also, of course, private health clubs abound in most of the country and can be joined for a fee.

3. *Follow a specific exercise plan.* Regardless of the form of exercise, the exercise session should start with a warm-up period, which is followed by the main intense (aerobic) exercise activity and ends with a cool-down phase. A 5- to 10-minute warm-up is used to stretch the muscles that will be used in the exercise session (e.g., leg muscles for jogging or tennis; arm and shoulder muscles for swimming). This reduces the risk of tendon and muscle injury. The main activity should consist of 20 to 30 minutes of aerobic exercise. (Brisk walking, jogging, bicycling, and swimming all are forms of aerobic exercise.) This is defined as exercise that requires the use of extra oxygen to meet the energy demands of the muscles. Less intense exercise (such as golf, strolling) is called *anaerobic,* and the energy demands are met without the utilization of extra oxygen. Aerobic exercise is the form associated with cardiovascular fitness, increased sensitivity to insulin, and improved health. This intensity of the aerobic exercise should be determined by the heart rate response (see Chapter 7 for exact calculation). The cool-down period should begin 2 to 3 minutes after the exercise is completed and should last for approximately 5 minutes. It consists of gently stretching the muscle groups used during the aerobic activity.

4. *Encourage commitment to the exercise program.* To achieve health benefits the aerobic activity must be performed a minimum of three times a week, for a continuous 20 to 30 minutes at each session.

Special Considerations and Risk Factors

FOOT PROBLEMS | Patients who have peripheral neuropathy may not be candidates for high-impact weight-bearing exercises such as jogging and high-impact aerobics. These may increase the risk of trauma to patients with insensitive feet. Swimming or cycling may be the best exercise.

PROLIFERATIVE RETINOPATHY | Patients with proliferative retinopathy should be evaluated on an individual basis. Some vigorous exercises can increase the blood pressure and put added stress on already weakened vessels in the retina, causing hemorrhage. In general, if recent photocoagulation procedures (laser) have been carried out, exercise may be contraindicated for several weeks. Exercise at any time that involves forceful holding of the breath (e.g., weightlifting) as well as jarring exercises (e.g., high-impact aerobics) may be contraindicated. Patients with proliferative retinopathy should check with their ophthalmologist for specific recommendations.

HYPERGLYCEMIA | Exercising when the blood glucose level is >250 to 300 mg/dl may lead to further increases in the blood glucose level. It may also lead to ketonuria in type 1 diabetic patients (see the exercise section in Chapter 7).

HYPOGLYCEMIA | For insulin-treated patients, hypoglycemia is a potential problem and *specific measures* should be taken to prevent hypoglycemia. Hypoglycemia may occur when unusual exercise is performed without adjustment in food intake or insulin dosage. This occurs primarily because of increased absorption of the injected insulin. To help prevent the development of hypoglycemia, the following suggestions should be followed:

1. Exercise after meals (45 to 60 minutes), when the meal carbohydrate has been absorbed into the bloodstream and glucose levels are higher.

2. Carry concentrated glucose preparations during exercise (e.g., glucose tablets or gels) to consume if symptoms of hypoglycemia develop.

3. For prolonged and high-intensity exercise, a snack food (e.g., fruit, fruit juice, skim milk, bread products) should be consumed just before and/or at intervals during the exercise to help prevent hypoglycemia.

4. Wear identification (medical alert bracelet or necklace) and exercise with someone else when possible.

5. Perform blood glucose monitoring before and after exercise to evaluate the blood glucose response to exercise and to check for impending hypoglycemia.

6. Be aware of the phenomenon of post-exercise late-onset hypoglycemia. This hypoglycemia occurs 6 to 15 hours after strenuous and prolonged activity and therefore may happen in the evening or overnight. If this proves to be a problem, a reduction in insulin doses that peak at these times may be

required. Increased frequency of blood glucose monitoring and food intake after exercise may also be indicated.

7. Exercise should be avoided at the time of the peak action of insulin unless food is also eaten just before exercise (e.g., if regular insulin is given before breakfast, do not exercise just before lunch).

8. Insulin should not be injected into the primary exercising part of the body (e.g., if jogging, do not use the leg for injection, especially for regular insulin). Injections given in the abdomen may not be as affected by exercise as injections given in other sites.

9. Insulin doses should not be omitted, but the dose may need to be decreased or food intake increased (see Chapter 3).

MEASUREMENTS OF GLYCEMIC CONTROL

Monitoring diabetes control means evaluating the therapeutic response to the treatment plan. In most illnesses, a physician monitors the results of the treatment and a patient is the passive consumer. In marked contrast, patients with diabetes must assume responsibility for management and control of their disease, and methods and tools such as self-monitoring of blood glucose (SMBG) or testing urine samples are required. Table 10–4 lists the ADA recommendations for treatment goals for diabetic patients.

Two basic methods for assessing diabetic control exist, both short-term tests (including SMBG, urine glucose testing, and blood glucose measurement in the laboratory) and longer-term tests (such as Hgb A_{1c} or fructosamine levels). The short-term tests, especially SMBG, are performed by patients in their own environment and can be used by patients (particularly patients taking insulin) to make immediate adjustments in insulin or diet. The longer-term tests are generally used by diabetes health care professionals (and the results shared with patients) to assess patients' progress and determine whether or

Table 10–4. Biochemical Indices of Glycemic Control

Biochemical Index	Normal	Goal	Action Suggested
Fasting/preprandial glucose	<115 mg/dl (<6.4 mM)	<120 mg/dl (<6.7 mM)	<80 or >140 mg/dl (<4.4 or >7.8 mM)
Bedtime glucose	<120 mg/dl (<6.7 mM)	100–140 mg/dl (5.6–7.8 mM)	<100 or >160 mg/dl (<5.6 or >8.9 mM)
Glycated hemoglobin[a]	<6%	<7%	>8%

[a]Referenced to a nondiabetic range of 4%–6% (mean 5%, SD 0.5%).

American Diabetes Association: Management of Non-Insulin-Dependent (Type II) Diabetes, 3rd ed. American Diabetes Association, Alexandria, VA, 1994.

not changes in the overall treatment plan need to be undertaken.

SELF-MONITORING OF BLOOD GLUCOSE

SMBG is one of the most significant developments in diabetes management since the discovery of insulin. It has allowed much greater interaction and teamwork between patients and health care providers in blood glucose management. For patients taking insulin, SMBG results are used to adjust insulin doses, and for patients with a sophisticated understanding of diabetes control, SMBG can help patients maintain a more flexible life style and diet without severely compromising glucose control.

For all diabetic patients (including those who do not use insulin), SMBG is a valuable tool in teaching the glycemic effects of various foods as well as increasing patients' involvement in overall evaluation of the diabetes treatment plan. In addition, SMBG has become a vital part of detecting and treating acute diabetic complications of hypoglycemia and hyperglycemia. This is especially important during times of diet or medication changes such as during illness, during the perioperative period, during fasting (e.g., for outpatient procedures), or after medication changes (e.g., changes in diabetic medication or drugs such as glucocorticoids that alter blood glucose levels).

Description

The three main categories of glucose-monitoring techniques are the visual strip, the meter with wipe technique, and the meter with nonwipe technique. In all techniques, patients must obtain a drop of blood and apply it to the reagent pad on a strip or on the sensor pad of an electrode-type strip. The blood stays on the strip for a certain amount of time, and a result is obtained either after the blood has been removed in a certain way (wipe) or after the blood has remained on the strip for a certain time (nonwipe).

In general, the less user technique–dependent methods of glucose monitoring (nonwipe) are thought to produce the most accurate, or at least the most consistent, results. However, with appropriate education, regular evaluation of technique, and regular laboratory assessment (e.g., glucose concentration measured simultaneously with the SMBG test), most methods of SMBG can yield clinically useful results.

Choosing a Glucose-Monitoring Technique

Assisting patients in selecting a glucose-monitoring technique can be a very complex aspect of diabetes education. It is easiest for a diabetes educator to have a simple choice of only one or two systems from which patients may select. This may indeed be the situation if institutional or insurance controls are imposed on the equipment patients may receive. However, to promote long-term commitment to glucose monitoring, it is important for patients to have as much choice as possible so that their goals and characteristics can be matched with the various glucose-monitoring systems. Diabetes educators can be of most help when they have personal experience using various techniques and have evaluated the results by testing the meters in the laboratory or at least have collected data from other patients who have checked meters against laboratory values.

Many patients prefer to use a meter because they have more confidence in the digital results than they do in visual interpretation of colors. Nonetheless, the use of visual strips, at least initially, should not be ruled out for patients under financial constraints. Even if patients cannot give an exact result using visual strips, most can give an approximate reading (low, medium, high) that could help guide some basic changes in medication or diet.

In terms of selecting a monitor, the following variables may be considered: accuracy, size, cost, memory, ease of use, coding, cleaning, computer compatibility, language capability, and company support. (For a detailed description of different monitoring systems, see *'97 Buyer's Guide to Diabetes Supplies* in the Appendix.)

Accuracy

Most of the monitors have the capability of giving results that are within 15% of a matching laboratory test, provided the following guidelines are observed:

- The general technique for using the monitor is accurate.
- Strips are current and have been stored properly (inside the vial or foil wrapping) at appropriate temperatures.
- The meter is calibrated to the correct lot number of strips.
- The meter is clean.
- A large, round drop of blood was applied.
- The patient was fasting.
- The finger was clean and dry before puncture.

Educators may receive information from various companies claiming improved accuracy of one system over another. It is best if educators can formulate their own opinions through personal experience with different systems. Most importantly, explain to patients that all systems are capable of producing accurate results and all systems are capable of producing erroneous results. Explain to patients that it is important to check their monitor and technique on a regular basis and that the best system is the one that they are most willing to use most often based on other characteristics.

Advantages and Disadvantages

The main advantage of SMBG is that it gives immediate feedback. Patients who are educated can make a decision in terms of insulin, diet, and/or exercise that immediately affects the glucose results. This, in turn, may give patients more of a sense of control over their diabetes and may allow them to adapt the diabetes treatment plan to their life style rather than vice versa.

Providing regular results to a physician allows more frequent adjustments of the medication and can thus improve symptoms and diabetic control more effectively, especially in an outpatient setting.

For less sophisticated patients, SMBG may promote greater awareness and acceptance of the diagnosis of diabetes, recognition of the impact of certain behaviors (eating, drinking, skipping medication), and more of a sense of personal responsibility. Diabetes can become less a condition for the doctor to manage and more of an issue calling for self-ownership.

The main disadvantages of SMBG are cost, discomfort, and inconvenience (e.g., having to interrupt one's usual activities to do it). In addition, some patients experience a feeling of frustration at seeing high blood glucose results when they expected lower readings based on adherence to the diabetes treatment plan or based on a sense of physical well-being. As some patients state, "The good thing about blood testing is that I know what my sugar is, and the bad thing about glucose testing is that I know what my sugar is. It can ruin my mood if I think I have a 'good' sugar and then I discover that my reading is high."

Patient Education

Introducing Patients to Self-Monitoring of Blood Glucose

To help patients feel comfortable with their decision to learn SMBG, it is important to illustrate how the information will be used. Adults are more inclined to try it if they believe that the information is relevant to them on an immediate basis. Show patients sample blood glucose records that illustrate the effects of food, exercise, and/or medication on blood glucose (see Fig. 10–4). Introducing SMBG in conjunction with diet education is very useful. If patients want to find out how much of a certain food they can consume, show them records of premeal and 2-hour postmeal SMBG. Supply examples from other patients in whom variations in glucose results directly correlated with changes in carbohydrate consumption. For patients starting insulin treatment, show a sample record illustrating gradual dose changes based on SMBG results.

For most patients, teaching all aspects of SMBG in one session is not advisable. If at all possible, educators should plan to meet with patients more than once, focusing first on obtaining a large drop of blood and on basic meter use. Then follow up with instruction on meter maintenance, calibration, and alarms.

If it is not possible to meet with patients a second time, it is still advisable to limit the information presented at one time, placing emphasis on drop size and on the importance of periodic meter checks in the laboratory. Patients can become overwhelmed with information on control solution and meter cleaning at the first session and may be disinclined to use the meter, assuming it is too confusing. All meters have a toll-free information line that patients can use to review questions.

Instruction in Self-Monitoring of Blood Glucose

Many patients have minimal difficulty learning basic meter functioning, especially with the newer, nonwipe meters. Each meter comes with its own set of instructions, which may include written guidelines and (sometimes) videotape instructions. However, regardless of the simplicity of the basic technique, hands-on instruction on obtaining the drop of blood is important in promoting accurate blood testing. (This type of instruction is often not provided at local pharmacies where patients may purchase glucose meters.)

Tips for Obtaining a Large Drop of Blood

The drop of blood needed frequently is larger than patients think. This is especially true if patients have selected a meter with the understanding that it requires significantly less blood than other meters. Patients may fear that if they squeeze out a large, hanging drop, it will bleed all over the machine or will fall. Because drop size is one of the most significant factors in accuracy and consistency of results, spending extra time discussing this is worthwhile (Fig. 10–5):

1. Encourage patients, especially beginners, to position their finger in such a way that the drop exits down toward the meter as it flows out of the puncture site and elongates like a teardrop as it forms on its own or with pressure on the finger.

2. Demonstrate how the drop typically clings to the finger and does not immediately fall so that they can continue to massage the finger as needed with the drop pointing

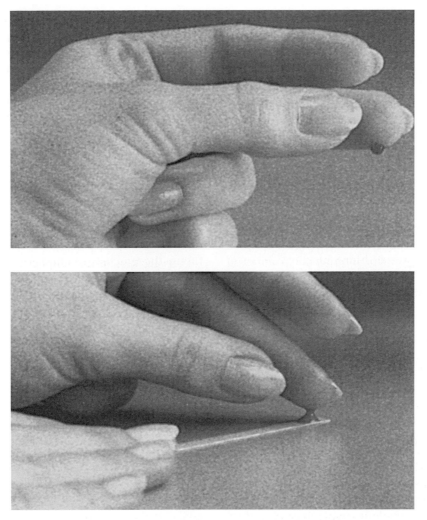

Figure 10–5. Technique of placing a drop of blood on the strip.

toward the strip before applying it to the strip.

3. If patients try to squeeze a drop of blood that comes up out of the finger toward their face (away from gravity), it may have a tendency to begin to roll down one surface of the finger or under the fingernail, and then a volume of blood that would have been sufficient becomes insufficient when finally applied (and sometimes smeared) onto the strip.

4. To promote greater blood flow, patients may be taught to wash and massage hands under warm water (finger must be dry for adequate drop size), shake the hand and hold it down at the side before performing the finger stick.

5. To increase drop size in patients who do not bleed easily, instruct patients to perform the finger stick and then immediately relax the arm and let the hand rest at the side for a few seconds without applying any pressure. Patients can wiggle their fingers while their hand hangs down to promote blood flow. After 5 to 10 seconds, teach patients to position the hand parallel to the

table with the puncture site facing downward and begin to apply pressure at the base of the finger (near the knuckle). Hold the pressure firmly and steadily for about 5 seconds. Then reposition the hand so that pressure is now applied to the middle of the finger—again with steady pressure for about 5 seconds. Advise patients that there may appear to be no results at all from this technique. The blood is moving toward the tip, and when pressure is finally applied at the tip of the finger, a larger drop forms.

6. Some patients may be impatient with this technique and may tend to milk the finger down repeatedly or may quickly apply pressure at the tip, limiting the volume of blood that flows out to the puncture site.

7. Encourage patients to try different surfaces of different fingers.

8. Encourage patients to try different finger-lancing devices and lancets.

9. Teach patients that most finger-stick devices come with different tips or gauges that allow for deeper puncture if needed.

Teaching Meter Maintenance and Calibration

Each monitoring system has a unique set of instructions for cleaning the meter, testing the meter with a check strip, and testing the strips and technique with glucose control (sugar-water) solutions. Some of the non-wipe meters require no special cleaning at all because the blood is applied on the end of a strip that has no direct contact with the meter. Other meters have a fairly simple cleaning routine that involves removing the part of the meter that holds the strip. Patients may mistakenly think that cleaning simply involves tidying up the outer surfaces of the meter and may be totally unaware that some meter parts are removable.

Many of the meters have an alarm indicating when the meter needs to be cleaned. In general, it is advisable to teach patients to clean the meter on a regular basis (according to the manufacturer's recommendations) rather than to wait for dust, lint, or blood to accumulate to such a degree that the alarm is triggered.

Most meters have a check strip or device that is included with the purchase of the meter. Patients need to use this regularly (e.g., once a week or as recommended by the manufacturer) to make sure that the meter gives an appropriate reading when the checking device is inserted. In addition, all meter purchases include glucose solutions, called *control solutions,* which can be used to check the accuracy of the strips, meter, and technique. Patients perform a test with the meter with the usual technique, substituting the glucose solution for blood. Provided on the container or strips or control solution is a range of glucose values within which the control solution test results should fall. If results are out of range, the educator should check for meter cleanliness, appropriate technique, and expiration date of the strips and control solution. Manufacturers provide a toll-free number for assistance in case problems with the meter have no obvious explanation.

Although usually done less frequently than a test using control solution, the most important and reliable test for meter accuracy is a meter comparison of a blood test result from the meter with a laboratory result obtained at the same time.

The manuals that are supplied with each meter contain a list of possible alarms that should be reviewed (e.g., for very high or very low values), but it is also important to explain that poor technique can sometimes bypass the alarms and give inaccurate results. Again, periodic (every 6 to 12 months) comparisons of the meter with laboratory results are important.

Working with a Veteran User of SMBG/ Evaluating Accuracy

The three main approaches to evaluating meter accuracy are (1) observation of patients' technique, (2) meter check (comparison with laboratory testing of glucose), and (3) Hgb A_{1c} level.

Observation of Patients' Technique

- Check the equipment for cleanliness—especially accumulation of dust, cotton, tissue fibers, or blood in the area where the strip is placed and read by the meter.
- Ask patients when they last cleaned the meter and watch their meter-cleaning technique.
- Check that the meter is programmed for the code number on the current batch of strips.
- Check the low-battery alarm.
- Check the expiration date of the strips and make sure the strips are securely stored in the vial or foil. Any exposure to light or air renders most strips inaccurate (falsely low readings result).
- Question patients about any extremes of temperature to which the strips or meter was exposed (e.g., leaving the equipment in a car on a hot day).
- Check meter and strip accuracy with the check strip and control solutions. Expected ranges are provided with all meter equipment.
- Observe patients' performing a test—pay close attention to drop size and placement (did the patient smear or mash the drop onto the strip?).

Meter Check

Have the patient bring the meter and strips to the laboratory to perform a finger stick (fasting blood sugar is recommended by most manufacturers) within a few minutes of a venipuncture for plasma glucose determination. Results should be within 15% of each other. (Note: It is possible for the check strip and control solution to be within the manufacturer's recommended range while meter comparison with laboratory results is >15%.) The laboratory meter check is the single most reliable test of meter and technique accuracy and should be performed at least every 6 to 12 months.

Glycated Hemoglobin

This test is described in more detail later. It reflects overall blood glucose control during the prior 8 to 12 weeks. If this test result is not consistent with reported SMBG results, one possibility is that the patient has a problem with the SMBG technique. The guidelines described earlier help detect possible errors in SMBG results. Another possibility is that only preprandial blood glucose values are being tested, and postprandial blood glucose values are too high, contributing to poor overall glucose control. In some cases, patients write down fabricated blood glucose levels, making blood glucose levels appear falsely normal. If a patient's meter has a memory, real values can be downloaded and compared with those written in the patient's SMBG record book.

Computer Downloading

Using various software programs (including some that are supplied by the meter manufacturers), it is now possible to download many meters into a computer, which can then print out lists of results, including various graphic representations of the blood glucose values. This information can be helpful in analyzing trends of blood glucose values. Patients often rely on the meter to store all of their blood glucose values instead of writing them down. This can be a problem if patients do not store their insulin doses and note changes in diet and exercise patterns in either their meter memory (if possible) or their written record as well.

Patient Situations/Questions

Situation 1—Fabricated Results

If fabricated results are suspected on the basis of a disparity between the meter memory and the results recorded in a patient's monitoring book, these differences should be discussed in as direct and nonjudgmental a manner as possible. Calmly instruct patients on using the memory. Have patients measure their blood glucose level and then immediately check the memory to provide reassurance that the memory is working properly. (Patients who have fabricated or deleted results typically feel guilty and uncomfortable when they realize that you are checking the memory. This makes a direct confrontation counterproductive.) A sensitive and understanding approach is best for most patients. Let them know that diabetes management is difficult and that the health care providers would prefer no information or high glucose results to results that are not authentic.

In certain circumstances, such as pregnancy, repeated problems with fabricated results, or repeated episodes of DKA, a more direct, confrontational approach may be necessary. However, this may undermine the rapport that has been established between the diabetes educator and the patient, and it may be advisable to enlist the help of the patient's physician in this process.

Situation 2—Patients Who Experience Discomfort Performing SMBG

Some patients are able to perform multiple daily tests with minimal discomfort, but others experience extreme discomfort with each test. There is not always a logical explanation for the difference. To help reduce discomfort, try the following:

- Use different finger-stick equipment.
- Try the techniques listed earlier for improving blood flow (especially allowing the hand to relax at the side for a few seconds after the puncture and before applying the pressure).
- Encourage use of the sides of the fingers that are used infrequently for activities of daily living.
- Try different rotation patterns; some pa-

tients prefer to use different surfaces of different fingers with each stick. Some prefer to use different surfaces of the same finger. Some prefer to use the same one or two fingers all the time.
- Reduce the number of tests requested. This may promote more long-term commitment to at least a limited SMBG schedule.
- Have open discussions with patients to help them come to terms with this uncomfortable but useful aspect of diabetes management (especially patients taking multiple insulin injections). Reinforce the usefulness of the results and discuss with patients the potential consequences of performing no glucose monitoring at all or of using only urine testing results.

Situation 3—Timing of Tests

Patients frequently inquire about the best time to test. They have often been taught that they simply need to test first thing in the morning, and they assume that if these results are in an acceptable range that overall control is adequate. Morning tests alone, however, do not reflect problems of postprandial hyperglycemia or preprandial hypoglycemia, especially in the late afternoon.

For patients taking insulin injections, physicians typically request specific times for blood tests throughout the day to help with ongoing evaluation of doses. For sophisticated patients, frequent premeal testing is used to help adjust daily insulin doses.

Patients who are taking oral medication and who have a Hgb A_{1c} level within the desired range may be instructed to alter the times of the tests—especially focusing on times at which hypoglycemia risk is the highest (before meals, after a long delay in meals, before and after exercise, before a long drive). Simply checking at different times on 3 or 4 days a week may be sufficient for patients to make sure that control is maintained. Other patients may prefer to test more often because it provides pressure or external motivation to stay on the diet and exercise routine.

*For patients who are on diet or oral agents and who have elevated Hgb A_{1c} re*sults, testing in premeal and postmeal pairs is useful for encouraging patients' awareness of the effect of various food combinations. Depending on the patient and the financial/insurance circumstances, testing around just three or four meals a week may be enough to provide knowledge and motivation. Other patients may opt to increase testing at a certain meal for a specified time while they experiment with different menus.

URINE TESTING

Urine testing by patients can be performed to assess the amount of glucose in the urine and to test for urine ketones. All patients with type 1 diabetes should have nonexpired strips for measuring urine ketones at home and should be educated about their use. Patients who are unwilling or unable to test their blood glucose levels at home may be willing to test their urine for glucose. Urine glucose testing is particularly helpful in showing patients that they are losing (spilling) glucose in their urine, indicating high circulating glucose levels. However, urine glucose testing does not distinguish between hypoglycemia, euglycemia, and mild hyperglycemia (the usual renal threshold in adults is approximately 180 mg/dl and even higher in older patients). Therefore, tight control is generally not possible when using urine glucose results. (See Chapter 7 for a more detailed description of the use of urine testing.)

TESTS OF LONG-TERM DIABETES CONTROL

The Hgb A_{1c} level test is a blood test that indicates the percentage of total hemoglobin to which glucose is attached. The higher the blood glucose level and the longer it has been elevated, the higher is the percentage of glucose that attaches to the hemoglobin. Hemoglobin is a substance (a protein) inside red blood cells that carries oxygen from the lungs to the body cells. On each hemoglobin molecule are several sites that attract sugar. An analogy is made with the product called Velcro. One side is smooth, and one is rough. The hemoglobin molecule could be compared to the rough side, the sugar to the smooth side. When the two attach to each other, they do not easily come apart. Therefore, the Hgb A_{1c} molecule has a memory that lasts for the life of the red blood cell. The memory remains until the red blood cells are replaced with new ones; this takes 2 to 3 months. Therefore, this test reflects the average blood glucose level during the preceding 2 months. Consequently, it serves as a reliable assessment of the overall control during this period. For teaching purposes, patients should know the difference between SMBG and the Hgb A_{1c} test. This has been described by Dr. Daniel L. Lorber, Assistant Professor of Clinical Medicine at the New York University School of Medicine in New York, as follows: "Imagine taking a train cross-country with all the curtains drawn except for one minute seven times a day, and trying to describe the countryside based on what you saw during those seven minutes. You can frequently come close, but not as close if you had had a panoramic view. The glycated hemoglobin is that panoramic view." Because laboratories use different assays, it is important to know which test your laboratory uses and what the normal range is. The best tests currently used include Hgb A_{1c} levels and total glycated hemoglobin levels (measured by affinity chromatography). Patients should have the test every 2 to 3 months. Seeing the Hgb A_{1c} level fall with treatment can be rewarding and motivating for patients (Fig. 10-6).

Glucose also attaches to other proteins in the circulation. Tests for these measure glycated albumin, glycated serum proteins,

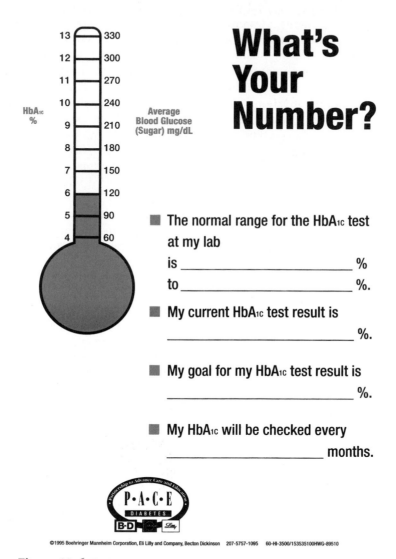

What's Your Number?

The normal range for the HbA1c test at my lab

is _____ %

to _____ %.

My current HbA1c test result is

_____ %.

My goal for my HbA1c test result is

_____ %.

My HbA1c will be checked every

_____ months.

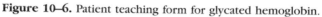

©1995 Boehringer Mannheim Corporation, Eli Lilly and Company, Becton Dickinson   207-5757-1095   60-HI-3500/153535100HWG-89510

Figure 10–6. Patient teaching form for glycated hemoglobin.

and fructosamine. They furnish the same information as the Hgb A_{1c} test but show changes over a 3- to 4-week period. Again, the normal range of these test results from each laboratory differ, and the appropriate values must be used to compare with patients' results. (See Chapter 7 for a more detailed discussion of Hgb A_{1c} and other proteins.)

USE OF ORAL ANTIDIABETIC MEDICATIONS

FOR THE DIABETES EDUCATOR

Clinical experience has shown that in general, patients who take oral antidiabetic medications lack knowledge about diabetes and do not appreciate the importance of these medications in the control of blood glucose. Some of these patients may not even consider themselves as having diabetes. Rather, they may assume that only people who require insulin injections actually have diabetes.

SULFONYLUREA AGENTS

These drugs are not insulin itself but act to stimulate the pancreas to secrete more insulin to lower blood glucose levels in patients with type 2 diabetes. By definition, they do not work in patients with type 1 diabetes, because these patients do not secrete any insulin. These drugs are often effective after diet therapy fails, although patients often gain some weight (4 to 6 pounds) when started on these agents. In addition, they sometimes cause the pancreas to secrete too much insulin, leading to hypoglycemia.

Table 10–5 lists the names of the currently available sulfonylurea agents. They all have similar mechanisms of action and therefore cannot be combined with each other. Tolbutamide is the least effective drug and must be given several times per day, but it is useful for patients in renal failure. Chlorpropamide

has a very long duration of action and can cause a low serum sodium level (especially in the elderly) and therefore should not be used in patients >65 years of age. Tolazamide (Tolinase), chlorpropamide (Diabinese), glyburide (Micronase, DiaBeta, or Glynase), and glipizide (Glucotrol or Glucotrol XL) all are similarly effective. Choosing which agent to use depends largely on cost, a patient's age (no chlorpropamide if >65 years of age), and compliance (some patients are more compliant with once-a-day medications such as chlorpropamide and Glucotrol XL).

Adverse Events

Side effects caused by sulfonylurea agents occur in <5% of patients. The first two listed below are by far the most common.

1. Skin rashes
2. Gastrointestinal symptoms (loss of appetite, nausea with occasional vomiting, heartburn, feelings of abdominal fullness)
3. Flushed feeling after drinking alcohol (chlorpropamide only)
4. Mental status changes due to low sodium level (chlorpropamide only)
5. Dark urine, light-colored stools, yellowing of eyes or skin (drug-induced liver damage—very rare)

Hypoglycemia can be a serious adverse effect of sulfonylurea agents. It is more likely to develop when patients (often elderly) eat irregularly or consume less food than usual. It is also more likely to occur in patients with renal insufficiency. Because of the duration of effect of the oral agents, patients with severe hypoglycemia must be monitored carefully for a recurrence. Patients who are taking oral agents and who develop severe enough hypoglycemia to cause mentation changes should be hospitalized to receive continuous intravenous dextrose. Patients taking oral agents need to be educated about the signs, symptoms, and treatment of hypoglycemia.

Table 10–5. Selected Characteristics of Oral Antidiabetic Medications

Generic Name	Trade Name	Tablet Size (mg)	Usual Daily Dose Range (mg)	Maximal Dose (mg)	Duration of Action (h)
Tolbutamide	Orinase[a]	250, 500	500–2,000 (divided)	3,000	6-12
Chlorpropamide	Diabinese[b]	100, 250	100–500 (single)	750	60
Acetohexamide	Dymelor[c]	250, 500	250–1,500 (single or divided)	1,500	12-24
Tolazamide	Tolinase[a]	100, 250, 500	100–750 (single or divided)	1,000	12-24
Glyburide	Micronase,[a] DiaBeta[d]	1.25, 2.5, 5.0	2.5–10 (single or divided)	20	12-24
	Glynase[a] (micronized glyburide)	1.5, 3.0, 6.0	1.5–6.0 (single or divided)	12	12-24
Glipizide	Glucotrol[e]	5, 10	5–20 (single or divided)	40	10-24
	Glucotrol XL (long-acting glipizide)[e]	5, 10	5–10 (single)	20	24-48
Glimepiride	Amaryl[d]	1, 2, 4	1–4	8	~24
Metformin	Glucophage[f]	500, 850	1,000–2,000 (divided)	2,500 (2,550)	6-12
Acarbose	Precose[g]	50, 100	75–150 (divided)	300	Not absorbed

[a]Upjohn Co., Kalamazoo, MI.
[b]Pfizer, Inc., New York, NY.
[c]Eli Lilly and Co., Indianapolis, IN.
[d]Hoechst-Roussel Pharmaceuticals, Somerville, NJ.
[e]Pratt Pharmaceuticals, New York, NY.
[f]Bristol-Myers Squibb Company, Princeton, NJ.
[g]Bayer Corp., Tarrytown, NY.

METFORMIN

Metformin lowers glucose concentrations without stimulating the pancreas to secrete more insulin. Its mechanism of action is still controversial but involves the liver (decreasing glucose output), muscle and fat (possibly increasing glucose utilization), and the gastrointestinal tract (decreasing absorption of glucose into the bloodstream). Because its action in the body differs from that of the sulfonylurea agents, it can be used in combination with a sulfonylurea agent when a patient is failing to respond to maximal doses of one agent and needs insulin therapy. Its benefits are that it does not cause weight gain (which often occurs with sulfonylurea agents) or hypoglycemia and it improves the lipid profile. However, it must be taken two to three times per day, gastrointestinal side effects are common, and lactic acidosis can

occur in patients with contraindications to its use (discussed later). Therefore, it must be used with careful consideration of its risks and benefits in each patient. An obese patient with elevated lipid levels is an appropriate candidate for metformin as a first-line drug.

Adverse Events

Patients taking metformin commonly experience gastrointestinal side effects such as cramping, diarrhea, nausea, vomiting, anorexia, metallic taste, and flatulence. These side effects usually are self-limited and improve after 1 to 2 weeks on the drug (or on the new dose). These side effects can be lessened by starting with small doses of the drug (500 or 850 mg/day), increasing the dose no more often than every other week, and giving the metformin with food. Lactic acidosis (a serious buildup of lactate levels in the blood) can occur in patients taking metformin, although only if the patient has a contraindication to its use. These contraindications include abnormal renal function (defined as a serum creatinine level >1.5 in males and >1.4 in females), liver function abnormalities, excessive alcohol use, chronic or acute acidosis, and situations of possible hypoxia (e.g., congestive heart failure, pulmonary insufficiency). Any serious medical situation, especially one in which renal function might deteriorate, such as during an angiographic dye study or during a myocardial infarction, requires that metformin use be temporarily discontinued. Furthermore, serum vitamin B_{12} and folate levels can fall, and therefore patients must be monitored to ensure that anemia secondary to the medication does not occur (which is rare).

ACARBOSE

Acarbose (Precose) is a new oral diabetic drug released in 1996. It works by a mechanism completely different from other oral medications for diabetes. This drug inhibits the action of gastrointestinal tract enzymes that digest carbohydrates—that is, the breakdown of the carbohydrates in the meal to glucose is delayed. (Fortunately, the enzyme that digests the carbohydrate in milk is not affected much, which means that lactose intolerance is not a problem.) When the delay of carbohydrate digestion in the gastrointestinal tract occurs, the rise of glucose in the circulation after the meal is blunted and less postprandial hyperglycemia is noted. Because of this mechanism of action, acarbose should be taken with the first bite of each meal. Some of the carbohydrate in the meal is not digested and reaches the large colon, where bacteria and other enzymes form gaseous products. Therefore, a common side effect of this drug is flatulence. However, if it is started in small doses and increased slowly, this side effect becomes less, although some patients choose not to take the

drug because of it. Acarbose can be used as initial therapy in type 2 diabetes or added to sulfonylurea agents or insulin. If patients are taking a combination of acarbose and a sulfonylurea agent or insulin, they must take a commercial preparation of glucose or milk to treat hypoglycemia. Because gastrointestinal side effects are also common with metformin, experience with the combination of acarbose and metformin is scarce. Because they work by different mechanisms, however, an additive effect should occur when they are used together. Finally, acarbose can be added to insulin therapy in type 1 diabetes.

DRUG INTERACTIONS

Patients should be told that whenever they take more than one medication, one medication might interact with another one. Some medications, such as sulfa-based antibiotics, can directly potentiate (increase) the effects of the sulfonylurea agents and lower blood glucose levels further. Other drugs affect glucose levels by themselves (i.e., not by interacting with sulfonylurea agents). These include thiazide diuretics, glucocorticoids (e.g., prednisone), estrogen compounds, and phenytoin (Dilantin), which may *increase* blood glucose levels, and salicylates, propranolol, and pentamidine, which may *decrease* blood glucose levels. (Propranolol and other β-blockers may also mask symptoms of hypoglycemia.)

PATIENT EDUCATION

Patients who start using oral antidiabetic medications need to be informed (1) about what type of diabetes they have (type 2); (2) about how to take the medications; (3) that they must be alert to any symptoms of hypoglycemia (if taking a sulfonylurea agent) and must report these episodes to their health care provider if they occur; (4) that these medications are not a substitute for a diabetic diet; (5) that they must be aware of the risks associated with the development of lactic acidosis (if on metformin—these include abnormalities of kidney or liver function, excessive use of alcohol, and any operation or medical test, which requires that metformin use be discontinued temporarily); and (5) that they must be monitored closely for their diabetic control and for side effects of the drug. As with insulin, the goal of therapy is to keep blood glucose levels close to the normal range, which means at least a fasting glucose level <140 mg/dl and an Hgb A_{1c} level $\leq 8.0\%$. SMBG may be helpful for detecting hypoglycemia and hyperglycemia (especially during illness).

Patients taking sulfonylurea agents should be advised to eat meals regularly to avoid hypoglycemia. The sulfonylurea agents can be taken just before, during, or after meals. Metformin, however, should always be taken with meals (after the patient has ingested some food) to decrease gastrointestinal side effects. Acarbose should be taken with the first bite of the meal to maximize its effectiveness.

PATIENT SITUATIONS/QUESTIONS

· If I am supposed to take my medication only once per day, does it matter when? (For sulfonylurea agents, no; for metformin and acarbose, yes.)
· If I have a low blood glucose reading on my meter, should I still take my medication? (Yes, but be sure to eat your meal.)
· If I have a treadmill test or gastrointestinal study and am told not to eat in the morning or to delay eating but am told to take all of my usual medications, should I take my diabetes pill? (Take it with the first meal that day.)
· Is it all right to take a combination of pills or to combine insulin and pills? (Yes, if your physician has prescribed a combination.)

INSULIN

FOR THE DIABETES EDUCATOR

Insulin is necessary to achieve blood glucose control in patients with type 1 diabetes and patients with type 2 diabetes who fail to respond satisfactorily to maximal doses of oral antidiabetic medications. The need to take insulin, especially daytime doses or mixed doses that affect meal timing, markedly increases the amount of information that a patient must master. In addition, the use of insulin in the diabetes treatment plan may be the focus of much fear and anxiety on the part of diabetes patients and their significant others.

Three main areas of instruction need to be addressed when patients start insulin treatment. These are practical issues (procedure for drawing up and injecting insulin); theoretic issues (how insulin works, timing of insulin, troubleshooting for missed or delayed doses); and emotional issues (dealing with the meaning of insulin treatment to the patient and significant others). In all three areas of discussion, it is important to assess and dispel any misconceptions about insulin treatment while respecting the unique set of experiences, expectations, and cultural beliefs that patients describe.

GENERAL ASSESSMENT

A helpful starting point when working with patients who need to learn about insulin is to allow patients to feel comfortable about expressing their fears: "Most people have fears or concerns about giving insulin shots. What concerns do you have about it?" Depending on the responses, an educator can begin instruction right away in the area of greatest concern to a patient. It is important for an educator to be flexible enough to allow discussion of information that may not necessarily follow a logical flow.

For example, if a patient's main concern

surrounds the injection itself, the educator can start the lesson by having the patient self-inject saline first. If a patient's main concern is about accuracy of doses, start the lesson by having the patient locate different doses with an empty syringe. If a patient expresses concern about insulin storage and travel, address these issues at the beginning of the lesson. It is often helpful to ask patients how they feel about starting insulin so that their fears can be expressed openly. Also helpful is inquiring about the reaction of the patient's family and friends because these people can offer patients important support.

If a patient seems totally overwhelmed or consumed with anxiety, it may be best for the educator simply to start the hands-on lesson—kindly but firmly guiding the patient through a practice injection. Once this is completed, a more open, patient-guided discussion can take place.

Table 10–6 lists some concerns or misconceptions that patients have when starting insulin.

MEDICAL ASSESSMENT

Determine the Type of Diabetes That Each Patient Has

Patients with type 1 diabetes are at risk for DKA and may even have experienced it. Issues of concern to patients must be addressed, but educators may need to exert more influence over the flow of information to ensure that the first lesson covers the basics of giving insulin and avoiding hypoglycemia.

For patients with type 2 diabetes in poor control complicated by infection, corticosteroid treatment, anticipated surgery, or worrisome symptoms, the educator may need to use an approach similar to that for type 1 patients. There may be less opportunity to address all of patients' concerns at the initial teaching session. However, reassure patients that the insulin treatment may be temporary and that further teaching sessions will address other information, including reverting to oral antidiabetic medications.

For patients with type 2 diabetes without symptoms or coexisting illness, an educator has more latitude in negotiating the insulin treatment plan with a patient. Perhaps a patient could be given the option of starting with one injection instead of two or postponing the insulin treatment or asked to agree to a trial of 1 or 2 months on insulin with the chance to discontinue the insulin at the end of the trial. Educators need to be sure that patients understand the consequences of their decision.

Determine Adequacy of Visual/Hearing Skills

Patients with decreased visual acuity need to be taught methods for magnifying the marks on the syringes (discussed later) and strategies for insulin administration (such as use of insulin pens or having a family member assist). Patients with significant hearing deficits need to be taught in a quiet room, and much of the information provided may need to be written down.

PATIENT EDUCATION

The following sections are divided into basic and comprehensive levels of information. A basic level of information is intended to provide patients with enough information to be safe users of insulin even if they never receive or are unable to comprehend more comprehensive insulin instruction. Focusing solely on the basic information is useful when working with patients who are very anxious, when time for the lesson is limited, and when patients have a limited capacity to comprehend complex information.

The educator can set up a follow-up appointment to review the basic information and to introduce the comprehensive information as appropriate. Some patients are able to receive comprehensive information from the beginning and wish to do so. The

Table 10–6. Misconceptions Related to Insulin

Misconception	Educator's Response
Once insulin injections are started (for treatment of type 2 diabetes), they can never be discontinued.	During periods of acute stress (such as illness, infection, or surgery) or when receiving certain medications that cause elevations in blood glucose, some patients with type 2 diabetes require insulin. If the diabetes had previously been well controlled with diet alone or diet with oral hypoglycemic agents, patients should be able to resume previous methods for control of diabetes when the stress is resolved. In addition, insulin is sometimes used to control blood glucose levels in obese type 2 diabetic patients who have been unsuccessful at weight loss. If patients are able to lose weight after insulin therapy is initiated, the insulin doses may be tapered and patients may be able to switch to diet and exercise alone or with oral hypoglycemic agents for control of blood glucose. (For patients with type 1 diabetes, insulin is needed on an ongoing basis. For thin patients with type 2 diabetes, once insulin has to be started, it is usually required permanently).
If increasing doses of insulin are needed to control the blood glucose, the diabetes must be getting "worse."	Explain to patients that unlike other medications that are given in standard doses, there is not a standard dose of insulin that is effective for all patients. Rather, the dose must be adjusted according to blood glucose test results. If the initial insulin dose prescribed for a patient does not adequately decrease the glucose level, the patient may assume that he or she has a "bad" case of diabetes or that the diabetes is getting worse. It is important to instruct patients that many different factors may affect the ability of insulin to lower the glucose, including obesity, puberty, pregnancy, illness, and certain medications. In addition, to avoid hypoglycemia, physicians frequently initiate insulin therapy with smaller doses than will eventually be needed. The doses are then increased in small increments until blood glucose levels are in the desired range.
Insulin causes blindness (or other diabetic complications).	When patients have a diabetic acquaintance in whom the initiation of insulin therapy happened to coincide with the onset of diabetic complications, the patient may view insulin as the cause of complications such as blindness or amputation. In these situations, the acquaintance probably had type 2 diabetes that was no longer controllable with diet and oral hypoglycemic agents. It must be explained to patients that factors such as elevated blood glucose and elevated blood pressure levels (and not insulin therapy) contribute to some of the diabetic complications. Furthermore, emphasize that insulin is a natural hormone present in every person's body, that it helps control blood glucose levels, and that it definitely does not cause long-term complications of diabetes.
Insulin must be injected directly into the vein.	When patients first learn that one area used for insulin injections is the arm, they may envision inserting the needle directly into a vein in the antecubital area as in blood withdrawal. Patients must be reassured that insulin is injected into the fat tissue on the *back* of the arm (or on the abdomen, thigh, or hip) and that the needle is much shorter than that used for venipuncture.
There is extreme danger in injecting insulin if there are any air bubbles in the syringe.	Patients may have a fear of dying if air bubbles are injected with a syringe. (This may be related to the misconception that insulin is injected directly into the vein). Reassure patients that the main danger in having air bubbles in the insulin syringe is that the amount of insulin being injected is less than the required dose. It is often difficult to remove every small "champagne" bubble from the syringe. Thus, patients should be reassured that injection of insulin when these bubbles are present does not cause any harm.

Table 10–6. Misconceptions Related to Insulin *Continued*

Misconception	Educator's Response
Insulin always causes people to have bad (hypoglycemic) reactions.	First, make sure that patients are aware that low blood sugar reactions are often related to an imbalance with the insulin, food, and activity and can often be avoided. Thus, before starting on insulin, patients should discuss their usual schedule of meals and activities as well as the content of meals with the health care team. Make sure that patients are aware that various different insulins and insulin schedules can be used to try to allow patients to maintain some of their usual life style habits. Reassure patients that avoiding hypoglycemic reactions is a high priority for the diabetes team. In addition, tell patients of the importance of reporting any hypoglycemic reactions to the health care team immediately so that early adjustments can be made in the insulin dosage. Focus early insulin education on treatment and prevention of hypoglycemia.
People who take insulin must travel only where there is a refrigerator to store the insulin.	Insulin bottles in use may be kept at room temperature. Therefore, for most business trips or vacations, keeping the insulin in a purse or brief case (or special diabetes supply case) is acceptable. If a prolonged trip is planned (more than 2 to 3 months), patients may want to consult the pharmacist or insulin manufacturer for suggestions. Most importantly, emphasize with patients that taking insulin should never deter them from pursuing activities they enjoy.

educator's assessment is helpful in determining the degree of difficulty of information to present.

Basic Insulin Instruction— Practical Issues

1. *Gather and identify supplies:* alcohol, insulin, syringe, and cotton or tissue. Locate on the insulin label the *letter* or *number* indicating the type of insulin (e.g., N, R, 70/30). Locate the word describing the *source*—human, beef, or pork. Note the *color* of the insulin (white or clear). Identify the *size* of the syringe by looking at the highest number of units that the syringe can hold (e.g., 25, 30, 50, 100). Explain that one bottle holds enough insulin (1,000 U) to last for 1 to 2 months.

At the basic level, it is not critical that a patient recite the full name for the insulin or identify the syringe by volume. Patients simply need to be able to correctly identify the insulin and syringes that they are supposed to be using.

2. *Open the supplies.* Flip off the cap on the insulin bottle. Carefully remove the needle cover and plunger cap (if present) from the syringe. At this point, patients can practice pulling and pushing the plunger of the syringe while locating different doses.

If patients are totally incapable of accurately positioning the plunger at this stage, the educator may need to make other arrangements for drawing up the insulin. For example, syringes can be prefilled by a member of the diabetes treatment team, a family member can be taught how to draw up the insulin, home health visits can be arranged, or the use of a prefilled insulin pen can be considered. Most patients can still be taught to give the injection, even if they are not able to draw up their own doses.

3. *Draw up the insulin* (Fig. 10–7).
   - Wipe the bottle top with alcohol.
   - Mix all cloudy insulin by gently shaking or rolling the bottle.
   - Insert the needle through the rubber stopper.

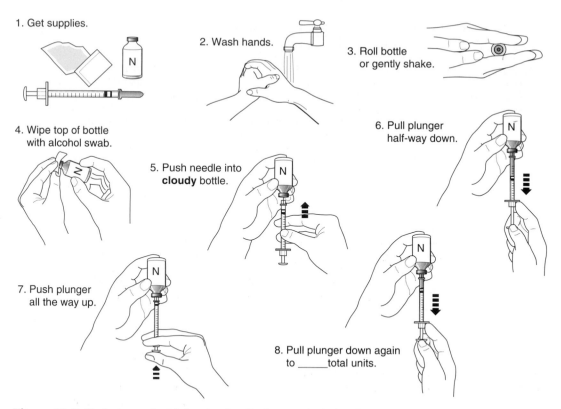

1. Get supplies.

2. Wash hands.

3. Roll bottle or gently shake.

4. Wipe top of bottle with alcohol swab.

5. Push needle into **cloudy** bottle.

6. Pull plunger half-way down.

7. Push plunger all the way up.

8. Pull plunger down again to _____total units.

Figure 10–7. Technique of withdrawing insulin from a single bottle. (Injecting air into bottle not shown.) (See text for description.)

- Position the bottle upside down, making sure the needle is completely covered with the insulin solution.
- Pull the plunger approximately half-way down the syringe and then push it all the way back up, squirting all the insulin back into the bottle.
- Pull the plunger down again and locate the prescribed number of units.
- Remove the syringe from the bottle—avoid touching the needle.

Holding the upside-down bottle and syringe in one hand while manipulating the syringe plunger with the other hand can be very awkward for new patients. They can be shown various bottle-holding devices such as the Becton Dickinson Magni-Guide or Diabetic Insulcap (see Appendix), or the educator can assist by holding the bottle for the patient at first. Another option is simply to tape the bottle to a vertical surface (e.g., a wall, refrigerator, or door) in an upside-down position.

4. *Give the injection* (Fig. 10–8).
   - Bunch up the skin of the abdomen (pinch up a fold about 1 inch thick).
   - Insert the needle straight in with a dart action.
   - Inject the insulin with slow, steady pressure on the plunger.
   - Remove the needle, let go of the pinch (can be done in reverse order), and apply pressure to the site with dry cotton or tissue.

Basic instruction need not cover elaborate injection site rotation patterns. It is simplest to teach one area for injection—preferably the abdomen, because it offers the most consistent absorption, is easy to reach, and typi-

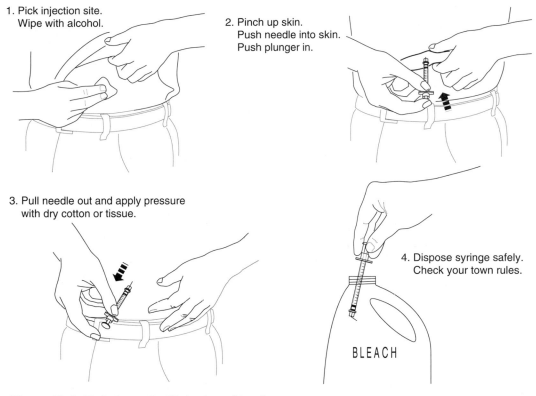

1. Pick injection site.
   Wipe with alcohol.

2. Pinch up skin.
   Push needle into skin.
   Push plunger in.

3. Pull needle out and apply pressure
   with dry cotton or tissue.

4. Dispose syringe safely.
   Check your town rules.

BLEACH

Figure 10–8. Technique of self-injection of insulin.

cally has the most subcutaneous tissue. In addition, patients who are taught to use only the arms or legs first are often quite fearful of trying the abdomen at a later date (whereas the reverse is not necessarily true).

Advise patients to use a new site about 1 inch away from the previous site—perhaps using up one horizontal row below the next, moving sites down and across the entire abdomen.

5. *Discard the syringe.* ADA and Environmental Protection Agency recommendations include placing the entire uncapped syringe into a puncture-proof container such as an empty bleach or detergent bottle. It is helpful to have patients discard the syringe in such a bottle during the teaching session. Once full, the bottle may be discarded with

the regular garbage—although the educator should check for any specific city or state regulations.

6. *Store the bottles of insulin.*

   · According to the insulin manufacturers, insulin bottles in use can be stored at room temperature for as long as 2 months.
   · Insulin bottles should be kept out of direct sunlight.
   · Unopened bottles should be refrigerated.
   · Open bottles should be refrigerated if the temperature is >75° in the room where the bottles are kept.
   · If bottles are refrigerated, they can be removed before the injection to allow them to return to room temperature. Be sure not to let the insulin freeze.

Comprehensive Insulin Instruction—Practical Issues

1. *Gather and Identify Supplies.* Rather than simply identifying the insulin by reading the label, patients prepared for more advanced instruction can be introduced to four main differentiating characteristics of insulin: type, species/source, manufacturer, and concentration.

   · *Type*—Short-acting insulin is regular [R] (for information on newer very rapid-acting insulin analogue, see Chapter 4), intermediate-acting insulins are NPH [N] or Lente [L], and long-acting insulin is Ultralente (UL). It is helpful to have sample bottles of different types of insulin available to show patients. Patients can be introduced to the approximate time course of action (Fig. 10-9), although it is often best to introduce this information from a practical perspective rather than having patients memorize onset, peak, and duration. For example, regular insulin goes to work on the meal consumed right after the injection, whereas NPH insulin is time released and goes to work on a later meal or overnight (Fig. 10-10). (For patients using premixed insulin, see the later discussion.)

   · *Species* (or origin)—Insulin sources include human (synthetic), beef, pork, or beef/pork combinations. Reassure patients that human insulin is produced in a laboratory to look just like human insulin and is not derived from humans, so there is no risk of being infected with hepatitis or AIDS.

   · *Manufacturer*—Eli Lilly and Novo Nordisk are the two companies currently supplying insulin in the United States. Teaching patients about

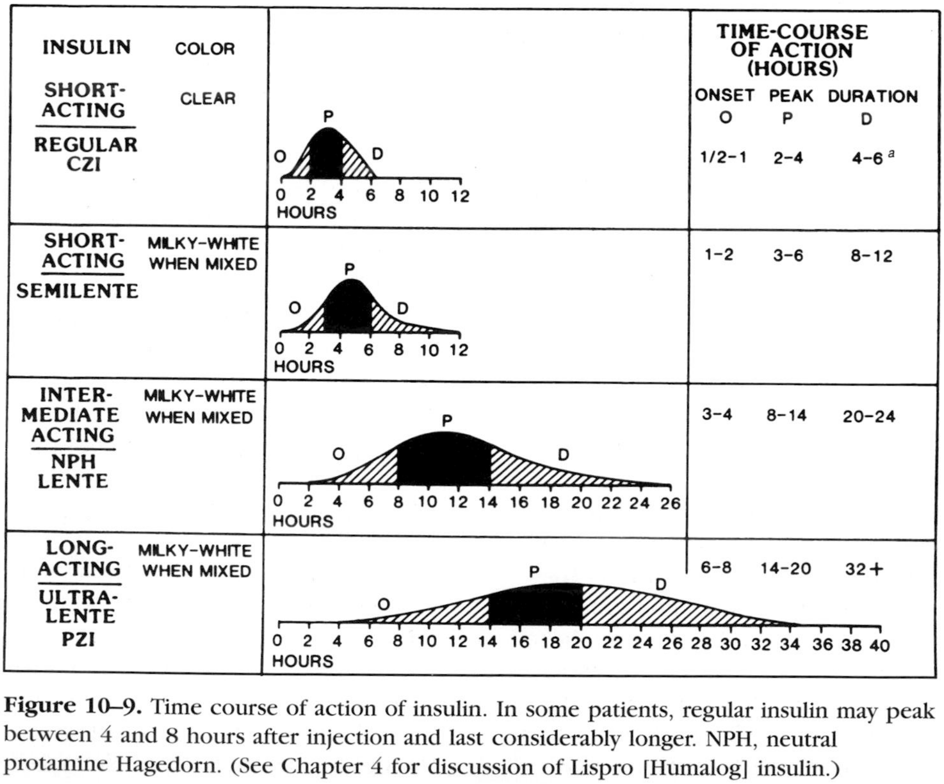

INSULIN	COLOR		TIME-COURSE OF ACTION (HOURS)		
			ONSET O	PEAK P	DURATION D
SHORT-ACTING REGULAR CZI	CLEAR		1/2–1	2–4	4–6 [a]
SHORT-ACTING SEMILENTE	MILKY-WHITE WHEN MIXED		1–2	3–6	8–12
INTER-MEDIATE ACTING NPH LENTE	MILKY-WHITE WHEN MIXED		3–4	8–14	20–24
LONG-ACTING ULTRA-LENTE PZI	MILKY-WHITE WHEN MIXED		6–8	14–20	32+

Figure 10–9. Time course of action of insulin. In some patients, regular insulin may peak between 4 and 8 hours after injection and last considerably longer. NPH, neutral protamine Hagedorn. (See Chapter 4 for discussion of Lispro [Humalog] insulin.)

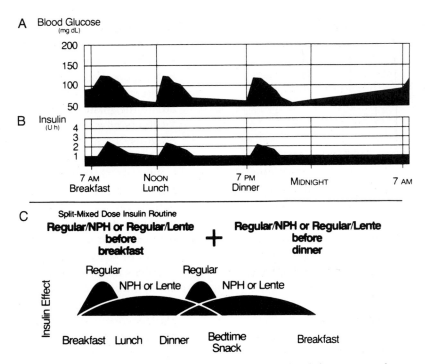

Figure 10–10. *A:* The normal rise in blood glucose level that occurs after meals. *B:* The normal increase in insulin release that occurs at mealtime. *C:* A twice-daily insulin injection regimen using two injections of NPH (or lente) mixed with regular; prebreakfast regular "covers" breakfast; prebreakfast NPH covers lunch and the afternoon snack; predinner regular covers dinner; predinner NPH covers bedtime snack and overnight.

the company names is helpful in terms of learning to differentiate insulins. Patients often identify their insulin type as simply Humulin or Novolin. They need to understand that these are simply trade names for the whole series of human insulins and do not describe the type of insulin used. Patients should be taught, for example, that the name Humulin N indicates the Lilly brand of human NPH or that Novolin R is the Novo Nordisk brand of human regular insulin (see *'97 Buyer's Guide to Diabetes Supplies*[3]).

· *Concentration*—Just one concentration of insulin is primarily available in the United States: U-100. Patients who travel, use insulin pumps, or are very inquisitive can be educated about different insulin concentrations such as U-40. Patients should be taught that this refers to the number of units of insulin per milliliter. Patients can be shown that the concentration noted on the bottle should match that noted on the syringe. Make patients aware that U-100 syringes are available in various sizes (e.g., 25 U, 30 U, 50 U, 100 U) and that syringe size does not denote a different concentration.

Show patients syringes of different sizes, pointing out that the main difference is that the 100-U (1-ml) syringes are typically marked in 2-U increments. Allow patients to practice drawing up insulin using different syringes so that they can appreciate the different sizes of syringes and are able to select the most appropriate size when new supplies are obtained.

2. *Equipment Issues: Flocculation and Syringe Reuse.* Patients prepared for more advanced information can be taught about insulin flocculation and syringe reuse.

   - *Flocculation.* White, cloudy insulins can develop a frosted appearance stuck to the inside of the insulin bottle, called *flocculation.* These white clumps may also appear in the insulin solution (Fig. 10-11). This is more common if the insulin has been kept at room temperature for a prolonged time (>2 to 3 months). Frosted insulin is inactive and should be discarded. However, reassure patients that if they inadvertently use insulin that has gone bad, they will not harm themselves but will have elevated blood glucose levels because their insulin is not working

properly. (It is helpful for the educator to have frosted bottles of insulin on display. The educator can keep one or two sample bottles of insulin at room temperature for a prolonged period to create the frosted appearance.)

   - *Syringe Reuse.* Studies that have been conducted have shown that reuse of insulin syringes is safe. The ADA Position Statement on Insulin Administration states, "For many patients, it appears both safe and practical for the syringe to be reused if the patient so desires. The syringe should be discarded when the needle becomes dull, has been bent, or has come into contact with any surface other than the skin; if reuse is planned, the needle must be recapped after each use."[2]

3. *Draw Up the Insulin.* In this stage of the insulin protocol, several variations in the technique are taught by diabetes

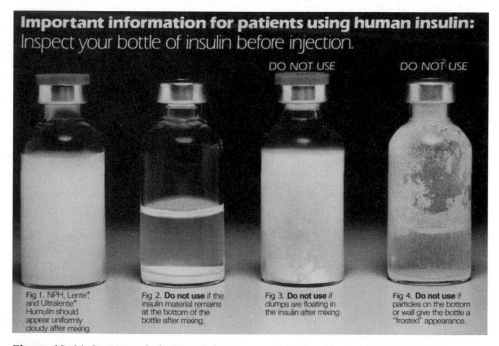

Important information for patients using human insulin: Inspect your bottle of insulin before injection.

DO NOT USE   DO NOT USE

Fig 1. NPH, Lente, and Ultralente Humulin should appear uniformly cloudy after mixing.

Fig 2. **Do not use** if the insulin material remains at the bottom of the bottle after mixing.

Fig 3. **Do not use** if clumps are floating in the insulin after mixing.

Fig 4. **Do not use** if particles on the bottom or wall give the bottle a "frosted" appearance.

Figure 10–11. Important information for patients using human insulin: Inspect your bottle of insulin before injection.

educators and promoted by printed instructional material. The steps described previously in the basic section represent one approach to drawing up insulin. Beginning learners are best served by being taught a simple technique that achieves the basic objective of getting insulin from the bottle into the syringe with as few steps as possible. Unfortunately, many diabetic patients harbor unwarranted anxiety about making any minor changes in the protocol that they were initially taught. At the more advanced level of teaching, diabetic patients can be exposed to several variations in the insulin protocol and allowed to select the steps that are most comfortable to them.

Injecting air into the vial—vacuum prevention: Injecting air into the vial of insulin is thought to eliminate the formation of a vacuum caused by repeated withdrawal of insulin from the closed vial. The most common technique is to inject air into the vial before each injection in a volume equivalent to the amount of insulin to be withdrawn. Variations are as follows:

· Inject an entire syringe full of air on a regular basis (e.g., every other day or once a week) rather than with each injection.
· Remove the plunger completely from a syringe and insert the empty syringe barrel into the insulin bottle, allowing the pressure inside the bottle to equalize for a few seconds.
· The simplest technique: completely eliminate all steps relative to injecting air.

Little if any scientific evidence shows that vacuum formation in insulin bottles is problematic. In fact, one study measured this phenomenon and found little support for the common and, for many patients, confusing steps of injecting exact quantities of air into bottles. Even if a vacuum does develop, it will not necessarily impair a patient's ability

to draw up an appropriate dose. Patients capable of learning more comprehensive insulin information can be given a demonstration of all the different approaches to dealing with the vacuum and can be allowed to select the technique of their choice. For patients who are not capable of comprehending more than the basic insulin information, it may be safer to risk vacuum formation than to risk confusion in preparing the dose.

4. *Give the injection.* Variations in injection technique can be introduced at the comprehensive level of education.

Injection sites (Fig. 10-12) | The first insulin instruction session can involve demonstration of just one injection area (preferably the abdomen). Follow-up comprehensive sessions can include information on the other possible sites, with discussion of site rotation and consequences of changing injection areas. *Abdominal* sites are located in a wide area from under the ribs, down to the hip line, and out to the side of the abdomen. *Arm* sites are located on the fleshy back surface of the upper arm, one hand's width down from the shoulder and one hand's width up from the elbow. A common error is for patients to use the deltoid area, just down from the shoulder, because the fleshy back surface is too hard to reach. This may cause inadvertent intramuscular injections, especially in a thin person. Intramuscular insulin injections may be more painful and can cause rapid absorption of the insulin. *Leg* sites are located one hand's width down from the groin and one hand's width up from the knee on the top surface of the thigh. *Hip* sites are located in the upper outer area of the buttocks. Research has shown that absorption is quickest from the abdomen and is progressively slower from the arm, leg, and hip sites.

Site rotation | Insulin should not be repeatedly injected in exactly the same site. If the same injection point is used, the skin may develop *lipohypertrophy,* a fatty, spongy area

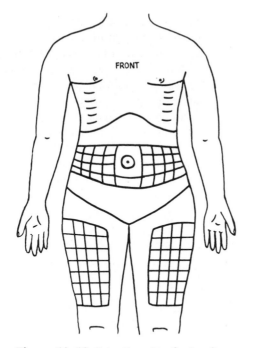
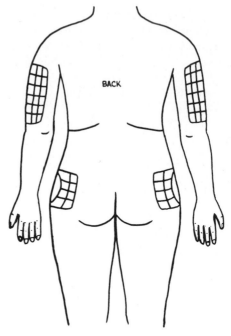

Figure 10–12. Injection sites for insulin.

of increased fat deposition, or *lipoatrophy,* a pitting or dimpling of the skin because subcutaneous fat is lost. Injections in these areas may lead to erratic absorption of the insulin.

Rotation of injection sites within one area is carried out by measuring one to two fingers' widths (1/2 to 1 inch) away from the most recent injection site. To avoid skin changes, patients should be advised to avoid injecting at the same site more than once in 2 to 3 weeks. If lipohypertrophy has occurred, it will resolve if no injections are given in the area until the skin resumes a normal contour.

Developing a systematic approach to site rotation, such as giving injections in a horizontal or vertical line pattern, helps to avoid repeated injections at the same site. Two different approaches that may be used for rotation of injection sites are as follows:

· Use injection sites on the abdomen exclusively (most patients can rotate

sites within the abdomen without using the same site in 2 to 3 weeks).
· Use injection sites in one area at the same time of day (e.g., use the abdominal area every morning and the arm every evening). Patients who are having problems with early peaking of intermediate-acting insulins (NPH or Lente) may benefit from using the leg or hip sites to prolong insulin action.

These approaches to rotation of injection areas provide the greatest consistency in absorption and effectiveness of insulin. They differ from previous methods of teaching rotation of injections, which included using a new area of the body for each injection. Patients who have been taking insulin for many years may need to be updated on this newer approach to injection rotation.

Stabilizing skin | Patients may choose between *bunching* the skin or *spreading* it before inserting the needle. Bunching the skin helps to avoid injection into the muscle, which is especially important in thin patients. Spreading the skin is helpful if the skin tends to give during needle insertion and for inserting the Teflon catheters used with insulin pumps.

Angle of insertion | A 90-degree angle is desirable in most patients to ensure delivery of insulin into the subcutaneous tissue instead of into the intradermal tissue. Also, injecting straight in promotes consistency from injection to injection. Very thin patients and children may prefer injecting at a 60- to 90-degree angle to avoid intramuscular injection. In general, patients can be reassured that if they can pinch an inch of fat between their fingers, they can inject straight in without a problem, because most needles are 1/2 inch or less in length.

Skin problems | Bruises, leaking, and lumps are the skin problems most commonly described by insulin users. Less commonly, insulin users describe burning, itching, or redness at the site. Potential causes and preventive measures are described next.

- *Bruises* may develop when the needle has nicked a superficial blood vessel or if the angle of the needle has shifted during insertion or withdrawal of the needle. Reassure patients that although bruises pose a cosmetic problem, they are not hazardous from a health standpoint. To prevent bruises, encourage the use of a 90-degree angle with swift, darting action used for needle insertion and swift, straight pulling outward for needle withdrawal. In addition, pressure should be applied to the injection site using dry cotton or tissue. Advise patients to avoid rubbing the area with cotton or an alcohol swab because this may promote bleeding or bruising.
- *Leaking or skin lumps* may result from injections that are too rapid, too large (volume), or too shallow. Encourage the use of a 90-degree angle

with slow injection of the insulin and release of the skin bunch as the injection is finishing. Patients using large doses of insulin may try dividing the injection and giving it in two different sites.
- *Burning, itching, and redness* may result from alcohol that is still wet at the time of needle insertion or from insulin that is too cold at the time of injection. Allowing the alcohol to dry on the skin before injection and using insulin at room temperature may resolve the problem. If not, patients may be having a reaction to the insulin preservative or to the needle. If the problem does not resolve with the use of different brands of insulin or syringes, patients may have an insulin allergy (see Chapter 4).

5. *Storing the bottles of insulin.* Patients who plan to carry insulin with them during the day or when traveling can consult the *'97 Buyer's Guide to Diabetes Supplies*[3] and other diabetes publications or stores for various tote bags and insulin or syringe carrying cases. For patients who want to carry one or two prefilled syringes for a planned meal away from home, a simple solution is to use a toothbrush holder or a long, thin box such as a necklace or a watch box.

6. *Combining two types of insulin—basic technique.* Before starting the procedure for drawing up two insulins, have patients write down or verbalize the two dose markings that will be used—the dose of the first insulin to be drawn up and then the *total* dose of both insulins (add the two individual doses together). Mixing the insulins is carried out as follows (Fig. 10-13):

- Wipe both bottle tops with alcohol.
- Insert the needle through the rubber stopper of the short-acting (clear, regular) insulin.

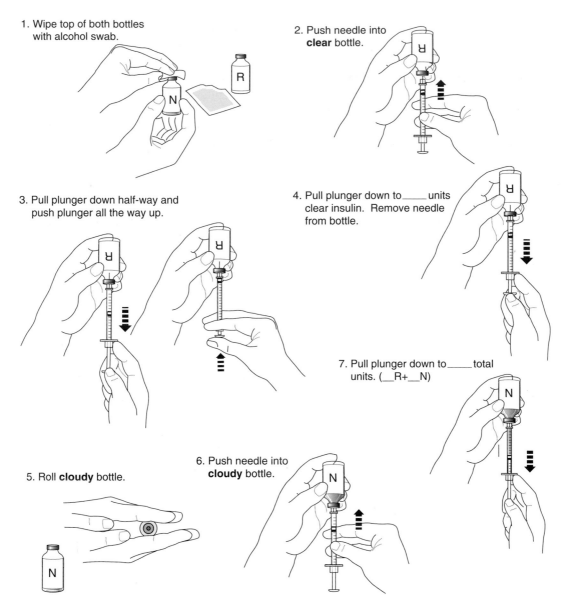

1. Wipe top of both bottles with alcohol swab.

2. Push needle into **clear** bottle.

3. Pull plunger down half-way and push plunger all the way up.

4. Pull plunger down to_____units clear insulin. Remove needle from bottle.

5. Roll **cloudy** bottle.

6. Push needle into **cloudy** bottle.

7. Pull plunger down to_____total units. (__R+__N)

Figure 10–13. Technique of withdrawing two different insulins from separate bottles into one syringe. (Injecting air into bottles not shown.) (See text for description.)

- Position the bottle upside down (and make sure the tip of the needle remains covered by solution).
- Pull the plunger approximately half-way down the syringe and then push it all the way back up, squirting all the insulin back into the bottle.

- Pull the plunger down again to the prescribed number of units of the regular insulin.
- Remove the syringe from the bottle.
- Mix the cloudy insulin by gently shaking or rolling the bottle.
- Insert the needle through the rubber

stopper of the longer-acting (cloudy, white, NPH or Lente) insulin.
- Pull the plunger down to the total dose calculated by adding the two doses together.
- Remove the syringe from the bottle.

Variations in the Technique of Combining Insulins

Troubleshooting for error in technique | Demonstrate for patients an error in technique in which the amount of the second insulin accidentally exceeds the correct total dose. Explain that the only option at that point is to squirt out all the insulin, discard it, and start over. Simply squirting out the excess insulin into the air or back into the bottle is not appropriate because it would result in an incorrect ratio of the two insulins.

Altering the order of insulin withdrawal | Generally, the regular (clear) insulin is drawn up first because accidental injection of a cloudy, delayed-acting insulin into the bottle of regular insulin may alter the time course of action of insulin remaining in the bottle. However, if patients have previously been taught to draw up the cloudy insulin first, they may continue to prepare the insulin this way provided the correct doses of both insulins are drawn up and the bottle of regular insulin appears clear and uncontaminated by cloudy insulin.

Premixed insulins | If a patient is unable to mix insulins, the physician may prescribe premixed insulins such as 70/30 or 50/50 with a set ratio of NPH and regular in the insulin bottle (provided the ratio of insulins appropriately matches the patient's insulin needs).

Prefilled syringes | Another option for patients unable to draw up insulin properly is to have family members or neighbors prefill 1 to 2 weeks' worth of syringes. These syringes can be stored in the refrigerator. Patients should be made aware that the insulin in the syringe settles and that rolling the syringe in the hands before the injection remixes the insulins and warms the syringe.

Adding regular insulin to the Lente series | Regular insulin added to NPH insulin has its usual time course of action. When regular insulin is added to Lente or Ultralente insulin, the time course of action is delayed. Patients having problems with blood glucose control because of delayed action of regular insulin mixed with a Lente insulin may need to take two separate injections rather than mix.

Basic Insulin Instruction—Theoretic Issues

The theoretic information about insulin that patients need to learn includes understanding how insulin works, how insulin relates to other variables that affect blood sugar control, and troubleshooting when there are changes in routine. This information can be quite complex and difficult for some patients to understand. Much of the information revolves around prevention of problems (such as hypoglycemia) that patients may never have experienced. The less well that patients seem able to comprehend theoretic information, the more practical and directed the information needs to be.

Start by asking questions such as, What does insulin do? If this is too broad, ask more specifically, Does insulin make your blood sugar go up or down? Can you name one thing that could make your sugar go down? (Answer: exercise, missed meal, delayed meal, too much insulin.) Can you name one thing that could make your sugar go up? (Answer: too much food, illness, too little insulin.) Alternatively, ask, Does food make your sugar go up or down? Does exercise make your blood sugar go up or down?

If patients are unable to answer the most basic questions, they need to be given very specific daily living and troubleshooting guidelines:

1. Take insulin at _____ (try to give a range of times).

2. Eat meals/snacks at _____ (again, give a range).

3. Don't skip meals—eat anything, even junk food, if you can't eat your normal meal on time.

4. If you miss your shot, just skip it. "When in doubt, leave it out."*

5. If you are supposed to skip a meal for medical reasons, call your doctor for advice. (If you can't reach your doctor, it is safer to miss one insulin shot.*)

Keep in mind that these recommendations are intended for the initial basic or survival education. During follow-up visits or phone calls, many patients can be taught a more flexible problem-solving approach to managing variations in schedule.

Comprehensive Insulin Instruction—Theoretic Issues

If patients seem comfortable describing the basic variables that cause an increase or decrease in blood glucose levels, they may then be ready to learn more sophisticated troubleshooting information.

Insulin timing | A practical approach to teaching the time course of insulin action is to identify which time periods during the day are covered by the different insulin doses (see Fig. 10-10). For example, for regular and NPH injections taken before breakfast and supper, the morning regular covers the

---

*These last recommendations may need to be altered for certain patients, especially those with type 1 diabetes. Usually, however, the acute complication of most concern with insulin-treated patients is hypoglycemia. Although hyperglycemia associated with missed doses is certainly a problem, one missed dose of insulin is less likely to cause DKA or hyperosmolar nonketotic syndrome than one poorly timed dose of insulin is to cause hypoglycemia.

breakfast to lunch time period, morning NPH the lunch to supper period, and evening regular the supper to bedtime snack period. Evening NPH works overnight.

If patients take only one or two of the four components of the insulin regimen listed earlier, the same information can be taught, making them aware of the time periods during the day that are not covered by the insulin taken.

To test patients' understanding of insulin timing and other variables, ask questions requiring application of knowledge, such as

- If you were going to exercise between breakfast and lunch, which insulin should be decreased? (Answer: morning regular.)
- If you got a low blood sugar reaction in the afternoon, which insulin would you blame? (Answer: morning NPH.)
- If you had to skip breakfast for a short morning dental appointment, which insulin could you skip? (Answer: morning regular.)
- To help reduce your high fasting blood sugars, which insulin dose should be increased? (Answer: evening NPH.)

TIMING OF MEALS AND INJECTIONS | More sophisticated patients can be given a more flexible routine in terms of insulin and meal timing. Rather than giving specific times always to eat or take injections, teach relationships between insulin timing and meals. For example, regular insulin is generally given 20 to 30 minutes before a meal. NPH insulin in the morning has a delayed and prolonged action that requires carbohydrate intake approximately every 4 to 5 hours during the day. NPH insulin in the evening helps control the body's own (liver) production of glucose during the night and is best taken approximately 8 to 10 hours before the anticipated time of arising in the morning. Thus, if patients plan to sleep late, the insulin could be given at a later time the night before. If the blood sugar is low at bedtime, a snack is usually required to prevent hypoglycemia in the middle of the night when the NPH starts to peak.

If patients stay up late or start their day later on days off, guidelines can be given for simply taking insulin doses at a later time, provided that the general guidelines for meal timing are followed. Patients who are taught how to vary their schedule need to understand clearly that avoidance of hypoglycemia is the main priority on days that follow a highly unusual pattern for them.

DELAYED/MISSED INSULIN DOSES | Teach patients what to expect if insulin doses are delayed or missed and how to adjust the insulin dosing. Refer to the original teaching approach of associating each insulin dose with a different time period of the day. It is important to avoid having two insulin doses that cover the sugar or peak during the same time period. For example, two NPH doses that are closer than 8 hours apart may overlap in terms of their hypoglycemic effect. Therefore, if a morning NPH injection is missed, it may be best to take regular alone at lunchtime rather than give the forgotten NPH dose at lunchtime because this late NPH dose may peak at night when the evening NPH and regular insulin doses are acting. A missed dose of regular insulin should generally be skipped entirely because postmeal regular insulin may cause hypoglycemia 3 to 4 hours after the injection.

INJECTING WHEN HYPERGLYCEMIC | To test patients' understanding, ask questions that require application of their knowledge—for example,

- If your blood sugar is high at the time of the injection, what could you do to help lower your blood sugar level? (Answer[s]: Delay the meal for 1 hour after the injection or take extra regular insulin according to your physician's guidelines or reduce the intake of carbohydrate at the meal.)

If patients are not able to answer such a broad question, specific situations can be discussed.

- If your sugar is high, do you think it's best to eat sooner than usual or to delay the meal longer than usual?
- If you cannot delay your meal more than usual, which of your usual breakfast foods might you eliminate from the meal?

Most importantly, explain to patients that all guidelines are personalized on the basis of frequent glucose monitoring, recording information, and reviewing information with their diabetes team.

INJECTING WHEN HYPOGLYCEMIC | Many patients assume that if their blood sugar is low (<100 mg/dl) before a meal, they do not need to take any insulin. To assess this, ask patients what they would do if their blood sugar were low and it was time to take insulin. Explain that it is normal for blood sugar levels to increase after meals. If patients are taking only NPH insulin, the prolonged nature of the insulin action gives them plenty of time to eat an extra snack or consume extra carbohydrate at the meal to prevent a decline in blood sugar level when the NPH insulin starts to work in 3 to 4 hours. If patients are taking regular insulin alone or combined with NPH insulin, they can either reduce their regular dose based on guidelines provided by their physician or eat a snack before the dose.

To help patients think of a solution, the following line of questioning may help: "At what blood sugar level do you feel comfortable taking your shot?" If patients cannot answer, be more specific. "If you had a blood sugar level of 150 mg/dl in the morning, would you take your usual shot? 130 mg/dl? 100 mg/dl?" Help patients identify the lowest blood sugar level at which they would take their injection. Then ask, "If you woke up with a reading of 75 mg/dl and you prefer to be over 120 mg/dl before taking your shot, what could you do to increase your blood sugar to 120 mg/dl?" This type of interaction helps patients to come up with their own solution and helps with applying this line of reasoning to other unexpected situations.

INJECTING FOR EXTRA FOOD INTAKE | Patients should be encouraged to find out which foods cause their highest blood glucose levels. Ask questions to help them discover their options for avoiding food-related hyperglycemia. Also, review the advantages and disadvantages of each option—for example,

Option 1 | Increase premeal regular insulin.
   Advantages. Allows more variable food intake with less hyperglycemia; gives patients a feeling of more flexibility.
   Disadvantages. Requires extra thinking and awareness with each meal; requires extra blood testing and documentation to test appropriateness of dose changes; may lead to weight gain owing to more relaxed approach to food intake.

Option 2 | Restrict or eliminate foods that cause excessive hyperglycemia.
   Advantages. Requires less thought and separate planning for different meals.
   Disadvantages. Feelings of deprivation; less enjoyment of meals.

Option 3 | Eat as desired; make no changes.
   Advantages. More flexibility, less preplanning, fewer feelings of deprivation.
   Disadvantages. Poor glucose control may lead to immediate symptoms such as fatigue or increased urination after the meal and may increase the chances of long-term diabetic complications.

The role of the diabetes educator within the empowerment approach is to help patients discover options available and to make sure patients are aware of the potential consequences of each course of action.

SPECIAL OCCASIONS | Holidays and family celebrations are frequently times when larger amounts of food and special desserts are eaten. More sophisticated patients can be guided through a series of questions to help them discover the various options available and the associated advantages and disadvantages as described earlier.

Less sophisticated patients are typically aware that avoidance of sweets and excess portions of fatty foods is advisable. If possible, direct patients to sources that can provide options for holiday foods that contain less fat and less sugar. Otherwise, patients can be greatly relieved of their anxiety and guilt by letting them know that one day of poor eating usually does not lead to immediate diabetic complications. Patients can be advised to attempt to take a walk and to increase water intake (to compensate for possible polyuria) after excessive food consumption. The educator may be able to advise a one-time insulin increase according to a physician's recommendation. Patients can be taught to reduce consumption of other carbohydrates, including healthy foods such as fruit or bread or potatoes, when a dessert is planned.

Some educators are concerned that teaching patients about this type of behavior and allowing it on special occasions may encourage more frequent dietary indiscretions. However, many diabetic patients choose to indulge whether or not they have discussed it with the diabetes team. An open discussion encourages better understanding of some immediate behaviors that help minimize the impact of dietary indiscretion and promotes more honesty and rapport in the relationship with patients and families.

INTENSIVE INSULIN THERAPY | For highly sophisticated patients who wish to have greater flexibility in meal timing and content, along with improved glycemic control, a number of intensive insulin regimens are available. Generally, the more injections per day and the more doses of regular insulin that are used, the more flexible a patient's life style can be. Another intensive insulin regimen involves use of an insulin pump (discussed later). It is outside the scope of this chapter to expand on the different intensive insulin regimens. Educators interested in this topic should read Chapter 4 and information located in books and magazines listed in the Appendix.

ALTERNATIVE METHODS OF INSULIN DELIVERY

Several devices have been developed in an attempt to simplify the procedures involved in drawing up and injecting insulin. These devices may be especially useful for patients injecting insulin several times per day.

INJECTION PORTS | These devices are similar in concept to intravenous ports used for intravenous piggyback medications in hospitalized patients. However, they are inserted by patients into the subcutaneous tissue and remain in place for 2 to 3 days. The Button Infuser has a 27-gauge needle attached to a resealable injection port. A newer device called the Insulfon has a flexible Teflon catheter with an injection port attached. Inside the Teflon catheter, this device has an introducer needle that is removed once the catheter is in place. Patients then give their insulin injections through the resealable port rather than puncture their skin many times daily.

INSULIN PENS | These devices use small (200-U) prefilled insulin cartridges that are housed in a penlike holder. A disposable needle is attached to the device for injection of the insulin. Insulin is delivered by dialing in a dose and/or pushing a button for every 1- or 2-U increment given. The insulin pen eliminates the need to draw up insulin before each injection. These devices are most useful for patients who need to inject only one type of insulin each time (e.g., premeal regu-

lar three times a day and bedtime NPH) or who can use premixed insulin (70% NPH/30% regular).

JET INJECTORS | As an alternative to needle injections, jet injection devices deliver insulin through the skin under pressure in an extremely fine stream. These devices are more expensive than the other alternative devices mentioned earlier and require thorough training and supervision when first used. In addition, patients should be cautioned that absorption rates, peak insulin activity, and insulin levels may be different when switching to a jet injector. (Insulin given by jet injector usually works faster.)

INSULIN PUMPS | Small, externally worn pump devices attempt to mimic the functioning of the normal pancreas by supplying insulin in a similar manner. Insulin pumps contain a syringe attached to a long (42-inch), thin, spaghetti-like tube with a needle or Teflon catheter attached to the end. Patients insert the needle or catheter into the subcutaneous tissue (usually on the abdomen) and secure it with tape or a transparent dressing. The needle or catheter is changed at least every 2 to 3 days. The pump is then worn either on a belt or in a pocket. Some women keep the pump tucked into the front or side of their bra or wear it on a garter belt on the thigh.

The pump delivers only regular insulin, which is delivered in two different ways. First, a continuous basal rate of insulin is typically infused at a rate of 0.5 to 2.0 U/h. Then, before each meal, patients activate the pump (through a series of button pushes) to deliver a bolus dose of insulin. Patients can decide on the amount of insulin bolus to give on the basis of blood glucose levels. For some patients, anticipated food intake and activity level also influence that decision.

Intensive training and follow-up are necessary for successful insulin pump therapy. Patients interested in this method of insulin administration should be referred to a diabetes program with a health care team experienced in the use of insulin pumps.

HYPOGLYCEMIA

FOR THE DIABETES EDUCATOR

Definition

Hypoglycemia is defined as a blood glucose level <50 to 60 mg/dl, often associated with symptoms (although some patients with diabetes lose their hypoglycemic warning signs, which is known as *hypoglycemia unawareness*). It can occur suddenly and is caused by an imbalance between the amount of insulin available (including increased insulin secretion caused by sulfonylurea agents), food eaten, and activity. Some patients, however, may experience signs and symptoms of hypoglycemia when the blood glucose level is much higher than 50 to 60 mg/dl. These patients have been in poor control previously and have accommodated to higher blood glucose levels. More normal glucose concentrations are perceived as too low. Patients may take several weeks to accommodate to these new, lower glucose levels. Other terms that patients may use to refer to hypoglycemia include *insulin shock* and *insulin reactions*. Insulin-treated patients who maintain near normal blood glucose levels may experience two to three mild (easily recognized and treated) episodes of hypoglycemia per week.

Signs and Symptoms (see Table 7–18)

The body has two main responses to hypoglycemia. First, several hormones (glucagon, epinephrine, growth hormone, and cortisol) are released into the bloodstream to help increase the amount of circulating glucose. The former two hormones act rapidly to bring blood glucose levels back up to normal. Epinephrine causes the autonomic (ad-renergic) symptoms of hypoglycemia, which include weakness, sweating, nervousness, anxiety, tachycardia, shakiness, tingling of the mouth or fingers, and hunger.

The second type of response to hypoglycemia results from a decreased level of glucose in the brain. These symptoms are called *neuroglucopenic* and may include headache, visual disturbances, mental dullness, confusion, amnesia, seizures, or coma. Patients who have had type 1 diabetes for ≥5 years have lost their ability to secrete glucagon in response to hypoglycemia, and some patients (after having diabetes for a longer duration) lose their ability to secrete epinephrine as well. Therefore, those patients who have lost both hormonal responses have no immediate defense against hypoglycemia, do not experience the autonomic symptoms of hypoglycemia, and develop only the much more serious neuroglucopenic symptoms. Tight control of blood glucose levels can lower the threshold for sensing hypoglycemia. In addition, hypoglycemia on one day can cause a decrease in hypoglycemic symptoms on the next day.

Causes

The main causes of hypoglycemia in diabetic patients include too much insulin (if taking insulin), sulfonylurea agents, too little food (carbohydrate), a delayed or missed meal, or excessive physical activity. Alcohol consumption may contribute to hypoglycemia if patients miss meals. In many cases, however, the exact reason why the hypoglycemia occurred is impossible to determine.

INADEQUATE FOOD INTAKE | When patients are initially started on insulin, the insulin doses are chosen to match their anticipated meal plan. Therefore, if patients' food intake decreases, that usual insulin dose may be excessive. This can occur when patients miss a meal, attempt to reduce their caloric intake, or choose to eat less for a given meal. Patients on intensive insulin regimens can reduce their premeal insulin dose, but those without this flexibility may develop hypoglycemia. If changes in the meal plan are persistent, the physician should alter the patient's insulin regimen (or sulfonylurea agent dose). If patients must delay a meal, they should be instructed to eat a small snack containing carbohydrate at the usual mealtime to prevent the occurrence of hypoglycemia.

INSULIN | Accidental injection of too much insulin may lead to hypoglycemia. Patients need to be as precise as possible in drawing up insulin. If visual problems develop, the patient's diabetes health care team should be notified. Additionally, any planned changes in diet or physical activity should be discussed with the physician so that insulin dose changes can be made.

The area into which insulin is injected may occasionally contribute to hypoglycemia. For example, exercise increases the blood flow to the area of the body being used. If insulin is injected into the thigh and the patient then performs exercises using the thigh (e.g., running), the increased blood flow to this area may cause insulin to be absorbed into the bloodstream more rapidly. Similarly, insulin injected into muscle rather than fat tissue may be carried into the bloodstream more rapidly, causing hypoglycemia.

EXERCISE | During exercise, the muscles use up glucose, which can decrease the level of glucose in the bloodstream, especially if preexercise glucose levels are normal to low. If patients using insulin do not eat extra carbohydrate before strenuous exercise, they may develop hypoglycemia. It is important to realize that any physical activities (including those not typically viewed as exercise) may cause hypoglycemia. These include gardening, cleaning, shopping, vacuuming, and moving furniture. Increasing food intake before these activities (or planning physical activity immediately after scheduled meals or snacks, when the glucose level is the highest) is important. A more detailed discussion

of how exercise causes hypoglycemia can be found in Chapter 7, and an approach to preventing exercise-induced hypoglycemia in Chapter 3.

ALCOHOL | Although a moderate amount of alcohol may be safely added to the diet if taken with meals, it can contribute to hypoglycemia if patients eat irregularly when drinking alcohol. Normally, when a person is not eating, the liver produces glucose to prevent hypoglycemia. Alcohol interferes with the ability of the liver to produce glucose (specifically, it inhibits gluconeogenesis). If a diabetic patient is taking insulin or a sulfonylurea agent, has not eaten for a while, and then drinks alcohol, hypoglycemia may occur if the individual does not eat for several more hours.

Treatment (Patient Conscious)

The treatment of hypoglycemia is to eat some form of sugar. The amount of sugar recommended for treating hypoglycemia varies from 10 to 20 g of glucose. Patients may use commercial preparations of glucose, such as glucose that comes in 3- and 5-g tablets. These are chewable tablets that dissolve rapidly when eaten, and some brands are available in various flavors. Also available are glucose gels. Other sources of concentrated sugar include juice, soda (nondiet), table sugar, honey, and LifeSavers (see Table 7-19). It is preferable to use commercial preparations of glucose because they provide a precise amount of glucose, are rapidly absorbed, and may offer less temptation to patients to overtreat hypoglycemia. *If patients are taking acarbose (Precose), an oral antidiabetic medication, they must take a commercial preparation of glucose or milk to treat hypoglycemia. Acarbose blocks the digestion of most carbohydrates such as table sugar, those in fruit and juice, and starches. Therefore, eating these carbohydrates does not correct low blood glucose levels.*

After taking approximately 10 to 15 g of glucose, patients should wait 10 to 15 minutes for the symptoms to resolve. If they have no improvement, they should take another 10 g of glucose. Once symptoms begin to resolve, a small snack should be eaten to prevent the recurrence of hypoglycemia. This snack should include a small amount of starch (one bread exchange) and 1 to 2 ounces of protein. Examples include cheese and crackers, milk and crackers, or half of a sandwich. If the next meal is to be eaten in 30 to 60 minutes, the snack is not necessary.

The use of dessert foods such as candy, cookies, and ice cream for treatment of hypoglycemia should be avoided. These foods are high in calories and may not work as rapidly to increase the blood glucose level because of the high fat content (which delays absorption of carbohydrate). In addition, it is difficult for many patients while experiencing hypoglycemic symptoms to limit the amount of sugar eaten in this form. From a psychologic perspective, dessert foods may be seen as a reward for experiencing hypoglycemia. This may limit patients' perception of the seriousness of this diabetic emergency and the importance of recognizing and treating hypoglycemia.

To avoid delays in treatment of hypoglycemia, patients should always carry some form of sugar and always wear and carry some form of identification (see Appendix). If patients taking insulin experience unusual symptoms at any time, it is always safer to treat the symptoms as if hypoglycemia has occurred rather than delay treatment because of uncertainty about the cause of symptoms. On the other hand, if they have the opportunity, patients may wish to measure the blood glucose level to document hypoglycemia. However, transient hyperglycemia does not create the same danger as worsening hypoglycemia.

Treatment (Patient Unconscious or Unwilling to Eat)

The commercial preparations and foods discussed earlier are effective only when swallowed. Therefore, they cannot be used if patients are unconscious.

An injection of glucagon (1 mg) should be given to persons who lose consciousness because of a severe hypoglycemic reaction or who, after repeated attempts, absolutely refuse to take sugar by mouth (the irrational behavior is usually a result of the hypoglycemia). As discussed earlier, glucagon (a hormone that is made by the α-cells in the islets of Langerhans in the pancreas) raises the blood glucose level by causing the liver to produce more glucose. It is sold as a prescription drug for emergencies and is a powder. A solution (diluent) to mix with the powder is provided in the package, either in a separate bottle or in a prefilled syringe. If in a bottle, draw up the liquid in the patient's (1 ml) insulin syringe. The liquid must be mixed with the powder until the resulting solution is clear (which occurs rapidly). All of the solution is then drawn up in the syringe provided or in the patient's (1 ml) insulin syringe and injected.

After the injection, turn the head of an unconscious patient to the side to avoid choking in case vomiting occurs when consciousness is regained. The glucagon may require 15 to 20 minutes to take effect. When patients regain consciousness, give them sugar and a snack for prevention of another hypoglycemic reaction. If no response occurs within 15 to 20 minutes, paramedics should be called.

The technique for drawing up and injecting glucagon should be taught to a family member, coworker, neighbor, or other person who spends time with the patient. It is sometimes helpful to encourage patients to allow this person to draw up and inject insulin on a periodic basis to maintain confidence in the skills required to use a syringe and give an injection under emergency conditions.

Hypoglycemia: Patient Education

Until patients actually experience hypoglycemic symptoms, it may be difficult for them to comprehend or memorize the symptoms and treatment for hypoglycemia. Simply giving patients a list or pamphlet describing the symptoms (especially if low and high blood sugar are addressed in the same pamphlet) does not usually ensure comprehension. Patients may be confused to find some similarities in the list of symptoms for low and high sugar (headache, fatigue, weakness, blurry vision). Patients may feel undue pressure to be able to differentiate hypoglycemia from hyperglycemia before treating themselves with carbohydrate consumption. Thus, for safety purposes, with new diabetic patients, it is important for the educator to emphasize the more serious nature of low sugar (as compared with high sugar) and to reassure patients that eating sugar when it was not really low does not have serious consequences for a hyperglycemic patient. Emphasize that problems resulting from low blood sugar can develop rapidly (minutes to 1 hour), whereas problems due to high blood sugar take much longer to develop (days to weeks).

Basic Teaching Guidelines

Listed next are some basic facts to address with both newly diagnosed diabetic patients and veteran diabetic patients, especially if a sulfonylurea agent or insulin has been added to the regimen. In addition to reviewing the symptoms, emphasize that

- Low blood sugar is an emergency.
- If you feel any unusual symptoms, eat sugar immediately.
- To treat low blood sugar, or hypoglycemia, we want you to eat the type of foods that you usually are supposed to avoid.
- Carry some form of sugar (sugar packets, LifeSavers, raisins, dextrose tablets) at all times.
- Don't worry about making a mistake. If you are not sure that you are having a low sugar reaction, eat sugar anyway.

- Low blood sugar is more of an emergency than high blood sugar.
- It's important to learn to avoid low blood sugar by eating snacks and extra food. Even though a low sugar reaction might not feel very serious, it can cause terrible problems if it happens in a dangerous place (like when you are driving).

Teaching Tips for All Patients

To reinforce the importance of carrying some form of sugar and identification, ask patients at each visit to show the nurse the sugar source being carried for treatment of hypoglycemia and identification tags/cards. If possible, keep a supply of sample glucose products available to give patients who are not carrying any sugar. Be sure to explain to patients that it is not safe to plan on purchasing soda or juice as needed whenever hypoglycemia occurs. Rather, encourage patients to carry the sugar constantly, especially when driving or participating in physical activity.

Prevention

Many patients may be tempted to increase their dose of oral agent or insulin on finding an elevated glucose result. They should not do this on the basis of one result only (unless given guidance on using extra amounts of regular insulin to compensate). In addition, patients taking medication need to understand that it is not safe to assume that they will always feel a low blood sugar reaction in an appropriate location and time frame to prevent a serious problem. Thus, rather than waiting until the symptoms occur, prevention is crucial.

1. Consistent technique of insulin injection and rotation of sites are important (see the earlier section on insulin).
2. Insulin dosage should be adjusted only according to a physician's guidelines.

3. If meals are going to be more than 4 to 5 hours apart, a snack should be eaten.

4. Eat extra food before engaging in some forms of exercise. (More experienced or sophisticated patients may be taught to lower the appropriate insulin dose.)

5. When patients are sick and normal intake of food is decreased (but the insulin dose remains the same), they should eat any form of carbohydrate (e.g., regular soda, Jell-O, ice cream) (see the later section on sick day rules).

HYPERGLYCEMIA

FOR THE DIABETES EDUCATOR

The syndromes of hyperglycemia (high blood sugar) are (1) diabetes out of control, (2) diabetic ketoacidosis (DKA), and (3) hyperosmolar nonketotic syndrome (HNKS).

Diabetic control is a term used to describe a patient's usual blood glucose concentrations. Poor control signifies marked hyperglycemia; strict or tight control implies glucose levels more near normal. Uncontrolled diabetes leads to the symptoms of polyuria, polydipsia, and nocturia. An explanation of both normal and abnormal glucose metabolism follows to provide a detailed understanding of the processes that lead to hyperglycemia.

Postprandial (After Eating)—Normal State

After gastrointestinal absorption of the carbohydrate contained in a meal, plasma glucose levels rise. This stimulates insulin secretion from the pancreatic β-cells located in the islets of Langerhans. After its release, insulin binds to specific receptors located on the cell surfaces of liver, muscles, and fat tissue, where it exerts an effect for several hours after its binding. This results in the storage of the carbohydrate from the meal largely as glycogen (the storage form of glu-

cose). In persons without diabetes, glucose levels rise between 20 and 50 mg/dl 1 to 2 hours after a meal and return to baseline before the next meal.

Postabsorptive (Fasting)—Normal State

In the postabsorptive state (i.e., after all of the food from meals has been absorbed and stored in the tissue); glucose concentrations are regulated within a narrow range (70 to 100 mg/dl). This is accomplished by very precise mechanisms by which the liver releases almost the exact amount of glucose that the tissues require. The glucose is produced by the liver through two separate pathways, *glycogenolysis* (breakdown of glycogen) and *gluconeogenesis* (synthesis of new glucose from other molecules). The control of glucose production by the liver is regulated by the balance between insulin (which inhibits production of glucose) and glucagon (which stimulates production of glucose).

Postprandial Hyperglycemia

When carbohydrate metabolism begins to deteriorate, diabetes starts to develop. Postprandial blood glucose concentrations fail to return to normal before the next meal. Once glucose levels exceed the kidneys' ability for glucose reabsorption, glucose is lost in the urine and urine test results for glucose become positive (glucosuria). This usually occurs at glucose levels >180 mg/dl. Patients often have minimal or no symptoms at this time, although they may complain of mild fatigue.

Fasting Hyperglycemia

The next stage of worsening carbohydrate metabolism is the loss of normal regulation of glucose production by the liver. This leads to fasting hyperglycemia, which leads to even higher preprandial and postprandial blood glucose levels. When blood glucose levels become higher, usually >180 mg/dl (or higher in older patients), they exceed the renal threshold for glucose. This means that sugar is lost in the urine. When glucose is in the urine, water is drawn out with it; hence, patients start to urinate frequently (polyuria)—especially noticeable at night (nocturia)—and drink increasing amounts of fluids (polydipsia). As insulin becomes increasingly unavailable and/or ineffective, the body is unable to utilize sufficient calories. This leads to weight loss even though patients usually have increased hunger (polyphagia).

The phenomenon of diabetes out of control can usually be treated in the outpatient setting with close follow-up. Patients with type 2 diabetes may either be relatively asymptomatic and may have had a blood glucose level measured for other reasons or may have sought medical attention for symptoms of poorly controlled diabetes (polyuria, polydipsia, nocturia, and/or unintentional weight loss). For type 2 diabetic patients, outpatient treatment may involve initiating diet measures and starting or increasing oral diabetes medication. It is imperative that patients be able to retain fluids. If patients are vomiting and/or unable to drink fluids, then hospitalization is often needed because they are at risk for developing severe dehydration, or HNKS (described later).

Diabetes out of control in type 1 diabetic patients may be a more serious situation because it can rapidly progress to DKA, which, if untreated, can render patients seriously ill. If patients are newly diagnosed with type 1 diabetes or are vomiting and unable to drink fluids, hospitalization is often needed.

Ketosis

In patients whose diabetes is out of control and in whom the amount of effective insulin becomes very low or absent (usually only in type 1 diabetes), an increase in ketone body formation, or ketosis, can occur. This occurs because without insulin, the body cannot utilize glucose effectively. Therefore, fat breakdown occurs to provide extra energy. A byproduct of increased fat breakdown is ketone body formation (by the liver). If patients do not receive insulin (and the pancreas is not able to produce insulin, as in type 1 diabetes), ketone body production increases, causing an acid-base imbalance called DKA.

Diabetic Ketoacidosis (DKA)

If a patient develops DKA and is not treated quickly and appropriately, coma and eventually death ensue. The biochemical hallmarks of DKA are electrolyte depletion, dehydration, and acidosis (see Chapter 6 for a detailed discussion of DKA).

Symptoms

The signs and symptoms of DKA result from the high levels of blood glucose and ketone bodies (Fig. 10-14). In an attempt to rid the body of the excess glucose, the kidneys excrete extra glucose and water. Both urination and thirst increase. In addition, high blood glucose levels and dehydration can lead to headache, weakness, and fatigue.

The acidosis caused by the ketone bodies produces an additional set of symptoms. Most importantly, patients often have abdominal pain, nausea, and vomiting and are unable to ingest the fluids necessary to prevent worsening dehydration. Symptoms of acidosis often include difficulty in catching one's breath, rapid or deep breathing, headache, and a sweet or fruity smell on the breath.

Causes

A common cause of DKA is illness. During illness, insulin resistance tends to increase, with a subsequent increase in blood glucose levels. It is important that patients do not omit insulin injections when ill, even if regular meals are not being eaten. Patients also

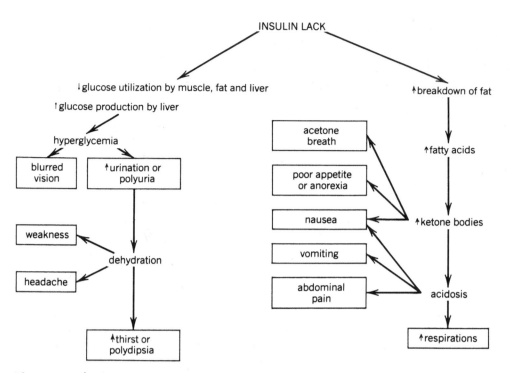

Figure 10–14. Abnormal metabolism that causes signs and symptoms of diabetic ketoacidosis. ↑, increased; ↓, decreased.

must receive prompt medical treatment for any infectious process that may develop, in order to avoid triggering DKA. Stopping insulin injections or inappropriately decreasing the dose of insulin can cause DKA in patients with type 1 diabetes. All of the causes of DKA listed earlier can largely be prevented if patients are treated appropriately with adequate insulin therapy throughout periods of illness as well as health. However, some patients (often children) who do not know they have diabetes first come to the attention of their physicians with DKA as the initial manifestation of their disease.

Treatment

In the early stages of DKA, treatment includes adjustment or initiation (if DKA is the initial sign of diabetes) of insulin therapy and drinking large quantities of salt-containing fluids. For more advanced cases, especially if nausea and vomiting prevent oral intake of fluids, hospitalization is necessary to institute treatment. In the hospital, patients are given a large volume of intravenous fluids for the first several hours, along with potassium and other electrolytes. In addition, insulin is given in an intravenous solution. DKA is usually resolved within 24 hours, although treatment sometimes takes longer. It is important to treat the underlying cause of the DKA if one is present. Once patients have recovered from their DKA, subcutaneous insulin injections must be started when the intravenous insulin infusion is stopped. Otherwise, patients could become insulin deficient again and have a another episode of DKA.

Prevention and Education

The most important way for patients to prevent DKA is to take insulin every day and to call their medical care provider if they become ill with elevated blood glucose levels. If a patient becomes ill, sick day rules (discussed later) should be followed to avert the development of DKA.

Hyperosmolar Nonketotic Syndrome (HNKS)

In patients with type 2 diabetes, some insulin is still being produced by the pancreas (even if patients have to take insulin to help control blood glucose levels) and prevents the development of ketoacidosis. However, symptomatic hyperglycemia can occur in patients with type 2 diabetes, especially during periods of illness or stress. In a few patients (often the elderly), the polyuria and polydipsia are ignored, and symptomatic hyperglycemia is tolerated for many weeks. In this situation, hyperglycemia can become so profound and prolonged that patients can experience extreme dehydration with glucose levels exceeding 1,000 mg/dl. This causes decreased mentation that can progress to coma. When this occurs, it is called *nonketotic hyperosmolar coma.*

Symptoms

The symptoms are similar to those of DKA, except that overbreathing and a fruity odor on the breath do not occur. The gastrointestinal symptoms (nausea, vomiting, abdominal pain) usually are less severe or are absent. Increased urination and thirst are most prominent. Patients may have seizures or symptoms similar to having a stroke (e.g., slurred speech, weakness of an arm or leg).

Causes

HNKS is often associated with an illness or infection. It is important for patients with type 2 diabetes to realize that illness can cause increases in blood glucose levels and that communication with a physician during times of illness is important. The general sick day rules should be followed, as indicated.

Patients with type 2 diabetes do not need to test their urine for ketones, but blood (or urine) glucose monitoring, eating and drinking properly, and notifying a physician of symptoms are important. Some patients with type 2 diabetes may temporarily require insulin during illness or other stressful situations, such as surgery, to avoid severe hyperglycemia or HNKS.

Treatment

The treatment of HNKS is similar to that of DKA, although the dehydration may be more severe and patients (who tend to be elderly) may tolerate vigorous fluid replacement poorly. Treatment of HNKS usually takes several days longer than treatment of DKA, because patients with HNKS tend to be sicker and to have more severe hyperglycemia. Unlike patients with DKA, however, patients with HNKS may not need insulin when they leave the hospital (i.e., they can be treated with diet alone or in combination with oral diabetes medications). It is very important to search for the cause of patients' HNKS because many have an underlying infection, myocardial infarction, or other illness that requires treatment in addition to the treatment of HNKS.

SICK DAY RULES

FOR THE DIABETES EDUCATOR

When teaching a patient about sick day rules, it is important to differentiate between patients with type 1 diabetes and type 2 diabetes (even though some may be treated with insulin). This is discussed earlier but is particularly important in this section because patients with type 1 diabetes can develop DKA in the absence of adequate intake of carbohydrate and injection of insulin whereas sick patients with type 2 diabetes with a decreased caloric intake may not require any insulin at all. In patients with type

How To Test

You can buy a ketone testing kit at your pharmacy. You don't need a prescription. Don't wait until you're sick to get one—keep one in your house and check the expiration date every six months.

Urine tests for ketones come in three forms: test strips, tapes, and tablets. To test:

1. Dip the strip or tape in your urine, or put drops of urine on a tablet.

2. Wait. The directions tell you how long—from 10 seconds to two minutes, depending on the brand you're using.

3. Match the color of the strip, tape, or tablet to the color chart on the package.

Results will be negative, trace, small, moderate, or large.

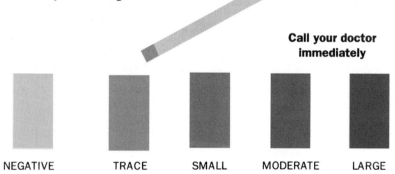

Call your doctor immediately

NEGATIVE   TRACE   SMALL   MODERATE   LARGE

Figure 10–15. Patient instructions for urine testing for ketones. (From Lebovitz HE: Keeping clear of ketoacidosis. Diabetes Forecast December:20-23, 1995.

1 diabetes, testing for urine ketones (Fig. 10-15) is necessary during periods of illness because hyperglycemia with negative urine ketones is not as serious a condition as hyperglycemia in the presence of small to moderate urine ketones, which could portend the development of DKA.

PATIENT EDUCATION: HYPERGLYCEMIA

Patients can become confused or forgetful if they are simply given a list of symptoms of hyperglycemia. They may notice that some of the symptoms are similar to those associated with hypoglycemia, such as fatigue, drowsiness, or blurred vision. To assist learning, the educator can provide an image or "anchor" with which patients can associate hyperglycemia. If patients have already had the experience of symptomatic hyperglycemia, ask them to describe the feelings in their own words. Make sure they are aware that these are the symptoms to associate with high blood glucose levels. For sophisticated patients, the educator could describe the progression of hyperglycemia as presented earlier in this section.

If patients have not experienced symptomatic hyperglycemia and need a simplified explanation, the educator could use an image such as, "When your blood sugar is high, the blood is filled with sugar and is very sweet and sticky. This makes you move slowly (like honey) and feel tired. Your body wants to get rid of the sugar or clean it out, so it pushes the sugar out into your urine and this makes you urinate a lot. Your body also tries to get more water to water down all the extra sugar, so it takes water from your tongue and mouth (dry mouth, thirst), and from your eyes (blurry vision)." Learning is most effective if the educator involves patients in the discussion by asking questions during the explanation (e.g., "When your body wants to get rid of the extra sugar, how can the sugar escape from your body? If your body takes a lot of water from your mouth and tongue, how does it make you feel?").

Hyperglycemia/Sick Day Rules— Type 2 Diabetes

1. *Hyperglycemia may not always cause dramatic (noticeable) symptoms.* Therefore, after diabetes is diagnosed, it is important to have regular doctor appointments and blood tests even if you feel well.

2. *Symptom education/recognition.* Symptoms of hyperglycemia include fatigue, thirst, excess urination, blurry vision, vaginal infections, and sores that heal slowly over a period of a few days or weeks. (At this point, have a discussion with patients in which they describe past experiences of hyperglycemia, or give patients an anchor story as described earlier.)

3. *Causes of hyperglycemia.* Blood sugar levels may increase in certain situations, such as increased stress, illness, or surgery. Certain medications, such as asthma medicine or steroids, may cause very high blood sugar levels. Increases in blood sugar levels may also result from an inadequate dose of diabetes medication, especially when combined with problems with diet recommendations or a decrease in exercise.

4. *Treatment of hyperglycemia.* Drink fluids, test your blood sugar level (if you have the equipment), and stay in touch with your diabetes health care professional. To avoid dehydration, *drink extra fluids* (at least one glass every hour) even if you are not thirsty. Good choices include water, broth, decaffeinated tea, diet soda, diet iced tea, diet Kool-Aid, and sugar-free Popsicles. *Take all diabetic medications.* However, sometimes the doctor may tell you to change the amount of medication. Also, the doctor may prescribe antibiotics if you have an infection—be sure to take all of the antibiotic pills, even if you are feeling better.

5. *Sick day rules: Appetite normal or slightly reduced.* If you are sick and your appetite is normal, be sure to take all of your diabetic medication and drink extra fluids. If you are sick and your appetite is less than normal, take all your diabetic medication and eat smaller meals every few hours, along with extra fluids. Avoid foods that are high in fat content and avoid dairy products if you have diarrhea.

6. *Sick day rules: Appetite poor or unable to eat solid foods.* In this situation, the ability to monitor blood glucose levels at home can be useful in making decisions about what to eat and what medication to take. It is important to continue drinking fluids and to communicate with your diabetes health care provider. If your blood sugar levels are high (>250 mg/dl), drink sugar-free fluids as listed earlier, and if they are low (<150 mg/dl), drink sugar-containing fluids. In some instances, it may be necessary to decrease your diabetes medication (especially if symptoms of low blood sugar levels develop). In other circumstances, no dose change should occur. Be sure to continue taking your diabetes medication as prescribed until you speak with your diabetes health care provider, who can give you advice and follow you through

your illness. It is particularly important to do this if your blood sugar levels remain >300 mg/dl or <100 mg/dl.

7. *Signs of severe dehydration.* If you become sick and unable to eat or drink, you can become dehydrated. If this occurs, you or your family must call your doctor or you must be taken to the hospital, especially if you become confused or sleepy or cannot be awakened.

Hyperglycemia/Sick Day Rules— Type 1 Diabetes

1. *Insulin: Never stop taking insulin.* Patients with type 1 diabetes should take their usual dose of insulin when they are ill (including sliding-scale regular insulin), unless instructed by their physician to do otherwise. For patients with type 1 diabetes, insulin is needed even if food intake is decreased. Illness tends to raise blood sugar levels, and thus the same dose or even more insulin usually is safe. Patients with type 2 diabetes who require insulin may be able to lower the dose if food intake is markedly decreased. A physician's guidance is often needed (see number 3 below for guidelines for eating).

2. *Monitoring: Check the blood (or urine) sugar* at least four times a day. In patients with type 1 diabetes, *urine testing for ketones* should occur several times per day, especially when blood sugar levels are >250 mg/dl in association with illness. *Notify your physician* if the urine ketones become more than trace positive and/or the blood glucose level is >300 mg/dl (or urine sugar levels are 1% to 2%).

3. *Eating:* If the normal meal pattern cannot be followed, eat soft foods or drink liquids instead. It may by necessary to eat soft foods or drink liquids that contain sugar in order to avoid hypoglycemia. Having food and liquids with salt and minerals is also important. Table 10–7 contains a list of foods commonly used for carbohydrate replacement during an illness. Some examples of soft foods include 1/3 cup regular gelatin, 1

cup cream soup, 1/2 cup custard, and three squares of graham crackers. Eat these six to eight times per day until the regular diet is resumed. Examples of liquids include 1/2 cup regular cola, 1/2 cup orange juice, 1 cup Gatorade, and 1/2 cup broth. Drink these every hour if you have vomiting, diarrhea, or a fever. It is important to drink liquids whenever you have an illness. However, if soft foods or the normal foods can be eaten, limit liquids to broth, tea, water, and diet drinks (i.e., limit the source of carbohydrates to the more slowly absorbable foods rather than the more rapidly absorbed liquids).

4. *Reporting symptoms: Keep your physician informed!* It may be possible to prevent ketoacidosis and avoid hospitalization. Report nausea, vomiting, and diarrhea to your physician, especially if it has not been possible to retain fluids for 3 to 4 hours. Also report any symptoms of possible DKA, such as abdominal pain, fruity breath, or inability to catch your breath. It is usually necessary for persons who have type 1 diabetes and who are unable to retain fluids to be hospitalized to avoid severe dehydration and ketoacidosis.

CHRONIC COMPLICATIONS

FOR THE DIABETES EDUCATOR

The long-term complications of diabetes are considered part of the diabetes syndrome, and in many cases, preventing these complications is the primary goal of diabetes treatment. The classification of the complications is summarized in Table 10–8 (see Chapter 8 for a more detailed discussion).

QUESTIONS TO TEST KNOWLEDGE/ STIMULATE THOUGHTS

When teaching patients about diabetic complications, it is helpful first to ask them if they are aware of any problems or complica-

Table 10–7. Sick Day Diet

Stage	Symptoms	Foods	Frequency
1	Severe nausea, vomiting, severe diarrhea, fever	Orange juice, grapefruit juice, tomato juice, broth, strong tea, coffee, cola, soft drinks.	Sip a tablespoon of liquid every 10 to 15 minutes. Advance to stage 2 when the nausea and the diarrhea have stopped or almost stopped and you are no longer vomiting.
2	Little or no appetite, occasional diarrhea, fatigue, fever	Cream soup, mashed potatoes, cooked cereal, plain yogurt, banana, ice cream, fruit-flavored gelatins, juice, broth, regular soft drinks.	Take 1/2 cup to 1 cup of food or liquid every 1 to 2 hours. Advance to stage 3 when you have eaten this amount of food several times and your symptoms are improving.
3	Limited appetite but can tolerate small meals, sluggish, slight fever, can be sitting up and walking	Food choices are selected using your diabetic meal plan (if you do not have one, talk to a dietitian or diet counselor). At this stage, you do not have to eat your protein and fat food choices. If you feel up to it, advance to stage 4.	Eat as many meals and snacks as planned in your meal plan. This usually means three meals plus an evening snack.
4	General sick feeling; heavy or spicy foods are upsetting	Use your food lists and follow your regular meal. Choose foods that do not give you problems (avoid spicy or high-fat foods). For protein choices, you might want to choose scrambled or soft boiled eggs, cottage cheese, broiled fish, or baked chicken. Eat fruit, vegetables, starch, and protein in moderate amounts according to your usual meal pattern.	Eat at regular meal and snack times. Advance to your regular diabetic meal plan if you have no problems with the easier-to-digest foods for a day. If at any stage your symptoms get worse and you cannot tolerate the described foods, drop back one stage until you feel better.

From Getting Started—Answers to Questions About Sick Days. Becton Dickinson Consumer Products, Becton Dickinson Company, Rochelle Park, NJ, 1995.

tions that can happen to people who have diabetes. The diabetes educator should take some time to find out if patients have any particular fears or worries based on past experiences with relatives or acquaintances who suffered a diabetic complication. It is important to try to instill a sense of hope and optimism about the ability of the patient and the health care team working together to prevent diabetic complications. The educator needs to acknowledge that this is not easy to do and requires some work and commitment.

Some patients may be confused by the seemingly unrelated list of problems that can result from diabetes. A simplified introductory explanation may help. Patients can be taught that high blood sugar can damage very small blood vessels of the body (such as those found inside the eyes and kidneys) and the nerves (such as those found in the feet and legs). The problem is that the dam-

Table 10–8. Long-Term Complications of Diabetes Mellitus

Macrovascular (large vessel or atherosclerosis)
  Coronary artery disease (angina, myocardial infarction)
  Cerebrovascular disease (stroke)
  Peripheral vascular disease
Microvascular (small vessel)
  Retinopathy (eye)
  Nephropathy (kidney)
Neuropathic
  Peripheral neuropathy
  Autonomic neuropathy

age does not show up immediately, and when damage to the eyes, kidneys, and nerves does begin, patients may not even know it because often there are no symptoms. People with diabetes can also develop problems with the large blood vessels in the body. Depending on the location of the damage, different problems can occur, such as damage to blood vessels in the heart (heart attack), in the brain (stroke), and in the legs (sores and possibly gangrene).

To prevent the complications, there are things that patients need to do at home and there are things that the health care professionals must do in the office. For example, patients have the job of working on control of blood sugar, blood pressure, and cholesterol levels through diet, exercise, medication, and monitoring. The health care team has the job of looking for any problems with the eyes, kidneys, heart, and so forth by performing certain laboratory tests, physical examinations, and check-ups. It is important to emphasize to patients that even if they have been feeling well or if they have had no problems in carrying out self-care activities at home, they will still benefit greatly from keeping appointments at which the health care team can monitor diabetic complications.

MICROVASCULAR COMPLICATIONS

Diabetic Retinopathy

Diabetic eye disease, commonly called *diabetic retinopathy* (although other structures are sometimes involved), is a potentially very serious complication. Although only 1% to 2% of diabetic patients become blind, diabetes is so common that it is the leading cause of blindness in persons between the ages of 20 and 74 years.

Background retinopathy, which is characterized by microaneurysms, hemorrhage, and exudates (see Chapter 8 for a description), usually takes approximately 10 years to occur after the onset of diabetes. As many as 80% of patients may eventually develop it. This form of retinopathy does not impair vision unless the area of the eye necessary for central vision (the macula) is involved, resulting in macular edema. Background retinopathy can progress to a more serious form, called *proliferative retinopathy*, in 5% to 10% of patients, most often the ones who maintain poor diabetic control. In this form of retinopathy, new vessels grow (proliferate) on the retina and extend toward the middle of the eye. If they break, the large amounts of blood released into the eye obscure vision, often resulting in permanent visual damage. Fortunately, laser treatment is helpful in forestalling visual loss in both macular edema and proliferative retinopathy. To be most effective, treatment must be given early to prevent damage. Therefore, the ADA recommends that type 1 diabetic patients be monitored yearly with a dilated funduscopic examination (usually performed by an ophthalmologist), beginning 5 years after the onset of diabetes. Patients with type 2 diabetes should be examined yearly from the time of diagnosis. As many as 25% of patients have some degree of retinopathy at the time of diagnosis owing to the hiatus of several years between the development of type 2 diabetes and its diagnosis.

The Lens

Visual impairment secondary to changes in the lens is also more common in patients with diabetes. The shape of the lens can be temporarily distorted owing to hyperglycemia, with resultant blurring of vision until blood glucose levels are normalized. The lens is also more prone to cataract formation in patients with diabetes. Although cataracts may not be more common in the diabetic population, they are approximately five times more likely to develop at a younger age than in the nondiabetic population. Diabetic control (as reflected in glucose levels) does not seem to have a role.

Patient Education

As part of teaching patients prevention of eye complications, the educator should encourage patients to keep a record of the dates of all eye examinations performed by the eye doctor. It should be emphasized that the eyes must be dilated and examined by a specialist. Clarify for patients that an optical examination for new prescription lenses or an examination by their regular physician (especially through undilated eyes) is not sufficient. Emphasize that permanent diabetic eye damage typically does not cause any symptoms in the early stages, when it could be treated. It is thus important to have yearly eye examinations even when vision is fine. It is possible, however, for very low or very high blood glucose levels to cause blurred vision temporarily, but this should resolve when levels become stable. Remind patients that in order to prevent eye damage, control of blood sugar and blood pressure are crucial.

Diabetic Nephropathy

Diabetic kidney disease (diabetic nephropathy) can be divided into five stages. *Stage I* occurs at the onset of the disease and is characterized by an increase in kidney size and function. These changes usually return to normal within a few weeks to a few months with treatment that lowers glucose levels.

In *stage II*, kidney size and function are normal (regardless of the duration of diabe-

tes). The kidneys normally excrete a very small amount of albumin (<30 mg/24 h). Neither the usual laboratory dipstick test for protein nor the more recently developed very sensitive ones detect this amount. Therefore, stage 2 is characterized by the urinary excretion of a tiny normal amount of albumin.

Stage III, or incipient diabetic nephropathy, is characterized by an amount of urinary albumin that is greater than normal but still less than the amount detected by the usual laboratory dipstick test for urinary protein. Patients who excrete this amount of albumin, between 30 and 300 mg/24 h, are said to have *microalbuminuria*. Sixty to 80% of these patients eventually progress to the next stage if they remain in poor control (e.g., Hgb A_{1c} >8% to 9%), compared with only 5% of those without microalbuminuria. Controlling elevated blood pressure, returning glucose levels to near normal, using angiotensin-converting enzyme (ACE) inhibitors, and/or ingesting a low-protein diet can decrease or possibly reverse microalbuminuria. Some evidence suggests that this may prevent progression of the kidney disease to the next stage.

Stage IV, or overt diabetic nephropathy, is characterized by clinical proteinuria (i.e., a level of urinary albumin [>300 mg albumin per 24 hours] that is detectable [dipstick positive] by tests routinely performed in clinical laboratories). Kidney function starts to decline during this stage, and hypertension is very common. Overt diabetic nephropathy is usually asymptomatic and can take years to progress to a point where symptoms of renal insufficiency (fatigue, nausea, vomiting) start to occur. Although returning glucose concentrations to near normal does not affect the rate of decrease of kidney function, controlling hypertension, use of ACE inhibitors, and possibly a low-protein diet help preserve kidney function during this stage.

Stage V, or end-stage renal disease, is similar to kidney failure due to any other cause.

Treatment is usually by hemodialysis or peritoneal dialysis. At present, one third of all patients starting dialysis have kidney failure secondary to diabetic nephropathy. An alternative to dialysis is kidney transplantation if a suitable donor can be found. Because diabetic patients generally fare worse on dialysis than nondiabetic patients, kidney transplantation is usually preferred, if possible.

Patient Education

As part of teaching patients how to prevent kidney damage, the educator should explain that it is important to accurately perform annual urine collection tests (either overnight or 24-hour) if ordered by the physician. If patients do not understand the directions or if they make a mistake and forget to save all the urine requested, encourage them to discuss the situation with the laboratory personnel or the doctor's office and to reperform the test if necessary. Remind patients that even though this type of urine collection is inconvenient, it is very important in detecting any signs of kidney damage before there are ever any symptoms of a problem. Emphasize that control of blood sugar and blood pressure are crucial for prevention of diabetic kidney damage.

Neuropathy

Diabetic neuropathy is a common long-term complication of diabetes and is the source of severe discomfort for many patients. The two types of neuropathy are peripheral and autonomic. Patients more commonly complain of symptoms associated with peripheral neuropathy than with autonomic neuropathy.

Peripheral Neuropathy

Symptoms of peripheral neuropathy consist of burning sensations, tingling, numbness, and pain in the lower extremities, especially starting in the feet. The pain can become very severe; it sometimes is relieved by walking and is often worse at night. Loss of feeling may occur eventually. This can be dangerous for patients because they cannot appreciate any external trauma to the feet, and they thus must take the appropriate measures either to prevent it from occurring or to treat the initial lesions. If skin breakdown should occur, infection is likely. If foot ulcers are not treated appropriately, amputation may be needed. The combination of a foot infection and impaired circulation due to peripheral vascular disease is extremely dangerous. Fifty to 75% of all lower extremity amputations in this country are performed on diabetic patients (who make up only 6% of the population). It is estimated that at least half of these amputations could have been avoided. Peripheral neuropathy can also involve the upper extremities. Patients may suffer burns, especially from cooking and smoking, because of the decreased sensation. Muscle atrophy (wasting), which also can occur in the feet, leads to weakness and impairs patients' ability to use their hands normally.

Patient Education

Working with patients suffering from the pain of peripheral neuropathy focuses mostly on pain relief measures. Patients first must understand that complete pain relief is often not possible, but measures can be taken to improve their ability to participate in normal activities. For some patients, the pain disappears spontaneously after 6 to 12 months. Persistent neuropathy pain may be treated with oral medications such as antidepressants or anticonvulsants. Another option is use of a topical cream derived from chili peppers (capsaicin). Some patients may benefit from a nondrug method of pain control using a transcutaneous electronic nerve stimulator (TENS) unit. TENS units work by stimulating pain-blocking nerves. In some patients, it may also be possible to improve the symptoms of peripheral neuropathy through improvement in blood glucose control.

Patients who have developed loss of sensation because of neuropathy must be instructed on safety measures for prevention of burns and injuries. Patients need to be made aware that normal daily activities such as driving, walking, and household chores all can be affected by decreased sensation of pressure and decreased ability to appreciate the location of limbs relative to other objects. A referral for occupational therapy is helpful for promoting independence and safety. (Specific education about avoidance of foot problems is discussed later.)

Diabetic Foot Lesions

Foot lesions in patients with diabetes occur frequently, especially in patients with peripheral neuropathy. Most foot lesions can be prevented by educated patients, and if they occur, early treatment is often effective. If the lesions are allowed to progress before therapy is started, the prognosis is much worse. Patients with diabetes are more vulnerable to foot lesions because of three contributory factors:

1. *Neuropathy:* A foot lesion develops when an injury occurs, causing a break in the skin. The skin is the first line of defense against infection, and if its integrity is altered, bacteria may invade and the infectious process is initiated. Neuropathy is often the inciting factor for repeated trauma. This is because of patients' inability to perceive pain or pressure or to distinguish temperatures. Loss of sensation can lead to burns by hot water soaks or baths. The inability to feel pain or pressure can cause patients to be unaware of such things as blisters caused by ill-fitting or new shoes or foreign objects in a shoe. Wounds can be caused by home surgery on corns, calluses, and toenails.

2. *Vascular disease:* Once an injury occurs, effective circulation is required for the delivery of nutrients and antibiotics. If patients have vascular disease, the healing process is compromised and the injury can worsen, progressing to ulceration, infection, or even gangrene.

3. *Hyperglycemia:* In addition to contributing to vascular problems, hyperglycemia itself can depress the body's defenses against invading bacteria, thus adding to the seriousness of the foot lesions.

Because of these three contributing factors, a minor injury can rapidly become a serious lesion, often eventually requiring some degree of amputation.

Foot Care

INSPECTION | The key to foot care is to look at the feet. Foot-care education can take place while performing a foot inspection. Shoes and stockings obviously must be removed. Some patients may need to use a mirror to see their feet completely. A foot inspection form (Fig. 10-16) provides a record for further visits. The office inspection should serve as a demonstration of self-inspection. In addition, the health care professional should assess patients for protective sensation using a 10-g monofilament (Fig. 10-17). If patients are unable to perform self-inspection (e.g., have visual impairment or are obese), it is advisable to involve a family member or other support person in foot-care education. The use of a home health service may be indicated. The following should be carried out during a daily foot inspection (by the health care professional or the patient). Foot care instructions for patients are summarized in Figure 10-18.

1. Inspect pressure points (Fig. 10-19) for corns, calluses, blisters, or redness.
2. Inspect between toes for cracks, signs of fungus, blisters, or discoloration.
3. Inspect the skin for dryness, especially the heels.
4. If a clawfoot (Fig. 10-20) or a hammertoe (Fig. 10-21) is present, inspect for calluses or blisters on the prominent joint(s).
5. Call the patient's physician about any

DIABETIC FOOT SCREEN   Date:

Patient's name (last, first, middle) _____ ID No.:

Fill in the following blanks with an R, L, or B to indicate positive findings on the right, left, or both feet.

Has there been a change in the foot since the last evaluation?	Yes _____	No _____
Is there a foot ulcer now or history of foot ulcer?	Yes _____	No _____
Does the foot have an abnormal shape?	Yes _____	No _____
Is there weakness in the ankle or foot?	Yes _____	No _____
Are the nails thick, too long, or ingrown?	Yes _____	No _____

Label sensory level with a plus sign in the circled areas of the foot if the patient can feel the 10-gram (5.07 Semmes-Weinstein) nylon filament and with a minus sign if he or she cannot feel the 10-gram filament.

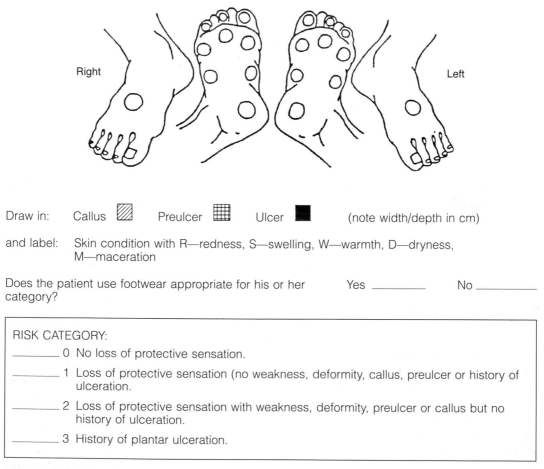

Draw in: Callus ▨   Preulcer ▦   Ulcer ■   (note width/depth in cm)

and label: Skin condition with R—redness, S—swelling, W—warmth, D—dryness, M—maceration

Does the patient use footwear appropriate for his or her category?   Yes _____   No _____

RISK CATEGORY:

_____ 0 No loss of protective sensation.

_____ 1 Loss of protective sensation (no weakness, deformity, callus, preulcer or history of ulceration.

_____ 2 Loss of protective sensation with weakness, deformity, preulcer or callus but no history of ulceration.

_____ 3 History of plantar ulceration.

Figure 10–16. Foot assessment record.

Filament Application Instructions

Note: The sensory testing device used with the foot screen is a nylon filament mounted on a holder that has been standardized to deliver a 10-gram force when properly applied. Our research has shown that a patient who can feel the 10-gram filament in the selected sites will not develop ulcers.

Instructions for sensory testing on the foot:
1. Use the 10-gram filament provided to test sensation.
2. The sites to be tested are indicated on the diabetic foot screen form.
3. Apply the filament perpendicular to the skin's surface (see diagram A, below).
4. The approach, skin contact, and departure of the filament should be approximately 1½ seconds in duration.
5. Apply sufficent force to cause the filament to bend (see diagram B, below).

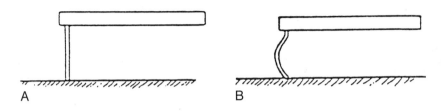

6. Do not allow the filament to slide across the skin or make repetitive contact at the test site.
7. Randomize the selection of test sites and time between successive tests to reduce the potential for a patient's guessing.
8. Ask the patient to respond "yes" when the filament is felt and record response on the diabetic foot screen form.
9. Apply the filament along the perimeter of and not on an ulcer site, callus, scar, or necrotic tissue.

Figure 10–17. Technique of use of 10-gram monofilament for foot assessment.

changes or signs of infection, such as tenderness, swelling, redness, or an injury that is not healing.

HYGIENE | All patients must keep their feet clean and dry. The guidelines listed next should be followed.

1. Wash your feet with mild soap as part of a daily shower or tub bath.
2. Water temperature must not be too hot (test with elbow).
3. Patients who do not shower or bathe daily may clean their feet in a foot basin (if a basin is used, do not soak the feet for more than 10 minutes).
4. Dry carefully between the toes with a soft cloth.
5. Prevent dryness of the skin by applying a skin lubricant daily (e.g., Vaseline Intensive Care, Nivea, Alpha-Keri, Eucerin). Do not apply between the toes.
6. Prevent fungus by removing excess moisture. A small amount of talcum powder may be used between the toes. If a fungal infection develops, an appropriate medication to treat the fungus should be prescribed.

PREVENTION OF FOOT INJURY | (It is most important to emphasize these measures for patients with loss of protective sensation—i.e., cannot feel the 10-g monofilament.) Prevent injury to the feet by being aware of potential injuries and practicing the following approaches in foot care:

1. Do not use hot water baths, heating

Foot Care for People with Diabetes

People with diabetes have to take special care of their feet.

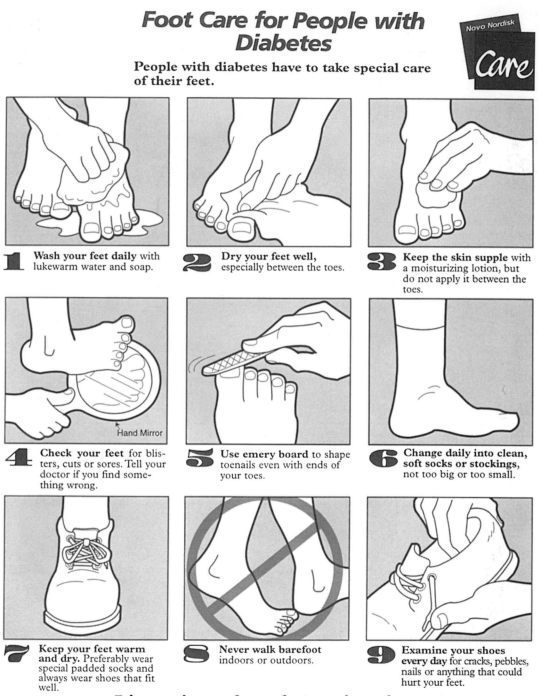

1. **Wash your feet daily** with lukewarm water and soap.

2. **Dry your feet well,** especially between the toes.

3. **Keep the skin supple** with a moisturizing lotion, but do not apply it between the toes.

4. **Check your feet** for blisters, cuts or sores. Tell your doctor if you find something wrong.

   Hand Mirror

5. **Use emery board** to shape toenails even with ends of your toes.

6. **Change daily into clean, soft socks or stockings,** not too big or too small.

7. **Keep your feet warm and dry.** Preferably wear special padded socks and always wear shoes that fit well.

8. **Never walk barefoot** indoors or outdoors.

9. **Examine your shoes every day** for cracks, pebbles, nails or anything that could hurt your feet.

Take good care of your feet - and use them.
A brisk walk every day stimulates the circulation.

Figure 10–18. Foot-care instructions for patients.

Figure 10–19. Pressure points on the bottom of the foot requiring daily inspection. (From Reed JK: Footwear for the diabetic. In Levin M: The Diabetic Foot, 3rd ed. CV Mosby, St. Louis, 1983, p. 360.)

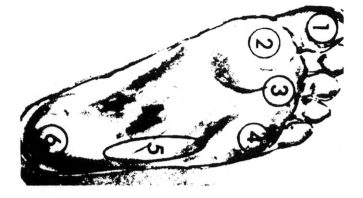

pads, or other heating techniques to warm the feet.

2. Try to avoid placing the feet on or near heat registers, car heaters, or heat lamps.

3. Avoid sunburn.

4. Do not walk barefooted on hot sand or pavement (sandals or water shoes may be necessary).

5. In general, shoes should be worn at all times to protect the feet. Seek medical advice if special shoes or foot appliances are necessary (e.g., cocked-up toe problems). The toe box (toes area) of the shoe should allow for toe expansion. Break in new shoes gradually—initially wear them for only 2 hours at a time.

6. Remove the shoes and inspect the feet for areas of redness or irritation.

7. Use the hand to feel and inspect the inside of the shoes for rough areas, foreign objects, exposed nails, or other protruding surfaces.

TOENAIL INJURIES | Toenail injuries are usually due to incorrect cutting. The following guidelines should be followed to prevent difficulty:

1. If vision is impaired or if patients are obese and unable to reach their feet, have a podiatrist, physician, or other trained person cut the nails.

2. Before cutting, soften the nails with soft brush, or cut after bathing.

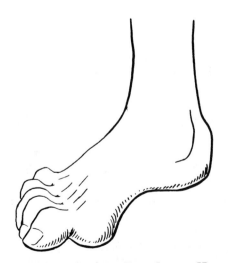

Figure 10–20. Clawfoot. (From Larson CB, Gould M: Calderwood's Orthopedic Nursing, 9th ed. CV Mosby, St. Louis, 1978, p. 346.)

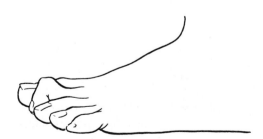

Figure 10–21. Hammertoe. (From Larson CB, Gould M: Calderwood's Orthopedic Nursing, 9th ed. CV Mosby, St. Louis, 1978, p. 346.)

3. Use a nail clipper to cut nails, not scissors, knives, or razor blades.

4. Cut nails straight across. Do not cut into the corners. File any sharp edges with an emery board.

5. Ingrown or thickened nails require special care and should not be self-treated.

CORNS AND CALLUSES | Corns and calluses indicate irritation and pressure on the skin and are potential areas for the development of an ulcer. Most ulcers start under a corn on the protruding part of a toe or under a callus on pressure areas of the foot. If the corn or callus is very prominent or if discoloration develops, seek medical advice. Otherwise, the following methods can be used to prevent buildup of a hard callus or cracking of the skin, which is a potential source of infection.

1. First, soften the corn or callus by soaking the feet in a foot basin filled with warm water (no longer than 10 minutes).

2. Rub the corn or callus gently with a soft brush, pumice, or cleansing sponge and then apply lubricating material. Do not use any tools or commercial preparations for removing corns or calluses (e.g., preparations that contain iodine, bichloride of mercury, or phenol, or corn remedies, corn pads, or adhesives).

3. If corns are caused by overlapping of the toes, place a small amount of lamb's wool between them.

4. Moleskin may be used for protecting any protruding parts of the foot that are subject to irritations.

CIRCULATION PROBLEMS | Improve circulation by walking or other physical activities that increase blood flow to the legs. Avoid behaviors or activities that decrease circulation, such as

1. Smoking
2. Sitting with legs crossed at the knees
3. Exposure to extremes in temperature

4. Wearing "gathers" or knee-high stockings that have a narrow elastic top

Autonomic Neuropathy

Autonomic neuropathy can involve the gastrointestinal, genitourinary, and cardiovascular systems. In addition, it may cause hypoglycemia unawareness.

Gastrointestinal Tract

1. *Gastroparesis diabeticorum:* This form of autonomic neuropathy causes delay in the emptying of stomach (gastric) contents, which may lead to unpredictable absorption of food and thus may interfere with diabetic control. Symptoms include feeling full after eating only a small amount of food (early satiety), nausea, and vomiting. It is common for the vomitus to contain food eaten many hours before. Small frequent feedings are helpful, as are metoclopramide (Reglan), cisapride (Propulsid), and erythromycin.

2. *Diabetic enteropathy:* Involvement of the nerves that control the intestinal function can cause either constipation or diarrhea. Constipation is more common. Some patients experience alternating constipation and diarrhea. The diarrhea may occur at night and may get better or worse for no apparent reason. Fecal incontinence occasionally occurs (especially at night) because the anal sphincter does not function normally. Treatment includes antibiotics and antidiarrheal drugs.

PATIENT EDUCATION—GASTROPARESIS | Education of patients with autonomic neuropathy affecting the gastrointestinal tract focuses on symptom recognition and explanation of treatments as listed earlier. In addition, encouraging frequent glucose monitoring is important for avoidance of unexpected hypoglycemia when food absorption and times of peak insulin action do not match. Patients need to understand that previously taught insulin dose adjustments based on patterns of blood glucose results and/or dose adjustments in anticipation of diet changes may need to be altered in response to inconsistent food absorption. Goals of blood glucose need to be less strict, with emphasis on avoidance of hypoglycemia.

Genitourinary Tract

1. *Neurogenic bladder:* When the bladder expands, autonomic nerves located in the muscle wall give the signal for the bladder to contract, resulting in urination. If these nerves are affected by diabetic autonomic neuropathy, the urge to urinate is delayed until the bladder becomes very full. This process is slow and insidious, but patients may eventually notice infrequent urination. In addition, the strength of contraction is weakened, causing incomplete emptying of the bladder. The urine that remains is a potential source for bacterial growth. Therefore, patients with neurogenic bladder often have urinary tract infections that start in the bladder but may ascend to the kidneys.

   Treatment involves drugs that promote bladder contraction, antibiotics, and in advanced cases surgery. Patients with neurogenic bladder should be instructed to

   - Void frequently (every 2 to 4 hours) on a scheduled basis; this may necessitate use of a watch or clock with an alarm.
   - Triple-void. This is a simple technique of voiding as much as possible, resting 1 minute and voiding again, and then repeating once again.
   - Perform Crede's maneuver. Press the hands against the lower abdomen to increase the pressure and thereby empty the bladder.

2. *Impotence:* Impotence is the inability to complete the act of sexual intercourse successfully because of failure either to initiate or sustain an erection. An erection results from a reflex action that traps blood in the penile shaft. The reflex is transmitted through a group of autonomic nerves originating in the lower part of the pelvic area. As a result of autonomic neuropathy, these nerves are unable to respond to the appropriate stimuli, and an erection can either not take place or if initiated cannot be sustained. Impotence is estimated to be four or five times more common in male diabetic patients older than 30 years than in nondiabetic individuals in the same age group. It may eventually affect as many as 50% of male diabetic patients.

In some diabetic patients, impotence may be due to macrovascular disease in the vessels supplying blood to the penis. Of course, nondiabetic causes of impotence (e.g., psychogenic, endocrine, drugs, alcohol) may also affect diabetic patients and must be ruled out. Impotence due to diabetes can be treated with vacuum tumescence devices, intrapenile injections, or penile implants.

PATIENT EDUCATION—IMPOTENCE | It is important to male diabetic patients that prevention of impotence involves general diabetes control measures. Thus, patients should make attempts with diet, exercise, medication, and monitoring to improve blood sugar, blood pressure, and cholesterol levels. In addition, a urologist may be consulted to discuss the various specific treatment options to assist with erections.

Cardiovascular Conditions

The autonomic nervous system is critically important for maintaining the blood pressure when one goes from lying down to standing up. A reduction in systolic blood pressure of 30 mm Hg 1 to 2 minutes after standing up defines orthostatic hypotension. Symptomatic orthostatic hypotension can be quite troublesome for diabetic patients with autonomic neuropathy. Treatment usually consists of administration of a salt-retaining hormone, but congestive heart failure is a possible side effect. In addition, diabetic patients are more likely to have silent myocardial infarction (i.e., heart attacks without pain). This is because of autonomic neuropathy of the nerves innervating the heart so that the chest pain of the heart attack is not felt by patients.

PATIENT EDUCATION—CARDIAC AUTONOMIC NEUROPATHY | Patients need to be taught that this type of nerve damage affects the ability of the heart and blood vessels to function normally. Patients with orthostatic hypotension should be taught to arise slowly from a standing or lying position (i.e., wait a minute or two at each position when moving from lying to sitting or from sitting to standing). Special elastic stockings that extend to the thigh or even waist may be used to help direct blood flow to the heart and brain and to prevent dizziness and falls. Some patients may need to use a wheelchair or walker to prevent falls. An evaluation of the home by an occupational therapist is important for promotion of safety and injury prevention.

Patients with cardiac autonomic neuropathy need to be taught to report any unusual symptoms such as shortness of breath, ankle swelling, or unusual fatigue. They may notice that they become short of breath during light physical activity. Explain to patients that these types of symptoms may be the only indication that they have had a heart attack. They need to understand the seriousness of the potential for a silent (painless) heart attack and the importance of immediately reporting these symptoms no matter how mild they may seem.

Hypoglycemia Unawareness

One of the causes of hypoglycemia unawareness is autonomic neuropathy. In this situation, failure of the autonomic nervous system leads to impairment of the epinephrine and norepinephrine response to hypo- glycemia. Therefore, the autonomic symptoms of hypoglycemia (see Table 7–18) are blunted or absent. Thus, patients with autonomic neuropathy may be unaware of their low blood glucose level and fail to take appropriate steps to correct it. As the hypoglycemia continues to worsen, they suffer from the more severe signs and symptoms (e.g., visual changes, behavioral changes, confusion, lethargy, and possibly seizures and coma) of neuroglycopenia (see Chapter 7 for a more detailed discussion of this topic).

PATIENT EDUCATION | Patients who no longer feel the adrenergic symptoms of hypoglycemia need to understand the serious danger this can pose. Patients may mistakenly enjoy the fact that they can tolerate much lower glucose levels than they used to without the inconvenient symptoms of sweating, shakiness, nervousness, and so forth. Explain to patients that without these warning signs to alert the patient or family to get something to eat, the blood sugar can drop so low that the brain no longer functions normally. Serious and possibly fatal damage can occur to patients or to people affected by patients if they are driving, operating machinery, walking alone, or supervising young children at the time of the low blood glucose level.

Prevention of low blood glucose levels is absolutely critical for these patients. Thus, goals for blood glucose control should be set higher than usual. Extra blood glucose testing is necessary—especially before driving and other types of activities listed earlier. If patients are unable or unwilling to test their glucose levels more often, then more frequent eating of snacks and meals (not more than about 3 hours between feedings) is required.

MACROVASCULAR COMPLICATIONS

Diseases of the large blood vessels are two (males) to four (females) times more common in diabetic patients than in persons without diabetes. These conditions include coronary artery disease, peripheral vascular disease, and cerebrovascular disease. Diabetes is only one of the six independent risk factors for macrovascular disease in the general population (Table 10-9). The first four of these risk factors are reversible ones—that is, once they are eliminated, the risk disappears. As difficult as it may be, patients can quit smoking. Hypertension and hyperlipidemia can be successfully treated by diet and drugs. Although obesity itself is associated with three other risk factors (hypertension, elevated triglyceride levels, and diabetes), it has been identified as an independent risk over and beyond the ones with which it is associated. Like smoking, the treatment of obesity requires a life style change, which, although difficult, can be successfully accomplished.

Everyone inherits a certain likelihood of acquiring large vessel diseases independent of the other risk factors. The best evidence of this genetic tendency for an individual is a history of atherosclerosis in first-degree male relatives (e.g., father, uncles, brothers). If such a relative suffered an early coronary event, the genetic tendency for macrovascular disease may be high. If these male relatives were free of coronary or other macrovascular disease until late in life, the inherited tendency is low. This risk factor is obviously an irreversible one.

Whatever the risk for macrovascular disease in an individual, the presence of diabetes approximately doubles it. Unfortunately, the available evidence does not suggest that strict diabetic control helps prevent or delay

these macrovascular diseases—that is, diabetes seems to be an irreversible risk factor. It may be that the presence of five other potential risk factors overrides the relationship between hyperglycemia and the large vessel diseases. Alternatively, the mechanism by which diabetes causes an acceleration of atherosclerosis does not involve glucose metabolism and is unchanged by achieving near euglycemia (nearly normal glucose concentrations). In any event, four important risk factors can be reversed, and diabetic patients must be vigorously encouraged to do so.

PATIENT EDUCATION | It is beyond the scope of this chapter to provide in-depth information on cardiovascular risk factor modification. A few general pointers are provided here to help patients understand that diabetes management means more than just blood sugar control.

Most diabetes education, especially for newly diagnosed diabetic patients, focuses on blood glucose control. Improvements in blood glucose levels are relatively easy to achieve in a short time and can easily be appreciated by patients. Patients may either feel immediate improvement in symptoms (if they had been experiencing hyperglycemic symptoms) or they will detect improvement in blood glucose results obtained at home or at the medical office. Once improvement in blood glucose control is achieved, it is important to emphasize (especially for type 2 diabetic patients) that the most common causes of death among people with diabetes are heart disease and stroke. These conditions require attention to matters other than blood glucose control—namely, blood pressure, cholesterol, and weight control.

To help patients deal with feeling overwhelmed by all the details of complications prevention, point out that the behaviors that improve blood glucose levels usually also improve cardiovascular conditioning—weight loss and exercise. Help patients identify whether they anticipate increased success with life style changes through small incre-

Table 10-9. Risk Factors for Macrovascular Disease

Reversible	Irreversible
Smoking	Family history (genetic)
Hypertension	Diabetes mellitus
Hyperlipidemia[a]	
Obesity	

[a]Elevated cholesterol and/or triglyceride levels.

mental changes or more drastic changes in health habits. Whatever approach patients choose, encourage them to celebrate successful behavior changes rather than focus solely on end results.

To promote a sense of empowerment and optimism, help patients to consider that the diagnosis of diabetes is forcing them to pay much needed attention to their diet and health. Many people who do not have diabetes suffer from the same cardiovascular problems but do not make attempts to improve their health until after their first heart attack or surgery. Patients with diabetes are given special opportunities through education and increased medical follow-up to prevent cardiovascular problems before they occur.

PERSONAL HYGIENE

The hygiene needs of diabetic patients do not differ from those of nondiabetic persons but must be attended to with more caution and diligence. Education should be directed toward preventive measures, especially during periods of high blood glucose levels, because this is the factor that interferes with the healing process. The three diseases discussed next require special care and are particular problems in diabetic patients.

URINARY TRACT INFECTIONS

Because urinary tract infections are common in diabetic females, special hygiene is indicated:

1. Clean the vagina and anus from front to back after urinating or defecating.
2. Urinate to empty the bladder after sexual intercourse.
3. If a patient has a neurogenic bladder, urinate on a schedule. It may be necessary to restrict fluids after midnight.
4. Report to the physician any symptoms of urgency, frequency, or painful urination.
5. Drink increased amounts of liquids and urinate every 3 to 4 hours during the day to help to irrigate the bladder and wash out bacteria.

CANDIDA SKIN INFECTIONS (FUNGUS OR YEAST INFECTION)

Fungus infections occur in warm, moist areas, particularly in the vagina and genital region. They can also occur under the breasts and between other overlapping skin folds. Therefore, this infection frequently affects overweight patients with blood glucose levels out of control. Instruct patients to look for a white, cheesy vaginal discharge with a peculiar yeasty odor, vaginal itching, and redness and swelling of the upper thighs, beneath the breasts, or in the creases between the legs and abdomen (the intertriginous area). If patients find evidence for a *Candida* infection, they should seek medical care. Topical medications are effective, but blood glucose control is also extremely important.

TEACH PREVENTIVE MEASURES | Patients should be taught the following:

1. Do not wear soiled underclothes.
2. Wear underclothing that does not promote or trap heat and moisture (e.g., wear cotton-crotch underwear, especially panty hose with a cotton crotch or cotton top).

During periods of high blood glucose levels, cleanse the perineal and vaginal areas after urination to wash away any residual glucose, which contributes to the *Candida* skin infection.

PERIODONTAL DISEASE

Diseases of the gums and surrounding tissues are estimated to occur three times more frequently in diabetic patients who have elevated blood glucose levels than in nondiabetic patients. Poor oral hygiene associated with hyperglycemia can cause gum (periodontal) infections. Teach patients to watch for

1. Inflammation of gum tissue (red and swollen gums)

2. Easy bleeding of gums

3. Dental plaque and calculus accumulation

4. Increased spacing between teeth, receding gums, and loose teeth

5. Early loss of teeth due to primary gum disease

TEACH PREVENTIVE MEASURES | Patients should be taught the following:

1. Achieving good control of blood sugar

2. Cleaning the teeth at least twice a day with a soft toothbrush and toothpaste; frequent use of dental floss

3. Not neglecting bleeding gums, poorly fitting dentures, or sores in the mouth

4. Examining the gums by pulling the lips apart and looking for inflamed tissue

5. Seeing a dentist on a routine basis (excess dental plaque may need to be removed more frequently) and when abnormalities develop

SPECIAL SITUATIONS

FASTING

The most important thing to remember whenever fasting is necessary (e.g., for a blood test, dental appointment, outpatient surgical procedure) is to speak to the diabetes health care professional who is assisting in the management of the diabetes. The main danger to be avoided is hypoglycemia, which may occur if the usual insulin or oral hypoglycemic medication is taken without eating. In general, having hyperglycemia for a few hours or for half a day is safer than risking hypoglycemia.

In type 2 diabetes, the body is still able to produce some of its own insulin. As discussed earlier, this prevents the development of DKA. If patients must fast for only a few hours or half a day, the physician may have them omit or delay taking the oral hypogly-

cemic agent until they are eating again. For type 2 diabetic patients taking insulin, the physician may have them decrease the dose or omit it entirely (and then resume insulin injections whenever the next dose is usually taken).

In type 1 diabetes, the body is not producing its own insulin, and omitting an insulin dose entirely may lead to DKA. Although delaying the dose for a few hours may be safe, the physician may also eliminate the short-acting (regular) insulin from the morning injection and have patients simply take a smaller dose of longer-acting (e.g., NPH) insulin alone. It is important to avoid injecting the usual morning dose of regular insulin when patients have no plans to eat for several hours. In addition, if the morning injection was not taken at all, it may be unsafe to take the usual full morning dose at a later point in the day because it may peak at a time not covered by appropriate food intake.

Communication with the physician involved in management of the patient's diabetes is crucial.

TRAVEL

To be a successful traveler, a diabetic patient needs to be prepared and well supplied. Travel that involves changing time zones requires that insulin-requiring patients consult with their physician to formulate a plan for insulin dose adjustments. Patients should contact the airlines and find out how many in-flight meals and snacks will be served. The timing of meals is not always predictable, however, and patients are thus advised to be prepared with their own snacks or meals. Some diabetes resources recommend a complex scheme for calculating insulin dosages to account for changing time zones. For many patients, this system may be too overwhelming and may discourage them from travel. Instead, they can be taught simply to keep their watches set to the time in the city of origin, changing to the local time only after the first 12 to 24 hours or on the morning of the first day in the new destination. They can then be instructed to try to eat meals and snacks according to their usual schedule, with the safety precaution that if meals are more than 4 hours apart, they should consume a snack. Patients must also rely on SMBG to evaluate changes in their blood glucose levels and to assess the need for food or insulin dose adjustments. Using supplemental regular insulin during periods of high blood glucose levels as the adjustment to the new time zone occurs or during periods of illness can be useful.

Patients should carry all of the supplies they need to care for their diabetes during the duration of the trip. A good rule of thumb is to carry twice the number of supplies necessary for the length of the trip to avoid running out. Many items cannot be purchased abroad. In some foreign countries, U-100 insulin is not available. All of the diabetes-related supplies (and any other medications) should be packed in a carry-on bag, not put in luggage that is checked. Also, obtain two copies of (1) a statement verifying the diabetic condition that requires insulin administration and (2) prescriptions for the insulin and syringes. Put one of each in a wallet or purse as well as in the luggage.

In the event that the insulin, syringes, or prescriptions are lost or stolen and U-100 insulin and syringes are not available, purchase U-40 or U-80 insulin with *syringes to match*. Give the *same number of units*. Do not try to compute insulin doses for a syringe that does not correspond (i.e., U-100 insulin in a U-40 syringe).

Patients taking oral diabetes medications must know the generic (chemical) name of the drug, because the brand name is different in foreign countries. This applies to all other medications as well. Medications should be transported in their original labeled bottles or in smaller bottles that are clearly labeled with the drug name and strength to avoid confusion. As with insulin,

take a liberal supply of all required oral medications.

In addition to a consultation with one's personal physician about diabetes management, other health care issues need to be addressed. If patients are going to a destination such as Africa or Asia, vaccinations must be updated (or given for the first time). Malaria prophylaxis may be required. For many destinations, it is useful to carry medication to treat nausea, vomiting, and diarrhea, should these symptoms develop. Sick day rules for food replacement in the event of gastrointestinal upset should be reviewed.

As recommended in general, it is particularly important to wear clear medical alert tags identifying the diabetic condition. It is important to prevent development of *hypoglycemia*. Patients should carry a fast-acting glucose preparation and a long-acting carbohydrate at *all* times (even on the airplane), especially if they plan much walking. (For more information, refer to the section on prevention and treatment of hypoglycemia.)

Appropriate *footwear* should be worn. Constant walking may cause blisters and other foot problems. Bring moleskin to apply to areas of redness that develop as a result of pressure from shoes. Change shoes and socks or stockings frequently. If shoes are new, break them in before traveling. As always, do not wear new shoes more than 2 hours at a time.

Diabetes Packing Checklist

The following items must be kept in the carry-on luggage so that they are available at all times. Luggage that is checked may be delayed, lost, or even stolen.

Medications

Insulins or oral diabetes medications
Antinausea suppositories
Other prescription medications
Antibiotic ointment
Glucagon emergency kit (for patients taking insulin)

Supplies

Urine ketone test strips (for type 1 diabetes)

Insulin syringes

Wallet medical identification card

Glucose meter with test strips and test strips for visual use (in case meter does not work)

Lancets

Blood-sampling device and a spare (spring may break)

Alcohol wipes

Extra batteries (if you use a meter)

Cotton or facial tissues

Food

Quick-acting glucose preparation for reactions

Convenient snacks, such as cheese and cracker packets, granola bars, trail mix, or dried fruit to eat as a longer-acting carbohydrate

For long journeys, especially in Third World countries, bring a spare meal to eat in case food isn't readily available or safe to eat

Resources

North America: contact the local ADA if problems occur.

Non–English-speaking countries:

1. Carry an index card with emergency phrases in the appropriate language. Essential phrases include "I have diabetes. Please call a doctor"; "I have diabetes and I am having a low-sugar reaction. Please give me sugar."

2. If possible, have the name of English-speaking physicians in each city/country on the itinerary. A list of physicians may be available from the local American Embassy or Consulate, from foreign tourism offices in the United States, or from the IAMAT (International Association for Medical Assistance to Travelers, 417 Center Street, Lewiston, NY 14092).

3. Know where the Diabetes Association is located in each country. The International Diabetes Federation (IDF; 10 Queen Street, London W1M OBD, England) can supply names and addresses. The IDF also has information on diabetes medications and supplies. Other sources are (1) the International Diabetes Federation at the International Association Center, 40 Washington Street, 1050 Brussels, Belgium, and (2) Intermedic 777, 3rd Avenue, New York, NY, 10017, telephone (212) 486-8976.

Useful Phrases in Foreign Languages

"I am diabetic."

French: "Je suis diabetique."

Spanish: "Yo soy diabetico."

German: "Ich bin zuckerkrank."

Italian: "Io sono diabetico."

"Please get me a doctor."

French: "Allez chercher un medecin, s'il vous plait."

Spanish: "Haga me el favor de llamar al medico."

German: "Rufen sie bitte einen Arzt."

Italian: Per favore chiami un dottore.

"Sugar or orange juice, please."

French: "Sucre ou jus d'orange, s'il vous plait."

Spanish: "Azucar o un vaso de jugo de naranja, por favor."

German: "Zuker oder orangesaft, bitte."

Italian: "Succhero or arancia succo, per favore."

SPECIAL POPULATIONS

VISUALLY IMPAIRED PATIENTS

Various degrees of visual impairment may affect diabetic patients. Causes range from blurred vision due to hyperglycemia, especially in newly diagnosed patients, to cataracts and, more seriously, diabetic retinopathy. Retinopathy can lead to marked decreases in a patient's sight, from diminished vision to blindness.

The educator's role may vary from simple explanations, such as the cause of blurred vision, to demonstrations and discussions of ways and aids to facilitate independence in diabetes management. One of the most important roles may be to direct patients to resources for special assistance. Many communities have centers for educating and treating partially sighted and totally blind patients, and a referral to one of these institutions is often helpful because they have the resources to fully evaluate and treat patients with all degrees of visual impairments.

Assessment

1. Determine the degree of independence that patients want and the support system that is available to them. For example, if the support system performs blood glucose monitoring and prefills syringes, education should be directed toward members of the support system to ensure accuracy in the procedures involved.

2. Determine patients' degree of visual impairment. Level 1 = blurred vision and visual fluctuation, usually transient and due to fluctuations in blood glucose levels in patients with new-onset diabetes; level 2 = usable vision, low vision, legally blind, or partially sighted; and level 3 = functionally blind, totally blind. Classifying patients' visual impairment is necessary so that the appropriate level of education can be provided (e.g., by a knowledgeable diabetes educator for levels 1 and 2 and by a center for the blind for level 3).

3. To assess the need for visual aids, check patients' vision in the following ways: Have patients use an insulin vial and insulin syringe. Can they read the labels on the insulin vial? Can they read the markings on the syringe? Can they insert the needle into the insulin vial without bending the needle? Can they read the blood glucose value seen on the meter?

Teaching Aids

Various aids can help patients with decreased vision. A discussion of these devices can be found in the *'97 Buyer's Guide to Diabetes Supplies* and *Diabetes and Visual Impairment: An Educator's Resource Guide* (see Appendix). To increase patients' function with diminished sight, the following may be helpful (see Appendix for more complete details):

- Emphasize strong lighting for insulin injections and SMBG procedures.
- Use the insulin syringe most closely suited for the insulin dose (e.g., for <30 U of insulin use a 30-U syringe).
- Magnifying devices that slip over the syringe (such as the Becton Dickinson Magni-Guide) can double the size of the numbers; some patients may prefer to use a small pocket magnifier.
- Use of prefilled syringes may be necessary.
- Some patients benefit from use of insulin pens.
- Blood glucose meters that have large displays or give audible instructions for the test procedure and that state the blood glucose result can be purchased.
- Needle guides and vial stabilizers can be used to help guide the needle into the vial.
- Devices are marketed for ensuring dose accuracy when a poorly sighted person is drawing up insulin into a syringe. It is helpful to mark the vials of insulin clearly if more than one type is used, with either a rubber band or a notch in the top.

PEDIATRIC PATIENTS

Educating children with diabetes and their families is a unique challenge. If at all possible, these families should be referred to a medical center, children's hospital, diabetes educator, and/or endocrinologist specializing in childhood and adolescent diabetes management. The specific information and diabetes treatment modalities are, for the most part, the same as those for adults with type 1 diabetes. However, a number of special issues must be considered in dealing with this population, such as dynamics of the relationship between parent-child, parent-parent, child-sibling, child-caretaker, child-school, and so on. When a child has recently been found to have diabetes, the parents may express a great deal of guilt, anger, or spousal blame in trying to understand "where the diabetes came from."

In the past, emphasis was placed on having the child or adolescent accomplish specific diabetes-related tasks by a certain chronologic age. Too much parental involvement was feared to foster lack of independence and poor control of diabetes. A child's inability to achieve certain tasks by a certain age could become a source of family conflict, cause parents to feel a sense of failure, and impede development of positive self-esteem in the child. Research now suggests promoting more of a parent-child team approach with flexible expectations. A child's ability to become more involved with diabetes management depends on cognitive and emotional maturity, external stressors (e.g., school, family, or social problems), and simple individual variations in growth and development. Table 10-10 provides a description of some general issues and tasks for parents and children with diabetes.

Special Considerations in Diabetes Treatment

Goals of Blood Glucose

The specific indices for control of blood glucose, lipids, Hgb A_{1c}, and so forth are similar for the pediatric population and the adult population. However, a more realistic approach promoting greater long-term involvement with the health care team might be setting blood glucose goals that are more flexible and that take into account other issues such as normally erratic eating habits, especially in very young children and adolescents. As with all diabetic patients, striving for the best possible blood glucose control

Table 10–10. Developmental Issues and Tasks in Children With Type I Diabetes

Infant (0-1 year)	Differentiate hypoglycemic reactions from "normal" distress Parents may be overwhelmed by demands of diabetes. Identify and train trustworthy babysitters
Toddler (1-3 years)	Differentiate misbehavior from hypoglycemia Expect dietary inconsistency as child begins to feed self Give child choices in food, injection, and finger-stick sites (avoid mealtime battles) Encourage child to report "funny" feelings (hypoglycemia) Let child begin to "help" with diabetes tasks
Preschool (3-6 years)	Teach child to report hypoglycemia to adults in charge Teach child what to eat when "low" Reassure child who may view finger sticks and injections as punishment and/or become overly fearful of procedures Teach preschool teachers about diabetes Encourage child to participate in simple diabetes tasks Involve child in menu planning
School age (6-12 years)	Teach all school personnel involved with child about diabetes Manage diabetes to minimize school absences Parents should foster age-appropriate independence Parents and child should learn to adjust insulin and regimen to encourage participation in social and sports events Encourage self-monitoring: recognize hypoglycemia, participate in meal planning, gradually learn to do own blood testing and injections—all activities to be supervised

Adapted from Schreiner B, Pontious S: Diabetes mellitus and the preschool child. In Haire-Joshu D (ed): Management of Diabetes Mellitus: Perspectives of Care Across the Life Span. Mosby-Year Book, St. Louis, 1992, pp. 362-398.

is of vital importance in preventing the long-term complications. If pursuit of unrealistic goals creates more parent-child tension and alienates the child or family from the diabetes team, however, the ultimate outcome may be worse than accepting less than optimum diabetic control.

Hypoglycemia

Hypoglycemia is of special concern to parents of young children who are not yet able to clearly recognize and report the symptoms of hypoglycemia. Special education and attention should be given to conditions that may predispose children to hypoglycemia (e.g., unusual activity, missed snack, smaller than usual meal). Parents concerned about possible overnight hypoglycemia need to be alerted to watch the child for nightmares and sweating and to test the blood glucose level during the night. Parents and caretakers must be taught to use injectable glucagon (see previous section on hypoglycemia). For small children, one half of the adult dose (0.5 mg) is usually sufficient.

Special attention to hypoglycemia is also important for adolescents learning to drive. Teaching adolescents to test their blood sugar and to take a snack as needed every time they plan to drive promotes safe practices as adolescents become more independent.

Diet

The current approach to diabetes diet education and treatment promotes greater flexibility for all patients. This is especially helpful in reducing conflict in families of children and adolescents with diabetes. Substitution of sucrose-containing foods for other carbohydrates and education on age-appropriate foods and snacks (e.g., pizza and other fast foods) help the family and child with diabetes deal with the normal social aspects of growth and development.

Injection Sites

Pediatric (older than toddler) and adolescent patients are encouraged to use the same injection sites as recommended for adults. In infants and toddlers, the sciatic nerve is not well stabilized and injection in the buttocks is discouraged until children are walking. If possible, use of the abdomen is encouraged for older children and adolescents, especially to avoid resistance to using this area later in life. If arms and legs are used, a consistent rotation pattern (as described in the earlier insulin section) is especially important in this physically active group of patients. As with adults, avoid injecting into a limb that will be used during an activity.

Organizations/Support Groups/Camps

The ADA and Juvenile Diabetes Foundation are good sources of information for parents of diabetic children. In addition, local hospitals or regional facilities specializing in the care of diabetic children could provide information on local support groups, camps, and ongoing classes. Parents are encouraged to obtain written materials from diabetes organizations and diabetes lay magazines (see Appendix) to use in educating teachers and school staff on basic diabetes information—especially symptoms, treatment, and prevention of hypoglycemia. Encouraging contact between families with diabetic children and participation with diabetes camps can provide much needed support and guidance for families and can prevent feelings of isolation, especially in communities that do not offer formal pediatric diabetes services.

DEALING WITH DIABETES IN THE ELDERLY

When dealing with elderly patients, assessment of patients' ability and willingness to learn diabetes self-management skills is important. With this group of patients, probably more than any other population, individualizing the treatment and teaching plans is essential for successful diabetes management and for assisting patients to maintain independence. Elderly patients represent a diverse population with self-care abilities that do not predictably correlate with a patient's age.

Factors that may impair elderly patients' ability to learn diabetes self-care skills include

Decreased vision and hearing
Decreased fine motor coordination
Tremulousness of hands
Decreased range of motion (impaired ability to perform foot care)
Impaired short-term memory

In addition, certain psychologic issues such as loneliness, depression, and an unwillingness to change long-standing habits may negatively affect patients' desire to learn about diabetes. Other medical illnesses, financial limitations, and decreased ability to travel (to the clinic or office) may limit the amount of time and effort patients may put into diabetes management.

If patients are resistant to learning new information or have difficulty attending to details, the teaching sessions must be kept brief and limited in scope. If necessary, written teaching materials should be in large print with dark-colored lettering. A flexible approach to teaching is essential. A well-prepared and organized teaching plan may need to be changed several times during the teaching session to ensure that the basic information is understood by patients.

A sensitive but firm approach must be taken when asking patients who have managed their diabetes for many years to demonstrate skills of preparing and injecting insulin or measuring capillary blood glucose. A fear of loss of independence or of embarrassment may lead patients to feel insulted when asked to demonstrate skills learned many years earlier. It may be helpful for educators to explain to patients that they would like to show them new equipment or new techniques. Giving the appearance of an information-sharing session rather than a teaching or evaluation session may help patients feel less threatened. Using shortcuts such as eliminating the injection of air into insulin vials,

using simpler blood glucose meters, or working with family members to prefill syringes is important in promoting continued independence in diabetes management.

Although the goal of diabetes control in the elderly may be less strict than in younger patients, careful monitoring for diabetes complications must not be neglected. Hypoglycemia may be especially dangerous because of cerebral or coronary artery disease. Importantly, it may result in falls in the elderly. Decreased appetite or irregular meals may increase the chances of hypoglycemia in this population. Dehydration is a concern in patients who have chronically elevated glucose levels because of the associated hyperglycemia-induced diuresis. Assessment for long-term complications such as eye and foot problems is important. Avoiding blindness and amputations through early detection and treatment of retinopathy and foot ulcers, respectively, may mean the difference between institutionalization and continued independent living for elderly patients with diabetes.

PREGNANCY

For a complete discussion of diabetes in pregnancy, see Chapter 9.

Diabetes Before Pregnancy

Strict control of blood glucose levels is essential for diabetic women at the time of conception and throughout the entire pregnancy. Fetal problems that have been associated with hyperglycemia include increased body fat (babies weighing >9 pounds at birth), often complicating vaginal delivery. After birth, these babies are at increased risk for neonatal hypoglycemia, hyperbilirubinemia, and hypocalcemia. In addition, hyperglycemia is thought to contribute to the increased rate of congenital malformations (noted in women with poor diabetic control during the first 2 months of pregnancy).

Women with diabetes should discuss plans

to become pregnant with the physician helping to manage their diabetes (as well as their obstetrician). Normalizing blood glucose levels before conception is important and may require several months of intensive monitoring, education, and diet counseling with follow-up. Women should also be counseled on the possible effects of pregnancy on maternal health. Women with advanced kidney and eye disease may experience worsening of these conditions during pregnancy and need to discuss these risks fully before becoming pregnant.

The goals of diabetic management during pregnancy are to maintain fasting blood glucose levels in the range of 60 to 90 mg/dl and 1-hour postmeal blood glucose values <140 mg/dl. Blood glucose levels must be monitored daily, usually at least four times per day. Insulin injections are taken a minimum of two and often three to four times per day. Because of the antiinsulin effects of the hormones of pregnancy, the insulin dose requirements may increase two- to threefold during the course of pregnancy. Women who have type 2 diabetes and who are taking oral hypoglycemic agents before pregnancy must stop taking the oral agents (some evidence in animals suggests that they can be harmful for a fetus) and use insulin during the pregnancy for control of blood glucose levels. Monitoring for urine ketones during pregnancy should be performed every morning as well as during any sudden elevation of blood glucose value or during minor illness. An elevation in ketone levels must be reported immediately, because ketosis poses a danger to the fetus.

Gestational Diabetes

Two percent to 5% of all (nondiabetic) women who become pregnant develop a temporary form of diabetes called *gestational diabetes*. During pregnancy, the amount of insulin produced by the pancreas of a pregnant woman normally increases. This occurs because the hormones that are produced by the placenta during pregnancy make it more difficult for the normal insulin in the body to control blood glucose levels. Therefore, more insulin needs to be produced to counteract the effect of these hormones. If a woman's body is not able to produce enough extra insulin, the blood glucose values become elevated. This occurs mostly during the latter part of pregnancy, when placental hormone levels increase. All pregnant women should be screened for gestational diabetes (with a 1-hour 50-g glucose challenge test) at 24 to 28 weeks of pregnancy or even earlier if they are at high risk.

Women most at risk for gestational diabetes are obese, are older than 30 years, have a family history of diabetes, and/or have previously given birth to a baby weighing more than 9 pounds. Treatment includes diet, monitoring blood glucose levels and urine ketones, and, for some women, insulin injections. Because gestational diabetes is not usually a problem until later in pregnancy, congenital malformations are not usually associated with gestational diabetes. However, the other problems related to hyperglycemia that were mentioned previously do occur more frequently if gestational diabetes is not well controlled.

The diabetes usually resolves after delivery, although approximately 50% of women who have gestational diabetes develop overt type 2 diabetes within 5 to 15 years (especially if they are obese).

The most important information to give to women dealing with pregnancy and diabetes is that (except for a slightly higher risk for congenital malformations) with close monitoring and teamwork on the part of these women and their health care providers, the chances of delivering a healthy baby are similar to those of any pregnant woman.

CONCLUSION

Working in the field of diabetes education can be a very challenging and rewarding experience. The most effective diabetes educators are those who keep abreast of new treatments and equipment available for diabetes care. In addition, successful diabetes education requires willingness to reevaluate teaching techniques and teaching tools continually to maximize patients' understanding and ability to apply concepts to daily living situations.

Helping patients and their families cope with the unrelenting and demanding routines and stresses of diabetes management is an important role of the diabetes educator. Diabetes educators are encouraged to read the literature available on motivation, coping, chronic illness, and relapse prevention.

Creative problem solving can be very useful in motivating patients who have strayed from the diabetes program. One helpful technique for prevention of burnout among diabetes patients is to suggest a monthly or biweekly diabetes vacation day—during which patients need not record blood glucose levels and can be more free with the diet (while maintaining basic safety precautions). Another suggestion is periodically to conduct a patient visit or at least a portion of the visit without looking at the blood glucose records or laboratory results. Simply allow patients to talk freely about how diabetes is affecting their life or about any other aspects of life. Spending some amount of time simply talking to patients helps them to appreciate that their personality and identity are not defined by the level of diabetes control and to learn to enjoy life no matter what their level of success with the diabetes program.

REFERENCES

1. American Diabetes Association: National standards for diabetes self-management education programs and American Diabetes Association review criteria. Diabetes Care 18:737, 1995.
2. American Diabetes Association: Clinical Practice Recommendations—Insulin Administration. Diabetes Care 19(suppl 1):31, 1996.
3. American Diabetes Association: '97 Buyer's Guide to Diabetes Supplies. Diabetes Forecast October:44-88, 1996.

APPENDIX

—

SELECTED ORGANIZATIONS AND COMPANIES THAT PRODUCE EDUCATIONAL MATERIALS, SUPPLIES, AND CATALOGS

Listed below are selected resources for diabetes educators. For a more complete list of products and companies involved with diabetes care, consult the annual American Diabetes Association '97 *Buyer's Guide to Diabetes Products* in *Diabetes Forecast* (October), your local drug company representatives, and local organizations.

American Association of Diabetes Educators
444 N. Michigan Avenue, Suite 1240
Chicago, IL 60611-3901
(800) 338-DMED

American Diabetes Association
1660 Duke Street
Alexandria, VA 22314
(800) 232-3472

American Heart Association
7272 Greenville Avenue, Box 45
Dallas, TX 75231-4596
(800) 242-8721

Bayer Corporation Diagnostics Division
511 Benedict Avenue
Tarrytown, NY 10591
(800) 348-8100

Becton Dickinson Consumer Products
One Becton Drive
Franklin Lakes, NJ 07417-1883
(800) 237-4554

Boehringer Mannheim Corporation
9115 Hague Road/P.O. Box 50100
Indianapolis, IN 46250-0100
(800) 858-8072

Chronimed Publishing
Ridgedale Office Center, Suite 250
13911 Ridgedale Drive
Minneapolis, MN 55305
(800) 444-5951

Diabetic Insulcap, Inc.
1606 Presidio Way
Roseville, CA 95661
(800) 781-3089

Health Journeys (guided imagery tapes)
Image Paths, Inc.
P.O. Box 5714
Cleveland, OH 44101-1714
(800) 800-8661

Hoechst-Marion-Roussel Pharmaceuticals, Inc.
P.O. Box 9627
Kansas City, MO 64134
(800) 552-3656

International Diabetes Center
3800 Park Nicollet Boulevard
Minneapolis, MN 55416-9963
(612) 993-3393

International Diabetic Athletes Association
1647 West Bethany Home Road #B
Phoenix, AZ 85015
(602) 433-2113

Joslin Diabetes Center
One Joslin Place
Boston, MA 02215
(800) 344-4501

Juvenile Diabetes Foundation
120 Wall Street
New York, NY 10005
(800) 223-1138

LEAP/Monofilaments (Lower Extremity Amputation Prevention)
Feet Can Last a Lifetime
National Diabetes Outreach Program
1 Diabetes Way
Bethesda, MD 20892-3600
(800) 438-5383

Lifescan, Inc.
100 Gibraltar Drive
Milpitas, CA 95035-6312
(800) 227-8862

Eli Lilly and Company
Lilly Corporate Center
Indianapolis, IN 46285
(800) 545-5979

National Diabetes Information Clearinghouse
Box NDIC
9000 Rockville Pike
Bethesda, MD 20892
(302) 654-3327

NCES Catalog (Nutrition Counseling
  Education Services)
1904 E. 123rd Street
Olathe, KS 66061
(800) 445-5653

Novo Nordisk Pharmaceuticals, Inc.
100 Overlook Center, Suite 200
Princeton, NJ 08540
(609) 987-5800

Pennsylvania Diabetes Academy
777 East Park Drive
Harrisburg, PA 17105-8820
(717) 558-7750, Ext. 271

Selected Diabetes Nutrition Education
  Resources: For the Diabetes Professional
Diabetes Care and Education
Practice Group of the American Dietetic
  Association
216 W. Jackson Blvd., Suite 800
Chicago, IL 60606-6995
(800) 877-1600

The Upjohn Company
7000 Portage Road
Kalamazoo, MI 49001
(800) 253-8600

JOURNALS FOR HEALTH PROFESSIONALS

Clinical Diabetes
Diabetes Care
Diabetes Spectrum
(Publications of the American Diabetes
  Association)
1660 Duke Street
Alexandria, VA 22314

Practical Diabetology
150 West 22nd Street
New York, NY 10011

The Diabetes Educator
(Publication of the American Association of
  Diabetes Educators)
444 N. Michigan Ave., Suite 1240
Chicago, IL 60611-3901

POSITION STATEMENTS: AMERICAN ASSOCIATION OF DIABETES EDUCATORS

(available by fax or mail; phone: 312-644-2233)

Blood Glucose Monitoring (1993)
Education for Continuous Subcutaneous
Insulin Infusion Pump Users (1986)
Effective Utilization of Blood Glucose Monitoring (1989)
Healthcare Reform (1993)
Implications of the DCCT for Diabetes Educators (1993)
Individualization of Diabetes Education
and Management (1995)
Medical Nutrition Therapy for People with
Diabetes Mellitus (1995)
Prevention of Transmission of Blood-Borne
Infectious Agents During Blood-Glucose
Monitoring
Special Considerations for the Aging in the
Education and Management of Persons with
Diabetes Mellitus (1993)

CLINICAL PRACTICE RECOMMENDATIONS: AMERICAN DIABETES ASSOCIATION (updated every January)

(in Diabetes Care, Vol 20 [suppl 1], Jan 1997)
Selected position statements, consensus
statements, and standards include:

Bedside Blood Glucose Monitoring in
  Hospitals

Continuous Subcutaneous Insulin Infusion

Diabetes Mellitus and Exercise

Foot Care in Patients With Diabetes Mellitus

Gestational Diabetes Mellitus

Hypoglycemia and Employment/Licensure

Insulin Administration

National Standards and Review Criteria for
  Diabetes Self-Management Education
  Programs

Nutritional Recommendations and Principles
  for People With Diabetes Mellitus

Preconception Care of Women With Diabetes

Self-Monitoring of Blood Glucose

Standards of Medical Care for Patients With Diabetes Mellitus

Tests of Glycemia in Diabetes

Translation of the Diabetes Nutrition Recommendations for Health Care Institutions

BOOKS FOR HEALTH PROFESSIONALS

Diabetes and Visual Impairment: An Educator's Resource Guide. American Association of Diabetes Educators, Chicago, 1995

Doak C, Doak L, Root J: Teaching Patients with Low Literacy Skills, 2nd ed. JB Lippincott Co, Philadelphia, 1995

Fredrickson L (ed): The Insulin Pump Therapy Book. Minimed Technologies, Los Angeles, 1995

Peragallo-Dittko V, Godley K, Meyer J (eds): A Core Curriculum for Diabetes Education, 2nd ed. American Association of Diabetes Educators, Chicago, 1993

Raskin P (ed): Medical Management of Non–Insulin-Dependent (Type II) Diabetes, 3rd ed. American Diabetes Association, Alexandria, VA, 1994

Santiago J (ed): Medical Management of Insulin-Dependent (Type I) Diabetes, 2nd ed. American Diabetes Association, Alexandria, VA, 1994

JOURNALS FOR CLIENTS

Diabetes Forecast
American Diabetes Association
1660 Duke Street
Alexandria, VA 22314

Diabetes Interview
3715 Balboa Street
San Francisco, CA 94121
(415) 750-1958

Diabetes Self-Management
P.O. Box 52890
Boulder, CO 80322-2890
(800) 234-0923

Diabetic Reader
Prana Publications
5623 Matilija Ave.
Van Nuys, CA 91401
(800) 735-7726

The Diabetic Traveler
P.O. Box 8223 RW
Stamford, CT 06905

The Health-O-Gram
4818 Starkey Road
Roanoke, VA 24014
(800) 847-4383

Kids' Corner. In Diabetes Forecast
American Diabetes Association
1660 Duke Street
Alexandria, VA 22314

BOOKS FOR CLIENTS

GENERAL

Beaser R: Outsmarting Diabetes. Chronimed Publishing, Minneapolis, MN, 1994

Biermann J, Toohey B: The Diabetic's Total Health Book, 3rd ed. G.P. Putnam's Sons, New York, 1992

Franz MJ, Etzwiler DD, Joynes JO, Hollander PM: Learning to Live Well with Diabetes. Chronimed Publishing, Minneapolis, MN, 1991

Henry L, Johnson K: Black Health Library Guide to Diabetes. Henry Holt & Co., New York, 1993

Jovanovic-Peterson L, Biermann J, Toohey B: The Diabetic Woman. Jeremy P. Tarcher, Los Angeles, 1987

Lodewick P, Biermann J, Toohey B: The Diabetic Man. Lowell House, Los Angeles, 1991

Milchovich S, Dunn-Long B: Diabetes Mellitus: A Practical Handbook. Bull Publishing Company, Palo Alto, 1994

Monk A, Pearson J, Hollander P, Bergenstal RM: Managing Type II Diabetes. Your

Invitation to a Healthier Lifestyle. IDC Publishing, Minneapolis, MN, 1996

Valentine V, Biermann J, Toohey B: Diabetes Type II and What to Do. Lowell House, Los Angeles, 1993

EMOTIONS/COPING

Feste C: The Physician Within, 2nd ed. Chronimed Publishing, Minneapolis, MN, 1993

Rubin R, Biermann J, Toohey B: Psyching Out Diabetes. Lowell House, Los Angeles, 1992

EXERCISE

Graham C, Biermann J, Toohey B: The Diabetes Sports and Exercise Book. Lowell House, Los Angeles, 1995

Hornsby W (ed): The Fitness Book for People with Diabetes. American Diabetes Association, Alexandria, VA, 1994

INTENSIVE INSULIN THERAPY AND INSULIN PUMPS

Brackenridge B, Dolinar R: Diabetes 101. Chronimed Publishing, Minneapolis, MN, 1993

Brackenridge B, Fredrickson L, Reed C: Counting Carbohydrates. Minimed Technologies, Sylmar, CA, 1995

Walsh J, Roberts R: Pumping Insulin. Torrey Pines Press, San Diego, 1994

Walsh J, Roberts R: The Pocket Pancreas; My Other Checkbook. Torrey Pines Press, San Diego, 1994

PEDIATRICS

Chase H: Understanding Insulin-Dependent Diabetes, 8th ed. Barbara Davis Center for Childhood Diabetes—The Guild of the Children's Diabetes Foundation, Denver, 1995

Loring G: Parenting a Diabetic Child. Lowell House, Los Angeles, 1991

MacCracken J: The Sun, the Rain, and the Insulin—Growing up with Diabetes. Tiffen Press of Maine, Orono, ME, 1996

Mulder L: Sarah and Puffle: A Story for Children About Diabetes. Magination Press, New York, 1992

Siminero L, Betschart J: Raising a Child with Diabetes. American Diabetes Association, Alexandria, VA, 1995

Wood Johnson R IV, Johnson S, Johnson C, Kleinman S: Managing Your Child's Diabetes. MasterMedia Limited, New York, 1992

Your School and Your Rights. American Diabetes Association, Government Relations, Alexandria, VA, 1996

PREGNANCY

Diabetes & Pregnancy: What to Expect, 3rd ed. American Diabetes Association, Alexandria, VA, 1995

Franz MJ, Davidson J, Reader D, Hollander P: Gestational Diabetes. Caring for Yourself and Your Baby. IDC Publishing, Minneapolis, MN, 1995

Gestational Diabetes: What to Expect. American Diabetes Association, Alexandria, VA, 1992

Jovanovic-Peterson L, Stone M: Managing Your Gestational Diabetes. Chronimed Publishing, Minneapolis, MN, 1994

INSULIN PUMPS

Disetronic Medical Systems, Inc.
5201 East River Road, Suite 312
Minneapolis, MN 55421-1014
(800) 688-4578

Minimed Technologies, Inc.
12744 San Fernando Road
Sylmar, CA 91342
(800) 933-3322

MEDICAL IDENTIFICATION

Medic Alert Foundation U.S.
P.O. Box 1009
Turlock, CA 95381-1009
(800) 432-5378

RESOURCES FOR VISUALLY IMPAIRED CLIENTS

(consult with local centers for the partially sighted)

'97 Buyer's Guide to Diabetes Supplies: Aids for People Who Are Visually Impaired. Diabetes Forecast, October, 54–55, 1996. (updated every October)

Jordan Medical Enterprises, Inc.
12555 Garden Grove Blvd., Suite 507
Garden Grove, CA 92643
(800) 541-1193

National Association for the Visually Handicapped
3201 Balboa St.
San Francisco, CA 94121
(415) 221-3201

INDEX

Note: Page numbers in *italics* refer to illustrations; page numbers followed by t refer to tables.

F

G

N

Q

R